RICOH CORP. CALIF. RESEARCH CENTER
LIBRARY
2882 Sand Hill Rd., Ste. 115
Menlo Park, CA 94025

1377

The IMAGE PROCESSING Handbook

John C. Russ

Materials Science and Engineering Department
North Carolina State University
Raleigh, North Carolina

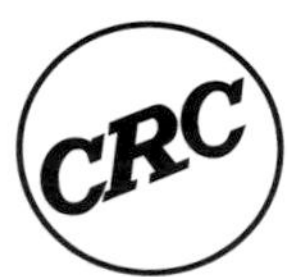

CRC Press
Boca Raton Ann Arbor London Tokyo

Library of Congress Cataloging-in-Publication Data

Russ, John C.
The image processing handbook/John C. Russ.
p. cm.
Includes index.
ISBN 0-8493-4233-3
1. Image processing. I. Title.
TA1632.R88 1992 92-4936
621.36'7—dc20 CIP

This book represents information obtained from authentic and highly regarded sources. Reprinted material is quoted with permission, and sources are indicated. A wide variety of references are listed. Every reasonable effort has been made to give reliable data and information, but the author and the publisher cannot assume responsibility for the validity of all materials or for the consequences of their use.

All rights reserved. This book, or any parts thereof, may not be reproduced in any form without written consent from the publisher.

Direct all inquiries to CRC Press, Inc., 2000 Corporate Blvd., N.W., Boca Raton, Florida 33431.

©1992 by CRC Press, Inc.

International Standard Book Number 0-8493-4233-3

Library of Congress Card Number 92-4936

Printed in the United States of America 3 4 5 6 7 8 9 0

Printed on acid-free paper

Introduction

Image processing is used for two somewhat different purposes:

a) improving the visual appearance of images to a human viewer and

b) preparing images for measurement of the features and structures present.

The techniques which are appropriate for each of these tasks are not always the same, but there is considerable overlap. This book covers methods which are used for both purposes.

To do the best possible job, it helps to know about the uses to which the processed images will be put. For visual enhancement, this means having some familiarity with the human visual process and an understanding of what cues the viewer responds to in images. It also is useful to know about the printing process, since many images are processed in the context of reproduction or transmission.

The measurement of images generally requires that features be well defined, either by edges or unique (and uniform) brightness or color. The types of measurements which will be performed on entire scenes or individual features are important in determining the appropriate processing steps.

It may help to recall that image processing, like food processing or word processing, does not reduce the amount of data present, but simply rearranges it. Some arrangements may be more appealing to the senses, and some may convey more meaning, but these two criteria may not be identical.

This handbook presents an extensive collection of image processing tools, so that the user of computer-based systems can both understand those methods provided in packaged software and program those additions which may be needed for particular applications. Comparisons are presented of different algorithms which may be used for similar purposes, using a selection of representative pictures from light and electron microscopes, as well as macroscopic, satellite, and astronomical images.

The reader is encouraged to use this book in concert with a real source of images and a computer-based system and to freely experiment with different methods to determine which are most appropriate for his or her particular needs. Selection of image processing tools to explore images when you do not know the contents beforehand is a much more difficult task than using tools to make it easier for another viewer or a measurement program to see the same things you have discovered. It places greater demand on computing speed and the interactive nature of the interface, but it particularly requires that you become a very analytical observer of images. If you can learn to see what the computer sees, you will become a better viewer and obtain the best possible images, suitable for further processing.

Acknowledgments

Most of the image processing and the creation of the resulting figures included in this book were performed on a Macintosh computer. Many of the images were acquired directly from various microscopes and other sources using color or monochrome video cameras and digitized directly into the computer. Others were digitized using a 24-bit color scanner, often from images supplied by many co-workers and researchers. These are acknowledged wherever the origin of an image could be determined. A few examples, taken from the literature, are individually referenced.

It happens that I use a Macintosh system and am most familiar with the software that runs on it. The particular programs and specialized hardware used in preparing the figures in this book are listed below, alphabetically by supplier. No single program can perform all of the operations discussed here. There are other programs for the Mac which in combination can perform many of these operations, and of course there are still others which can do so on other platforms, such as the PC, Sun, DEC or Silicon Graphics systems. However, this list may give interested readers a starting point.

Software

Adobe Systems Inc., 1585 Charleston Rd., Mountain View, CA 94039 (Photoshop)

Analytical Vision, Inc., 213 Merwin Road, Raleigh, NC 27606 (Prism)

Ranfurly Microsystems, 170B Clark St., Airdrie ML6 6DZ, Scotland (MacStereology)

Wayne Rasband, NIH, Research Services Branch, NIMH, Bethesda, MD (Image)

Signal Analytics, 374 Maple Ave. East, Suite 200, Vienna, VA 22180 (IP Lab)

Spyglass, Inc., 701 Devonshire Drive, C-17, Champaign, IL 61820 (Dicer, Transform)

Vital Images, Inc., 505 N. Third St., Suite 205, Fairfield, IA 52556 (VoxelView)

Hardware

Data Translation, Inc., 100 Locke Dr., Marlboro, MA 01752 (Model 2255 frame grabber)

LaCie Ltd, 19552 Southwest 90th Court, Tualatin, OR 97062 (Silverscanner color scanner)

Microtek Lab. Inc., 680 Knox St., Torrance CA 90502 (Scanmaker color slide scanner)

Perceptics, Inc., P.O. Box 22991, Knoxville, TN 37933 (Pixelgrabber frame grabber)

RasterOps, Inc., 2500 Walsh Ave., Santa Clara, CA 95051 (Model 24 XLTV color digitizer)

The book was produced by directly making film with a Linotype connected to a Macintosh, without intermediate hard copy, negatives, or prints of the images, etc. Among other things, this means that the author must bear full responsibility for any errors, since no typesetting was involved. However, it also shortens the time needed in production and helps to keep costs down, while preserving the full quality of the images.

Special thanks are due to Chris Russ (Analytical Vision, Raleigh, NC), who helped to program many of these algorithms, and to Helen Adams, who proofread many pages, endured many discussions, and provided the moral support which makes writing projects such as this possible.

John C. Russ
Raleigh, North Carolina

Contents

Chapter 1 **Acquiring Images** **1**

Chapter 2 **Correcting Imaging Defects** **53**

Chapter 3 **Image Enhancement** **101**

Chapter 4 **Processing Images in Frequency Space** ... **165**

Chapter 5 **Segmentation and Thresholding** **225**

Chapter 6 **Processing Binary Images** **277**

Chapter 7 **Tomography** **339**

Chapter 8 **Three-Dimensional Imaging** **375**

References **435**

Index **443**

The IMAGE PROCESSING Handbook

1

Acquiring Images

Humans are primarily visual creatures. Not all animals depend on their eyes, as we do, for 99% or more of the information received about their surroundings. Bats use high-frequency sound, cats have poor vision but a rich sense of smell, snakes locate prey by heat emission, and fish have organs that sense (and in some cases generate) electrical fields. Even birds, which are highly visual, do not have our eye configuration. Their eyes are on opposite sides of their heads, providing nearly 360-degree coverage but little in the way of stereopsis, and they have four or five different color receptors (we have three, loosely described as red, green, and blue). It is difficult to imagine what the world "looks like" to such animals. Even the word "imagine" contains within it our bias towards images, as does much of our language. People with vision defects wear glasses, because of their dependence on this sense. We tolerate considerable hearing loss, however, before resorting to a hearing aid, and there are, practically speaking, no prosthetic devices for the other senses.

This bias in everyday life extends to how we pursue more technical goals as well. Scientific instruments commonly produce images to communicate results to the operator, rather than generating an audible tone or emitting a smell. The space missions to other planets and to Comet Halley included cameras as major components, and we judge the success of those missions by the quality of the images returned. This suggests a few of the ways in which we have extended the range of our natural vision. Simple optical devices, such as microscopes and telescopes, allow us to see things that are vastly smaller or larger than we could otherwise. Beyond the visible portion of the electromagnetic

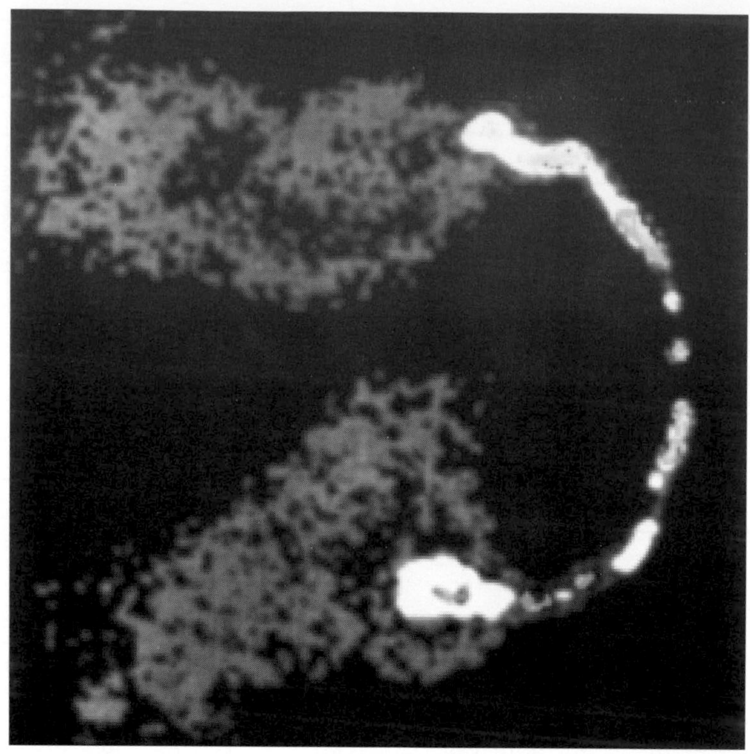

Figure 1. *Radio astronomy produces images such as this view of NGC1265. These are often displayed with false colors to emphasize subtle variations in signal brightness.*

spectrum (a narrow range of wavelengths between 400 and 700 nanometers) we now have sensors capable of detecting infrared and ultraviolet light, X-rays, and radio waves. In **Figure 1**, an image presenting radio telescope data uses grey scale brightness to represent radio intensity. Such enhancements further extend our imaging capability.

Signals other than electromagnetic radiation can be imaged, as well. Acoustic waves at low frequency produce sonar images, while at gigahertz frequencies the acoustic microscope produces images with resolution similar to that of the light microscope. Image contrast is produced by local variations in the attenuation

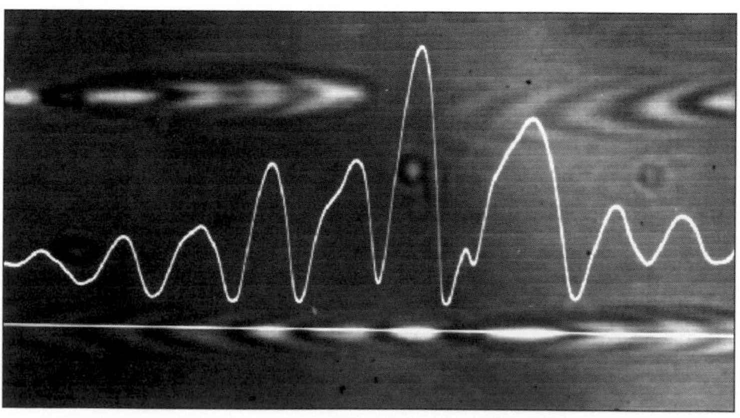

Figure 2. *Scanning acoustic microscope image (with superimposed brightness profile along one scan line) of a polished cross section through a composite. The central white feature is a fiber intersecting the surface at an angle. The arcs on either side are interference patterns which can be used to measure the fiber angle.*

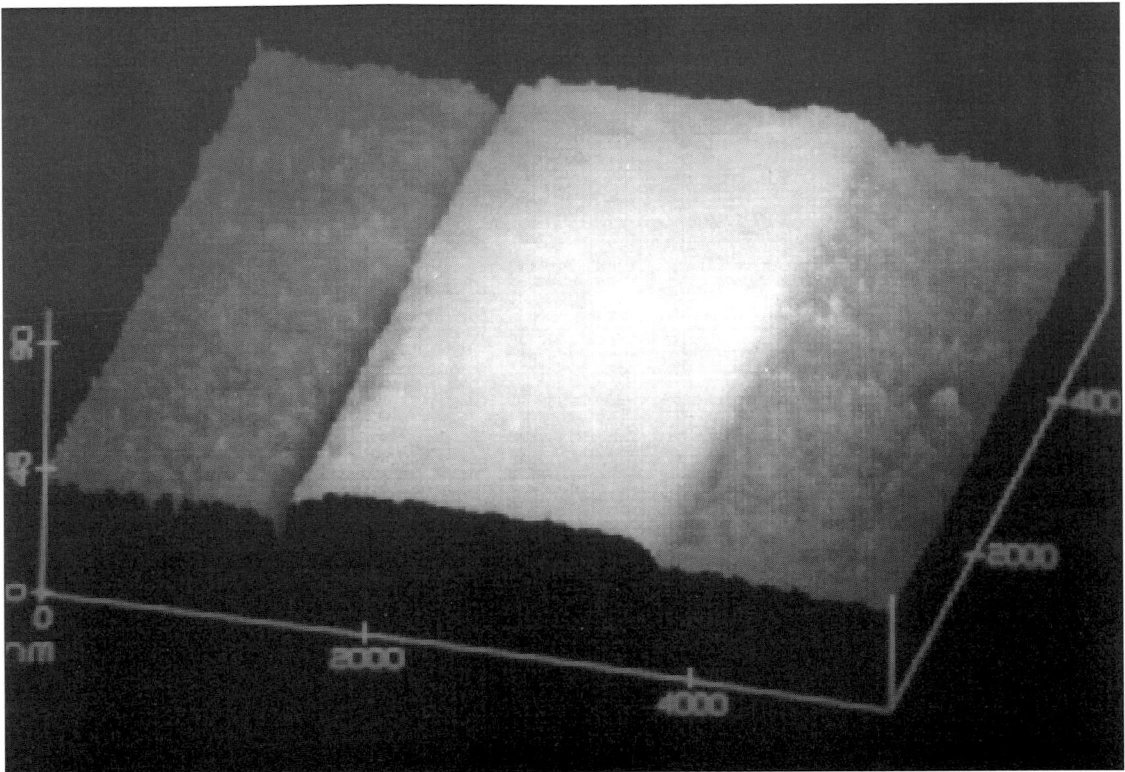

Figure 3. *Scanning tunneling microscope (STM) image.The specimen actually is flat surfaced silicon, with apparent relief showing altered electron levels in a 2-µm-wide region with implanted phosphorus. (Image courtesy of J. Labrasca, North Carolina State University, and R. Chapman, Microelectronics Center of North Carolina.)*

and refraction of sound waves, rather than light. **Figure 2** shows an acoustic microscope image of a composite material.

Surfaces are imaged by scanning profilometers or scanning tunneling microscopes. Operating on entirely different principles, they produce signals that we understand as representations of the surface when appropriately presented. In **Figure 3**, the apparent step in surface elevation reveals something different: the surface is actually flat, but the electronic properties of the sample (a junction in a microelectronic device) produce the variation in signal.

Some images, such as holograms or electron diffraction patterns, are recorded in terms of brightness as a function of position, but are unfamiliar to the observer. **Figure 4** shows an electron diffraction pattern that reveals the atomic spacings in the sample. Other kinds of data, including weather maps with isotherms, elaborate graphs of business profit and expenses, and charts with axes that are time, family income, cholesterol level, or even more obscure parameters, have become part of our daily lives. **Figure 5** shows a few examples. The latest developments in computer interfaces and displays rely extensively on graphics, again to take advantage of the large bandwidth of the human visual pathway.

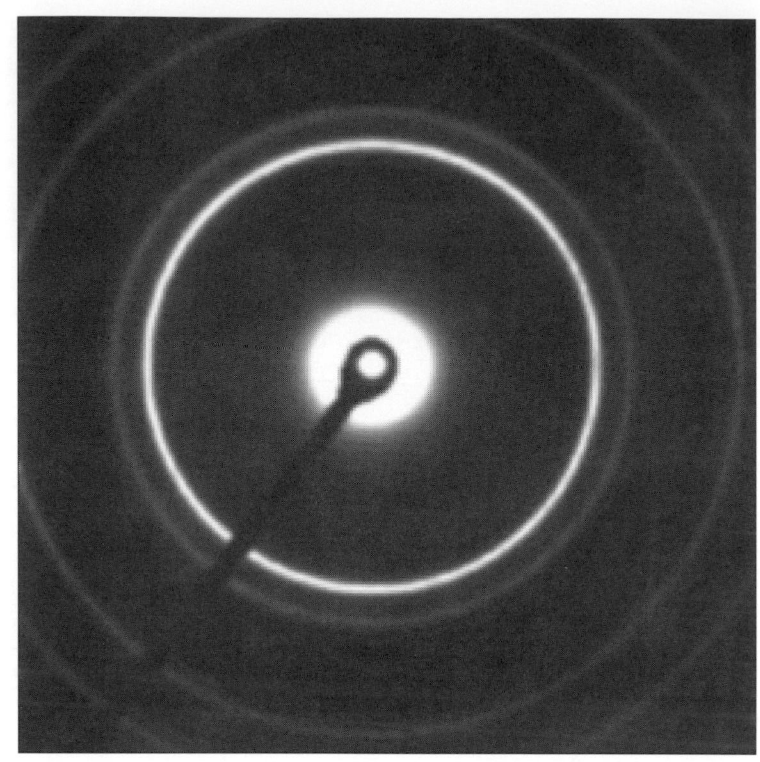

Figure 4. *An electron diffraction pattern from a thin foil of gold. The rings correspond to diffraction angles which identify planes of atoms in the crystal structure.*

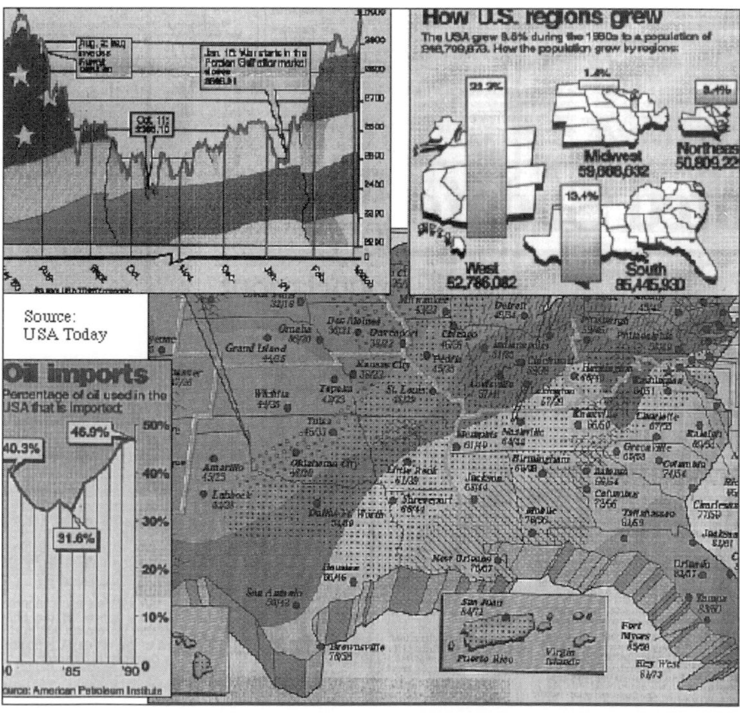

Figure 5. *Typical graphics used to communicate news information. (Source: USA Today.)*

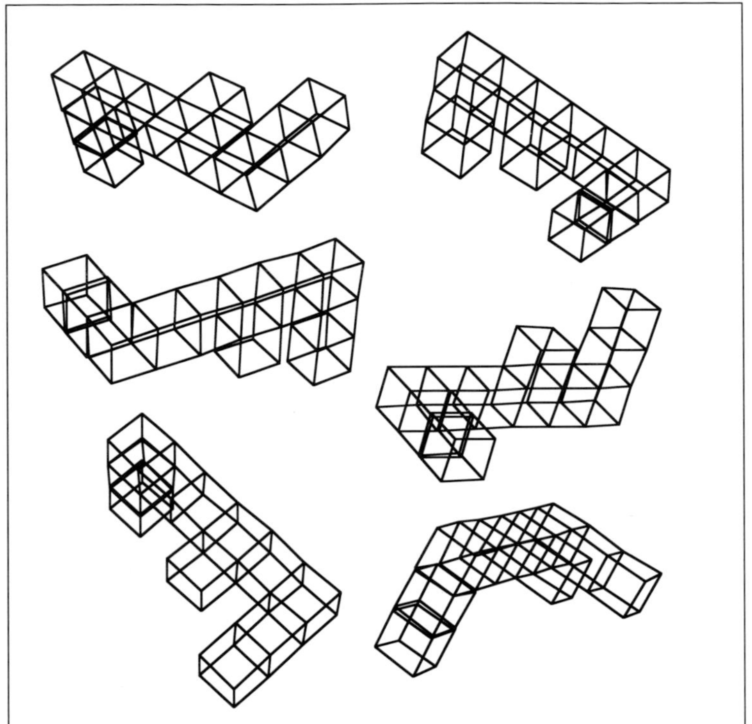

Figure 6. *Several views of a complex three-dimensional figure. Which of the representations is/are identical and which are mirror images? The time needed to decide is proportional to the mis-alignment, indicating that we literally "turn objects over" in our minds to compare them.*

There are some important differences between human vision, the kind of information it yields from images, and the ways in which it seems to do so, compared to the use of imaging devices with computers for technical purposes. Human vision is primarily qualitative and comparative, rather than quantitative. We judge the relative size and shape of objects by mentally rotating them to the same orientation, overlapping them in our minds, and performing a direct comparison. This has been shown by tests in which the time required to recognize features as being the same or different is proportional to the degree of misorientation or intervening distance. **Figure 6** shows an example.

Humans are especially poor at judging color or brightness of features within images unless they can be exactly compared by making them adjacent. Gradual changes in brightness are generally ignored as representing variations in illumination, for which the human visual system compensates automatically. This means that only abrupt changes in brightness are easily seen. It is believed that only these discontinuities, which usually correspond to physical boundaries or other important structures in the scene being viewed, are extracted from the raw image falling on the retina and sent up to the higher-level processing centers in the cortex.

These characteristics of the visual system allow a variety of visual illusions (**Figure 7**). Some of these illusions enable researchers to

Figure 7. A few common illusions:
a) *the two horizontal lines are identical in length, but appear different because of grouping with the diagonal lines;*
b) *the diagonal lines are parallel, but the crossing lines cause them to appear to diverge due to grouping and inhibition;*
c) *the illusory triangle may appear brighter than the surrounding paper and is due to grouping and completion;*
d) *the two inner squares have the same brightness, but the outer frames cause us to judge them as different due to brightness inhibition.*

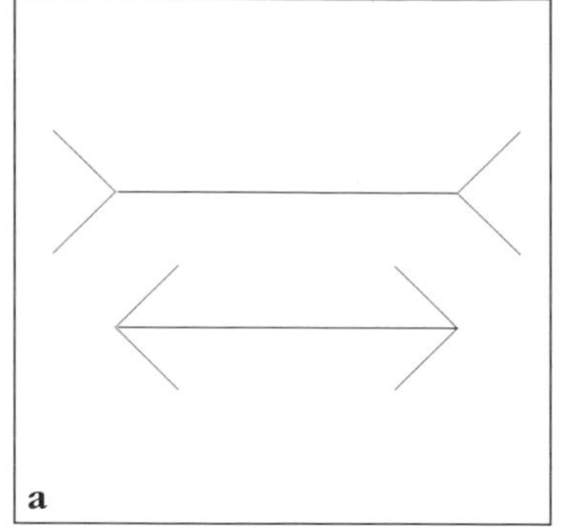

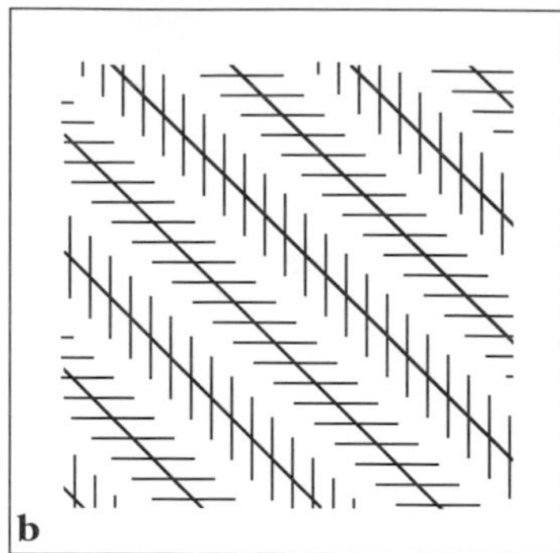

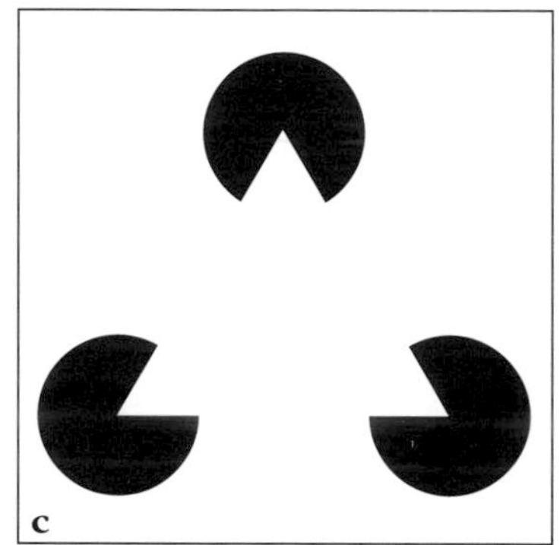

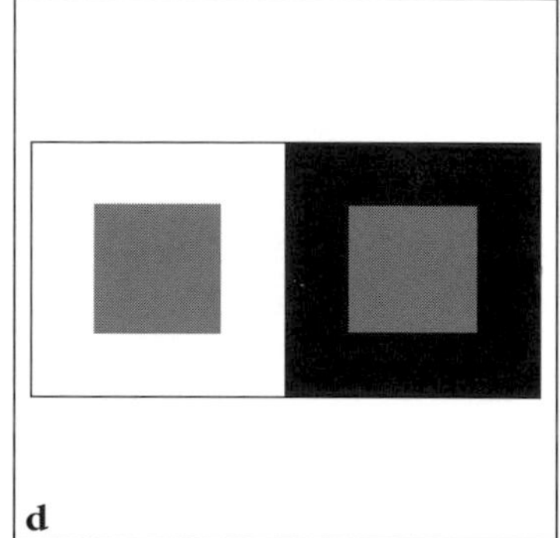

study the visual system itself, and others suggest ways that computer-based systems can emulate some of the very efficient (if not always exact) ways that our eyes extract information. Gestalt theory says that this is done by dealing with the image as a whole, not breaking it down into constituent parts. The idea that grouping parts within images is done automatically by our vision system–and is central to our understanding of scenes–has been confirmed by many experiments. This offers important insights into human physiology and psychology. One of the things it explains is why camouflage works (**Figure 8**). Our purpose is not to study the human visual pathway, but it obviously helps to understand how we see things in order to become better observers. The interested reader may want to read Frisby, 1980; Marr, 1982; Rock, 1984; and Hubel, 1988. Computer-based image processing and analysis use algorithms based on these methods when possible, but also employ other methods that seem not to have counterparts in human vision.

Using video cameras to acquire images

The first important difference between human vision and computer-based image analysis lies in the ways images are acquired. The most common sensor is a standard video camera, but there are several important variations available. Solid-state cameras use a chip with an array of individual "pixel" (picture element) sensors. With current technology, it is possible to place arrays of more than 300,000 devices in an area of less than 1 square cen-

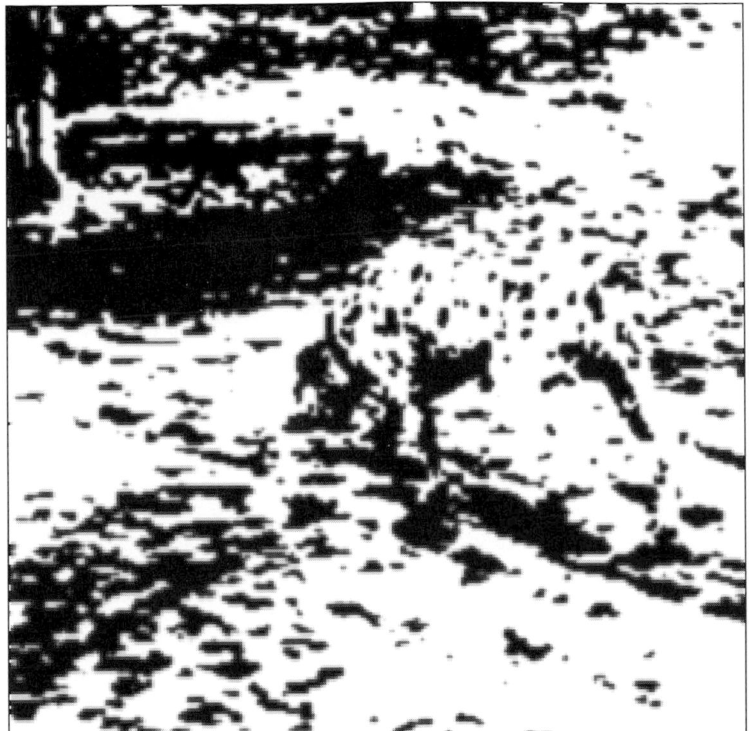

Figure 8. An example of camouflage, grouping together of many seemingly distinct features in the image, and ignoring apparent similarities between others, allows the eye to find the real structures present.

timeter. Each detector functions as a photon counter, as electrons are raised to the conduction band in an isolated well. The signal read out from each line of detectors then produces the analog voltage. **Figure 9** shows a schematic diagram of a typical device.

Several different types of circuitry are used to read the contents of the detectors, giving rise to CCD (charge coupled device), CID (charge injection device), and other designations. **Figure 10** shows an example. The most important effect of these differences is that some camera designs allow dim images to be accumulated for extended periods of time in the chip and be read out nondestructively, while others can only function with continuous scanning. Cameras used to store the very low-intensity

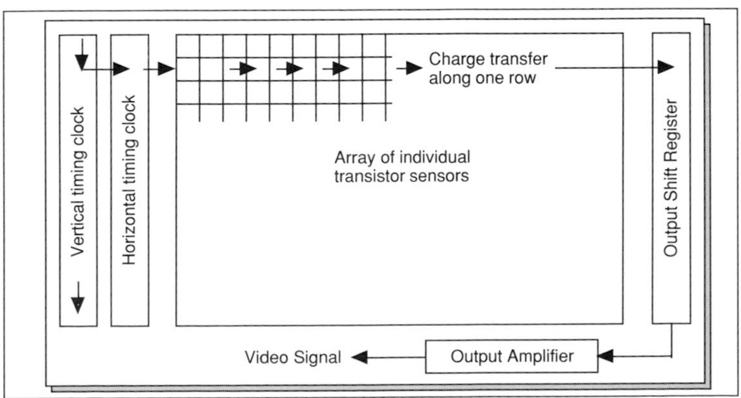

Figure 9. Diagram of a typical CCD camera chip. The vertical timing clock selects each line of pixel detectors in turn. Then the horizontal clock shifts the contents from each detector to its neighbor, causing the line to read out sequentially into a shift register and amplifier which produces an analog voltage as a function of time.

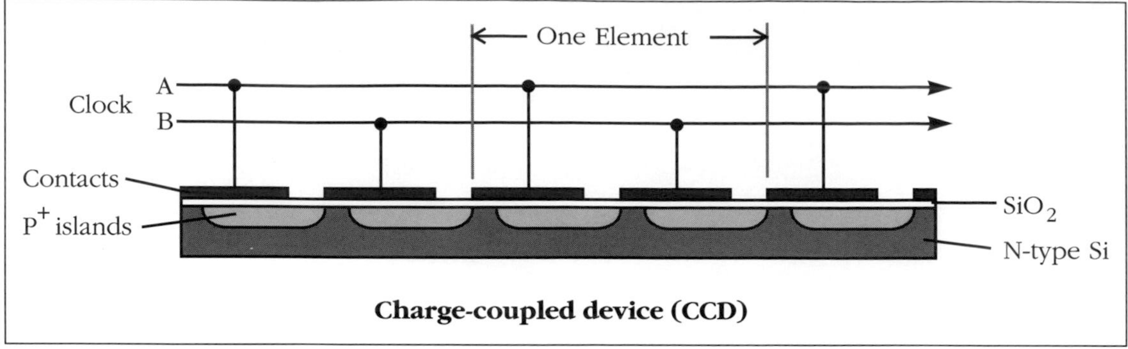

Figure 10. *Schematic diagram of the chip in a solid-state camera. Each sensor records the incident illumination; the signals are read out sequentially to form the raster scan.*

images encountered in astronomy, fluorescence microscopy, and some X-ray imaging devices are usually cooled to keep the electronic noise down. Integration times totaling many minutes are not uncommon.

The older type of camera uses a vacuum tube. Light passes inside the glass envelope to strike a coating, whose conductivity is altered by the photons. A scanning electron beam strikes this coating, and the change in resistance is converted to the image signal. Many varieties of tube design are used, some with intermediate cathode layers or special coatings for low-light-level sensitivity. The simple vidicon shown in **Figure 11** is the least expensive and most common type and can serve as a prototype for comparison to solid-state cameras.

Electronic cameras are similar to film in some respects. Film is characterized by a response to light exposure which (after chemical development) produces a density vs. exposure curve such as that shown in **Figure 12**. The low end of this curve represents the fog level of the film–the density which is present even without exposure. At the high end, the film saturates to a maximum

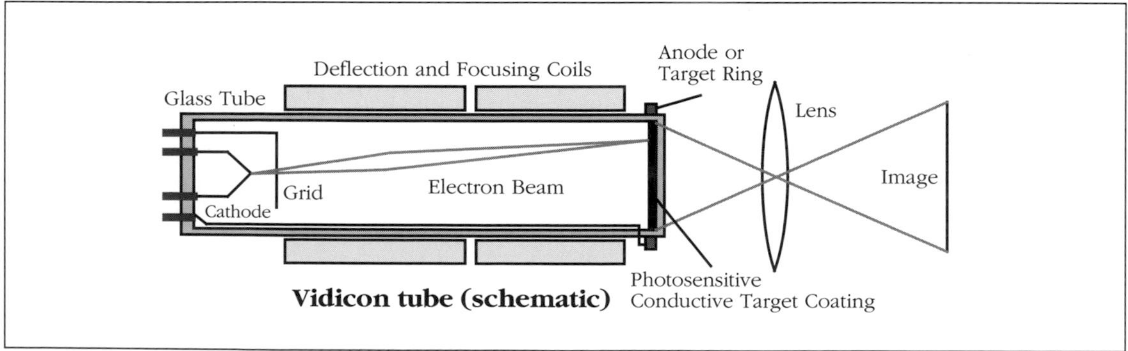

Figure 11. *Functional diagram of a vidicon tube. Light striking the coating changes its resistance, and hence the current that flows as the electron beam scans in a raster pattern.*

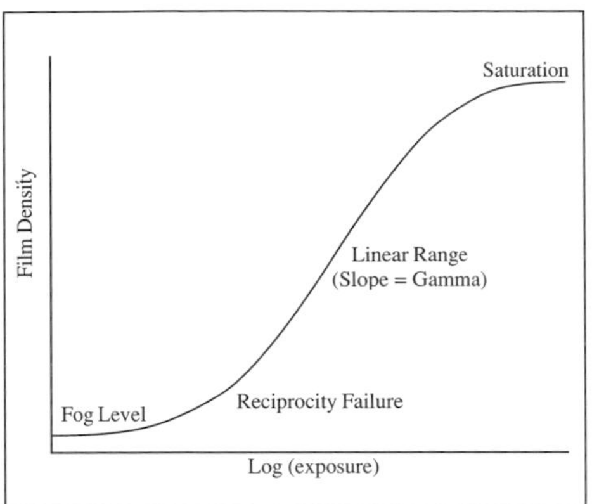

Figure 12. *Response of photographic film. The "H&D" curve includes the linear response range in which the slope distinguishes high- and low-contrast films. High contrast means that a small range of exposure causes a large change in film density. Density is defined as the base-ten logarithm of the fraction of incident light that is transmitted.*

density, for instance based on the maximum density of silver particles. In between, it has a linear relationship whose slope represents the contrast of the film. A high slope corresponds to a high-contrast film, which exhibits a large change in density with a small change in exposure. Conversely, a low-contrast film has a broader latitude, to record a scene with a greater range of brightnesses. A value of gamma greater or less than one indicates that the curve is not linear, but instead compresses either the dark or bright end of the range, as indicated in **Figure 13**.

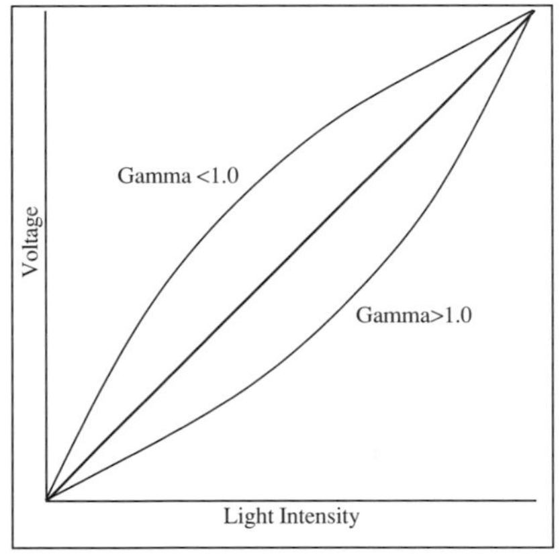

Figure 13. *Response of a light sensor. Gamma values greater or less than 1.0 expand or compress the contrast range at the dark or light end of the range.*

Both solid-state and tube-type cameras are characterized by contrast and latitude and may have values of gamma that are not equal to one. Sometimes, special electronics circuits are used to vary gamma intentionally. Solid-state cameras are inherently linear. Some tube-type cameras are also linear, but the most common type, the vidicon, is quite nonlinear when the average illumination level is low and varies to linear for bright scenes. **Figure 14** shows images of a grey scale wedge (as used in the photographic darkroom) obtained with a CCD camera and with a vidicon. The CCD response is linear, while that for the vidicon changes with the overall brightness level. This variability introduces some problems for image processing.

Solid-state cameras have both advantages and drawbacks compared to tube-type cameras. Tube cameras may suffer from

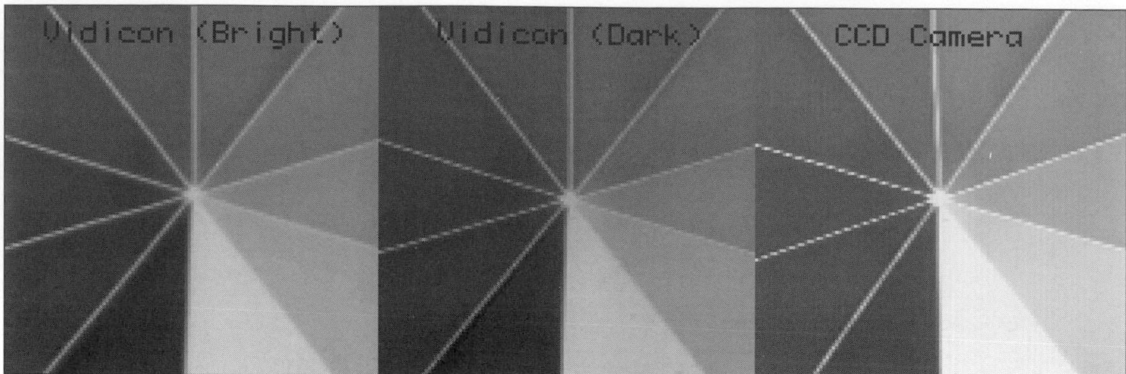

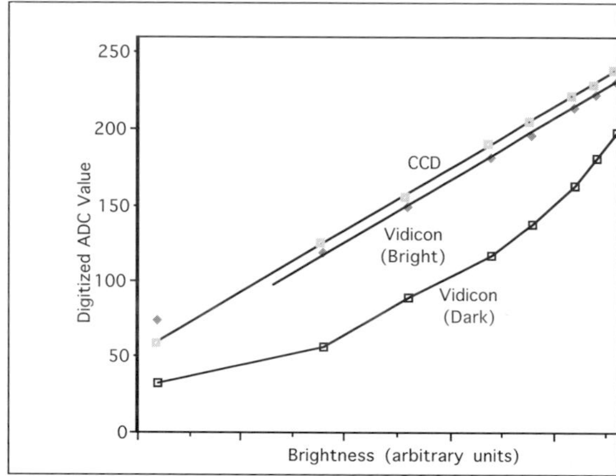

Figure 14. *Camera response curves determined by measuring an image of a series of photographic density steps shown at the top. The CCD camera is linear (gamma = 1) while the vidicon varies with overall illumination level.*

blooming, in which a bright spot is enlarged due to the spreading of light or electrons in the coating. Dissipation within the coating also makes integrating dim images impractical, while the time lag required for the phosphor to respond causes "comet tails" behind moving bright spots. **Figure 15** shows examples of blooming and comet tails. These cameras may also exhibit distortion in the raster scan, producing either pincushion or barrel distortion (**Figure 16**) or more complicated effects, especially if used with instruments that generate stray magnetic fields. Keeping the two interlaced fields within each full frame in exact alignment can also be a problem.

Defocusing of the electron beam at the corners of the tube face may cause the corners and edges of the image to degrade in sharpness, while light absorbed passing through the thicker glass near edges may cause the corners and edges to be dim. **Figure 17** shows an example of this vignetting. The most simply designed tube cameras, such as the vidicon, have a relationship between output signal and illumination that varies as the average brightness level varies, which confuses absolute measurements of brightness or density. Tube cameras also degrade with time when installed in a vertical orientation (such as mounted on the top of a microscope), as internal contaminants settle onto the coating. They are physically larger and heavier than solid-state cameras.

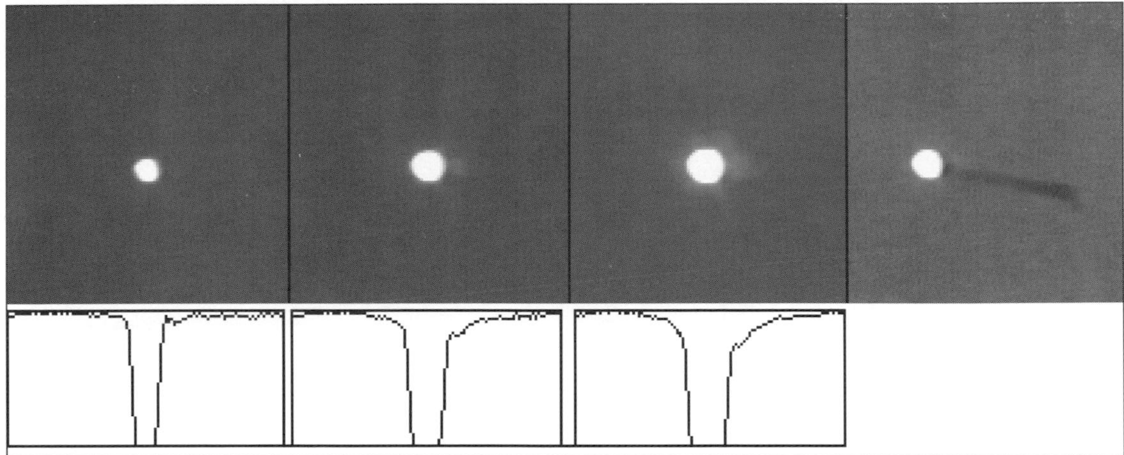

Figure 15. *Blooming in a vidicon camera. The bright spot is of constant actual size, but appears to grow larger as its brightness increases. There is also tailing on the right side (shown in the brightness profiles) due to the recovery time of the tube electronics. The fourth image at the right shows a dark comet tail when the spot is moved, due to the long recovery time of the phosphor coating.*

On the other hand, solid-state cameras rely on each of the 300,000 or more sensors to be identical, which is difficult even with modern chip fabrication techniques. Variations in sensitivity show up as noise in the image. Chip cameras are also most sensitive at the red end of the visible spectrum, as shown in **Figure 18**. Many are also sensitive to infrared light, which, if not eliminated in the optics, can produce an overall blur or fogging–since it is unlikely to be correctly focused. For some astronomical and remote sensing applications in which extended infrared sensitivity is desired, the spectral response of the CCD can be extended even further. One way is to thin the substrate and illuminate the chip from the back side so that light can reach the active region with less absorption in the overlying metal or silicide gate contacts. Another way is to use other semiconductors, such as In-Sb, instead of silicon. By comparison, tube cameras can use phosphors that duplicate the spectral sensitivity of the human eye or may be tailored to selected parts of the spectrum.

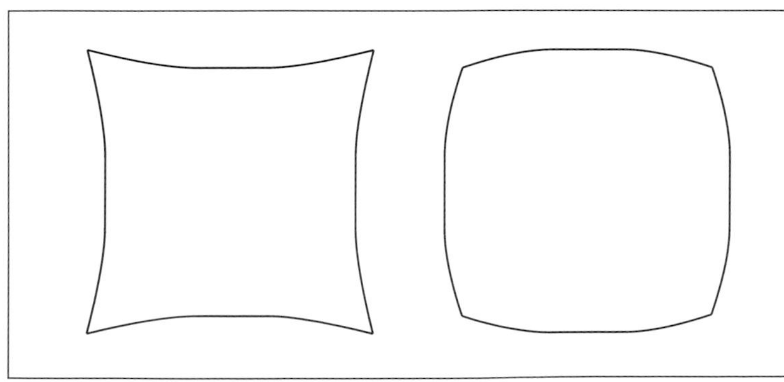

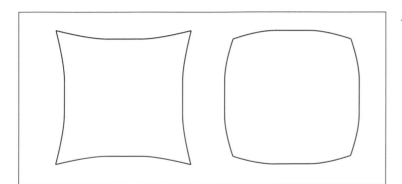

Figure 16. *Pincushion and barrel distortion. The ideal raster scan is rectilinear, but the use of magnetic deflection, and the curvature of the front face of the camera tube, may cause distortion. The variation in the distance from the electron gun to the front face may also require dynamic focusing to keep the edges and corners from blurring.*

Figure 17. *Darkening of edges and corners of an image of a blank grey card acquired with a vidicon, shown as originally acquired and with the contrast expanded to make the vignetting more obvious. Printing technology causes the apparent stepped or contoured variation in brightness, which is actually a smoothly varying function of position.*

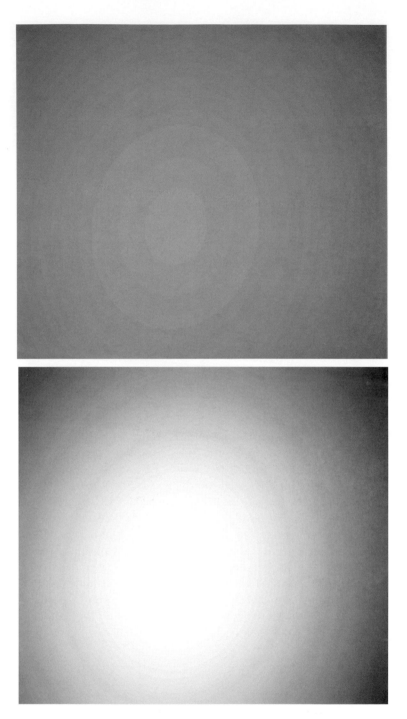

The trend, though, is clearly toward solid-state cameras, which are continually improving in resolution (number of individual sensors), uniformity, and cost. It remains to be seen whether the commercial development of high-definition television (HDTV) will result in a significant improvement of cameras, which are not the weakest link in the imaging chain used for commercial television.

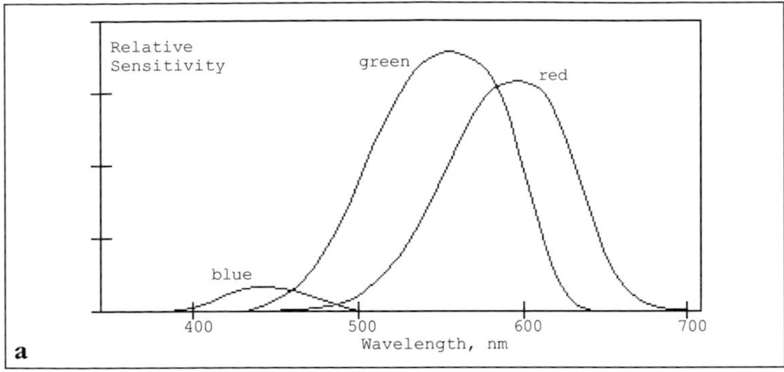

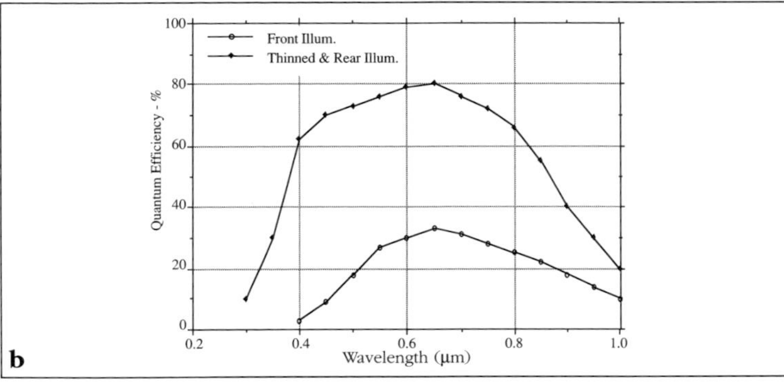

Figure 18. Spectral response:
a) *sensitivity of the cones in the human retina; while they are commonly identified as red, green, and blue sensitive, each actually responds to a wide range of wavelengths;*
b) *response of a solid-state detector for the normal case of front illumination, and rear illumination after thinning the support, showing greater red and infrared sensitivity.*

Electronics and bandwidth limitations

Cameras of either the solid-state or tube type produce analog voltage signals corresponding to the brightness at different points in the image. In the standard RS-170 signal convention, voltage varies over a 0.7-volt range from minimum to maximum brightness, as shown in **Figure 19**. The scan is nominally 525 lines per full frame, with two interlaced 1/60th second fields combining to make an entire image (**Figure 20**). Only about 480 of the scan lines are actually useable, with the remainder lost during vertical retrace. In a typical broadcast television picture, more of these lines are lost due to overscanning, leaving fewer than 400 lines in the actual viewed area. The time duration of each scan line is 62.5 μs, part of which is used for horizontal retrace. This leaves 52 μs for the image data, which must be subdivided into the horizontal spacing of discernible pixels. For PAL (European) television, these values are slightly different based on a 1/25th second frame time and more scan lines, but the resulting resolution is not significantly different.

Broadcast television stations are given only a 4-MHz bandwidth for their signals, which must carry color and sound information as well as the brightness signal we have so far been discussing. This limits the number of separate voltage values that can be distinguished along each scan line to about 330. Even this value is reduced if the signal is degraded by the electronics or by recording using standard videotape recorders. Many consumer-quality

Figure 19. *Composite video signal used in US television. Each scan line duration is 63.5 μsec, of which 52 μsec contains one line of the image. The remainder contains the 5-μsec horizontal sync pulse, plus other timing and color calibration data.*

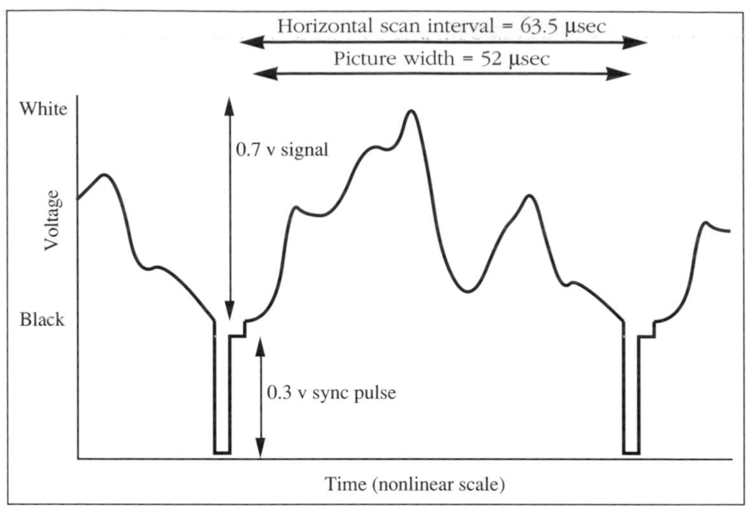

videotape recorders reduce this value to 200 points per line. In "freeze frame" playback, they display only one of the two interlaced fields, so that only 240 lines are resolved vertically. Therefore, using such equipment as part of an image analysis system makes choices of cameras or digitizer cards on the basis of resolution quite irrelevant.

Even the best system can be degraded in performance by such simple things as cables, connectors, or incorrect termination impedance. Another practical caution in the use of standard cameras is to avoid automatic gain or brightness compensation circuits. They can change the image contrast or linearity in response to bright or dark regions that do not even lie within the digitized portion of the image and can increase the gain and noise for a dim signal.

Figure 21 shows a micrograph with its brightness histogram. This is an important tool for image analysis, which plots the number of pixels as a function of their brightness values. The histogram is initially well spread-out over the available 256 brightness levels, with peaks corresponding to each of the

Figure 20. *The interlaced raster scan used in standard video equipment records the even-numbered scan lines comprising one half-field in 1/60th of a second, and then scans the odd-numbered lines comprising the second half-field in the next 1/60th of a second, giving a complete frame every 30th of a second. European TV is based on 1/50th of a second, corresponding to the 50-Hz frequency of their power grid.*

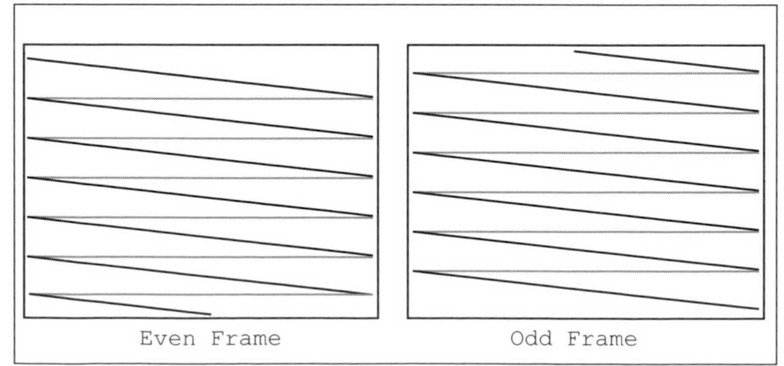

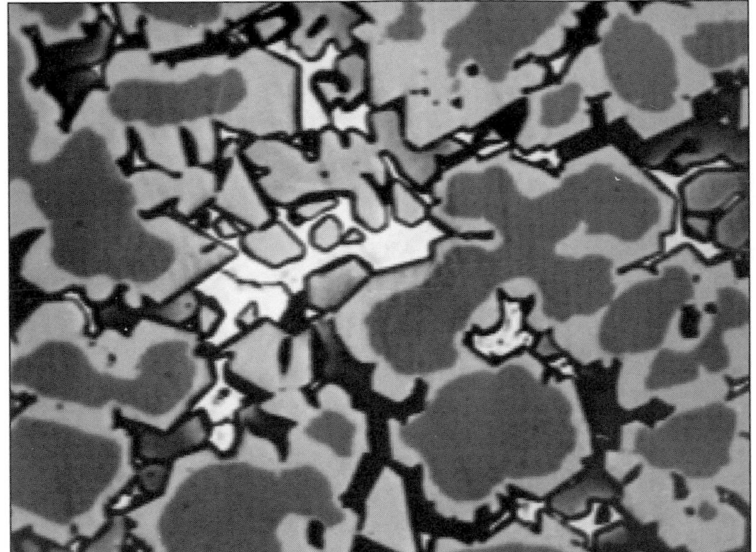

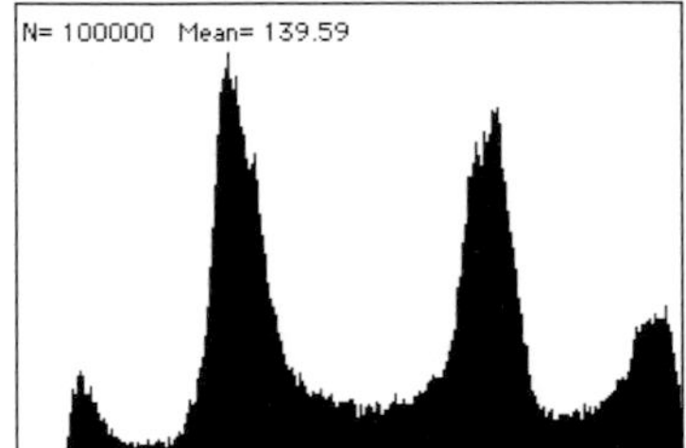

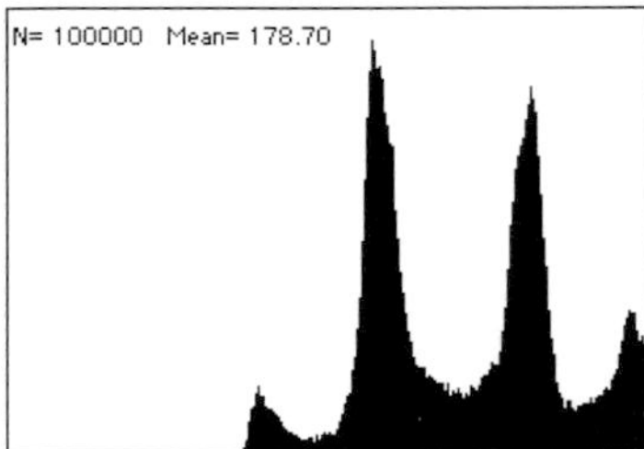

Figure 21. *A grey scale image digitized from a metallographic microscope and its brightness histogram (white at the left, dark at the right). A bright reflection within the camera tube causes the automatic gain circuit to shift the histogram, even though the bright spot is not within the digitized area. This would cause the same structure to have different grey values in successive images.*

phases in the metal sample. When an internal reflection in the microscope causes a bright light to fall on a portion of the detector in the solid-state camera that is not part of the digitized image area, the automatic gain circuits in the camera alter the brightness-voltage relationship so that the image changes, as shown in the second histogram. This same effect occurs when a white or dark mask is used to surround images placed under a camera on a copy stand. The relationship between structure and brightness is changed, making subsequent analysis more difficult.

Issues involving color will be dealt with later, but obtaining absolute color information from video cameras is nearly impossible considering the variation in illumination color (e.g., with slight voltage changes on an incandescent bulb) and the way the color information is encoded.

The analog voltage signal is usually digitized with an 8-bit "flash" ADC (analog-to-digital converter). This is a chip using successive approximation techniques to rapidly sample and measure the voltage in less than 100 ns, producing a number value from 0 to 255 that represents the brightness. This number is immediately stored in memory, and another reading made, so that a

Figure 22. Digitization of an analog voltage signal such as one line in a video image (top) produces a series of numbers that represent a series of steps equal in time and rounded to integral multiples of the smallest height increment (bottom).

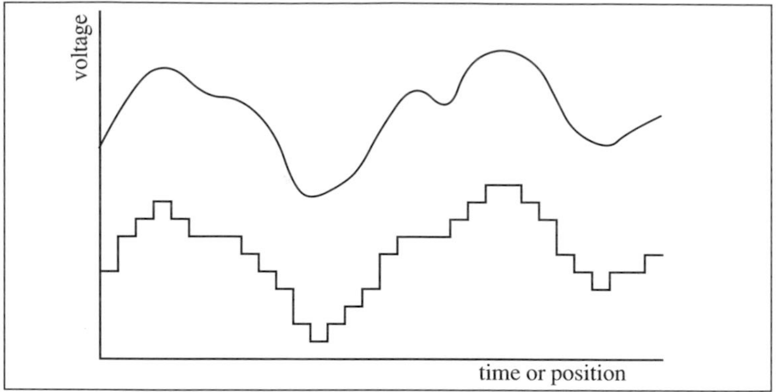

series of brightness values are obtained along each scan line. **Figure 22** illustrates the digitization of a signal into equal steps in time and value. Additional circuitry is needed to trigger each series of readings on the retrace events, so that positions along successive lines are consistent.

Degraded signals, especially from videotape playback, can cause the even and odd fields of a full frame to be offset from each other, producing significant degradation of the image. **Figure 23** shows the consequences of offset in the interlace correction, which can occur if the horizontal retrace signal is imprecise or difficult for the electronics to lock onto. This is a particular problem with signals played back from video recorders. Digitizing several hundred points along each scan line, repeating the process for each line, and storing the values into memory while adjusting for the interlace of alternate fields produces a digitized image for further processing or analysis.

It is most desirable to have the spacing of the pixel values be the same in the horizontal and vertical directions (i.e., square

Figure 23. Example of interlace tearing when horizontal sync pulses between half-fields are inadequate to trigger the clock in the ADC correctly. Even and odd lines are systematically displaced.

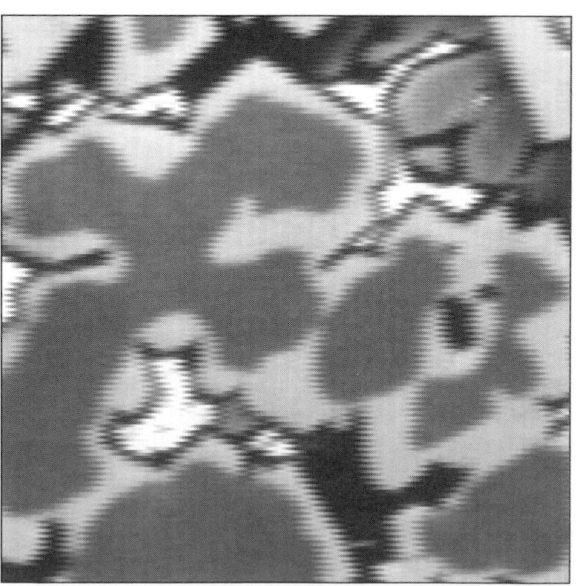

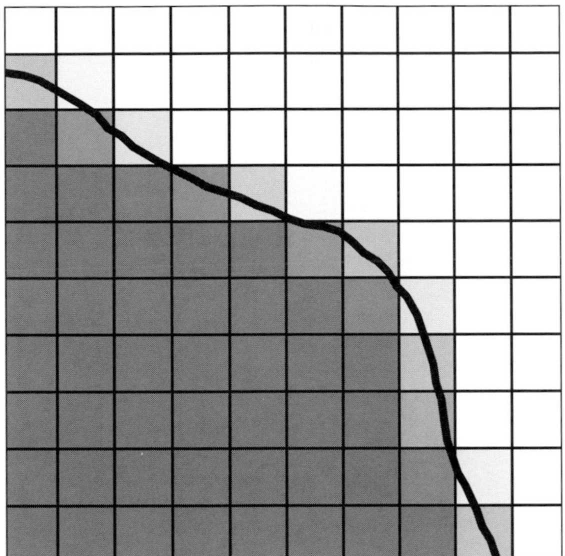

Figure 24. *Pixels have a finite area, and those straddling the boundary of a feature or region will have an intermediate brightness value resulting from averaging of the two levels. Accurate definition of the location of the boundary requires that the pixels be small and the number of grey values be large.*

pixels), as this simplifies many processing and measurement operations. This requires a well-adjusted clock to control the acquisition. Since the standard video image is not square, but has a width-to-height ratio of 4:3, the digitized image may represent only a portion of the entire field of view. Digitizing boards, also known as frame grabbers, were first designed to record 512 × 512 arrays of values, since the power-of-two dimension simplified design and memory addressing. Many of the newer boards acquire a 640 wide by 480 high array, which matches the image proportions while keeping the pixels square.

Of course, digitizing 640 values along a scan line that, as limited by electronic bandwidth, only contains 300+ meaningfully different values produces an image with unsharp or fuzzy edges and "empty" magnification. Cameras capable of resolving more than 600 points along each scan line can sometimes be connected directly to the digitizing electronics to reduce this loss of horizontal resolution. Other camera designs bypass the analog transmission altogether, sending digital values to the computer, but these are generally much slower than standard video systems. They are discussed below.

Since pixels have a finite area, those which straddle a boundary effectively average the brightness levels of two regions and have an intermediate brightness that depends on how the regions lie with respect to the boundary. **Figure 24** illustrates this schematically. This means that a high lateral pixel resolution and a large number of distinguishable grey levels are needed to accurately locate boundaries. **Figure 25** shows several examples of an image with varying numbers of pixels across its width, and **Figure 26** shows the same image with varying numbers of grey levels.

In addition to defining the number of sampled points along each scan line, and hence the resolution of the image, the design of

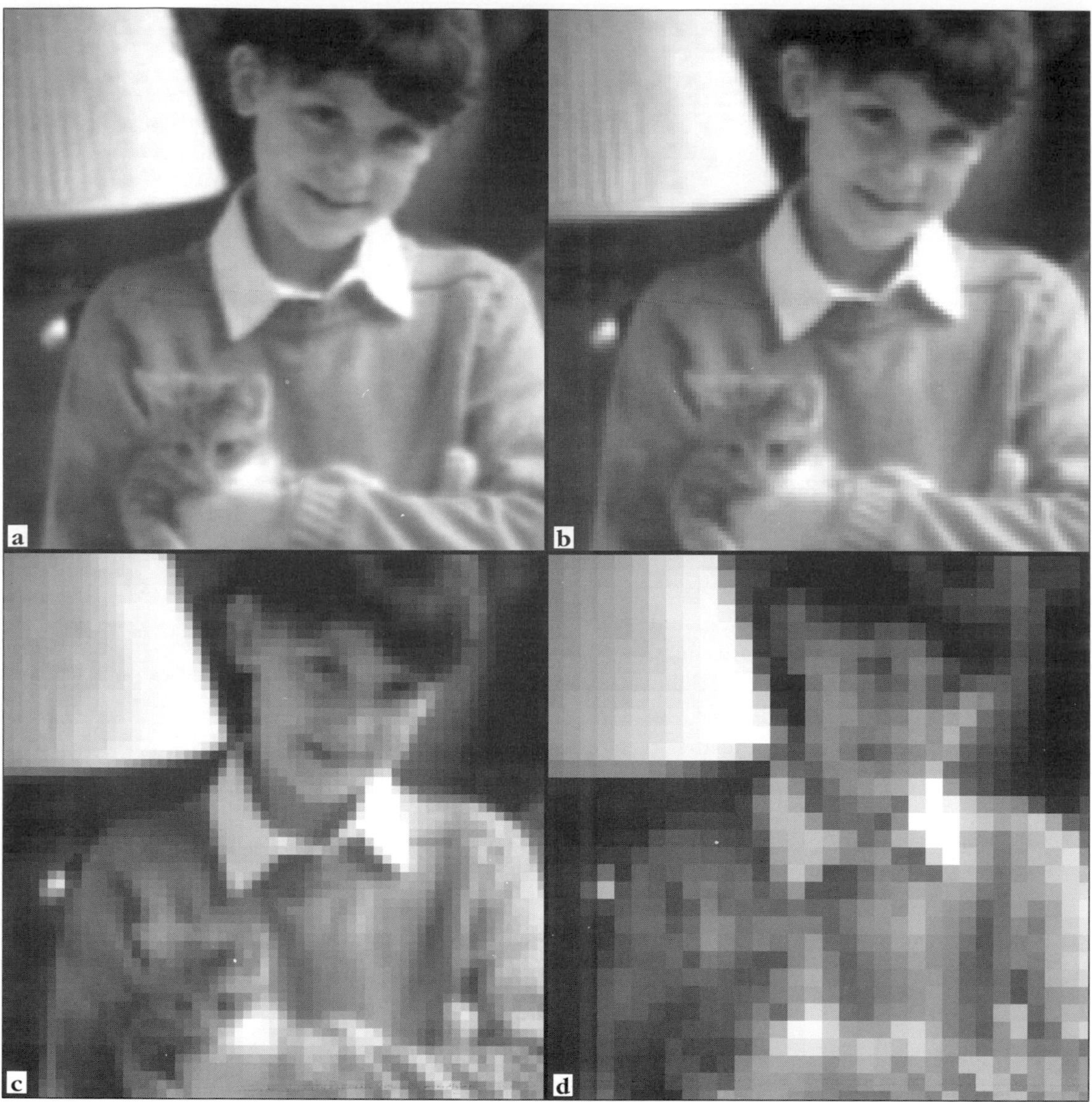

Figure 25. Four representations of the same image, with variation in the number of pixels used:
a) *256×256;* ***b)*** *128×128;* ***c)*** *64×64;* ***d)*** *32×32.*
In all cases, a full 256 grey values are retained. Each step in coarsening of the image is accomplished by averaging the brightness of the region covered by the larger pixels.

the ADC board also controls the precision of each measurement. Inexpensive commercial flash analog-to-digital converters usually measure each voltage reading to produce an 8-bit number, from 0 to 255. This range may not entirely be used for an actual image, since it may not vary from full black to white. Also, the quality of most cameras and other associated electronics rarely produces voltages that are free enough from electronic noise to justify full 8-bit digitization anyway. However, 8 bits corresponds nicely to the most common organization of computer memory

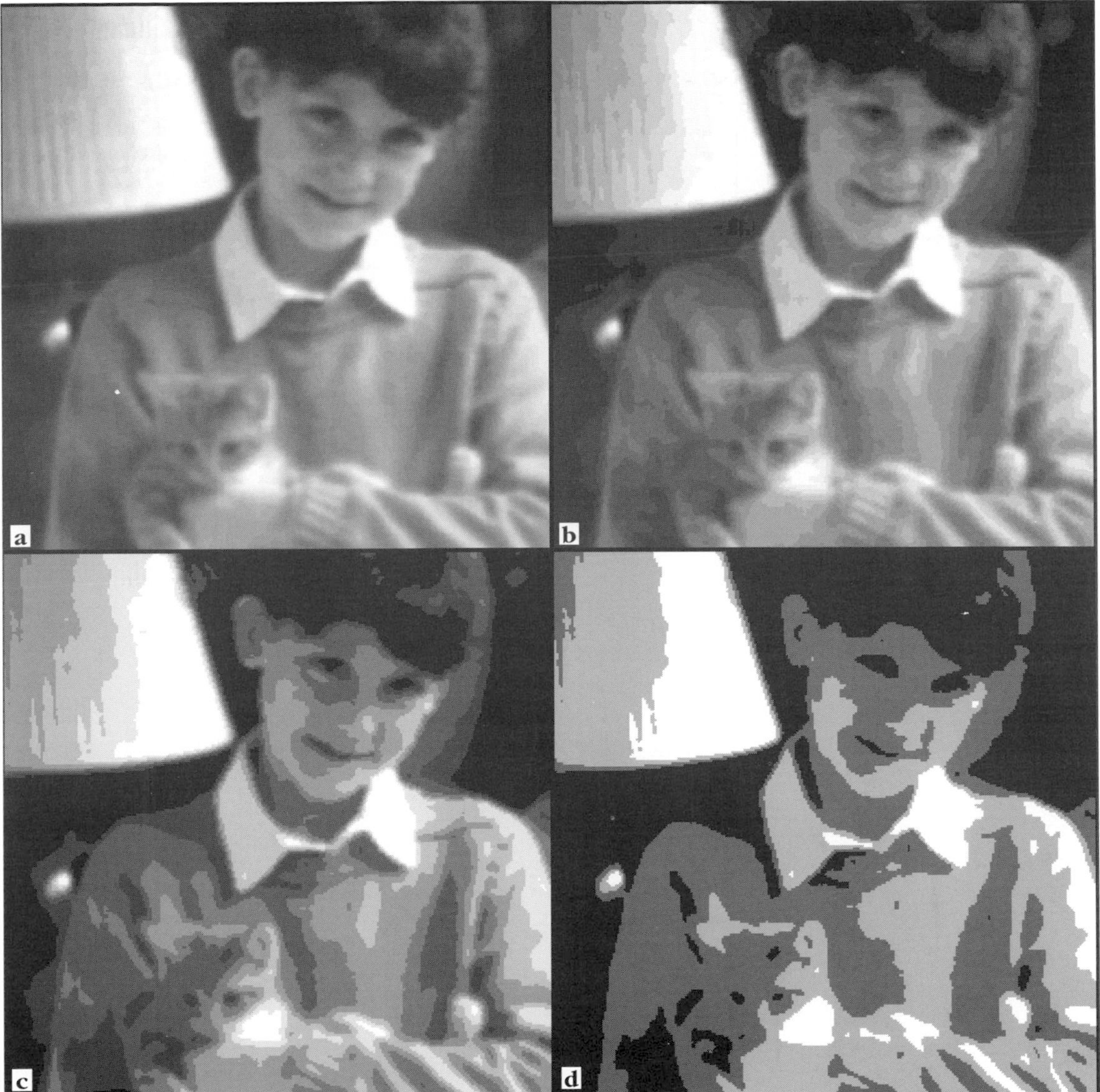

Figure 26. Four representations of the same image, with variation in the number of grey levels used: a) *32;* ***b)*** *16;* ***c)*** *8;* ***d)*** *4.*

In all cases, a full 256×256 array of pixels are retained. Each step in the coarsening of the image is accomplished by rounding the brightness of the original pixel value.

into bytes, so that one byte of storage can hold the brightness value from one pixel in the image.

Figure 27 shows an image that appears to be uniformly grey. When the contrast range is expanded, we can see the faint lettering present on the back of this photographic print. Also evident is a series of vertical lines which are due to the digitizing circuitry–in this case electronic noise from the high-frequency clock used to control the time base for the digitization. Nonlinearities in the ADC, electronic noise from the camera itself, and

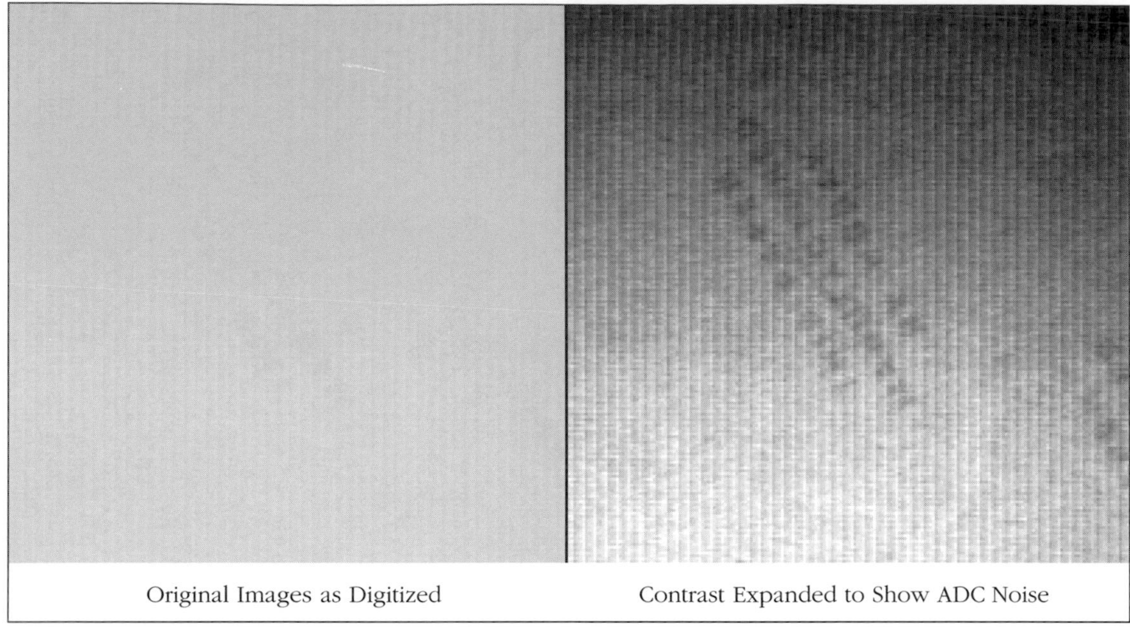

Figure 27. *Digitized camera image of the back of a photographic print, showing the periodic noise present in the lowest few bits of the data from the electronics (especially the clock) in the analog to digital converter.*

degradation in the amplifier circuitry combine to make the lowest two bits of most standard video images useless, so that about 64 grey levels are actually distinguishable in the data. Higher performance cameras and circuits exist, but do not generally offer "real time" speed (30 frames per second).

When this stored image is subsequently displayed from memory, the numbers are used in a digital-to-analog converter to produce voltages that control the brightness of a display, often a cathode ray tube (CRT). This process is comparatively noise-free and of high resolution, since computer display technology has been developed to a high level for other purposes. A monochrome (black/grey/white) image displayed in this way, with 640×480 pixels, each of which can be set to one of 256 brightness levels (or colors using pseudo-color techniques to be discussed below), can be used with many desktop computers.

The human eye cannot distinguish all 256 different levels of brightness in this type of display, nor can the levels be successfully recorded photographically or printed using affordable technology, such as ink-jet or laser printers. About 30 grey levels can be visually distinguished on a CRT or photographic print, suggesting that the performance of the digitizers in this regard is more than adequate, at least for those applications where the performance of the eye was enough to begin with.

Images acquired in very dim light, or some other imaging modalities such as X-ray mapping in the scanning electron microscope, impose another limitation of the grey scale depth of the image.

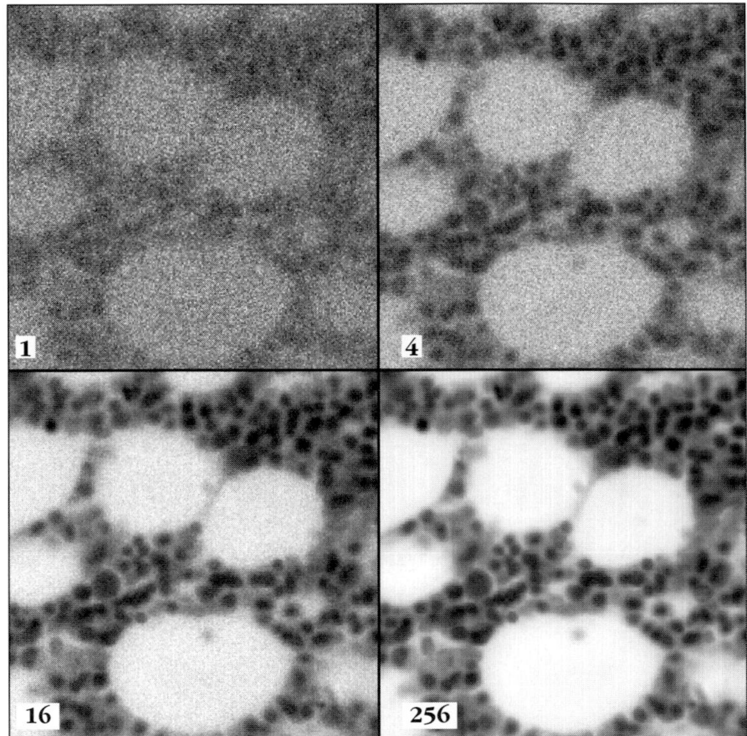

Figure 28. *Averaging of a noisy (low photon intensity) image (light microscope image of bone marrow): one frame; addition of 4, 16, and 256 frames.*

When the number of photons (or other particles) collected for each image pixel is low, statistical fluctuations become important. **Figure 28** shows a fluorescence microscope image in which a single video frame illustrates extreme statistical noise, which would prevent distinguishing or measuring the structures present.

Images in which the pixel values vary even within regions that are ideally uniform in the original scene can arise either because of limited counting statistics for the photons or other signals or due to electronic noise in the amplifiers or cabling. In either case, it is generally referred to as noise, and the ratio of the contrast which is actually due to structural difference to the noise level is the signal-to-noise ratio. When this is low, the features present may be invisible to the observer. **Figure 29** shows an example in which several features of different size and shape are superimposed on a noisy background with different signal-to-noise ratios. The ability to discern the presence of the features is generally proportional to their area and is independent of shape.

In the figure, a smoothing operation is performed on the image with the poorest signal-to-noise ratio, which somewhat improves the visibility of the features. The methods available for smoothing noisy images by image processing are discussed in the chapters on spatial and frequency domain methods. However, the best approach to noisy images, when it is available, is simply to collect more signal and improve the statistics.

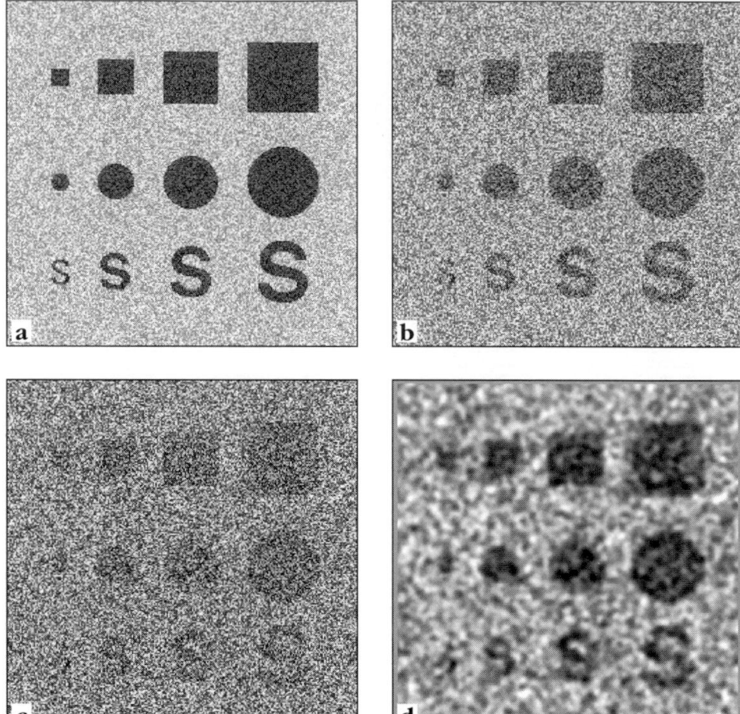

***Figure 29*. Features on a noisy background:**
a) *signal-to-noise ratio 1:1;*
b) *signal-to-noise ratio 1:3;*
c) *signal-to-noise ratio 1:7;*
d) *image c after spatial smoothing.*

Adding together more video frames is shown in **Figure 28**. The improvement in quality is proportional to the square root of the number of frames (**Figure 30**). Since each frame is digitized to 8 bits, adding together up to 256 frames as shown requires a total image storage capability that is 16 bits deep. Acquiring frames and adding together the pixels at video rates generally requires specialized hardware, and performing the operation in a general-purpose computer limits the practical acquisition to only a few of the video frames per second. This discards a large percentage of the photons that reach the detector. It is more efficient to use a camera capable of integrating the signal directly for the appropriate length of time, and then read the final image to the computer. Cameras with this capability, and cooled chips to reduce electronic noise during long acquisitions of many minutes, are available. They are intended primarily for use in astronomy, where dim images are often encountered, but are equally suitable for other applications.

Acquiring images from a video camera is sometimes referred to as "real time" imaging, but of course this term should properly be reserved for any imaging rate which is adequate to reveal temporal changes in a particular application. For some situations, time-lapse photography may only require one frame to be taken at periods of many minutes. For others, very short exposures and high rates are needed. Special cameras which do not use video frame rates or bandwidths can achieve rates up to ten times that of a standard video camera for full frames, and even higher for

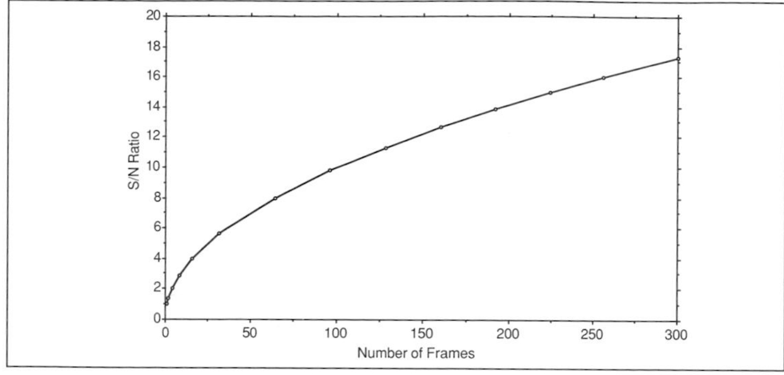

Figure 30. *Signal-to-noise ratio of averaged image improves as the square root of the number of frames summed.*

small image dimensions. These typically use a single line of detectors and optical deflection to cover the image.

For many applications, the repetition rate does not need to be that high. Either stroboscopic imaging or simply a fast shutter speed may be enough to stop the important motion to provide a sharp image. Electronic shutters can be used to control solid-state imaging devices, instead of a mechanical shutter. Exposure times under 1000th of a second can easily be achieved, but of course this requires plenty of light.

High-resolution imaging

The use of commercial video cameras as sources of images for technical purposes such as industrial quality control, scientific or medical research, etc. seems rather limiting. Much better cameras exist, and avoiding the use of an analog signal path for the information can reduce degradation and improve resolution. Chips with 1000 × 1000, 2000 × 2000, and even 4000 × 4000 arrays of sensors are available. The cost of these cameras rises extremely rapidly, because the market is small, the yield during fabrication of these devices is small, and only a few will fit on a single wafer. However, they are used for some rather specialized imaging purposes, such as astronomical cameras. It seems unlikely that either the number of sensors will increase dramatically or the cost will drop sharply in the near future.

It is also possible to increase the "depth" of the display, or the number of grey levels that can be distinguished at each point. Whereas an 8-bit ADC gives $2^8 = 256$ brightness levels, using 12 bits gives $2^{12} = 4096$ levels, and 16 bits gives $2^{16} = 65536$ levels. Such great depth is needed when the brightness range of the image is extreme (as for instance in astronomy), in order to acquire enough signal to show detail in dark regions of the image without bright areas saturating so that information is lost. These depths are achievable, although they require cooling the camera to reduce electronic noise, and permit much slower image acquisition and digitization than the 1/30 second per full frame associated with "real time" video.

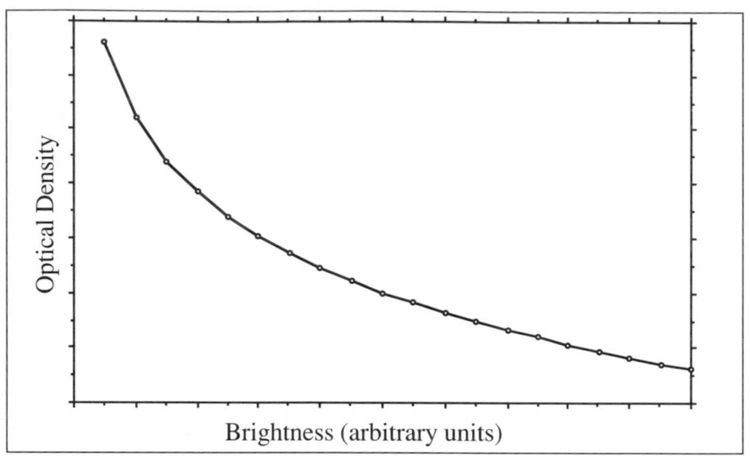

Figure 31. *Optical density is a logarithmic function of brightness.*

In some cases, the entire 12- or 16-bit depth of each pixel is stored. However, since this exceeds the capabilities of most CRTs to display, or of the user to see, reduction is often appropriate. If the actual brightness range of the image does not cover the entire possible range, scaling (either manual or automatic) to select just the range actually used can significantly reduce storage requirements. In other cases, especially when performing densitometry, a nonlinear conversion table is used. For densitometry, the desired density value varies as the logarithm of the brightness, as shown in **Figure 31**. A range of 256 brightness steps is not adequate to cover a typical range from 0 to greater than 2 in optical density with useful precision, because at the dark end of the range, 1 part in 256 represents a step of more than 0.1 in optical density. Using a digitization with 12 bits (1 part in 4096) solves this problem, but it is efficient to convert the resulting value with a logarithmic lookup table to store an 8-bit value (occupying a single computer byte) that is the optical density.

Lookup tables (LUTs) may be implemented either in hardware or software. They simply use the original value as an index into a stored or precalculated table, which then provides the derived value. This process is fast enough that acquisition is not affected. The context for LUTs discussed here is for image acquisition, converting a 12- or 16-bit digitized value with a nonlinear table to an 8-bit value that can be stored. LUTs are also used for displaying stored images, particularly to substitute colors for grey scale values to create pseudo-color displays. This is discussed in Chapters 2 and 3.

Many images do not have a brightness range that covers the full dynamic range of the digitizer. The result is an image whose histogram covers only a portion of the available values for storage or display. **Figure 32** shows a histogram of such an image. The flat regions indicate brightness values at both the light and dark ends that are not used by any of the pixels in the image. Expanding the brightness scale by spreading the histogram out to

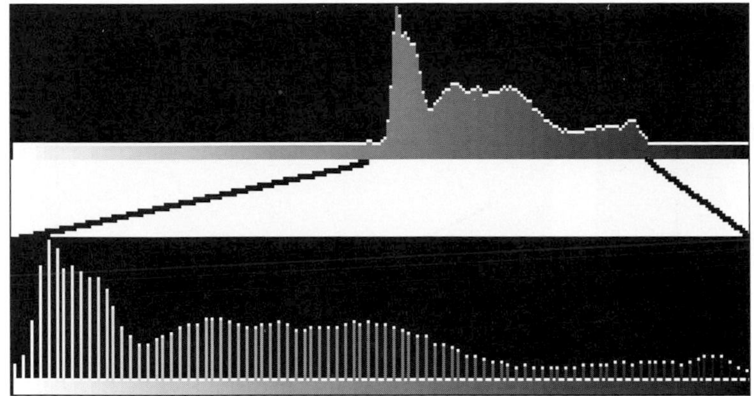

Figure 32. Linear expansion of a histogram to cover the full range of storage and/or display.

the full available range, as shown in the figure, may improve the visibility of features and the perceived contrast in local structures. The same number of brightness values are missing from the image, as shown by the gaps in the histogram, but now they are spread uniformly throughout the range. Other ways to stretch the histogram nonlinearly are discussed in Chapter 2.

Because the contrast range of many astronomical images is too great for photographic printing, special darkroom techniques have been developed. "Unsharp masking" (**Figure 33**) increases the ability to show local contrast by suppressing the overall brightness range of the image. This is done by first printing a "mask" image, slightly out of focus, onto another negative. The negative is developed and then placed on the original to make the final print. This reduces the exposure in bright areas so that the detail can be shown. The same method can also be used in digital image processing, either by subtracting a smoothed version of the image or by using a Laplacian operator (both are discussed in Chapter 3 on spatial domain processing). When the entire depth of a 12- or 16-bit image is stored, this may be needed in order to display the image for viewing on a CRT.

Some perspective on camera performance levels is needed. While a standard video camera has about 300,000 sensors, and a high-performance camera may have a few million, the human eye has about $1.5 \cdot 10^8$. These are clustered particularly tightly in the fovea, the central area where we concentrate our attention. While it is true that only a few dozen brightness levels can be distinguished in a single field, the eye adjusts automatically to overall brightness levels covering nine orders of magnitude to select the optimal range (although color sensitivity is lost in the darkest part of this range).

It is also interesting to compare video technology to other kinds of image-acquisition devices. The scanning electron (SEM) or scanning tunneling microscopes (STM) typically use from a few hundred to about 1000 scan lines, and those that digitize the signals use 8 or sometimes 12 bits, and so are similar in image res-

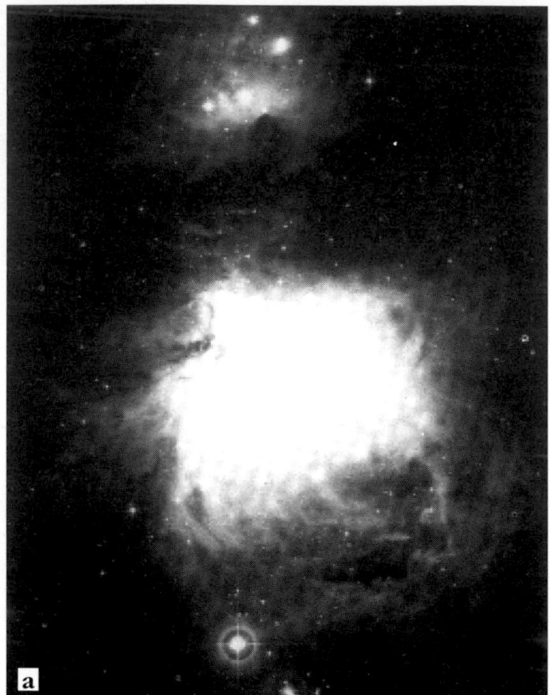

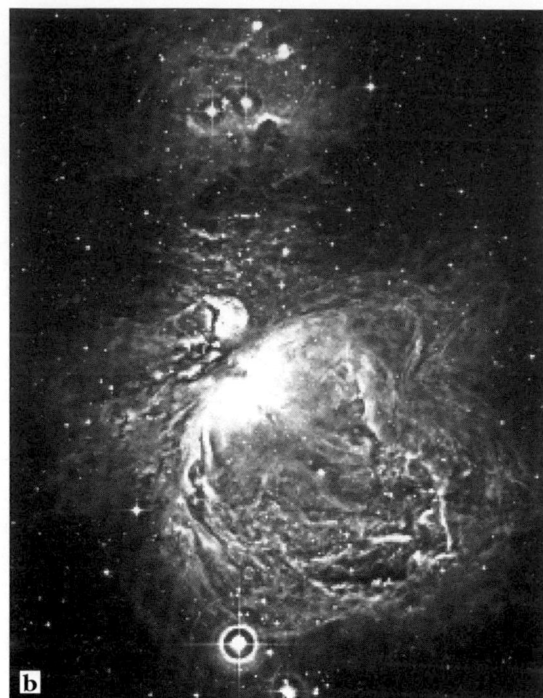

Figure 33. Unsharp masking:
a) *A telescope image originally recorded on film of the Orion nebula.*
b) *The same image using unsharp masking. An out-of-focus photographic print is made onto negative material, which is then placed on the original to reduce the exposure in bright areas when the final print is made. This reduces the overall contrast so that local variations show. Laplacian filtering performs the same function in digital image analysis.*

olution and size to many camera systems. **Figure 34** shows schematically the function of an SEM. The focused beam of electrons is scanned over the sample surface in a raster pattern while various signals generated by the electrons are detected. These include secondary and backscattered electrons, characteristic X-rays, visible light, and electronic effects in the sample.

Other point-scanning microscopes, such as the STM, the confocal scanning light microscope (CSLM), and even contact profilometers, produce very different signals and information. All provide a time-varying signal that is related to spatial locations on the sample by knowing the scanning speed and parameters, which allows storing the data as an image.

Significantly larger arrays of pixels are available from flat-bed scanners. These devices use a linear solid-state detector array which offers from 300 to 600 pixels per inch and can typically scan areas at least 8×10 inches and sometimes up to four times that size. While primarily intended for the desktop publishing market, they are readily adapted to scan electrophoresis gels used for protein separation or photographic prints or negatives. A high-quality negative can record several hundred discrete brightness levels and several hundred points per inch (both val-

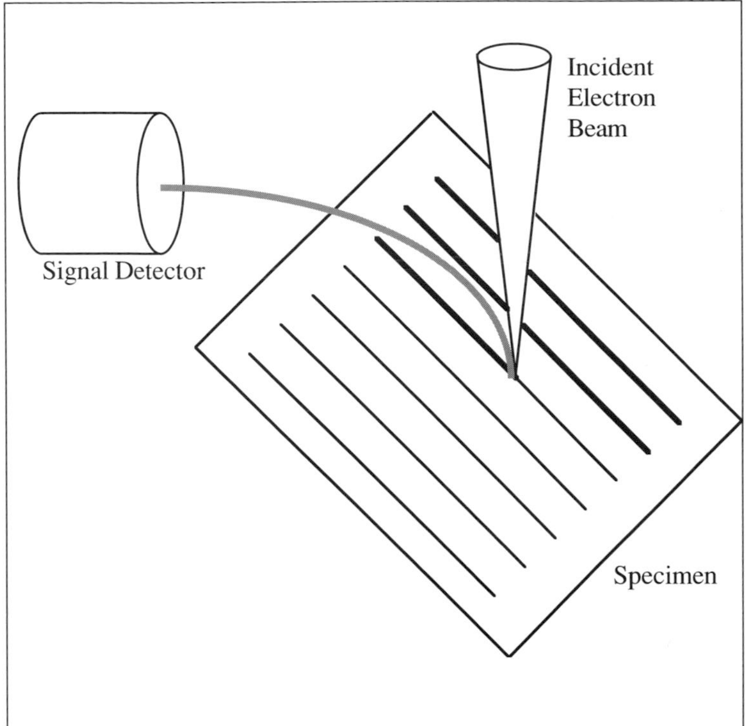

Figure 34. *The scanning electron microscope (SEM) focuses a fine beam of electrons on the specimen, producing various signals which may be used for imaging as the beam is scanned in a raster pattern.*

ues are much better than prints), which means that these scanners are quite suitable for digitizing photographic negatives, such as medical X-rays. Many can also digitize color (RGB) images, which are discussed below. These devices are quite stable and inexpensive, but rather slow, taking tens of seconds to digitize the scan area.

Hardcopy recordings of images, once they are stored in the computer, can also make use of hardware intended primarily for the desktop publishing market. Typical inexpensive laser printers or ink-jet printers have stated resolutions of 300 points per inch, but these are black, not grey points. These points must be collected to form halftone cells to print grey scale images. A 6×6 block of these small black dots can provide more than 30 distinct grey levels by printing all, some, or no dots. This reduces the lateral resolution to about 50 cells per inch. The lateral resolution can be increased to about 75 cells per inch by reducing the number of dots per cell to 4×4, which gives 17 different grey levels–about the quality of newspaper halftone printing. **Figure 35** shows the relationship between printer dots and halftone cells, for the case of 4×4 dots per cell and 17 grey levels, using one possible arrangement of the dots. Other configurations for turning on the dots within a cell, including random patterns, are also used.

Figure 36 shows several examples of halftone output from a 300-dot-per-inch laser printer, in which the number of halftone

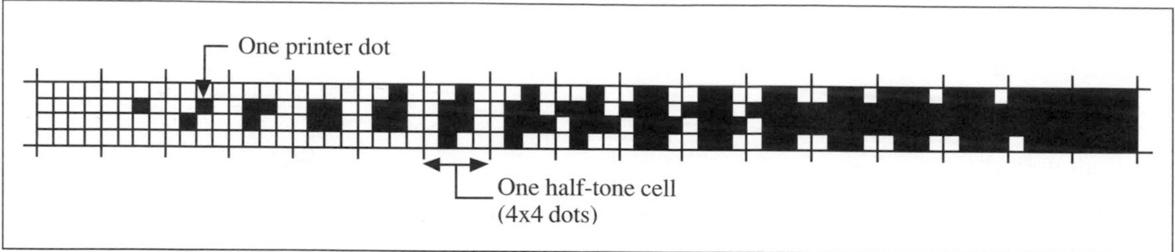

Figure 35. *Example of the relationship between printer dots and halftone cells. Groups of dots (in this example 4×4) are printed or not to produce 17 different grey levels. For a printer resolution of 300 dots per inch, the halftone resolution would be 75 cells per inch.*

cells is varied to trade off grey scale vs. lateral resolution. The output from the current generation of laser printers is adequate for some reports. Similar resolution is available with ink-jet or dye transfer printers primarily intended for color printing. Publication-quality printing requires higher resolution, such as a Linotype. These printers are becoming more readily available, but are hardly standard office or laboratory equipment as yet.

Color imaging

Most "real world" images are not monochrome, of course, but full color. The light microscope produces color images, and many tissue specimen preparation techniques make use of color to identify structure or localize chemical activity in novel ways. Even for inorganic materials, the use of polarized light or surface oxidation produces color images to delineate structure. The SEM would seem to be a strictly monochromatic imaging tool, but color may be introduced based on X-ray energy or backscattered electron energy. **Figure 37** shows individual grey scale images from the electron and X-ray signals. Assigning several of these arbitrarily, e.g., to the red, green, and blue planes of a display, may aid the user in judging the alignment of regions. This is not "true color" of course, but substitutes distinct visible colors for different signals. Colored X-ray maps are now fairly common with the SEM, but other uses of color, such as energy loss in the transmission electron microscope (TEM), are still experimental.

Similar use of color is potentially useful with other kinds of microscopes, although in many cases these possibilities have not been exploited in commercial instruments. This is also true for macroscopic imaging tools. A simple example is the use of color to show altitude in air traffic control displays. This use of color increases the bandwidth for communicating multidimensional information to the user, but using it effectively will require user education and would benefit from some standardization.

This use of color to encode richly multidimensional information must be distinguished from the very common use of false-color or pseudo-color to substitute colors for brightness in a monochrome image. Pseudo-color is used because of the limitation mentioned before in our visual ability to distinguish subtle differences in brightness. Although we can only distinguish about 30 shades of grey in a monochrome image, we can distinguish hundreds of different colors. Also, it is easier to describe a particular feature of interest as "the dark blue one" rather than "the medium grey one."

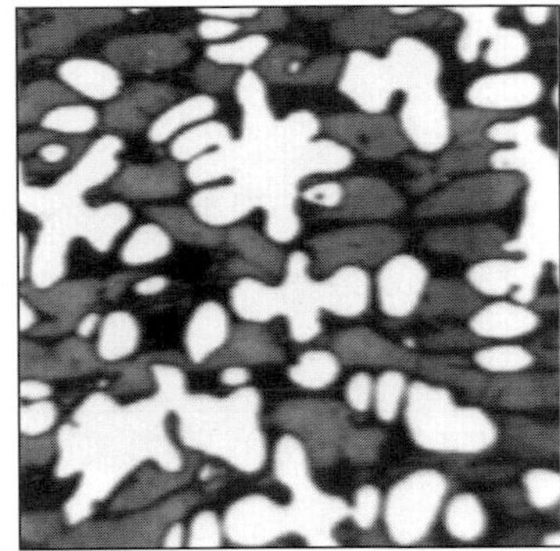

Plate 1. *See color plate, page I. Color plates appear following page 246.*

The use of color scales as a substitute for brightness values lets us show and see small changes locally and identify the same brightness values globally in an image. This should be a great benefit, since these are among the goals for imaging discussed below. Pseudo-color has been used particularly for many of the images returned from space probes. It would be interesting to know how many people think that the rings around Saturn really are brightly colored or that Comet Halley really is surrounded by a rainbow-colored halo! The danger in the use of pseudo-color is that it can obscure the real contents of an image. Colors force us to concentrate on the details of an image and to lose the gestalt information.

Pseudo-color displays as used in this context simply substitute a color from a stored or precalculated table for each discrete stored brightness value. As shown in **Plate 1**, this should be distinguished from some other uses of color displays to identify structures or indicate feature properties. These also rely on the use of color to communicate rich information to the viewer, but require considerable image processing and measurement before this information becomes available.

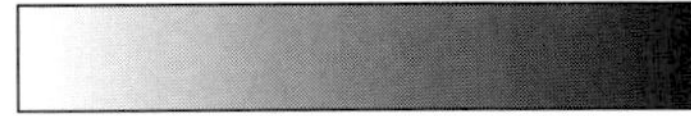

Plate 2. *See color plate, page I.*

Color can be used to encode elevation of surfaces (see Chapter 8 on 3D imaging). In scientific visualization it is used for velocity, density, composition, and many less obvious properties. These uses generally have little to do with the properties of the image and simply take advantage of the human ability to distinguish more colors than grey scale values.

Most computer-based imaging systems make it easy to substitute various LUTs of colors for the brightness values in a stored image. These work in the same way as input LUTs, described previously. The grey scale stored value is used to select a set of red, green, and blue brightnesses in the LUT which are the voltages sent to the display tube. Many systems also provide utilities for creating tables of these colors, but there are few guidelines to assist in constructing useful ones. All we can do here is advise caution. One approach is to systematically and gradually vary color along a path through color space. Examples (**Plate 2**) are a rainbow spectrum of colors or a progression from brown through red and yellow to white and then blue, the so-called heat scale. This helps to organize different parts of the scene. Another approach is to rapidly shift colors, for instance by varying the hue sinusoidally. This enhances gradients and makes it easy to see local variations, but may completely hide the overall contents of some images (**Plate 3**).

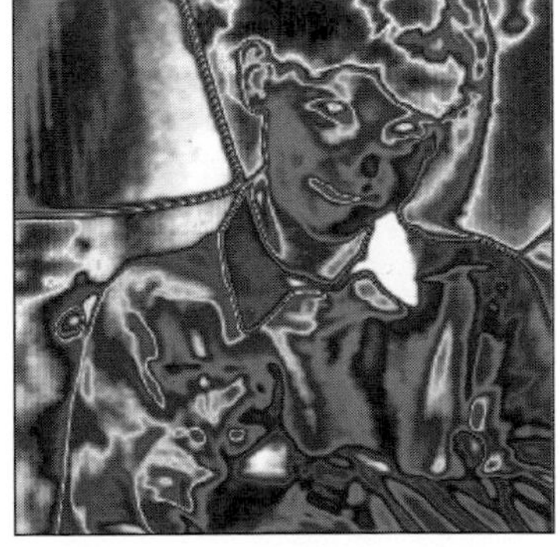

Plate 3. *See color plate, page II.*

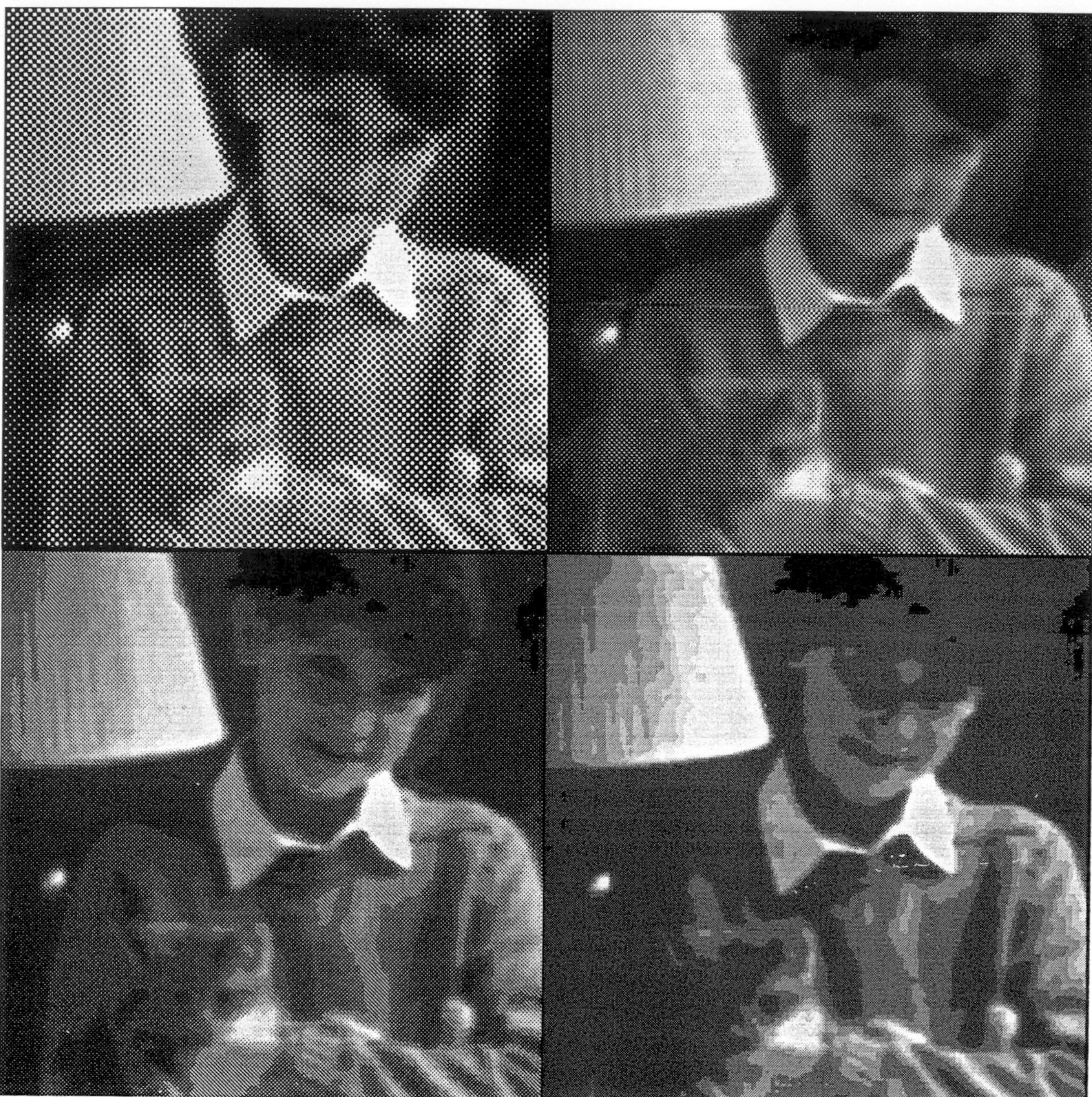

Figure 36. *Printed halftone images of the same image from Figures 25 and 26 using a 300-dot-per-inch Postscript laser printer, with halftone grids of 32, 50, 75, and 100 cells per inch. Increasing the number of cells improves the lateral resolution at the expense of the number of grey levels which can be shown, which in this example are 82, 37, 17, and 10, respectively.*

Some image sources may use color to encode a variety of different kinds of information, such as the intensity and polarization of radio waves in astronomy. However, by far the most common type of color image is that produced by recording intensity at three different wavelengths of visible light. Video deserves consideration as a suitable medium for this type of image, since standard broadcast television uses color effectively. The National Television Systems Committee (NTSC) color encoding scheme used in the U.S. was developed as a compatible add-on to existing monochrome television broadcasts. It adds the color information within the same, already narrow bandwidth limitation. The result is that the color has even less lateral resolution than the brightness information.

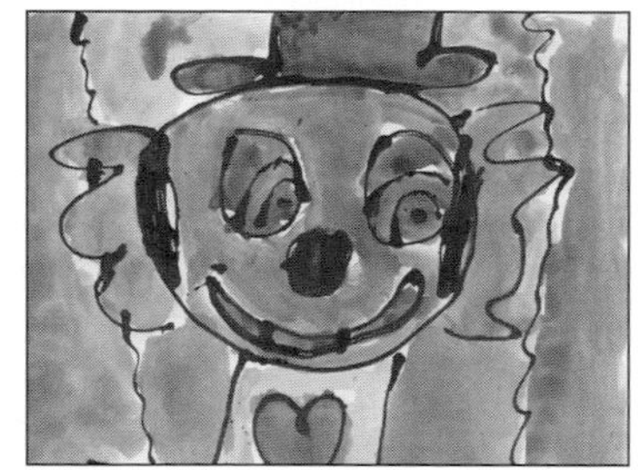

Plate 4. *See color plate, page II.*

This is acceptable for television pictures, since the viewer tolerates colors that are less sharply bounded and uses the edges of features defined by the brightness component of the image where they do not exactly correspond. The same tolerance has been used effectively by painters and may be familiar to parents whose young children have not yet learned to color "inside the lines." **Plate 4** shows an example in which the bleeding of color across boundaries or variations within regions is not confusing to the eye.

The poor spatial sharpness of NTSC color is matched by its poor consistency in representing the actual color values (a common joke is that NTSC means "Never The Same Color"). Videotape recordings of color images are even less useful for analysis than monochrome ones, but the limitations imposed by the broadcast channel do not necessarily mean that the cameras and other components may not be useful. An improvement in the sharpness of the color information in these images is afforded by Super-VHS or S-video recording equipment, in which the brightness or luminance and color or chrominance information are transmitted and recorded separately.

The least expensive color cameras, developed in response to consumer demand, are solid state. Chips are identical to those used in monochrome cameras, except that vertical rows of sensors are alternately made sensitive to red, green, and blue light. This may be done either by adjusting the electrical band gap in the semiconductor or more commonly by simply applying a filter coating to absorb the complementary colors. The detection of the red, green, and blue primary colors allows the camera electronics to produce the encoded color signal. This particular encoding scheme (YIQ) is discussed below, along with others.

Beyond the fact that the camera electronics may limit sharpness, since the expected use of the encoded signal is for videotape recording, the use of a single chip for recording has caused a loss in lateral resolution by a factor of three–because it now takes three sensors to record the information from each point. Higher quality cameras, including the ones used for broadcast TV, use a beam splitter to send the image, through appropriate color filters, to three separate monochrome cameras (which may be three solid-state chips or three tube-type cameras). These are, of course, much more expensive.

Some color cameras intended for technical purposes bring out the red, green, and blue signals separately, so they can be individually digitized. Recording the image in computer memory would then involve simply treating each signal as a monochrome

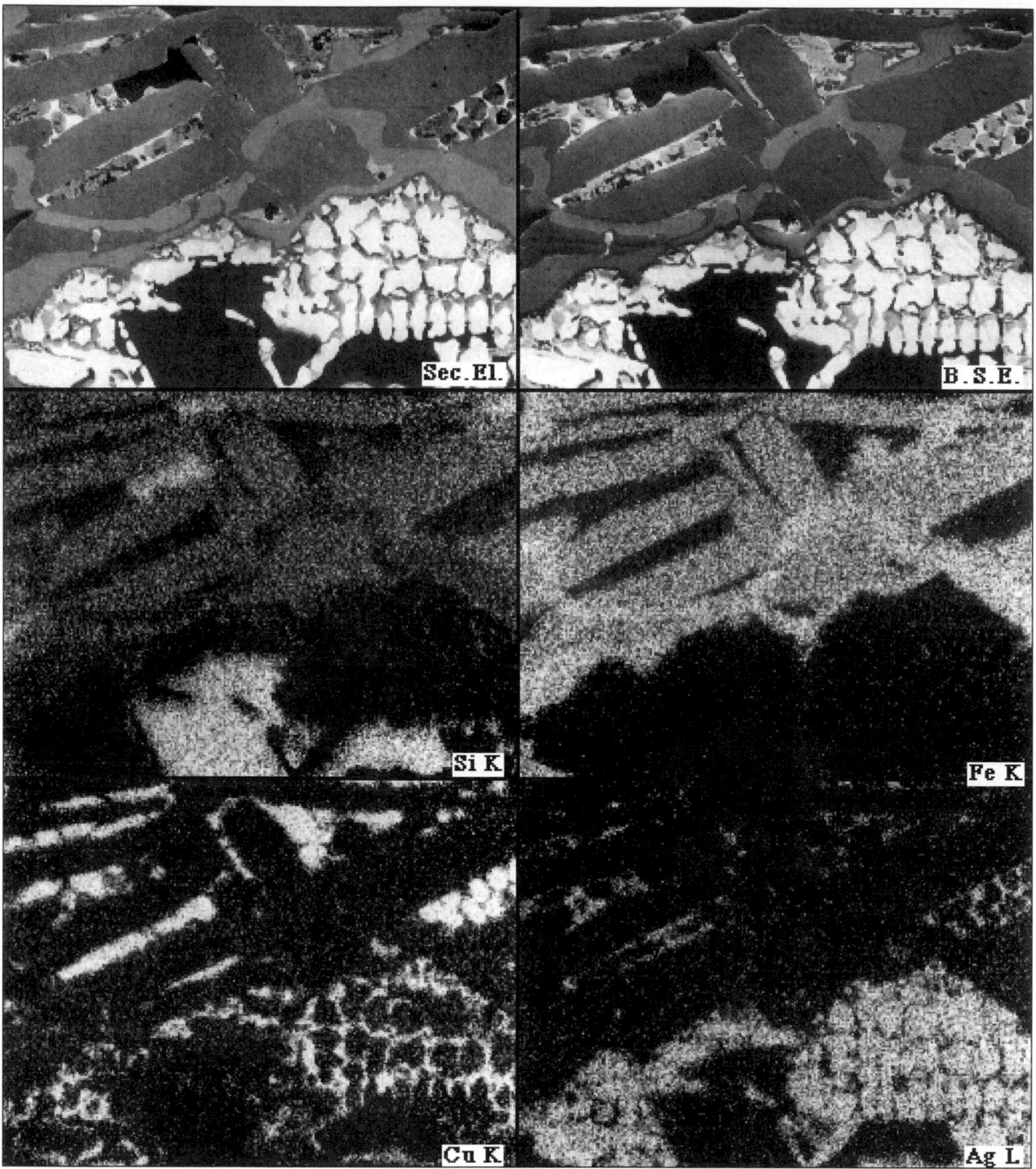

Figure 37. *Scanning electron microscope images of a mineral. The secondary and backscattered electron images delineate the various structures, and the silicon, iron, copper, and silver X-ray images show which structures contain those elements. (From Amray Corp., Bedford, MA.)*

one, converting it into a set of numbers, and storing it in memory. If the signals have first been combined, the encoding scheme used is likely to be YIQ, which is closely related to the NTSC broadcasting scheme.

Conversion from RGB (the brightness of the individual red, green, and blue signals at defined wavelengths) to YIQ and to the other color encoding schemes is straightforward and loses no information. Y, the "luminance" signal, is just the brightness of a panchromatic monochrome image that would be displayed by a black and white television receiver. It combines the red, green, and blue signals in proportion to the human eye's sensitivity to them. The I and Q components of the color signal are chosen for compatibility with the hardware used in broadcasting; the I signal is essentially red minus cyan, while Q is magenta minus green. The relationship between YIQ and RGB is shown in **Table 1**. An inverse conversion from the encoded YIQ signal to RGB simply requires inverting the matrix of values.

Table 1. Interconversion of RGB and YIQ color scales

Y	=	0.299 R	+	0.587 G	+	0.114 B		R	=	1.000 Y	+	0.956 I	+	0.621 Q
I	=	0.596 R	–	0.274 G	–	0.322 B		G	=	1.000 Y	–	0.272 I	–	0.647 Q
Q	=	0.211 R	–	0.523 G	+	0.312 B		B	=	1.000 Y	–	1.106 I	–	1.703 Q

RGB (and the complementary CMY subtractive primary colors used for printing) and YIQ are both hardware-oriented schemes. RGB comes from the way camera sensors and display phosphors work, and YIQ comes from broadcast considerations. **Figure 38** shows the "space" defined by RGB signals: it is cubic, since the red, green, and blue signals are independent and can be added to produce any color within the cube. There are other encoding schemes that are more useful for image processing, since they are more closely related to human perception.

The oldest of these is the CIE (Commission Internationale de L'Éclairage) chromaticity diagram. This is a two-dimensional plot defining color, shown in **Figure 39**. The third axis is the luminance, which corresponds to the panchromatic brightness, which, like the Y value in YIQ, would produce a monochrome (grey scale) image. The other two primaries, called x and y, are always positive–unlike the I and Q values–and combine to define any color that we can see.

Instruments for color measurement assess the CIE primaries, which define the dominant wavelength and purity of any color. Mixing any two colors corresponds to selecting a new point in the diagram along a straight line between the two original colors. This means that a triangle on the CIE diagram with its corners at the red, green, and blue locations of emission phosphors used in a CRT defines all of the colors that the tube can display. Some colors cannot be created by mixing these three phosphor colors, shown by the fact that they lie outside the triangle. The range of possible colors for any display or other output device is the gamut; hardcopy printers generally have a much smaller gamut

Figure 38. *RGB color space, showing the additive progression from black to white. Combining red and green produces yellow, green plus blue produces cyan, and blue plus red produces yellow. Greys lie along the cube diagonal. Cyan, yellow, and magenta are subtractive primaries used in printing, which if subtracted from white leave red, blue, and green, respectively.*

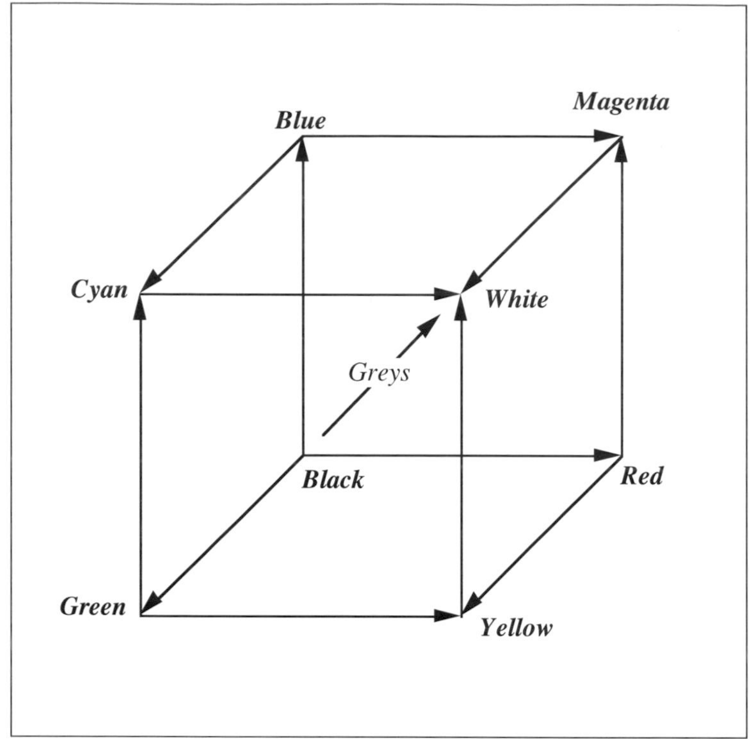

than display tubes. The edge of the bounded region in the diagram corresponds to pure colors and is marked with the wavelength in nanometers.

Complementary colors are shown in the CIE diagram by drawing a line through the central point, which corresponds to white light. Thus, a line from green passes through white to magenta. One of the drawbacks of the CIE diagram is that it does not indicate the variation in color that can be discerned by the eye. Sometimes this is shown by plotting a series of ellipses on the diagram. These are much larger in the green area, where small changes are poorly perceived, than elsewhere.

The CIE diagram provides a tool for color definition, but corresponds neither to the operation of hardware nor directly to human vision. Another approach, which does, is embodied in the HSV (hue, saturation, and value), HSI (hue, saturation, and intensity), and HLS (hue, lightness, and saturation) systems. These are closely related to each other and to the artist's concept of tint, shade, and tone. In this system, hue is the color as described by wavelength–for instance, the distinction between red and yellow. Saturation is the amount of the color that is present–for instance, the distinction between red and pink. The third axis (variously called lightness, intensity, or value) is the amount of light–the distinction between a dark red and light red or between dark grey and light grey.

The space in which these three values is plotted can be shown

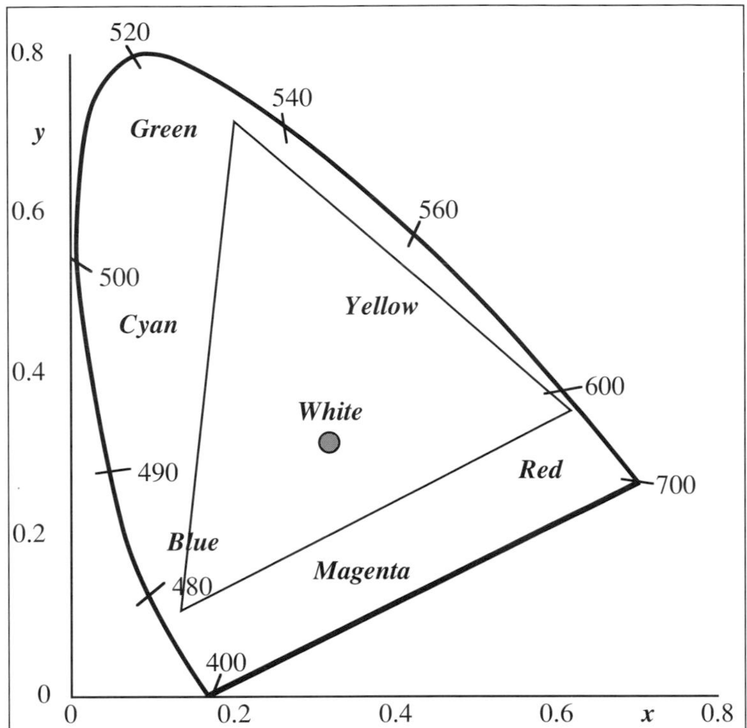

Figure 39. *The CIE chromaticity diagram. The dark outline contains visible colors, which are fully saturated along the edge. Numbers give the wavelength of light in nanometers. The inscribed triangle shows the colors that typical color CRTs can produce by mixing of red, green, and blue.*

as a circular or hexagonal cone or double cone, all of which can be stretched to correspond. It is straightforward to imagine the space as a double cone, in which the axis of the cone is the grey scale progression from black to white, distance from the central axis is the saturation, and the direction is the hue. **Figure 40** shows this schematically. The relationship between RGB and HSI is shown in **Table 2**.

Table 2. Conversion from RGB color coordinates to HSI coordinates

H	=	$[\pi/2 - \arctan\{(2 \cdot R - G - B)/\sqrt{3} \cdot (G - B)\} + \pi; G < B] / 2\pi$
I	=	$(R + G + B) / 3$
S	=	$1 - [\min(R,G,B) / I]$

This space has many advantages for image processing. For instance, if the algorithms discussed in Chapter 2, such as spatial smoothing or median filtering, are used to reduce noise in an image, applying them to the RGB signals separately will cause color shifts in the result, but applying them to the HSI components will not. **Plate 5** shows an example of processing to sharpen an image with a high-pass filter. Also, the use of hue (in particular) for distinguishing features in the process called segmentation (Chapter 5) often corresponds to human perception and ignores shading effects. On the other hand, because the HSI

Figure 40. *Bi-conic representation of Hue-Saturation-Intensity Space. Greys lie along the central axis. Distance from the axis gives the Saturation, while direction specifies the Hue.*

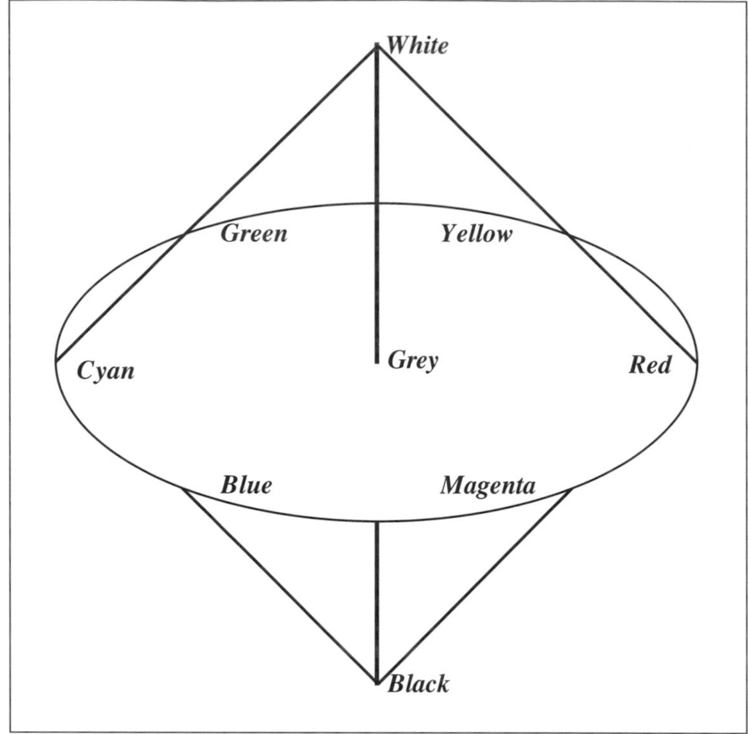

components do not correspond to the way that most hardware works (either for acquisition or display), it requires a significant amount of computation or custom hardware to convert RGB-encoded images to HSI and back.

Hardware for digitizing color images accepts either direct RGB signals from a special camera or a composite signal (e.g., NTSC) and uses filters to separate the individual components and extract the red, green, and blue signals. As for the monochrome case discussed above, these are then digitized to produce values, usually 8-bit ones ranging from 0 to 255 each for R, G, and B. This takes 3 bytes of storage per pixel, so a 640×480 pixel image would require nearly 1 megabyte of storage space in the computer. With most cameras and electronics, the signals do not contain quite this much information, and the lowest 2 or more bits are noise. Consequently, some systems keep only 5 bits each for R, G, and B, which can be fit into 2 bytes. This is often adequate for desktop publishing work, but when packed this way, the color information is difficult to get at for any processing or analysis operations.

In many situations, although color images are acquired, the "absolute" color information is not useful for image analysis. Instead, it is the relative differences in color from one region to another that can be used to distinguish the structures and features present. In such cases, it may not be necessary to store the entire color image. Various kinds of color separations are available. Calculating RGB components (or complementary CMY values) is commonly used in desktop publishing, but as we have seen is not often useful for image analysis. Separating the image into hue, saturation, and intensity components can also be performed; **Plate 6** shows an example.

Finally, it is possible to compute the amount of any color (hue) in the image. This is equivalent to the physical insertion of a transmission filter in front of a monochrome camera. The filter can be selected to absorb a complementary color (for instance, a blue filter will darken yellow regions by absorbing the yellow light) and transmit light of the same color, so that the resulting image contrast can be based on the color distribution in the image. Photographers have long used yellow filters to darken blue sky and produce monochrome images with dramatic contrast for clouds, for example. The same color filtering can be used to convert color images to monochrome (grey scale). **Plates 7 and 8** show examples in which the computer is used to apply the filter. This offers greater flexibility than physical filters, since the desired wavelength can be specified, and a drawer full of physical filters (some very difficult to make) is not needed.

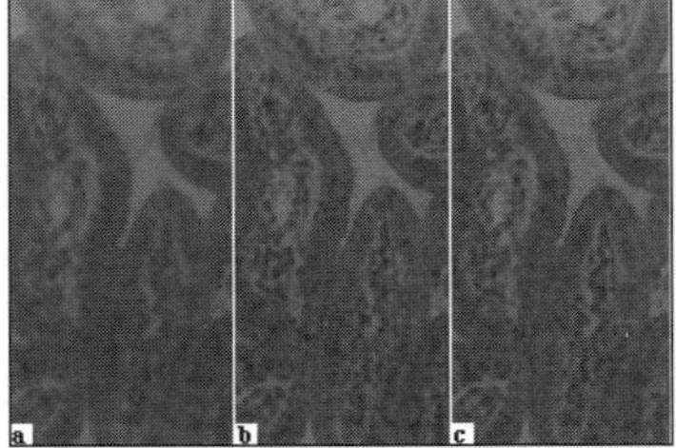

Plate 5. *See color plate, page III.*

In terms of computer storage, the old Chinese adage that a picture is worth a thousand words is clearly a vast understatement. Monochrome images may vary from 300,000 to several million bytes, and full-color images occupy about three times as much space. One of the consequences of this large size is the time needed to address each pixel, which must sometimes be repeated many times to perform processing operations. Another is the requirement for storage and transmission. Even with the continuing decline in the costs of memory and storage media, the large amounts of storage space afforded by optical disk technology, and higher speed networks for communication, images tax the resources of computer systems.

Compaction schemes attempt to reduce the size of images for storage and transmission. The time needed to accomplish compression and decompression is one criterion for judging this approach. The other is the degree of image preservation. Methods of current interest include the JPEG (Joint Photographic Experts Group) algorithm based on a discrete cosine transform. They can be implemented in either hardware or software on small computers, offering compression ratios of more than 50 times. This obviously reduces the storage and transmission costs for the image, but it is accomplished by discarding some of the small differences between pixels. Methods that are quite adequate when the images are simply to be printed in a desktop publishing application are not acceptable when the images are to be processed or analyzed. Common problems include variations in colors (especially near boundaries), broadening of edges, and loss of subtle texture information.

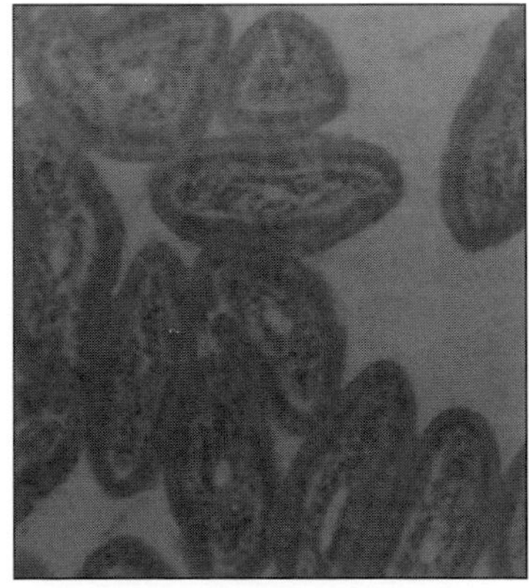

Plate 6. *See color plate, page III.*

The JPEG compaction scheme has several parts. First, the image

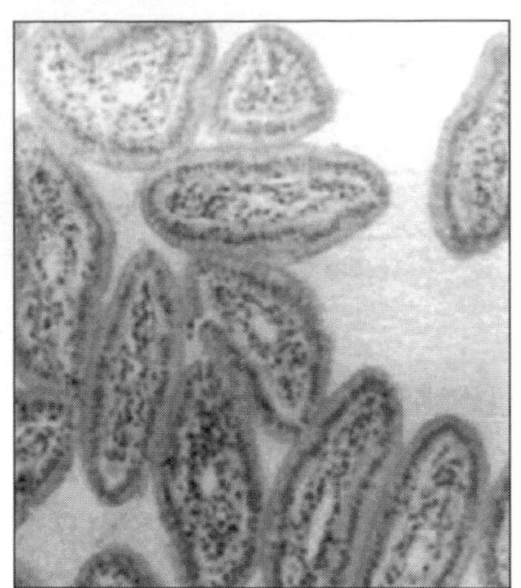

Plate 7. *See color plate, page IV.*

is transformed from RGB to a video-based encoding scheme, in which the grey scale image (the luminance) and the color information (the chrominance) are separated. Each of these is compacted separately, since for visual purposes it is possible to lose more of the color information than grey scale. This is because the eye uses the grey scale edges to indicate boundaries and allows color to bleed across boundaries without confusion.

Next, square subregions in the image are processed with a discrete cosine transform. This is similar to the FFT discussed in Chapter 4, except that the terms in the expansion are real valued (the FFT uses complex numbers). For a spatial image $f(x,y)$ the two-dimensional transform $F(u,v)$ is given by

$$F(u,v) = \frac{4c(u,v)}{N^2} \sum_{x=0}^{N-1} \sum_{y=0}^{N-1} f(x,y) \cos \frac{(2x+1)\pi u}{2N} \cos \frac{(2y+1)\pi v}{2N}$$

where N is the width of the image, the range for u and v is from 0 to N–1, and the function $c(u,v) = 1$ (except when u or v is 0–it is then equal to 0.5). The magnitude of these terms drops very rapidly as u and v increase, and the compression is achieved by keeping only some of them, starting from 0 and working up. The fewer the terms kept, the greater the compression (and the greater the loss of high-frequency information). This may be done separately for different areas within the image, so that the amount of color or detail preservation is varied according to the actual image contents.

Finally, additional compression is achieved by truncating the precision of the terms and then using a coding scheme that looks for repeated characters and stores them only once, along with the number of repeats. From all of these operations, compression ratios in excess of 100:1 are possible, although much lower ratios of the order of 10:1 are more typical (and still very useful). **Plate 9** shows an example of a color image that has been compressed by 16:1. There is some detectable loss of detail and sharpness which would be objectionable for measurement purposes, but it is not visually distracting. Depending on whether hardware or software is used to perform the transform (and its inverse, which is required to retrieve the image for display), the time required to perform the compression and decompression can vary up to tens of seconds.

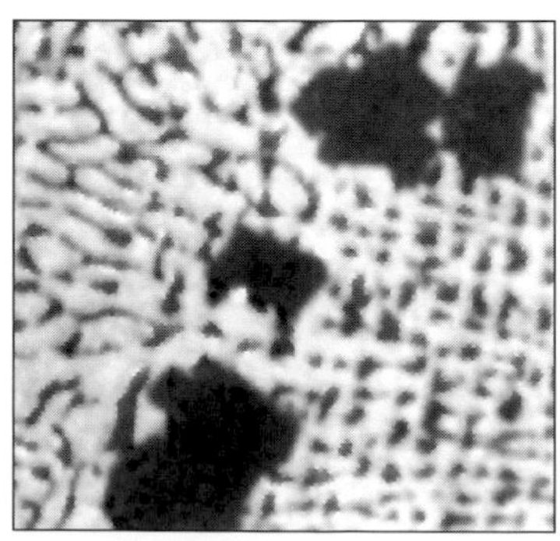

Plate 8. *See color plate, page IV.*

Other encoding schemes may also be used. One that is often employed in image analysis, image storage in computers, and for telephone facsimile transmission (fax) is chord encoding or run-length encoding (**Figure 41**). This works best for images with only a few grey scale values or, ideally, black-and-white or binary images. Each raster line of the image is reduced to a series of horizontal lines of uniform brightness. For each line segment, the brightness, line number, horizontal position of the start of the line, and its length are listed. For images that have large uniform areas, this produces a significant reduction in the size of the record. For grey scale or color images of natural scenes there is unfortunately little redundancy, so this method is not useful.

Another quite new approach to image compression uses fractal generators to reconstruct images from an iterated equation. Compaction ratios as great as 500:1 have been reported, but these methods also discard the low-level and fine-detail information in the image. They are also extremely slow both for compaction and restoration. Consequently, they are not useful for images that are to be used for subsequent processing and analysis.

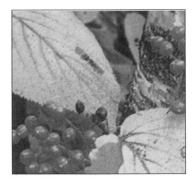

Plate 9. *See color plate, page V.*

Multiple images

For many applications, a single image is not enough. Multiple images may constitute a series of views of the same area, using different wavelengths of light or other signals. Examples include the images produced by satellites, such as the various visible and infrared wavelengths recorded by the Landsat Thematic Mapper (LTM), and images from the SEM in which as many as a dozen different elements may be represented by their X-ray intensities. These images may each require processing; for example, X-ray maps are usually very noisy. They are then often combined either by using ratios, such as the ratio of different wavelengths used to identify crops in LTM images, or Boolean logic, such as locating regions that contain iron and sulfur in an SEM image of a mineral. **Plate 10** and **Figure 42** show an example in which two satellite color photographs of the same region–one covering the usual visual range of wavelengths and one extending into the near infrared–are combined by constructing the ratio of infrared to green intensity. Combinations reduce, but only slightly, the amount of data to be stored.

Another multiple image situation is a time sequence. This could be a series of satellite images used to track the motion of weather systems or a series of microscope images used to track the motion of cells or the beating of cilia. In all of these cases, the need is usually to identify and locate the same features in each of the images, even though there may be some gradual changes in feature appearance from one image to the next. If the images can be reduced to data on the location of only a small number of features, then the storage requirements are greatly reduced.

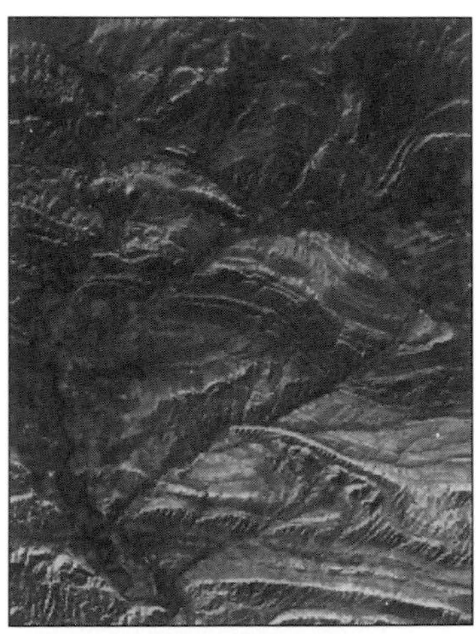

Plate 10. *See color plate, page V.*

A technique known as motion flow works at a lower level, in which matching of pixel patterns by a correlation method is used to create a vector field showing the motion between successive images. This method is used particularly in machine vision and robotics work, in which the successive images are very closely spaced in time. Simplifying the vector field can again result in modest amounts of data, and these are usually processed in real time so that storage is not an issue. The principal requirement is

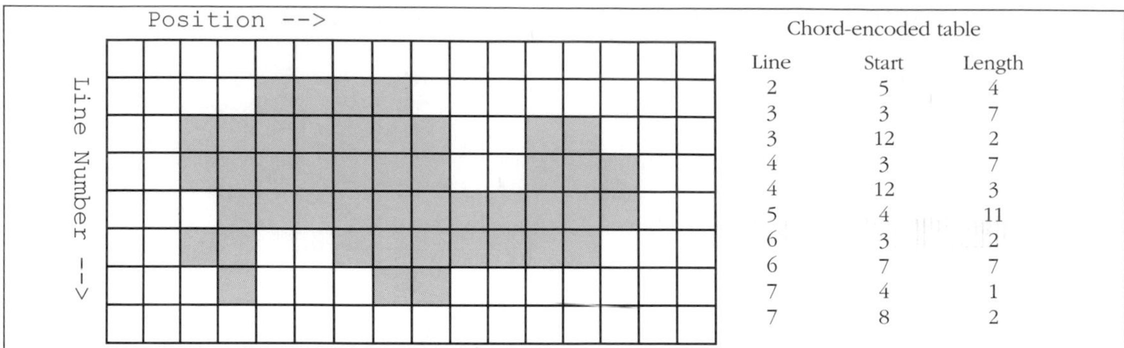

Line	Start	Length
2	5	4
3	3	7
3	12	2
4	3	7
4	12	3
5	4	11
6	3	2
6	7	7
7	4	1
7	8	2

Figure 41. *Chord encoding or run-length coding is particularly useful with binary (black and white) images. The line number, start, and length are listed for each horizontal line of pixels.*

that the local texture information needed for matching is present. Therefore, the images must be low in noise and each image should contain simple and distinctive surfaces with consistent illumination. Matching is performed using cross-correlation matching, in either the spatial or frequency domain.

A set of images can also produce three-dimensional information. These are usually a series of parallel-slice images through a solid object (**Figure 43**). Medical imaging methods such as tomography and magnetic resonance images can produce this sort of data. So can some seismic imaging techniques. Even more common are various serial section methods used in microscopy. The classical method for producing such a series of images is to microtome a series of sections from the original sample, image each separately in the light or electron microscope, and then align the images.

Optical sectioning, especially with the CSLM, which has a very shallow depth of field and can collect images from deep in partially transparent specimens, eliminates the problems of alignment. **Figure 44** shows several focal section planes from a CSLM. Some imaging methods such as the SIMS (secondary ion mass spectrometer) produce a series of images in depth by physically eroding the sample, which also preserves alignment. **Figure 45** shows an example of SIMS images. Sequential polishing of harder samples, such as metals, also produces new surfaces for imaging, but it is generally difficult to control the depth to space them uniformly.

The ideal situation for three-dimensional interpretation of structure calls for the lateral resolution of serial section image planes to be equal to the spacing between the planes. This produces cubic "voxels" (volume elements), which have the same advantages for processing and measurement in three dimensions that square pixels have in two. However, it is usually the case that the planes are spaced apart by much more than their lateral resolution, and special attention is given to interpolating between the

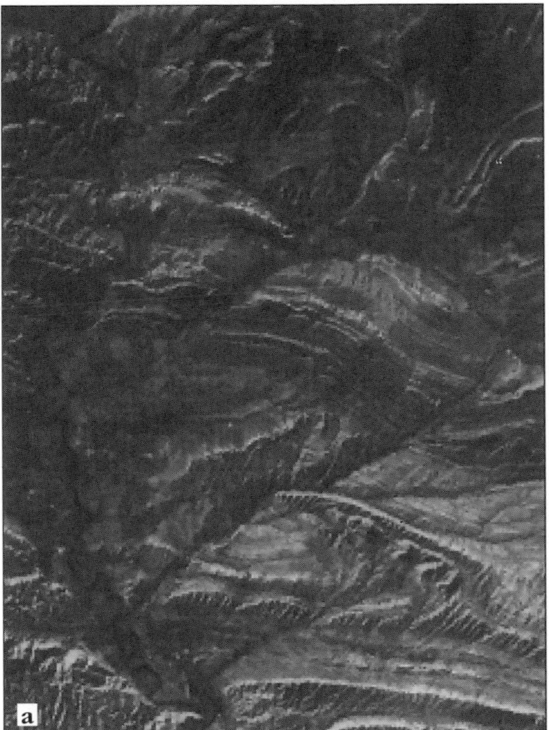

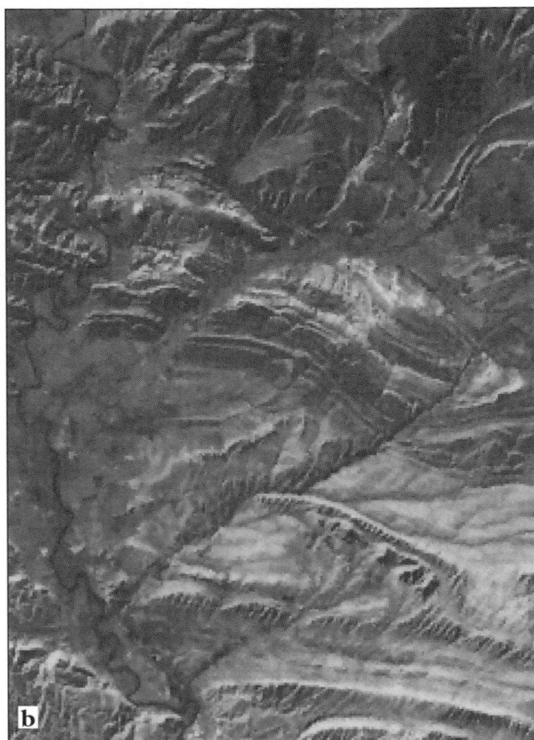

Figure 42. Monochrome images from color Landsat data:
a) *visible wavelengths;*
b) *infrared wavelengths. Compare to the colored, filtered, and ratioed images in Plate 10.*

planes. In the case of the SIMS, the situation is reversed and the plane spacing (as little as a few atom dimensions) is much less than the lateral resolution in each plane (typically about 1 μm).

There are techniques that directly produce cubic voxel images, such as three-dimensional tomography. In this case, a series of projection images, generally using X-rays or electrons, are obtained as the sample is rotated to different orientations, and then mathematical reconstruction calculates the density of each voxel. The resulting large, three-dimensional image arrays may be stored as a series of planar slices. When a three-dimensional data set is available, a variety of processing and display modes are

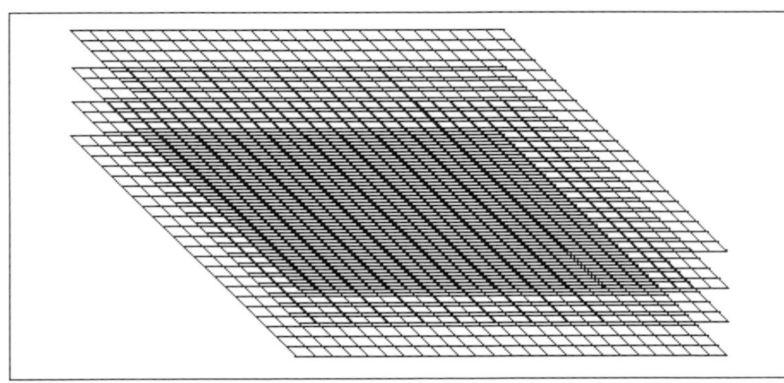

Figure 43. *Multiple planes of pixels fill three-dimensional space. Voxels (volume elements) are ideally cubic for processing and measurement of three-dimensional images.*

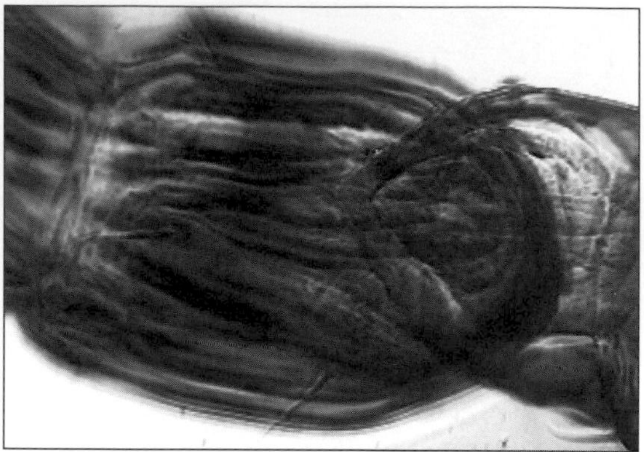

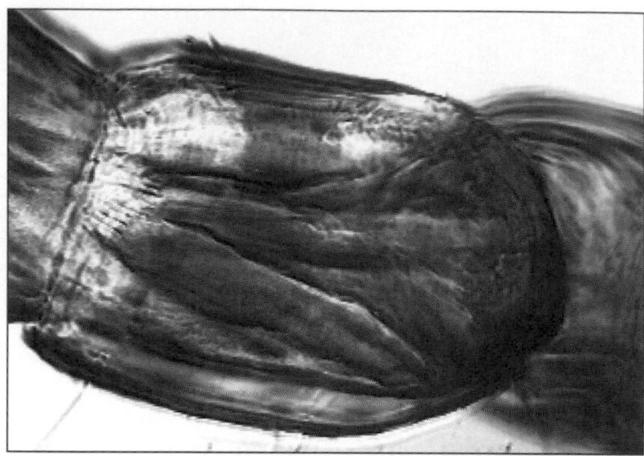

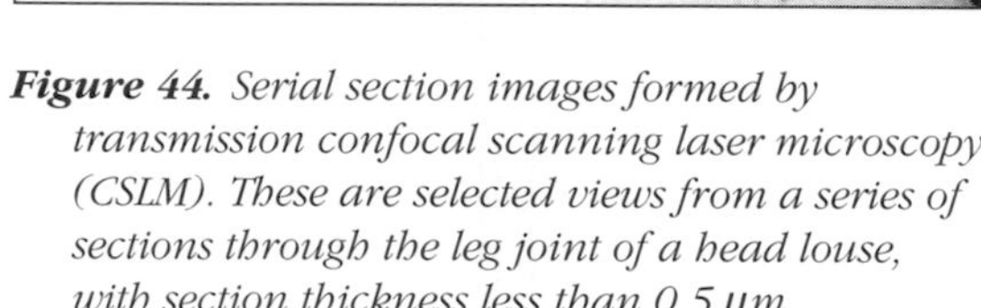

Figure 44. *Serial section images formed by transmission confocal scanning laser microscopy (CSLM). These are selected views from a series of sections through the leg joint of a head louse, with section thickness less than 0.5 μm.*

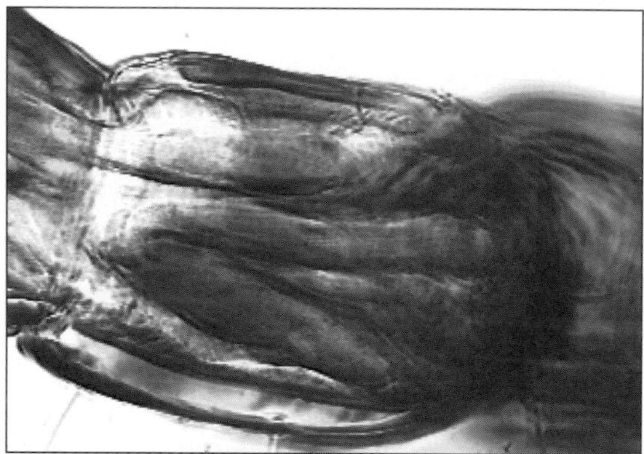

available. They are discussed in more detail in the final chapter of this book. **Figure 46** shows an example of sectioning through a series of magnetic resonance images (MRI) in the X, Y, and Z planes.

Three-dimensional information can also be obtained from two images of the same scene, taken from slightly different viewpoints. Human stereoscopy gives us depth perception, although we also get important data from relative size, precedence, perspective, and other cues. Like other aspects of human vision, stereoscopy is primarily comparative: the change of vergence angle of the eyes as we shift attention from one feature to another indicates to the brain which is closer. **Figure 47** shows schematically the principle of stereo fusion, in which the images from each eye are compared to locate the same feature in each view. The eye muscles rotate the eye to bring this feature to the fovea, and the muscles provide the vergence information to the brain.

Not all animals use this method. The owl, for instance, has eyes that are not movable in their sockets. Instead, the fovea has an elongated shape along a line that is not vertical, but angled toward the owl's feet. The owl tilts his head to accomplish fusion–bringing the feature of interest to the fovea–and judges the relative distance by the angle required.

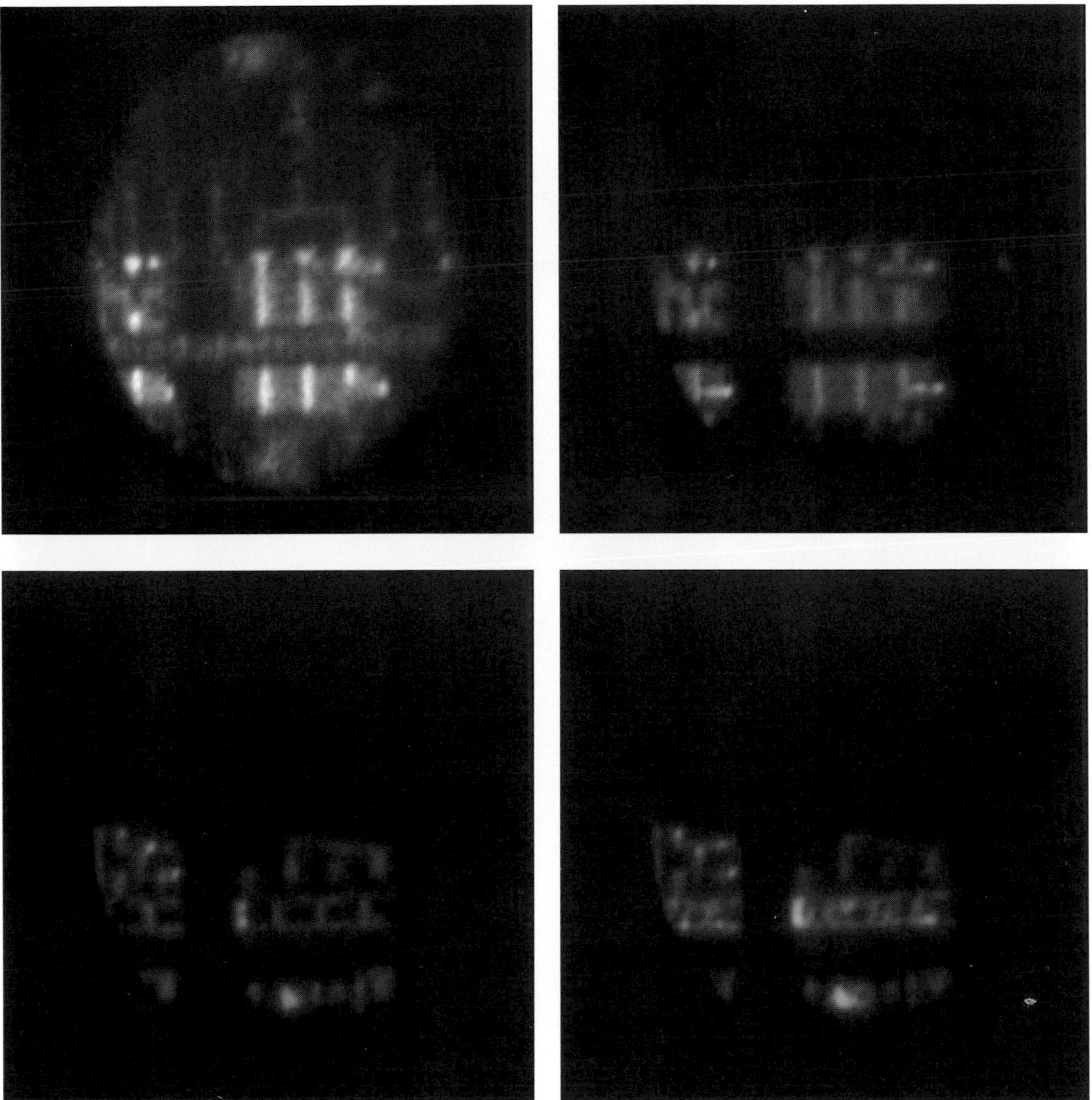

Figure 45. *SIMS (Secondary Ion Mass Spectrometer) images of boron implanted in a microelectronic device. The images are selected from a sequence of 29 images covering a total of about 1 µm in depth. Each image is produced by physically removing layers of atoms from the surface, which erodes the sample progressively to reveal structures at greater depth.*

Computer fusion of images is a difficult task, requiring the location of matching points in the images. Brute force correlation methods that try to match many points based on local texture are fundamentally similar to the motion flow approach. This produces many false matches, but these are assumed to be removed by subsequent noise filtering. The alternate approach is to locate selected points in the images that are "interesting" based on their representing important boundaries, or feature edges, which can then be matched more confidently. However, the areas be-

***Figure 46*. Examples of three-dimensional data sets formed by a series of planar images:**

a) *A sintered ceramic imaged by X-ray tomography (CAT), with a characteristic dimension of μm: the dark regions are voids. The poorer resolution in the vertical direction is due to the spacing of the image planes, which is greater than the lateral pixel resolution within each plane.*

b) *A human head imaged by magnetic resonance (MRI), with characteristic dimension of cm. The section planes can be positioned arbitrarily and moved to reveal the internal structure.*

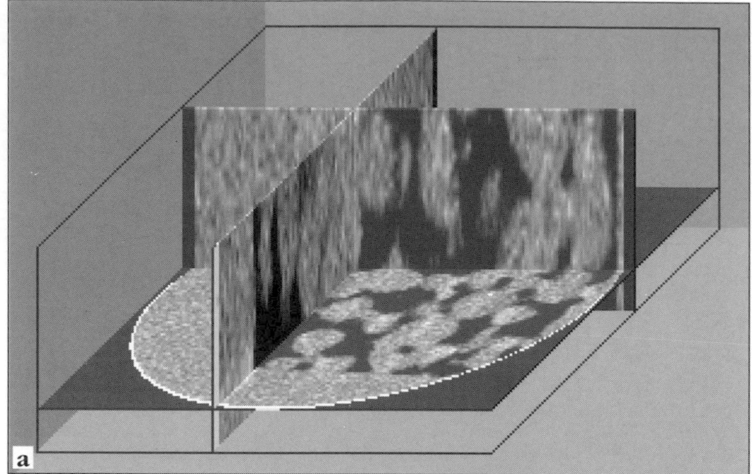

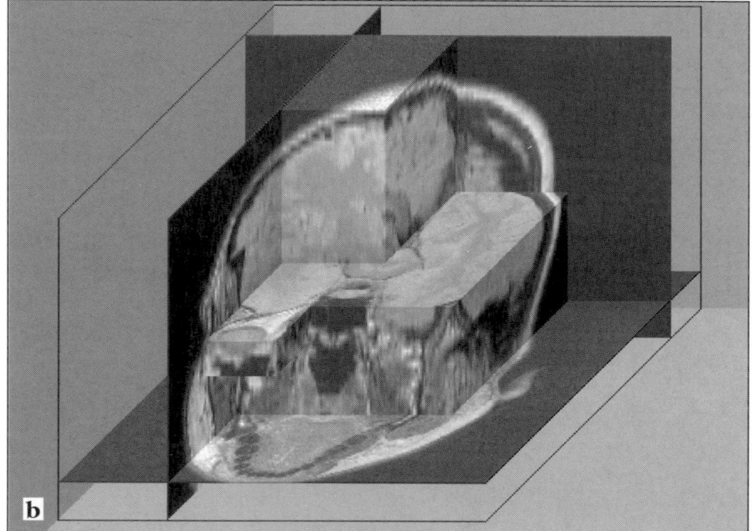

tween the matching points are then assumed to be simple planes.

However fusion is accomplished, the displacement of the points in the two images, or parallax, gives the range. This method is used for surface elevation mapping, ranging from satellite or aerial pictures used to produce topographic maps (in which the two images are taken a short time apart as the satellite or airplane position changes) to SEM metrology of semiconductor chips (in which the two images are produced by tilting the sample). **Figure 48** shows an example of a stereo pair from an SEM, and **Figure 49** shows two aerial photographs and a complete topographic map drawn from them.

Imaging requirements

Given the diversity of image types and sources described above,

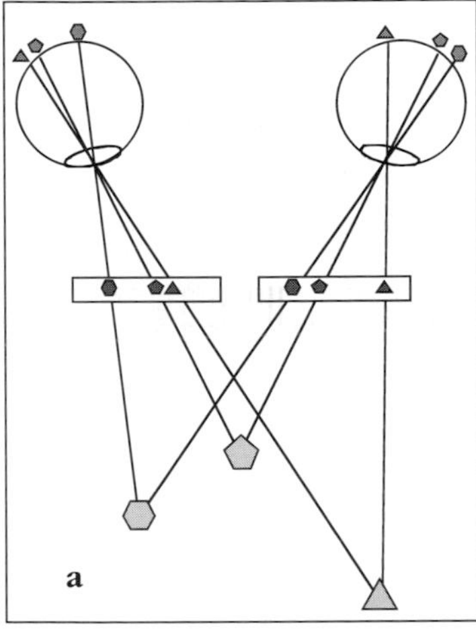

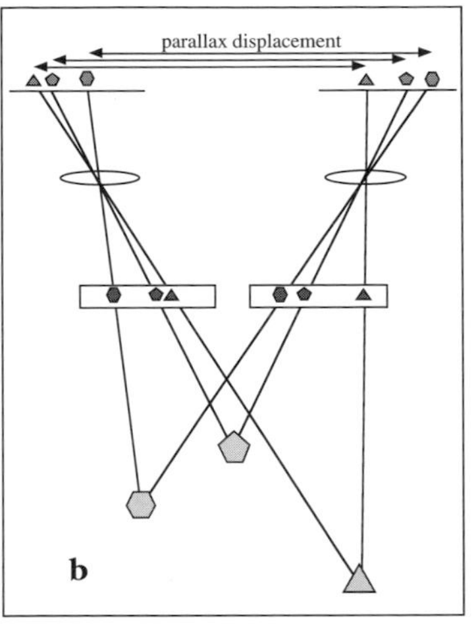

Figure 47. Stereoscopic depth perception:

a) *The relative distance to each feature identified in both the left and right eye views is given by differences in the vergence angles by which the eyes must rotate inward to bring each feature to the central fovea in each eye. This is accomplished one feature at a time. Viewing stereo pair images provides the same visual cues to the eyes and produces the same interpretation.*

b) *Measurement of images to obtain actual distances uses the different parallax displacements of the features in two images. The distance between the two view points must be known. Identifying the same feature in both images is the greatest difficulty for automated analysis.*

there are several general criteria we can prescribe for images intended for computer processing and analysis. The first is the need for global uniformity. The same type of feature should look the same wherever it appears in the image. This implies that brightness and color values should be the same and, consequently, that illumination must be uniform and stable for images acquired at different times. When surfaces are nonplanar, such as the earth as viewed from a satellite or a fracture surface in the microscope, corrections for the changing local orientation may be possible, but this usually requires extensive calculation and/or prior knowledge of the surface and source of illumination.

Figure 50 shows an example of a microscope image with nonuniform illumination. Storing a "background" image with no specimen present (by moving to a clear space on the slide) allows this nonuniformity to be leveled. The background image is either subtracted from or divided into the original (depending on whether the camera has a linear or logarithmic response). This type of leveling is discussed in Chapter 2 on correcting image defects, along with other ways to obtain the background image when it cannot be acquired directly.

The requirement for uniformity limits the kinds of surfaces that are normally imaged. Planar surfaces, or at least simple and known ones, are much easier to deal with than complex surfaces. Simply connected surfaces are much easier to interpret than ones with arches and loops that hide some of the structure. Features that have precedence problems, in which some feature hides entirely or in part behind others, present difficulties for interpretation or measurement. Illumination that casts strong shadows, especially to one side, is also undesirable in most cases. The exception occurs when well-spaced features cast shadows that do not interfere with each other: their lengths can be used to geometrically calculate feature heights. **Figure 51** shows an example in aerial photography. One form of sample preparation for the TEM deposits a thin film of metal or carbon from a point

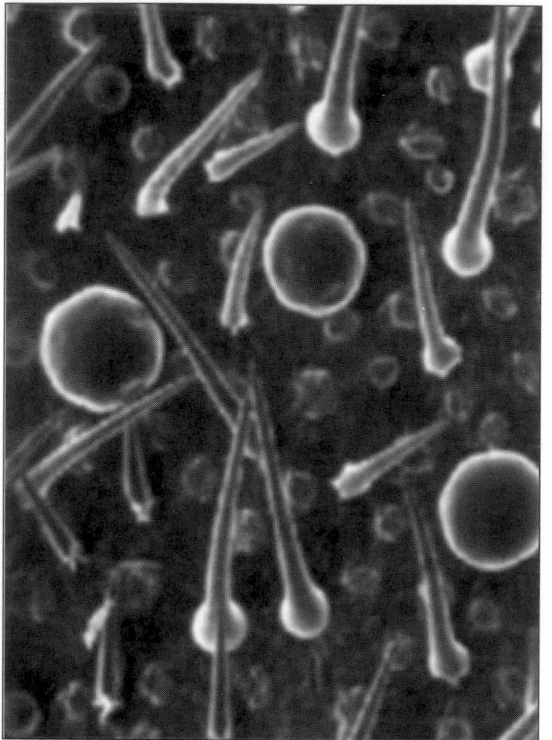
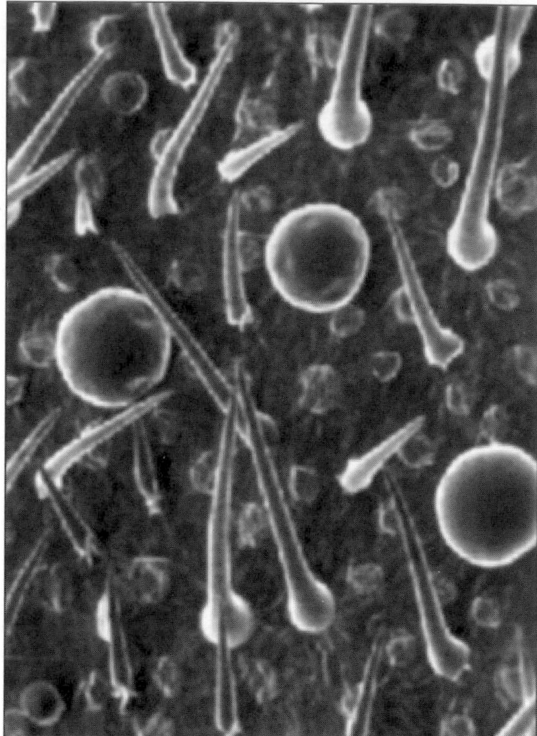

Figure 48. *Stereo pair images from the scanning electron microscope (SEM). The specimen is the surface of a leaf; the two images were obtained by tilting the beam incident on the specimen by 8° to produce two points of view.*

source, which also leaves shadow areas behind particles or other protrusions that can be used in the same way.

In addition to global uniformity, we generally want local sensitivity to variations. This means that edges and boundaries must be well delineated and accurately located. The resolution of the camera sensor was discussed above. Generally, anything that degrades high frequencies in the signal chain will disturb the subsequent ability to identify feature boundaries or locate edges for measurement. On the other hand, such simple problems as dust on the optics can introduce local variations that may be mistaken for image features, causing serious errors.

Dimension measurement requires that the geometry of the imaging system be well known. Knowing the magnification of a microscope or the altitude of a satellite is usually straightforward. Calibrating the lateral scale can be accomplished either by knowledge of the optics or by using an image of a known scale or standard. When the viewing geometry is more complicated, either because the surface is not planar or the viewing angle is not perpendicular, measurement is more difficult and requires determination of the geometry first.

Figure 52 shows the simplest kind of distortion when a planar surface is viewed at an angle. Different portions of the image

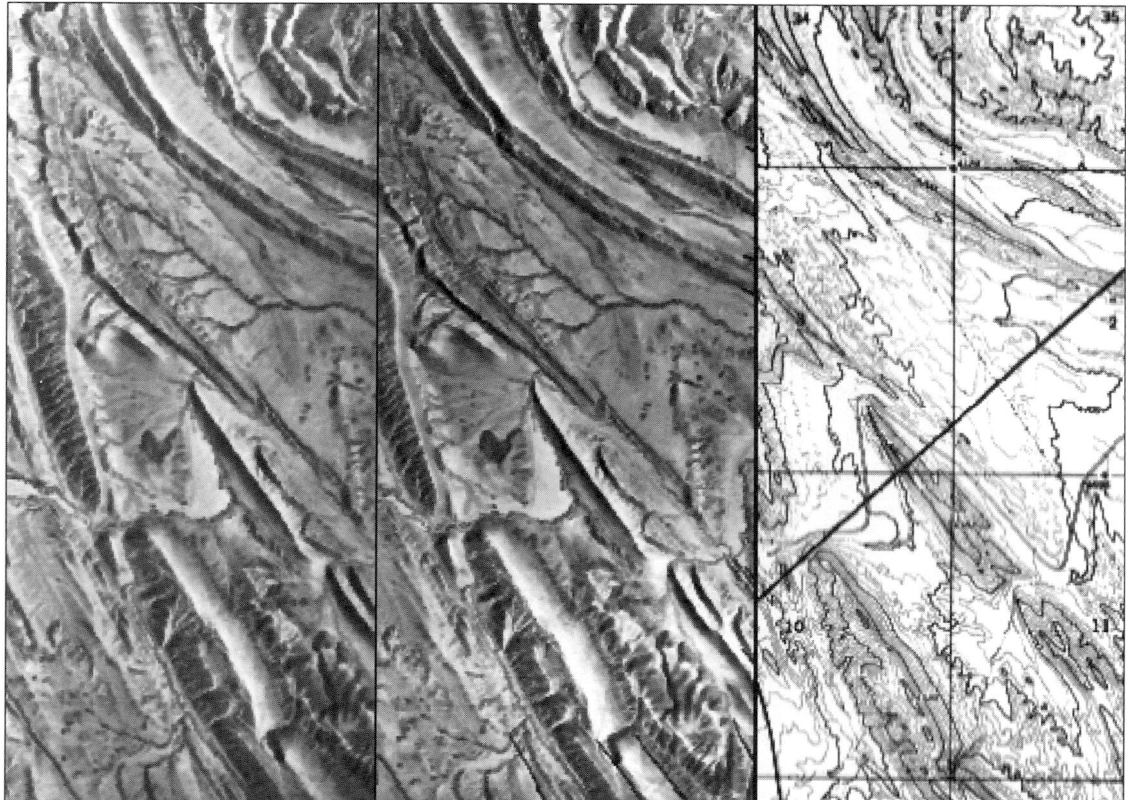

Figure 49. *Stereo pair images from aerial photography, and the topographic map showing iso-elevation contour lines derived from the parallax in the images. The scene is a portion of the Wind River in Wyoming. (From Sabins, 1987.)*

have different magnification scales, which makes subsequent analysis difficult. It also prevents combining multiple images of a complex surface into a mosaic. This problem is evident in two applications at very different scales. Satellite images of the surface of planets are assembled into mosaics covering large areas only with elaborate image warping to bring the edges into registration. This type of warping is discussed in Chapter 2. SEM images of rough surfaces are more difficult to assemble in this way, because the overall specimen geometry is not so well known, and the required computer processing is more difficult to justify.

Measuring brightness information, such as density or color values, requires a very stable illumination source and sensor. Color measurements are easily affected by changes in the color temperature of an incandescent bulb, due to minor voltage fluctuations or as the bulb warms up. Fluorescent lighting, especially when used in light boxes with X-ray films or densitometry gels, may be unstable or may introduce interference in solid-state cameras, due to the high-frequency flickering of the fluorescent tube. Bright specular reflections may cause saturation, blooming, or shifts in the camera gain.

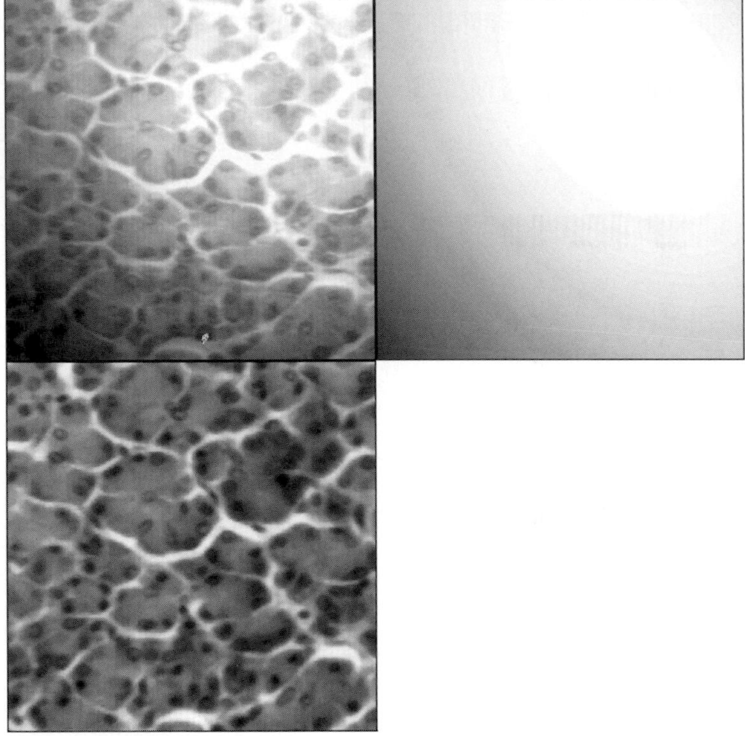

Figure 50. *A microscope image obtained with nonuniform illumination (due to a misaligned condenser). The "background" image was collected under the same conditions, with no sample present (by moving to an adjacent region on the slide). Subtracting the background image and expanding the contrast of the difference produces a "leveled" image with uniform brightness values for similar structures.*

It will help to bear in mind what the purpose is when digitizing an image into a computer. Some of the possibilities are listed below, and these place different restrictions and demands on the hardware and software used.

Storing and filing images becomes more attractive as massive storage devices, such as optical disks, drop in price or where multiple master copies of images may be needed in more than one location. In many cases, this application also involves hard-copy printing of the stored images and transmission of images to other locations. If further processing or measurement is not required, then image compression is worthwhile. The advantage of electronic storage is that the images do not degrade with time and can be accessed by appropriate filing and cross-indexing routines. On the other hand, film storage is far cheaper and offers much higher storage density and higher image resolution.

Image enhancement for visual examination requires a large number of pixels and adequate pixel depth so that the image can be acquired with enough information to perform the filtering or other operations with fidelity and then display the result with enough detail for the viewer. Uniformity of illumination and control of geometry are not of great importance. When large images are used, and especially for some of the more time-consuming processing operations, or when interactive experimentation with many different operations is intended, this application may benefit from very fast computers or specialized hardware.

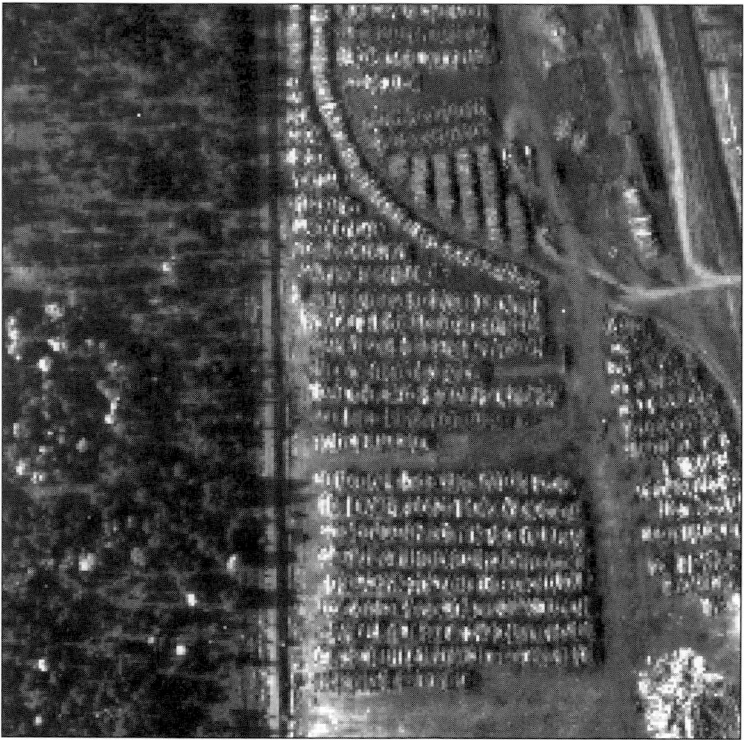

Figure 51. *Aerial photograph in which length of shadows and knowledge of the sun position permit calculation of the heights of trees and the height of the piles of logs in the lumberyard, from which the amount of wood can be estimated.*

Measurement of dimensions and density values can often be performed with modest image resolution if the magnification or illumination can be adjusted beforehand to make the best use of the image sensor. Processing may be required before measurement–for instance derivatives are often used to delineate edges for measurement–but this can usually be handled completely by software. The most important constraints are tight control over the imaging geometry and the uniformity and constancy of illumination.

Quality control applications usually do not involve absolute measurements so much as watching for variations. In many cases, this is handled simply by subtracting a reference image from each acquired image, point by point, to detect gross changes. This can be done with analog electronics, at real-time speeds. Preventing variation due to accidental changes in the position of camera or targets, or in illumination, is a central concern.

Structural research in either two or three dimensions usually starts with image measurement and has the same requirements as noted above, plus the ability to subject the measurement values to appropriate stereological and statistical analysis. Image interpretation in terms of structure is different for images of planar cross sections or projections (**Figure 53**). The latter are familiar to human vision, while the former are not. However, section images, such as the one in **Figure 54**, contain rich information for three-dimensional measurement, which can be revealed by sta-

Figure 52. *Geometric distortion occurs when a surface is viewed from a position away from the surface normal. Correcting this distortion to obtain a rectilinear image which can be properly processed and measured, or fitted together with adjoining images, requires knowing the viewing geometry and/or including some known fiducial marks in the scene which can be used to calculate it.*

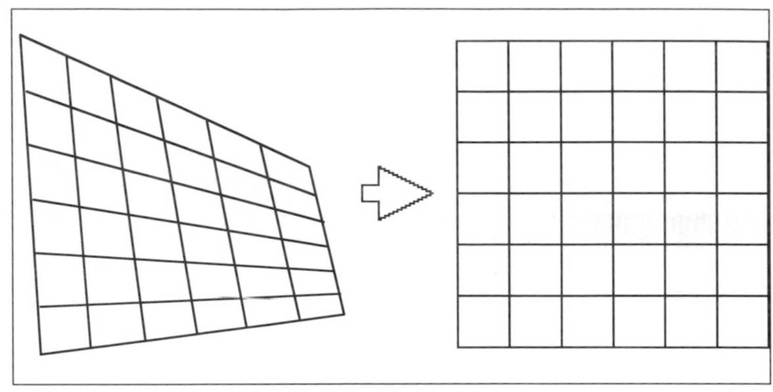

tistical analysis. Projection images, such as the one in **Figure 55**, present greater difficulties for interpretation.

Three-dimensional imaging utilizes large data sets, and in most cases the alignment of two-dimensional images is of critical importance. Some three-dimensional structural parameters can be inferred from two-dimensional images. Others, principally topological information, can only be determined from the full three-dimensional data set. Processing and measurement operations in three dimensions place extreme demands on computer storage and speed. Displays of three-dimensional information in ways interpretable by, if not familiar to, human users are improving, but need further algorithm development. They also place considerable demand on processor and display speed.

Pattern recognition is generally considered to be the high-end task for computer-based image analysis. It ranges in complexity from locating and recognizing isolated objects belonging to a few well-established classes to much more open-ended problems. Examples of the former are locating objects for robotic manipulation or recognizing targets in surveillance photos. An ex-

Figure 53. *Projection images, such as the spheres shown at left, are familiar, showing the external surfaces of features. However, some features are partially or entirely obscured and it is not possible to determine the number or size distribution. Cross-section images, as shown at right, are unfamiliar and do not show the maximum extent of features, but statistically it is possible to predict the size distribution and number of spheres.*

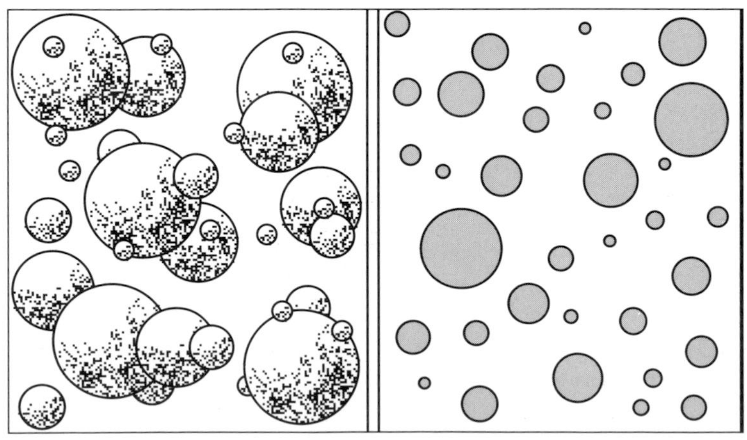

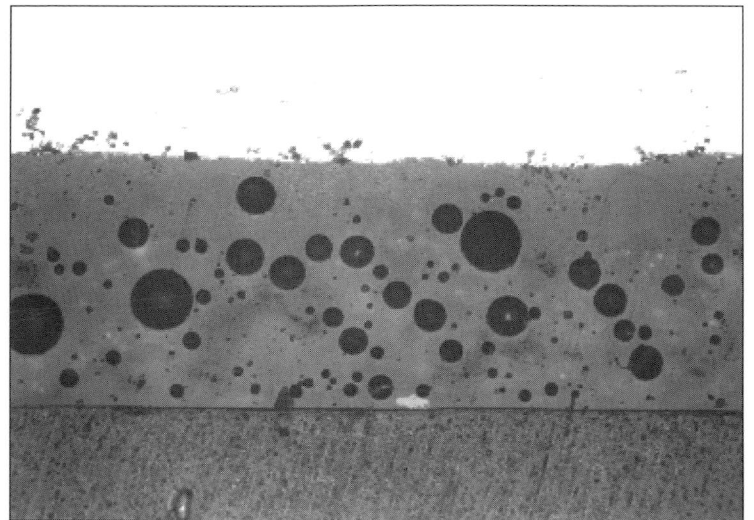

Figure 54. *Light microscope image of section through a colored enamel coating applied to steel (courtesy V. Benes, Research Inst. for Metals, Panenské Brezany, Czechoslovakia). The spherical bubbles arise during the firing of the enamel. They are sectioned to show circles whose diameters are smaller than the maximum diameter of the spheres, but since the shape of the bubbles is known, it is possible to infer the number and size distribution of the spheres from the data measured on the circles.*

ample of the latter is medical diagnosis, in which much of the important information comes from sources other than the image itself. Fuzzy logic, expert systems, and neural nets are all being applied to these tasks with some success. Extracting the correct information from the image to feed the decision-making process is more complicated than simple processing or measurement, because the best algorithms for a specific application must themselves be determined as part of the logic process.

These tasks all require the computer-based image processing and analysis system, and by inference the image acquisition hardware, to duplicate some operations of the human visual system. In many cases, they do so in ways that copy the algorithms we believe are used in vision, but in others quite different approaches are used. While no computer-based image system can come close to duplicating the overall performance of human vision in its flexibility or speed, there are specific tasks at which the computer surpasses any human. It can detect many more imaging signals than just visible light; is unaffected by outside influences, fatigue or distraction; performs absolute measurements rather than relative comparisons; can transform images into other spaces that are beyond normal human experience (e.g., Fourier or Hough space) to extract hidden data; and can apply statistical techniques to see through the chaotic and noisy data that may be present to identify underlying trends and similarities.

These attributes have made computer-based image analysis an important tool in many diverse fields. The image scale may vary from the microscopic to the astronomical, with substantially the same operations used. For the use of images at these scales, see especially Inoue (1986) and Sabins (1987). Familiarity with computer methods also makes most users better observers of images,

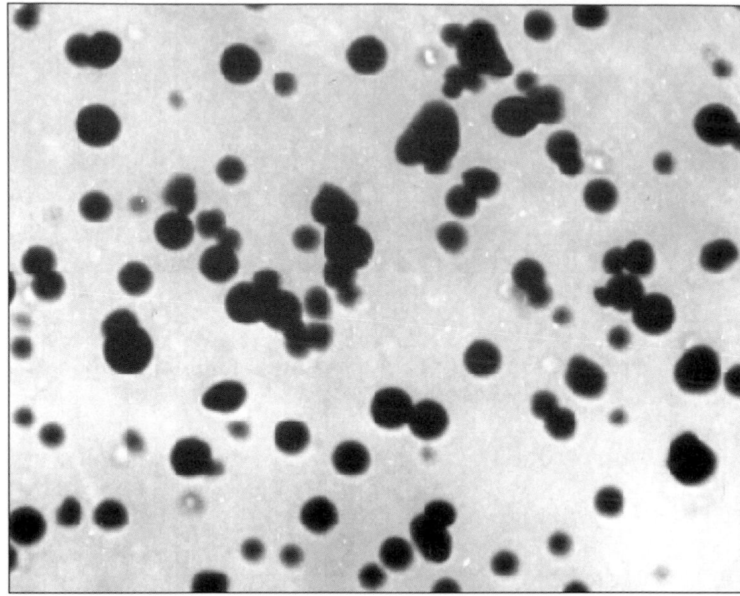

Figure 55. *Transmission electron microscope image of latex spheres in a thick, transparent section. Some of the spheres are partially hidden by others. If the section thickness is known, the size distribution and volume fraction occupied by the spheres can be estimated, but some small features may be entirely obscured and cannot be determined.*

who are able to interpret unusual imaging modes (such as cross sections) that are not encountered in normal scenes and who are conscious of both the gestalt and details of images and their visual response to them.

2

Correcting Imaging Defects

The first class of image processing operations considered here are those applied to correct some of the defects in as-acquired images. Defects may be present due to imperfect detectors, inadequate or nonuniform illumination, or an undesirable viewpoint. It should be emphasized that these are corrections that are applied *after* the image has been digitized and stored, and therefore will be unable to deliver the highest quality result that could have been achieved by optimizing the acquisition process in the first place.

Of course, optimizing image acquisition is sometimes impractical. If the camera can collect only a small number of photons in a practical time or before the scene changes, then the noise present in the image cannot be averaged out by acquiring and adding more frames, so other noise reduction means are needed. If the source of illumination cannot be controlled to be perfectly centered and normal to the viewed surface (for instance, the sun) or if the surface is curved instead of planar, then the image will have nonuniform illumination that must be corrected afterward. If the viewpoint cannot realistically be adjusted (for instance the path of a space probe or satellite) or if the surface is irregular (as in the case of a metal fracture), then some parts of the scene will be foreshortened and must be taken into account when comparing sizes or measuring distances. Even in typical laboratory setups, such as the light microscope, it may be very time-consuming to keep the instrument in ideal alignment or difficult to achieve adequate stability to collect dim fluorescence images for a long time. Therefore, it becomes more practical to trade off some of the ultimately achievable image quality for convenience and speed, and utilize image processing methods to perform corrections. When the first space probe pictures were collected and the need for these kinds of corrections was first appreciated, lengthy computations on moderate-sized computers were required to apply them. Now, it is possible to implement image corrections on desktop machines in times measured in seconds or minutes, making corrections practical for even routine imaging needs.

Noisy images

In Chapter 1, improving image quality (technically, signal-to-noise ratio) by averaging the number of frames was demonstrated. The most common source of noise is counting statistics in the image detector caused by incident particles (photons, electrons, etc.). This is particularly the case for X-ray images from the SEM, where the ratio of incident electrons to detected X-rays may vary from 10^5 to 10^6. In fluorescence light microscopy, the fluoresced light photons in a narrow wavelength range from a dye or activity probe may also produce very dim images, an effect compounded by the need to acquire a series of very short duration images to measure activity as a function of time.

Noisy images may also occur because of instability in the light source or detector during the time required to scan or digitize an image. The pattern of this noise may be quite different from Gaussian noise (random-intensity variations due to counting statistics), but it still shows up as a variation in brightness in uniform regions of the scene. One common example is the noise in field emission SEM images due to the variation in field emission current at the tip. With a typical time constant of seconds, the electron emission may shift from one atom to another, producing a change of several percent in the beam current. The usual approach to minimizing the effects of this fluctuation in the viewed image is to use scan times that are either much shorter or longer than the fluctuation time.

Similar effects can be seen in images acquired using fluorescent lighting, particularly in light boxes used to illuminate film negatives. This results from an interference, or beat, between the camera and the flickering of the fluorescent tube (which is much greater than that of an incandescent bulb, whose thermal inertia smooths out the variation in light emission caused by the alternating current). When the noise has a characteristic that is not random in time and does not exhibit "normal" statistical behavior, it is more difficult to place numeric descriptors on the amount of noise. However, many of the same reduction techniques can be used, though usually with somewhat less efficacy.

Assuming that an image represents the best quality that can practically be obtained, this chapter will deal with ways to suppress noise to improve the ability to visualize and demarcate for measurement the features that are present. The underlying assumption in all of the noise suppression methods is that the pixels in the image are much smaller than any of the important details and most of the pixels' neighbors represent the same structure. This permits the application of various averaging and comparison.

This assumption is very much the same as that inherent in classical image averaging, which assumes that pixel readings at different times represent the same structure in the viewed scene. This directly justifies averaging (or integrating) pixel readings over time to reduce random noise. When the signal varies in some of the other ways described above, other methods, such as median filtering, can be used that are directly analogous to the spatial comparison methods discussed here, except that they utilize the time sequence of measurements at each location.

Neighborhood averaging

The simplest form of spatial averaging is simply to add together the pixel brightness values in each small region of the image, divide by the number of pixels in the neighborhood, and use the resulting value to construct a new image. **Figure 1** shows that this method essentially produces an image with a smaller number of pixels. The block size in **Figure 1b** is 4×4, so that 16 pixel values are added. Since the noise in this image is random due to the counting statistics of the small number of photons, the improvement in image quality, or signal-to-noise ratio, is just the square root of 16, or a factor of 4. However, the image lateral resolution is seriously impacted and the small structures in the image can no longer be separately discerned.

A more common way to accomplish neighborhood averaging is to replace each pixel with the average of itself and its neighbors. This is often described as a "kernel" operation, since implementation can be generalized as the sum of the pixel values in the region multiplied by a set of integer weights.

$$P^*_{x,y} = \frac{\sum_{i,j=-m}^{+m} W_{i,j} \cdot P_{x+i,\,y+j}}{\sum_{ij=-m}^{+m} W_{i,j}} \qquad (1$$

The equation above shows the calculation performed over a square of dimension $2m + 1$, which is odd. The neighborhood sizes thus range from 3×3 to 5×5, 7×7, etc. It is also possible, although uncommon, to use non-square regions. The array of weights W for a simple neighbor averaging contains only 1s, and for a 3×3 region could be written as

Figure 1. Smoothing by averaging:

- ***a)*** *a noisy original image (fluorescence light microscopy of bone marrow);*
- ***b)*** *each 4×4 block of pixels averaged;*
- ***c)*** *each pixel replaced by the average of itself and its 8 neighbors in a 3×3 square block;*
- ***d)*** *each pixel replaced by the average of itself and its 120 neighbors in an 11×11 square.*

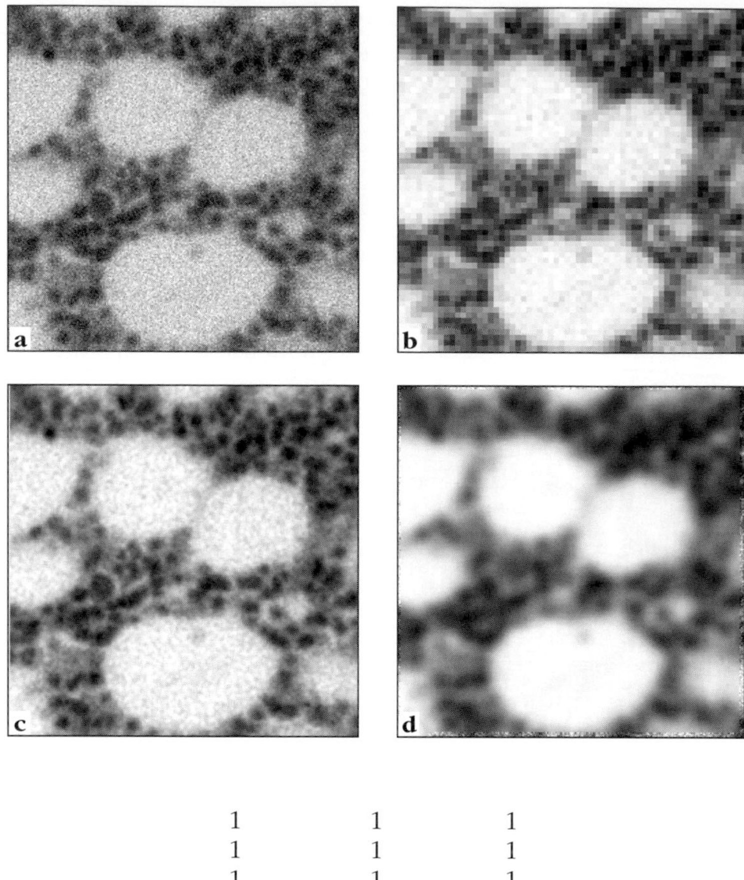

$$\begin{matrix} 1 & 1 & 1 \\ 1 & 1 & 1 \\ 1 & 1 & 1 \end{matrix}$$

where we understand the convention that these coefficients are to be multiplied by pixels that surround the central pixel and sum normalized by dividing by the sum of the weights, then the value written to the location of the central pixel to form a new image.

As a matter of practicality (since storage space is never unlimited), it is common to write the new image back into the same memory as the original. When this is done, however, it is important to use the original pixel values for the summation, not those new ones that have already been calculated for some of the neighbors. This requires keeping a copy of a few lines of the image during the process.

Neighborhood operations that employ kernel multiplication are usually applied symmetrically around each pixel. This creates a problem for pixels nearer to the edge of the image than the half-width of the neighborhood. Various approaches are used to deal with this, including designing special asymmetrical kernels or rules along edges or in corners; assuming that the image edges are mirrors, so that each line of pixels within the image is duplicated beyond it; or assuming that the image wraps around, so that the left and right edge, and the top and bottom edges, are continuous. In the examples shown here, an even simpler approach is used: the processing is restricted to that portion of the image where no edge conflicts arise. This leaves lines of unprocessed pixels along the edges of the images, equal in width to half the dimension of the neighborhood.

Figure 1 shows the effect of smoothing using a 3×3 neighborhood average, and also an 11×11 neighborhood size. The noise reduction is much greater with the larger region, but is accompanied by a significant blurring of the feature edges.

By using weight values that are not 1, the amount of blurring can be reduced and more control exerted over the neighborhood averaging procedure. For example, the values

1	2	1
2	4	2
1	2	1

have several attractive characteristics. First, the central 4 that multiplies the original pixel contents is the largest factor, causing the central pixel to dominate the average and reduce blurring. The values of 2 for the 4 orthogonally touching neighbors and 1 for the 4 diagonally touching neighbors acknowledge the fact that the diagonal pixels are in fact further away from the center of the neighborhood (actually by the factor $\sqrt{2}$). Finally, these weights have a total value of 16, which is a power of 2 and is consequently very easy to divide by quickly in a computer implementation of this averaging procedure.

Similar sets of ad hoc weight values can be devised in various sizes. Integers are used to speed implementation, and storage requirements are modest. We will see in Chapter 4, in the context of processing images in frequency space, that these kernels can be analyzed quite efficiently in that domain to understand their smoothing properties. It turns out that one of the very useful shapes for a weight kernel is Gaussian. This is a set of integers that approximates the profile of a Gaussian function along any row, column, or diagonal through the center. It is characterized by a standard deviation expressed in terms of pixel dimensions. The size of the kernel is generally made large enough that adding another row of terms would insert negligibly small numbers (ideally zeroes) into the array. Some zero values will be present anyway in the corners, though, since they are farther from the central pixel.

Choosing the actual integers is something of an art, at least for larger kernels. The goal is to approximate the smooth analytical curve of the Gaussian, while generally keeping the total of the weights smaller than some practical limit to facilitate the computer arithmetic. Several Gaussian kernels are shown below, with standard deviations that increase in geometric proportions from much less than one pixel to many pixels. The standard deviation for these kernels is the radius (in pixels) containing 68% of the integrated magnitude of the coefficients, or the volume under the surface if the kernel is pictured as a three-dimensional plot of the integer values. This is a two-dimensional generalization of the usual definition of standard deviation; for a one-dimensional Gaussian distribution, 68% of the area under the curve lies within plus or minus one standard deviation.

```
σ=0.391 pixels (3x3)
  1  4  1
  4 12  4
  1  4  1

σ=0.625 pixels (5x5)
 1  2  3  2  1
 2  7 11  7  2
 3 11 17 11  3
 2  7 11  7  2
 1  2  3  2  1

σ=1.0 pixels (9x9)
 0  0  1  1  1  1  1  0  0
 0  1  2  3  3  3  2  1  0
 1  2  3  6  7  6  3  2  1
 1  3  6  9 11  9  6  3  1
 1  3  7 11 12 11  7  3  1
 1  3  6  9 11  9  6  3  1
 1  2  3  6  7  6  3  2  1
 0  1  2  3  3  3  2  1  0
 0  0  1  1  1  1  1  0  0

σ=1.6 pixels (11x11)
 1  1  1  2  2  2  2  2  1  1  1
 1  2  2  3  4  4  4  3  2  2  1
 1  2  4  5  6  7  6  5  4  2  1
 2  3  5  7  8  9  8  7  5  3  2
 2  4  6  8 10 11 10  8  6  4  2
 2  4  7  9 11 12 11  9  7  4  2
 2  4  6  8 10 11 10  8  6  4  2
 2  3  5  7  8  9  8  7  5  3  2
 1  2  4  5  6  7  6  5  4  2  1
 1  2  2  3  4  4  4  3  2  2  1
 1  1  1  2  2  2  2  2  1  1  1

σ=2.56 pixels (15x15)
 2  2  3  4  5  5  6  6  6  5  5  4  3  2  2
 2  3  4  5  7  7  8  8  8  7  7  5  4  3  2
 3  4  6  7  9 10 10 11 10 10  9  7  6  4  3
 4  5  7  9 10 12 13 13 13 12 10  9  7  5  4
 5  7  9 11 13 14 15 16 15 14 13 11  9  7  5
 5  7 10 12 14 16 17 18 17 16 14 12 10  7  5
 6  8 10 13 15 17 19 19 19 17 15 13 10  8  6
 6  8 11 13 16 18 19 20 19 18 16 13 11  8  6
 6  8 10 13 15 17 19 19 19 17 15 13 10  8  6
 5  7 10 12 14 16 17 18 17 16 14 12 10  7  5
 5  7  9 11 13 14 15 16 15 14 13 11  9  7  5
 4  5  7  9 10 12 13 13 13 12 10  9  7  5  4
 3  4  6  7  9 10 10 11 10 10  9  7  6  4  3
 2  3  4  5  7  7  8  8  8  7  7  5  4  3  2
 2  2  3  4  5  5  6  6  6  5  5  4  3  2  2

σ=4.096 pixels (21x21)
  5  6  7  8  9 10 11 12 13 13 13 13 13 12 11 10  9  8  7  6  5
  6  7  9 10 11 12 14 15 15 16 16 16 15 15 14 12 11 10  9  7  6
  7  9 10 12 13 15 16 17 18 18 19 18 18 17 16 15 13 12 10  9  7
  8 10 12 13 15 17 18 20 21 21 21 21 21 20 18 17 15 13 12 10  8
  9 11 13 15 17 19 21 22 23 24 24 24 23 22 21 19 17 15 13 11  9
 10 12 15 17 19 21 23 25 26 27 27 27 26 25 23 21 19 17 15 12 10
 11 14 16 18 21 23 25 27 28 29 29 29 28 27 25 23 21 18 16 14 11
 12 15 17 20 22 25 27 29 30 31 31 31 30 29 27 25 22 20 17 15 12
 13 15 18 21 23 26 28 30 32 33 33 33 32 30 28 26 23 21 18 15 13
 13 16 18 21 24 27 29 31 33 34 34 34 33 31 29 27 24 21 18 16 13
 13 16 19 21 24 27 29 31 33 34 34 34 33 31 29 27 24 21 19 16 13
 13 16 18 21 24 27 29 31 33 34 34 34 33 31 29 27 24 21 18 16 13
 13 15 18 21 23 26 28 30 32 33 33 33 32 30 28 26 23 21 18 15 13
 12 15 17 20 22 25 27 29 30 31 31 31 30 29 27 25 22 20 17 15 12
 11 14 16 18 21 23 25 27 28 29 29 29 28 27 25 23 21 18 16 14 11
 10 12 15 17 19 21 23 25 26 27 27 27 26 25 23 21 19 17 15 12 10
  9 11 13 15 17 19 21 22 23 24 24 24 23 22 21 19 17 15 13 11  9
  8 10 12 13 15 17 18 20 21 21 21 21 21 20 18 17 15 13 12 10  8
  7  9 10 12 13 15 16 17 18 18 19 18 18 17 16 15 13 12 10  9  7
  6  7  9 10 11 12 14 15 15 16 16 16 15 15 14 12 11 10  9  7  6
  5  6  7  8  9 10 11 12 13 13 13 13 13 12 11 10  9  8  7  6  5
```

Of course, the kernel size increases with the standard deviation, as well. In the largest examples below, only the upper left quadrant of the symmetrical array is shown. Repeated application of a small kernel or the sequential application of two or more kernels is equivalent to the single application of a larger one, which can be constructed as the convolution of the two kernels (applying the weighting factors from one kernel to those in the other as if they were pixel values, then summing and adding them to generate a new, larger array of weights).

```
σ=6.536 pixels (29x29)
  7  8  9 10 10 11 12 13 13 14 14 15 15 15 15 ...
  8  9 10 11 11 12 13 14 15 15 16 16 16 17 17 ...
  9 10 11 12 13 13 14 15 16 17 17 18 18 18 18 ...
 10 11 12 13 14 15 16 17 17 18 19 19 20 20 20 ...
 10 11 13 14 15 16 17 18 19 20 20 21 21 21 21 ...
 11 12 13 15 16 17 18 19 20 21 22 22 23 23 23 ...
 12 13 14 16 17 18 19 20 21 22 23 24 24 24 24 ...
 13 14 15 17 18 19 20 22 23 24 24 25 25 26 26 ...
 13 15 16 17 19 20 21 23 24 25 26 26 27 27 27 ...
 14 15 17 18 20 21 22 24 25 26 27 27 28 28 28 ...
 14 16 17 19 20 22 23 24 26 27 28 28 29 29 29 ...
 15 16 18 19 21 22 24 25 26 27 28 29 30 30 30 ...
 15 16 18 20 21 23 24 25 27 28 29 30 30 30 31 ...
 15 17 18 20 21 23 24 26 27 28 29 30 30 31 31 ...
 15 17 18 20 21 23 24 26 27 28 29 30 31 31 31 ...
```

```
σ=10.486 pixels (43x43)
  6  6  6  7  7  7  8  8  8  9  9  9  9 10 10 10 10 10 10 10 11 11 ...
  6  6  7  7  7  8  8  8  9  9  9 10 10 10 10 11 11 11 11 11 11 11 ...
  6  7  7  7  8  8  9  9  9 10 10 10 11 11 11 11 11 12 12 12 12 12 ...
  7  7  7  8  8  9  9  9 10 10 10 11 11 11 12 12 12 12 12 12 12 13 ...
  7  7  8  8  9  9  9 10 10 11 11 11 12 12 12 12 13 13 13 13 13 13 ...
  7  8  8  9  9 10 10 10 11 11 12 12 12 13 13 13 13 13 14 14 14 14 ...
  8  8  9  9  9 10 10 11 11 12 12 12 13 13 13 14 14 14 14 14 14 14 ...
  8  8  9  9 10 10 11 11 12 12 13 13 13 14 14 14 15 15 15 15 15 15 ...
  8  9  9 10 10 11 11 12 12 13 13 14 14 14 15 15 15 15 15 16 16 16 ...
  9  9 10 10 11 11 12 12 13 13 14 14 14 15 15 15 16 16 16 16 16 16 ...
  9  9 10 10 11 12 12 13 13 14 14 15 15 15 16 16 16 16 17 17 17 17 ...
  9 10 10 11 11 12 12 13 14 14 15 15 15 16 16 16 17 17 17 17 17 17 ...
  9 10 11 11 12 12 13 13 14 14 15 15 16 16 17 17 17 17 18 18 18 18 ...
 10 10 11 11 12 13 13 14 14 15 15 16 16 17 17 17 18 18 18 18 18 18 ...
 10 10 11 12 12 13 13 14 15 15 16 16 17 17 17 18 18 18 18 19 19 19 ...
 10 11 11 12 12 13 14 14 15 15 16 16 17 17 18 18 18 19 19 19 19 19 ...
 10 11 11 12 13 13 14 15 15 16 16 17 17 18 18 18 19 19 19 19 19 19 ...
 10 11 12 12 13 13 14 15 15 16 16 17 17 18 18 19 19 19 19 19 20 20 ...
 10 11 12 12 13 14 14 15 15 16 17 17 18 18 18 19 19 19 19 20 20 20 ...
 10 11 12 12 13 14 14 15 16 16 17 17 18 18 19 19 19 19 20 20 20 20 ...
 11 11 12 12 13 14 14 15 16 16 17 17 18 18 19 19 19 20 20 20 20 20 ...
 11 11 12 13 13 14 14 15 16 16 17 17 18 18 19 19 19 20 20 20 20 20 ...
```

```
σ=16.777 pixels (55x55)
  5  5  5  5  5  5  5  6  6  6  6  6  6  6  6  7  7  7  7  7  7  7  7  7  7  7  7  7 ...
  5  5  5  5  5  6  6  6  6  6  6  6  6  7  7  7  7  7  7  7  7  7  7  7  7  7  7  7 ...
  5  5  5  5  6  6  6  6  6  6  6  6  7  7  7  7  7  7  7  7  7  7  7  7  7  7  7  7 ...
  5  5  5  6  6  6  6  6  6  6  7  7  7  7  7  7  7  7  7  7  7  8  8  8  8  8  8  8 ...
  5  5  6  6  6  6  6  6  6  7  7  7  7  7  7  7  7  7  8  8  8  8  8  8  8  8  8  8 ...
  5  6  6  6  6  6  6  6  7  7  7  7  7  7  7  7  8  8  8  8  8  8  8  8  8  8  8  8 ...
  5  6  6  6  6  6  6  7  7  7  7  7  7  7  8  8  8  8  8  8  8  8  8  8  8  8  8  8 ...
  6  6  6  6  6  6  7  7  7  7  7  7  7  8  8  8  8  8  8  8  8  8  8  8  8  8  8  8 ...
  6  6  6  6  6  7  7  7  7  7  7  8  8  8  8  8  8  8  8  8  8  9  9  9  9  9  9  9 ...
  6  6  6  6  7  7  7  7  7  7  8  8  8  8  8  8  8  8  8  9  9  9  9  9  9  9  9  9 ...
  6  6  6  7  7  7  7  7  7  8  8  8  8  8  8  8  8  9  9  9  9  9  9  9  9  9  9  9 ...
  6  6  6  7  7  7  7  7  8  8  8  8  8  8  8  8  9  9  9  9  9  9  9  9  9  9  9  9 ...
  6  6  7  7  7  7  7  7  8  8  8  8  8  8  9  9  9  9  9  9  9  9  9  9  9  9  9  9 ...
  6  7  7  7  7  7  7  8  8  8  8  8  8  9  9  9  9  9  9  9  9  9  9  9  9 10 10 10 ...
  6  7  7  7  7  7  8  8  8  8  8  8  9  9  9  9  9  9  9  9  9  9 10 10 10 10 10 10 ...
  7  7  7  7  7  7  8  8  8  8  8  8  9  9  9  9  9  9  9  9 10 10 10 10 10 10 10 10 ...
  7  7  7  7  7  8  8  8  8  8  8  9  9  9  9  9  9  9 10 10 10 10 10 10 10 10 10 10 ...
  7  7  7  7  7  8  8  8  8  8  9  9  9  9  9  9  9 10 10 10 10 10 10 10 10 10 10 10 ...
  7  7  7  7  8  8  8  8  8  8  9  9  9  9  9  9 10 10 10 10 10 10 10 10 10 10 10 10 ...
  7  7  7  7  8  8  8  8  8  9  9  9  9  9  9  9 10 10 10 10 10 10 10 10 10 10 10 10 ...
  7  7  7  7  8  8  8  8  8  9  9  9  9  9  9 10 10 10 10 10 10 10 10 10 10 10 10 10 ...
  7  7  7  8  8  8  8  8  9  9  9  9  9  9  9 10 10 10 10 10 10 10 10 10 10 10 10 10 ...
  7  7  7  8  8  8  8  8  9  9  9  9  9  9 10 10 10 10 10 10 10 10 10 10 10 10 10 11 ...
  7  7  7  8  8  8  8  8  9  9  9  9  9  9 10 10 10 10 10 10 10 10 10 10 11 11 11 11 ...
  7  7  7  8  8  8  8  8  9  9  9  9  9  9 10 10 10 10 10 10 10 10 10 11 11 11 11 11 ...
  7  7  7  8  8  8  8  8  9  9  9  9  9 10 10 10 10 10 10 10 10 10 10 11 11 11 11 11 ...
  7  7  7  8  8  8  8  8  9  9  9  9  9 10 10 10 10 10 10 10 10 10 10 11 11 11 11 11 ...
  7  7  7  8  8  8  8  8  9  9  9  9  9 10 10 10 10 10 10 10 10 10 11 11 11 11 11 11 ...
```

Figure 2. Isometric plots of the integers used as weight values in the Gaussian smoothing kernels:
a) *5×5, σ = 0.625 pixels;*
b) *43×43, σ = 10.486 pixels*

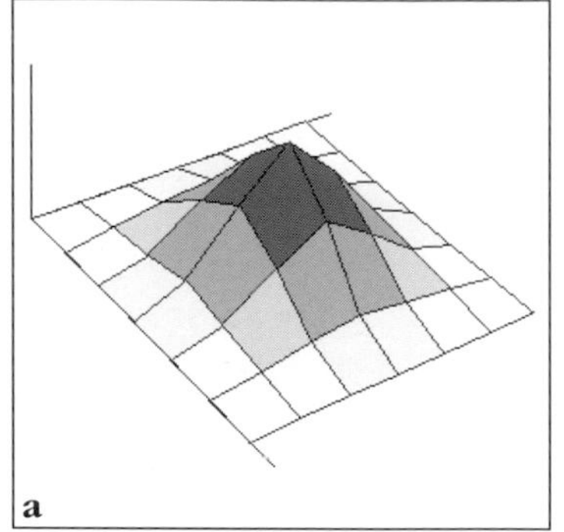

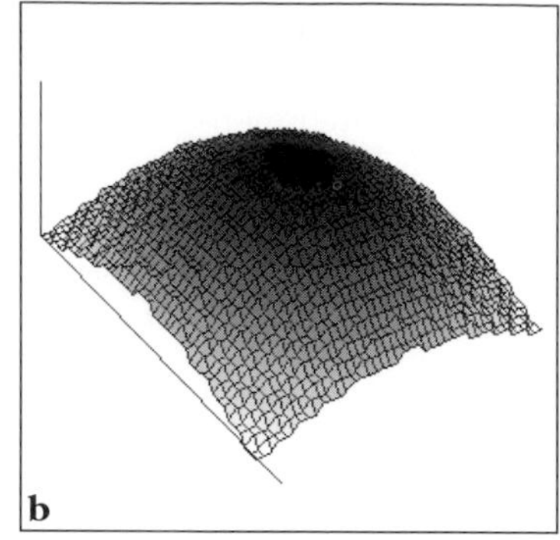

Figure 2 shows two examples, the 5×5 and 43×43 Gaussian kernels, plotted as an isometric view. Notice that even with the large kernel, quantizing the weights using integers produces some distortion.

In subsequent sections on image processing, we will see other uses for these kernels in which the weights are not symmetrical in magnitude, or not all positive. The implementation of the kernel will remain the same, except that when negative weights are present, the normalization is usually performed by dividing by the sum of the positive values only (because in these cases the sum of all the weights is usually zero). For the present, our interest is restricted to the smoothing of noise in images.

Figure 3. Test image for several neighborhood smoothing operations:
a) *original light microscope fluorescence image of bone marrow, obtained by averaging four video frames;*
b) *enlargement of a portion of image a to show individual pixels;*
c) *an image of the same specimen area with reduced noise obtained by averaging 256 video frames;*
d) *the same enlargement of image c.*

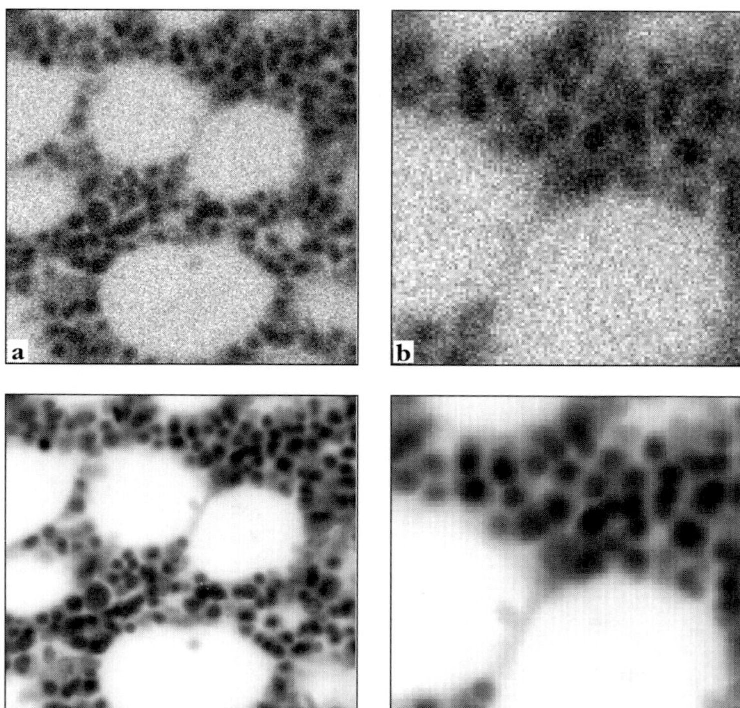

Figure 3 shows the same noisy image as **Figure 1,** along with an image of the same region using image averaging to reduce statistical noise, as was shown in Chapter 1. The figure also shows an enlargement of a portion of the image in which the individual pixels can be discerned, as an aid to judging the pixel-to-pixel noise variations in uniform regions and the sharpness of boundaries between different structures. Applying smoothing with the 5×5 kernel corresponding to a Gaussian shape with a standard deviation of 0.625 pixels produces the improvement in quality shown in **Figure 4** (for two applications of the kernel). Using a larger kernel (the 9×9 kernel with a standard deviation of 1.0 pixels, applied once) produces the result shown.

Though kernel averaging can reduce visible noise in the image, it also blurs edges, displaces boundaries, and reduces contrast. It can even introduce an artefact, often called "pseudo resolution," when two nearby structures are averaged together in a way that creates an apparent feature between them. **Figure 5** shows an example, in which the lines of the test pattern are blurred by the 11×11 averaging window, causing false lines to appear.

Smoothing one-dimensional signal profiles, such as X-ray diffraction patterns, spectra, or time-varying electronic signals, is often performed using a Savitsky and Golay (1964) fitting procedure. Tables of coefficients published for this purpose (and intended for efficient application in dedicated computers) are designed to be used in the same way as the weighting coefficients discussed

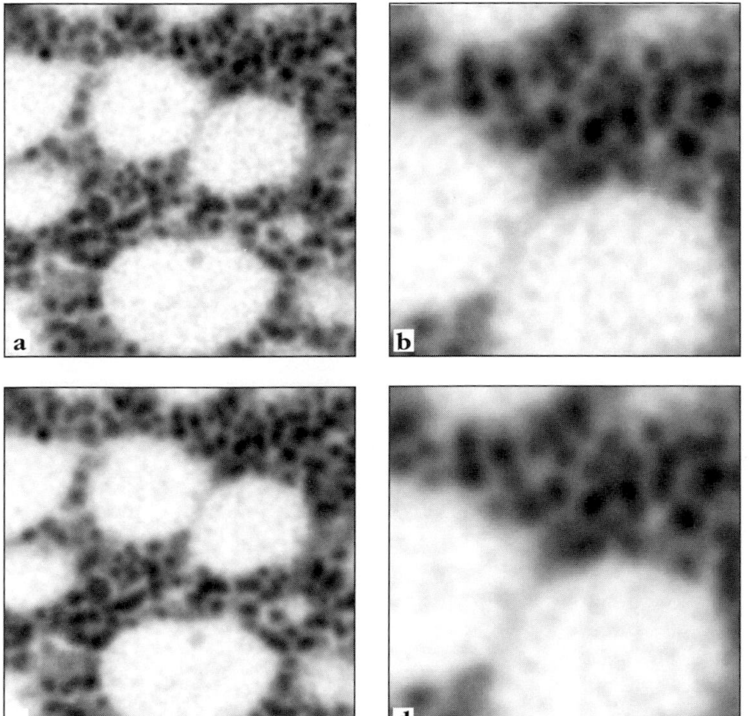

Figure 4. Neighborhood smoothing with Gaussian kernels:

- ***a)*** *two applications of a 5×5 kernel with standard deviation of 0.625 pixels;*
- ***b)*** *enlargement of image a to show pixel detail;*
- ***c)*** *one application of a 9×9 kernel with standard deviation of 1.0 pixels;*
- ***d)*** *the same enlargement of image b.*

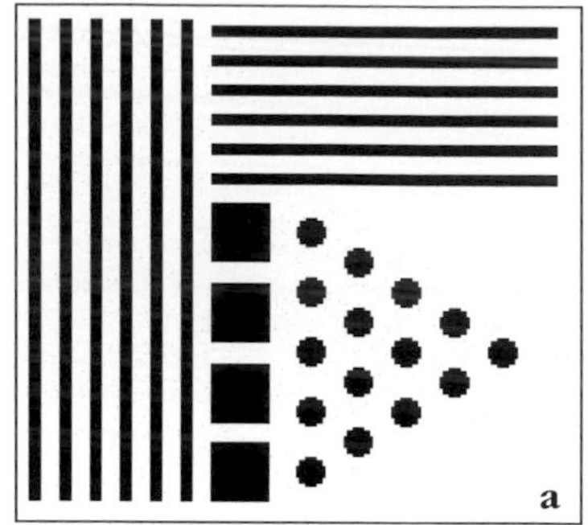

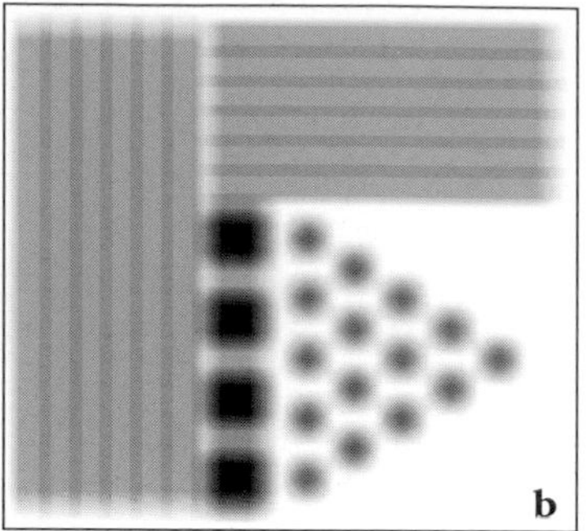

Figure 5. *Pseudo-resolution due to smoothing. Applying an 11 × 11 unweighted smoothing kernel to the test pattern in image a produces apparent lines between the original ones, as shown in image b.*

above, except that they operate in only one dimension. The process is equivalent to performing a least-squares fit of the data points to a polynomial. The smoothed profiles preserve the magnitude of steps while smoothing out noise. **Table 1** lists these coefficients for second (quadratic) and fourth (quartic) power poly-

Table 1. Savitsky and Golay fitting coefficients

Quadratic polynomial fit

5	7	9	11	13	15	17	19
0	0	0	0	0	0	0	−.0602
0	0	0	0	0	0	−.065	−.0226
0	0	0	0	0	−.0706	−.0186	.0106
0	0	0	0	−.0769	−.0118	.0217	.0394
0	0	0	−.0839	0	.038	.0557	.0637
0	0	−.0909	.021	.0629	.0787	.0836	.0836
0	−.0952	.0606	.1026	.1119	.1104	.1053	.0991
−.0857	.1429	.1688	.1608	.1469	.133	.1207	.1101
.3429	.2857	.2338	.1958	.1678	.1466	.13	.1168
.4857	.3333	.2554	.2075	.1748	.1511	.1331	.119
.3429	.2857	.2338	.1958	.1678	.1466	.13	.1168
−.0857	.1429	.1688	.1608	.1469	.133	.1207	.1101
0	−.0952	.0606	.1026	.1119	.1104	.1053	.0991
0	0	−.0909	.021	.0629	.0787	.0836	.0836
0	0	0	−.0839	0	.038	.0557	.0637
0	0	0	0	−.0769	−.0118	.0217	.0394
0	0	0	0	0	−.0706	−.0186	.0106
0	0	0	0	0	0	−.065	−.0226
0	0	0	0	0	0	0	−.0602

Quartic polynomial fit

5	7	9	11	13	15	17	19
0	0	0	0	0	0	.0464	−.0343
0	0	0	0	0	.0464	−.0464	−.0565
0	0	0	0	.0452	−.0619	−.0619	−.039
0	0	0	.042	−.0814	−.0636	−.0279	.0024
0	0	.035	−.1049	−.0658	−.0036	.0322	.0545
0	.0216	−.1282	−.0233	.0452	.0813	.0988	.1063
.25	−.1299	.0699	.1399	.1604	.1624	.1572	.1494
−.5	.3247	.3147	.2797	.2468	.2192	.1965	.1777
1.5	.5671	.4172	.3333	.2785	.2395	.2103	.1875
−.5	.3247	.3147	.2797	.2468	.2192	.1965	.1777
.25	−.1299	.0699	.1399	.1604	.1624	.1572	.1494
0	.0216	−.1282	−.0233	.0452	.0813	.0988	.1063
0	0	.035	−.1049	−.0658	−.0036	.0322	.0545
0	0	0	.042	−.0814	−.0636	−.0279	.0024
0	0	0	0	.0452	−.0619	−.0619	−.039
0	0	0	0	0	.0464	−.0464	−.0565
0	0	0	0	0	0	.0464	−.0343
0	0	0	0	0	0	0	.0458

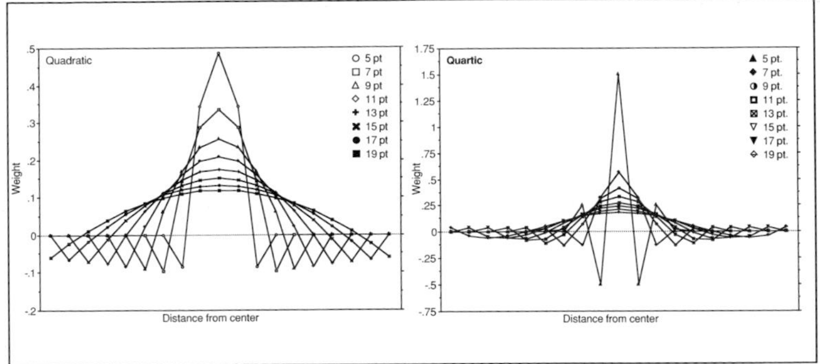

Figure 6. *Savitsky and Golay linear smoothing weights for least-squares fitting to quadratic and quartic polynomials.*

nomials for fits extending over neighborhoods ranging from 5 to 19 points. These profiles are plotted in **Figure 6.**

The Savitsky and Golay method can be extended to two dimensions, of course (Edwards, 1982). This can be done either by first applying the coefficients in the horizontal direction and then in the vertical direction, or by constructing a full two-dimensional kernel. Since the points in the kernel are not all at integer distances from the center, it is necessary to fully calculate additional weight values for each specific two-dimensional case. **Figure 7** shows the application of a 7×7 Savitsky and Golay quadratic polynomial to smooth the image from **Figure 3.**

It is interesting to compare the results of this spatial-domain smoothing to that which can be accomplished in the frequency domain. As discussed in Chapter 4, multiplying the frequency transform by a convolution function is equivalent to applying a kernel in the spatial domain. The most common noise filtering method is to remove high-frequency information, which represents pixel-to-pixel variations associated with noise. This may be performed by setting an aperture on the two-dimensional transform, eliminating higher frequencies, and retransforming. **Figure 8** shows the result of applying this technique to the same image as in **Figures 1** and **3.** A circular low-pass filter with a radius of 35 pixels and a 10-pixel-wide cosine edge shape (the importance of these parameters is discussed in Chapter 4) was applied. The smoothing is quite similar to that accomplished in the spatial domain.

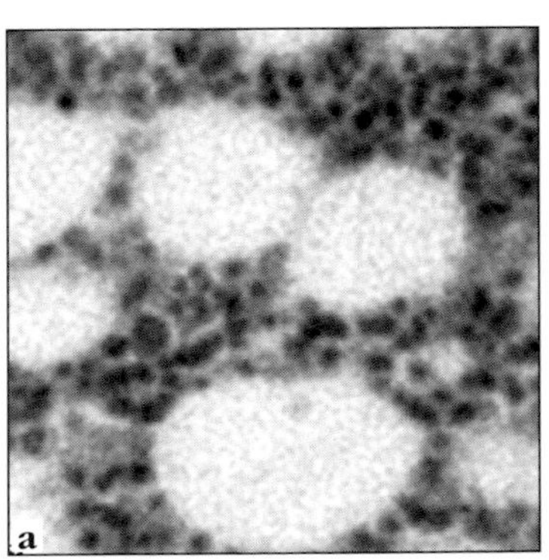

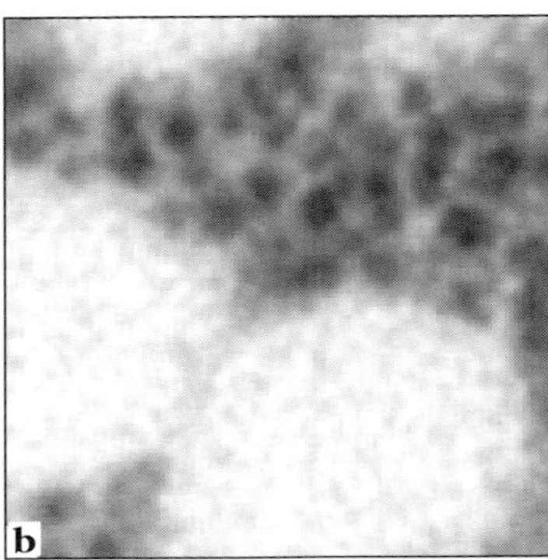

Figure 7. Smoothing with a 7-point-wide, quadratic Savitsky and Golay fit:
a) *applied to same image as Figure 3;*
b) *enlarged to show pixel detail.*

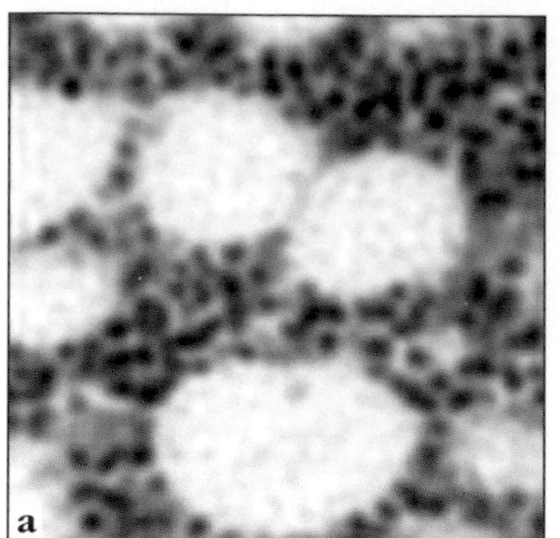
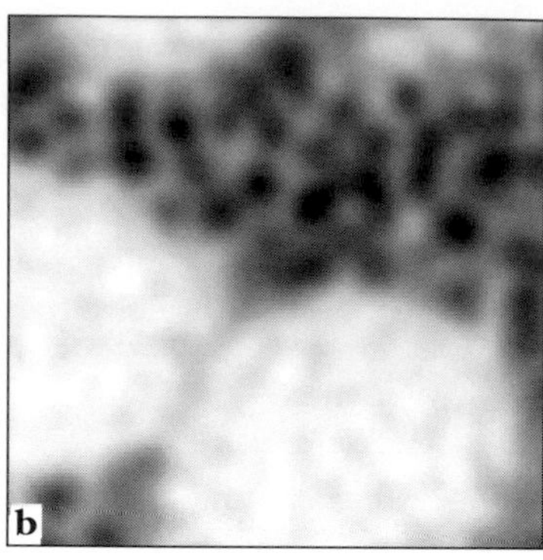

Figure 8. Smoothing in frequency space, using a circular low-pass filter with radius = 35 pixels and a 10-pixel-wide cosine edge shape:
a) *application to image in Figure 3;*
b) *enlargement to show pixel detail.*

Neighborhood ranking

The use of weighted kernels to average together pixels in a neighborhood is a convolution operation, which has a direct counterpart in frequency-space image processing. It is a linear procedure in which no information is lost from the original image. There are other processing operations that can be performed in neighborhoods in the spatial domain that also provide noise smoothing. However, they are not linear and do not utilize or preserve all of the original data.

The most widely used of these additional methods are based on ranking the pixels in a neighborhood according to their brightness. Then, for example, the median value in the ordered list can be used as the brightness value for the central pixel. As in the case of the kernel operations, this is used to produce a new image. Only the original pixel values are used in the ranking for the neighborhood around each pixel.

The so-called median filter is an excellent rejector of certain kinds of noise, such as "shot" noise, in which individual pixels are corrupted or missing from the image. If a pixel is accidentally changed to an extreme value, it will be eliminated from the image and replaced by a reasonable value–the median value in the neighborhood.

Figure 9 shows an example of this type of noise. Ten percent of the pixels in the original image (selected randomly) are set to black, and another ten percent to white. This is a rather extreme amount of noise. However, a median filter is able to remove the noise and replace the bad pixels with reasonable values while causing minimal image distortion or degradation. Two different neighborhoods are used: a 3×3 square containing a total of 9 pixels, and a 5×5 octagonal region containing a total of 21 pixels. **Figure 10** shows several of the neighborhood regions often used for ranking. Of course, the computational effort required rises quickly with the number of values to be sorted. This is true even using specialized methods that keep partial sets of the pixels ranked separately, so that only a few additional pixel comparisons are needed as the neighborhood is moved across the image.

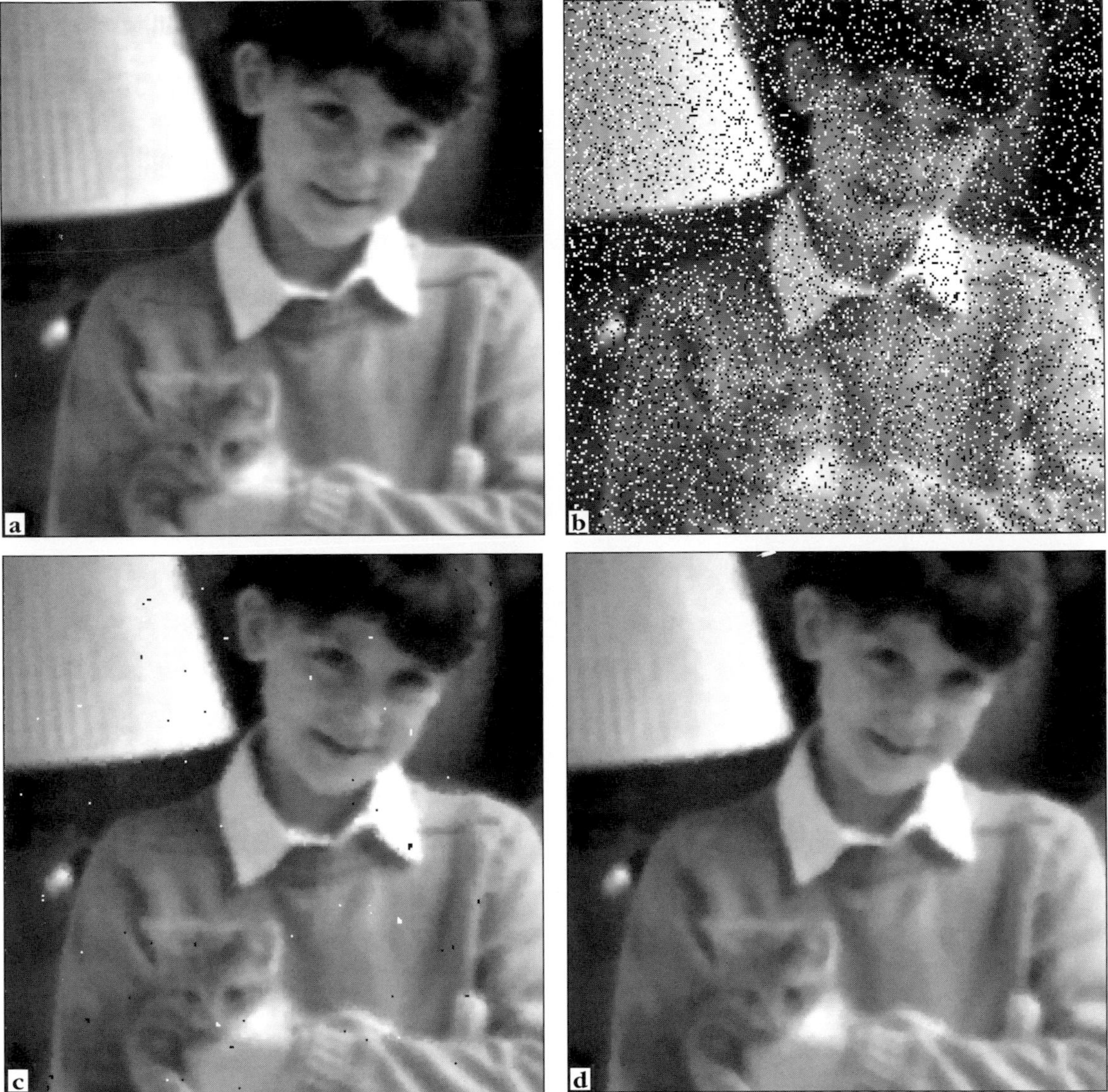

Figure 9. Removal of shot noise with a median filter:
a) *original image;*
b) *image a with 10% of the pixels randomly selected and set to black, and another 10% randomly selected and set to white;*
c) *application of median filtering to image b using a 3×3 square region;*
d) *application of median filtering to image b using a 5×5 octagonal region.*

A median filter can also be used to reduce the type of random noise shown before in the context of averaging. **Figure 11** shows the same image as in **Figures 1** and **3,** but with a 5×5 octagonal median filter applied. There are two principal advantages to the median filter compared to multiplication by weights. First, the method does not reduce the brightness difference across steps, because the available values are only those present in the neighborhood region, not an average between those values. Second, unlike averaging, median filtering does not shift bound-

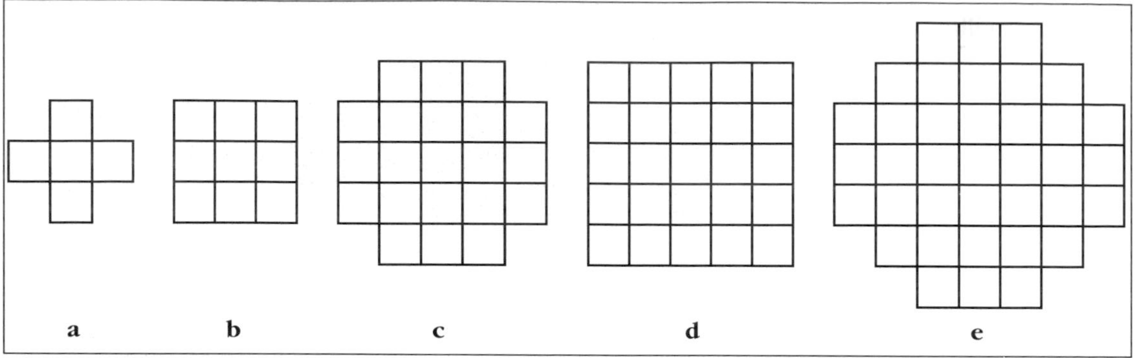

Figure 10. Neighborhood patterns used for median filtering:
a) *4 nearest-neighbor cross;* ***b)*** *3×3 square containing nine pixels;* ***c)*** *5×5 octagonal region with 21 pixels;* ***d)*** *5×5 square containing 25 pixels;* ***e)*** *7×7 octagonal region containing 37 pixels.*

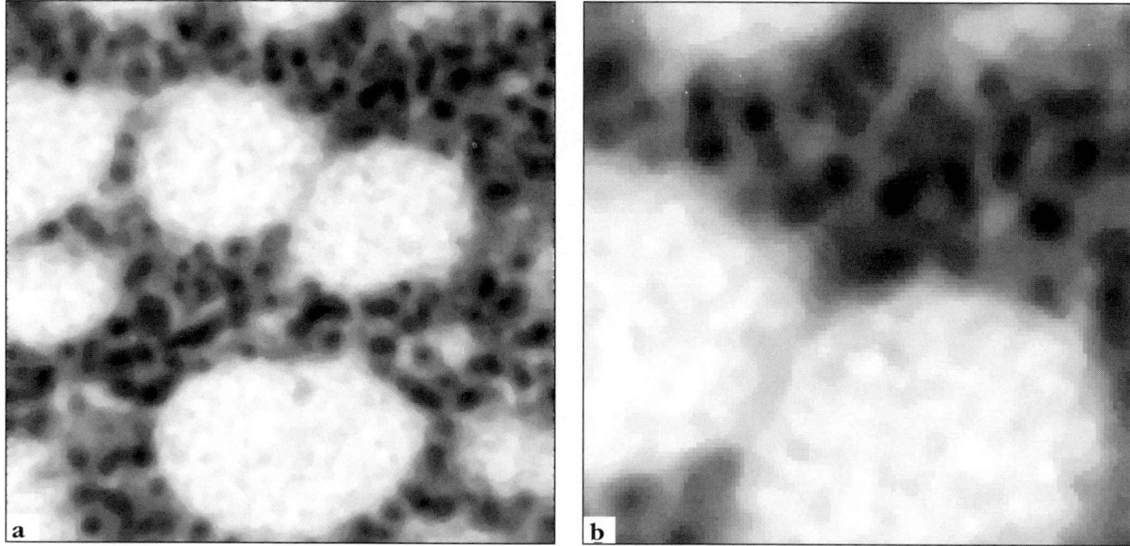

Figure 11. Smoothing with a median filter:
a) *the same image as in Figure 3 after application of a 5×5 octagonal median filter;*
b) *enlargement of image a to show individual pixels.*

aries–depending on the relative magnitude of values present in the neighborhood. The ability to overcome these problems makes the median filter preferable for both visual examination and measurement of images (Huang, 1979; Yang & Huang, 1981).

The minimal degradation to edges in median filtering allows the method to be repeatedly applied. **Figure 12** shows an example of a 5×5 octagonal median filter applied 12 times to an image. The fine detail is erased in this process, and large regions take on the same brightness values. However, the edges remain in place and well-defined. This type of brightness leveling due to repeated median filtering is sometimes described as contouring or posterization.

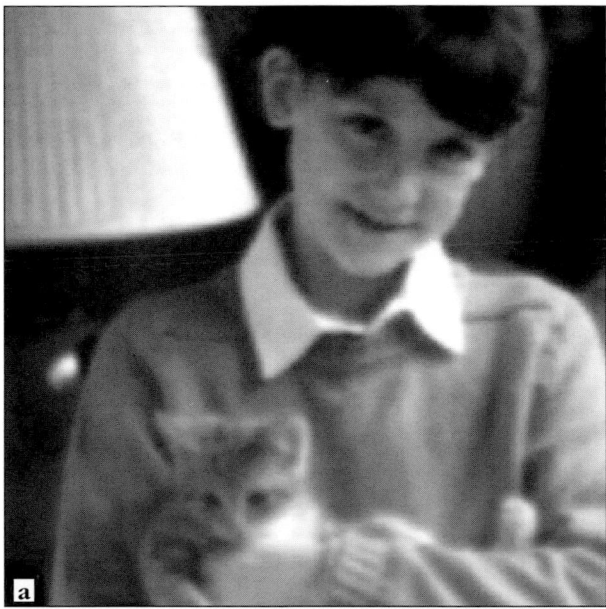

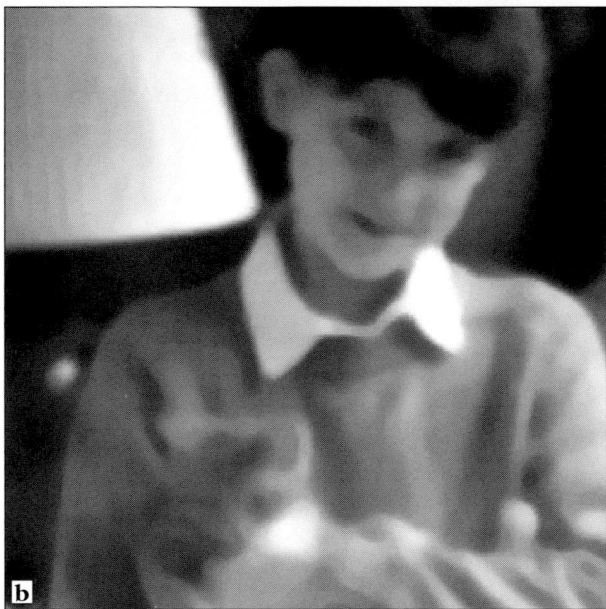

Figure 12. Repeated application of a 5×5 octagonal median filter:
a) *original image;*
b) *after 12 applications–the fine details have been erased and textured regions leveled to a uniform shade of grey, but boundaries have not shifted.*

Edge sharpening can be improved even more with a mode filter (Davies, 1988). The mode of the distribution of brightness values in each neighborhood is, by definition, the most likely value. For a small neighborhood, however, the mode is poorly defined. An approximation to this value can be obtained with a truncated median filter. For any asymmetric distribution, such as would be obtained at most locations near (but not precisely straddling) an edge, the mode is the highest point and the median lies closer to the mode than the mean value. This is illustrated in **Figure 13.** The truncated median technique consists of discarding a few values from the neighborhood so that the median value of the re-

Figure 13. *Schematic diagram of an asymmetric histogram distribution of brightness values, showing the relationship between the mode, median, and mean. The truncated median filter works by discarding the values in the distribution which are farthest from the mean, and then using the median of the remainder as an estimate for the mode. For a symmetrical distribution values are discarded from both ends and the median value does not change (it is already equal to the mode).*

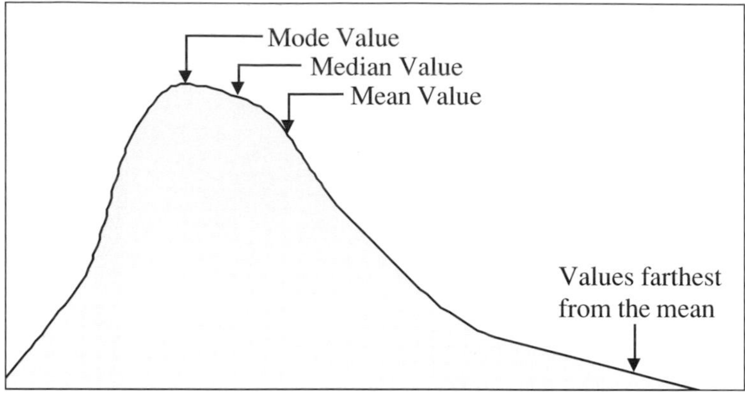

maining pixels is shifted toward the mode. In the example shown in **Figure 14**, this is demonstrated for a 3×3 neighborhood by skipping the two pixels whose brightness values are most different from the mean, ranking the remaining seven values, and assigning the median to the central pixel. This has the effect of sharpening steps and produces posterization when it is applied repeatedly.

Another modification to the median filter is used to overcome its tendency to erase lines that are narrower than the half-width of the neighborhood and to round corners. The so-called hybrid, or edge-preserving median, is actually a three-step ranking operation (Nieminen et al., 1987). In a 5×5 pixel neighborhood, pixels are ranked in two different groups, as shown in **Figure 15.** The median values of the "X" and "+" groups (both of which include the central pixel) are compared to the central pixel. The median value of that set is then saved as the new pixel value. As in **Figure 16,** this preserves lines and corners that are erased or rounded off by the conventional median–even one of smaller size, which does a poorer job of eliminating noise.

If the hybrid median filter is applied repeatedly, it also produces posterization. Because the details of lines and corners are better preserved by the hybrid median than by a conventional neighborhood median, the shapes of regions are not smoothed as much, although the brightness values across steps are still sharpened and posterized. This is illustrated in **Figure 17.**

The fact that the hybrid median involves three ranking operations, first within each of the two groups of pixels and then to compare those medians to the central pixel, does not impose a serious computational penalty. Each of the ranking operations is for a much smaller number of values than used in a square or octagonal region of the same size. For example, the 5-pixel-wide neighborhood used in the examples contains either 25 (in the square neighborhood) or 21 pixels (in the octagonal neighborhood), which must be ranked in the traditional method. In the hybrid method, each of the two groups contains only 9 pixels, and the final comparison involves only 3 values. Even with the

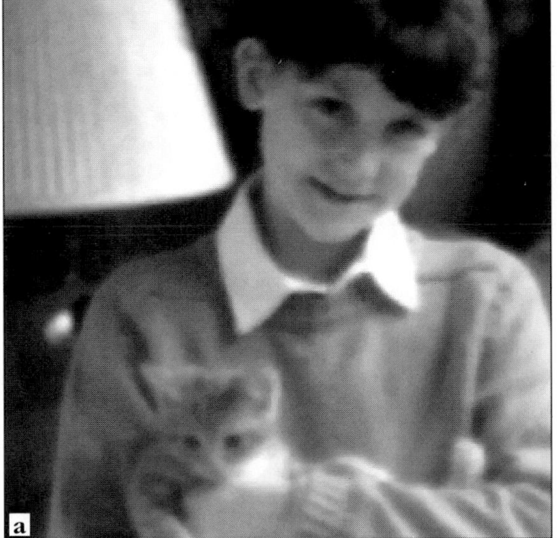

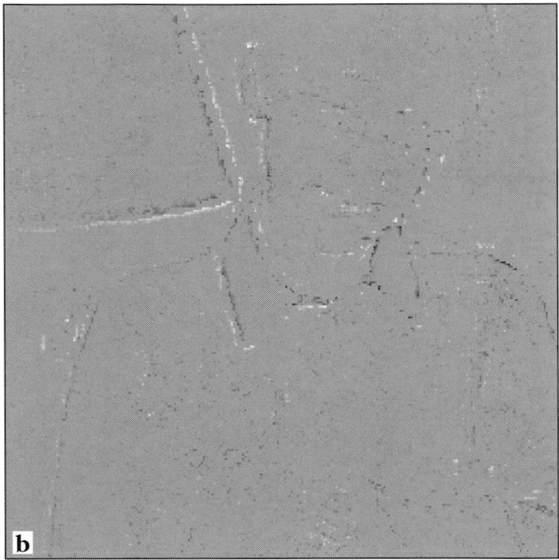

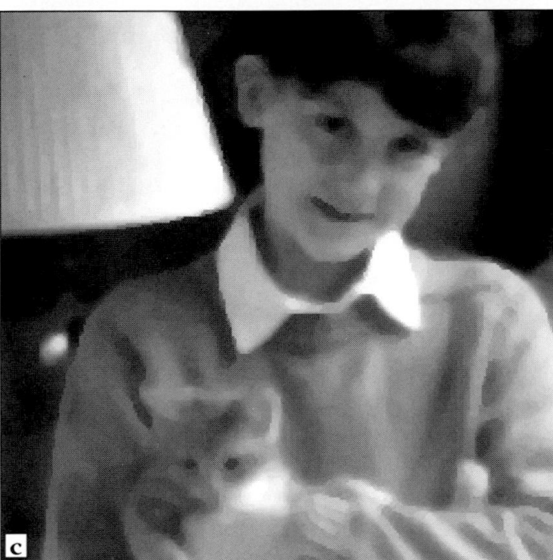

Figure 14. Application of the truncated median filter to posterize the image from Figure 9:

a) *one application of the 3×3 truncated median;*

b) *difference between Figure a and a conventional 3×3 median filter, showing the difference in values along edges;*

c) *12 applications of the truncated median filter.*

additional logic and manipulation of values, the hybrid method is at least as fast as the conventional median.

Posterizing an image, or reducing the number of grey levels so that regions become uniform in grey value and edges between regions become abrupt, falls more into the category of enhancement than defect correction. It is included here as a side effect of median filtering. Other methods can also produce this effect. One that is related to the median is the extremum filter, which replaces each pixel value with either the minimum or maximum value in the neighborhood, whichever is closer to the mean value. **Figure 18** shows this operator applied to the image from **Figure 16.** The extremum filter is not edge-preserving and may shift boundaries.

Figure 15. Diagram of pixels in a 5×5 neighborhood to show the groups used in the hybrid median filter. The two separately ranked groups are those in the two medium shaded diagonal lines and those in the lightly shaded horizontal and vertical lines. Both groups include the dark central pixel. The white pixels are not used in the operation.

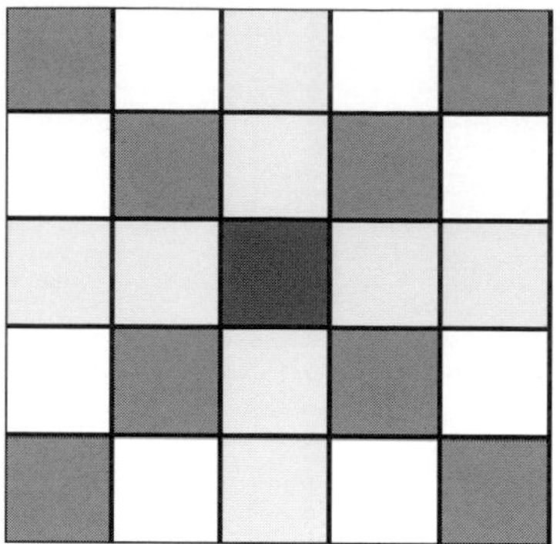

Other neighborhood noise reduction methods

A modification to the simple averaging of neighborhood values which attempts to achieve some of the advantages of the median filter is the so-called Olympic filter. The name comes from the system of scoring used in some events in the Olympic games, in which the highest and lowest scores are discarded and the remainder averaged. The same thing is done with the pixel values in the neighborhood. By discarding the extreme values, shot noise is rejected. Then the average of the remaining pixel values is used as the new brightness.

Figure 19 shows an application of this method to the image from **Figures 1** and **3,** containing Gaussian noise. Because it still causes edge blurring, is not easily adapted to weighting values that take into account the original pixel locations, and requires

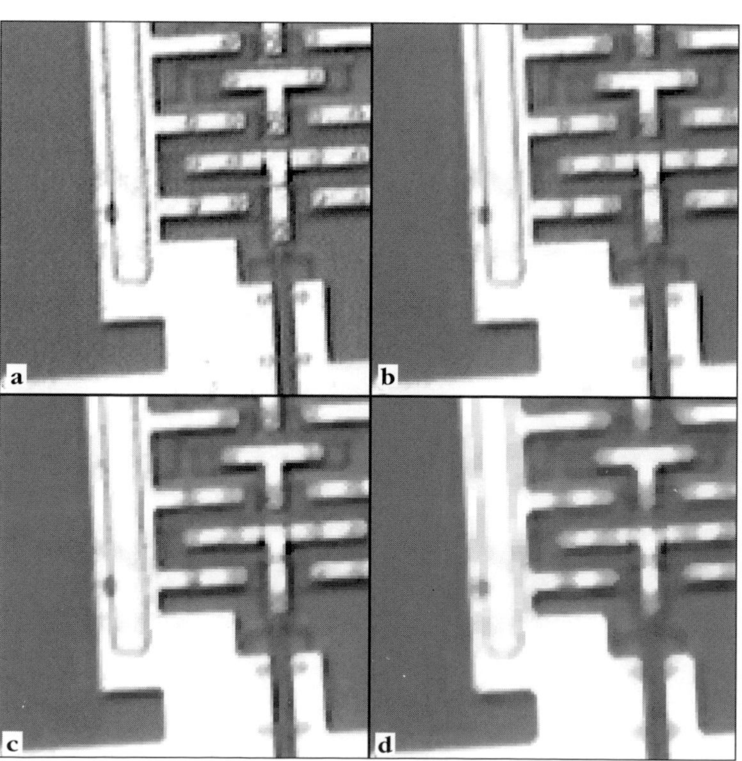

Figure 16. Application of the hybrid median filter to a light microscope image of an integrated circuit, showing the improved retention of lines and corners:

- ***a)*** *original image with noise;*
- ***b)*** *application of the 5×5 hybrid median filter;*
- ***c)*** *application of a conventional 3×3 median, which does not remove all of the noise but still degrades corners and edges somewhat;*
- ***d)*** *application of a conventional 5×5 filter, showing its effect on corners and edges.*

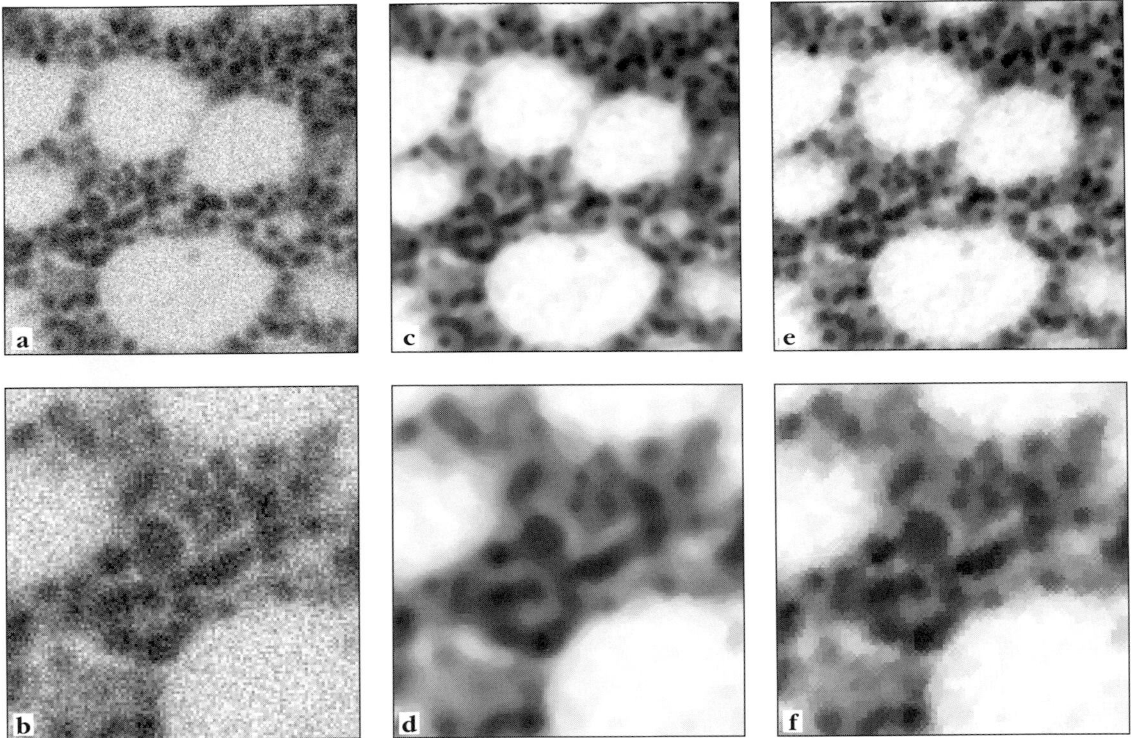

Figure 17. Repeated application of the hybrid median filter to the noisy image in Figure 1:
a) *original image;*
b) *zoomed portion of Figure a showing individual pixels;*
c) *repeated application of a conventional 5-pixel-wide median filter;*
d) *zoomed portion of Figure c showing individual pixels;*
e) *repeated application of the hybrid 5-pixel-wide median filter;*
f) *zoomed portion of Figure e showing individual pixels.*
Notice that the brightness values are posterized and smoothed and edge contrast is sharpened, but the shapes of features and edges are not smoothed.

sorting of the brightness values, this method is generally inferior to the others discussed and is not often used. **Figure 20** shows an application to the shot noise introduced in **Figure 9.** The performance is quite poor; the features are blurred and yet the noise is not entirely removed.

There are other, more complicated combinations of operations that are used for very specific types of images. For instance, synthetic aperture radar (SAR) images contain speckle noise, which varies in a known way with the image brightness. To remove the noise, the brightness of each pixel is compared to the average value of a local neighborhood. If it exceeds it by an amount calculated from the average and the standard deviation, then it is replaced by a weighted average value. Using some coefficients determined by experiment, the method reportedly (Nathan & Curlander, 1990) performs better at improving signal-to-noise than a simple median filter. This is a good example of an ad hoc processing method. In general, any filtering method that chooses

Figure 18. *Posterization of the image from Figure 16, produced by applying a 3×3 extremum filter which replaces each pixel value with either the minimum or maximum value in the neighborhood, whichever is closer to the mean value.*

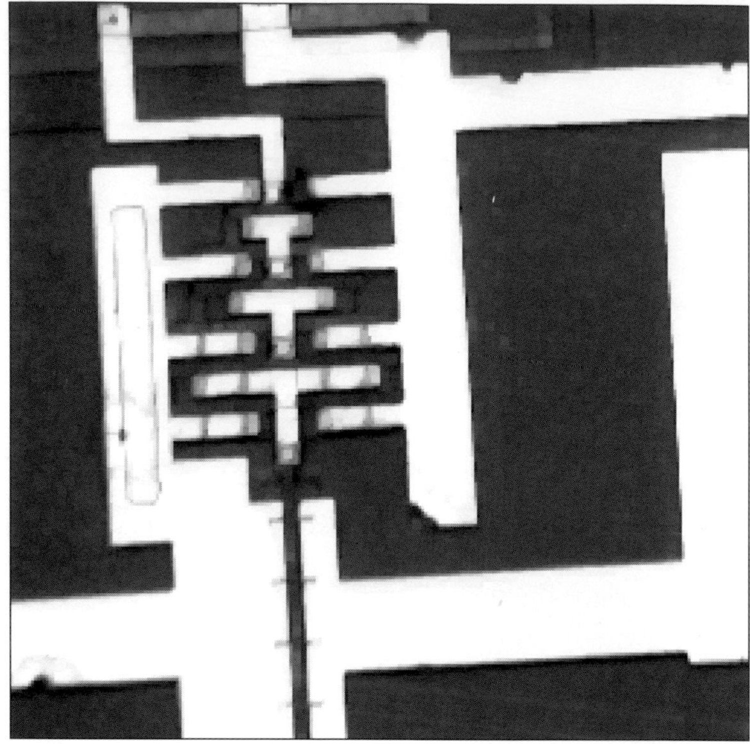

between several algorithms, or modifies its algorithm based on the actual contents of the image or the neighborhood, is called an adaptive filter (Mastin, 1985).

There is still another method of ranking, using the maximum and minimum brightness rather than the median. **Figure 21** shows the results of a two-step operation. First, the brightest pixel value in each region (a 5×5 octagonal neighborhood) was used to replace the original pixel values. Then, in a second transformation, the darkest pixel value in each region was selected. This type of combined operation requires two full passes through the image, and during each pass only the previous pixel brightness values are used to derive the new ones.

For reasons that will be discussed in more detail in Chapter 6, this type of operation is often described as a grey scale erosion

Figure 19. Application of an Olympic filter to Gaussian noise. The 4 brightest and 4 darkest pixels in each 5×5 neighborhood are ignored and the remaining 17 averaged to produce a new image:

a) *application to image in Figure 3;*

b) *enlargement to show pixel detail.*

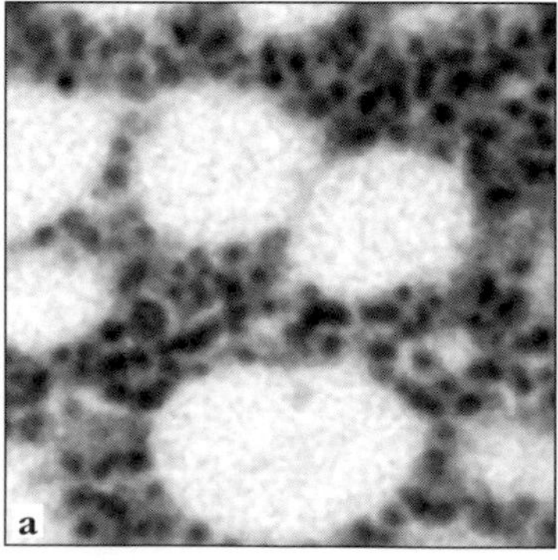

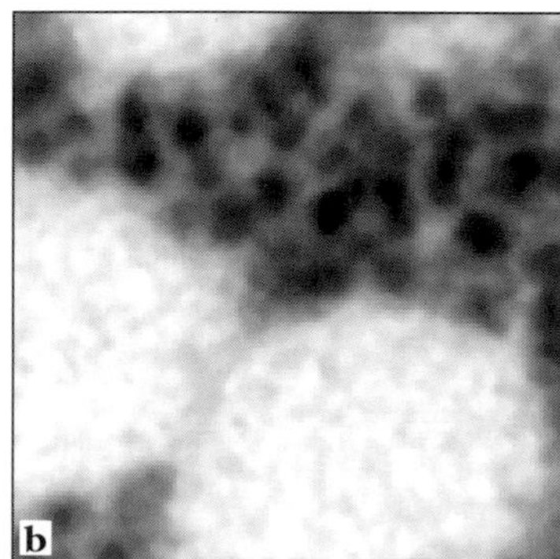

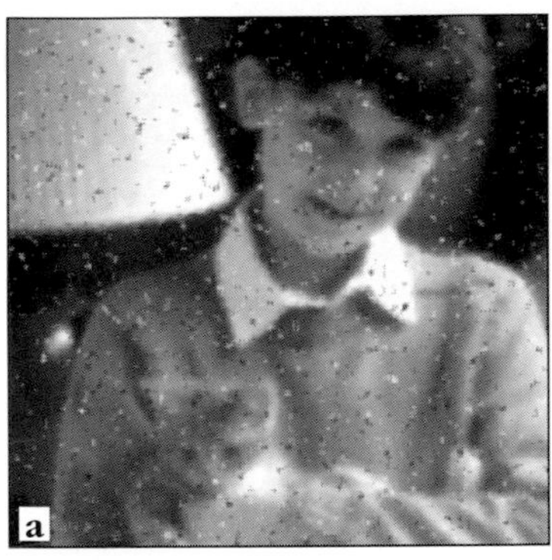

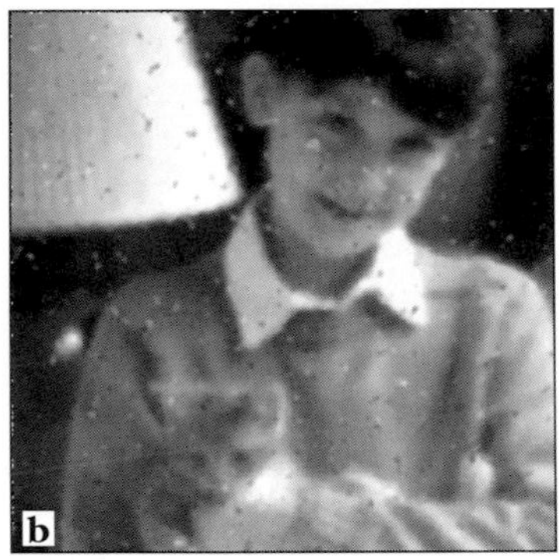

Figure 20. Application of Olympic filter to shot noise. The original image is the same as in Figure 12:
a) *the 2 brightest and 2 darkest pixels in each 3×3 neighborhood are ignored and the remaining 5 averaged;*
b) *the 4 brightest and 4 darkest pixels in each 5×5 neighborhood are ignored and the remaining 17 averaged.*

and dilation, by analogy to the erosion and dilation steps performed on binary images. The sequence is also called an opening, again by analogy to operations on binary images. By adjusting the sizes of the neighborhoods (which need not be the same) used in the two separate passes to locate the brightest and then the darkest values, other processing effects are obtained. These are described in Chapter 3.

As a method for removing noise, this technique would seem to be the antithesis of a median filter, which discards extreme values. It may be helpful to visualize the image as a surface in which the brightness represents an elevation. **Figure 22** shows a one-dimensional representation of such a situation. In the first pass, the brightest values in each region are used to construct a new profile which follows the "tops of the trees." In the second pass, the darkest values in each region are used to bring the pro-

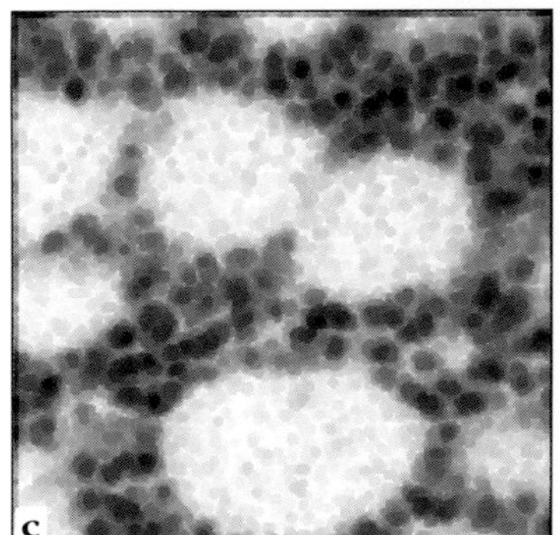

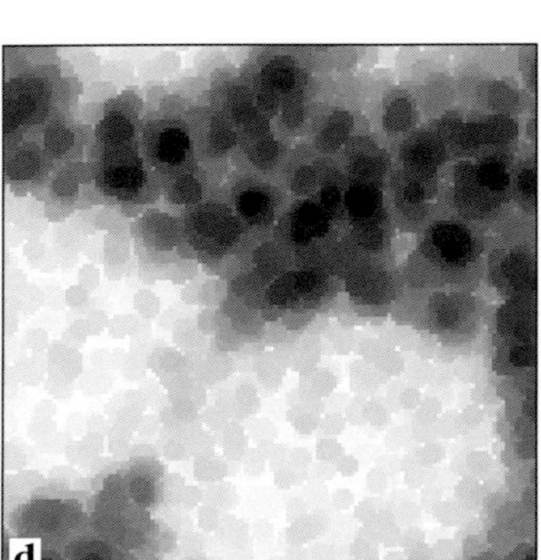

Figure 21. Grey scale opening, or erosion and dilation. Two separate ranking operations are performed on the original image from Figure 3. First each pixel value is replaced with the brightest value in the neighborhood; then using this image, each pixel value is replaced by the darkest value in the same size neighborhood:
a) *application using a 3×3 square neighborhood;*
b) *enlargement to show pixel detail;*
c) *application using a 5×5 octagonal neighborhood;*
d) *enlarged to show pixel detail.*

Figure 22. *Schematic diagram of the operation of grey scale erosion and dilation in one dimension, showing (starting from the top): the original profile with result of first (maximum) pass, producing a new profile through brightest points; the second step in which a new profile passes through the darkest (minimum) points in the result from step 1; comparison of the final result to the original profile, showing rejection of noise and dark spikes.*

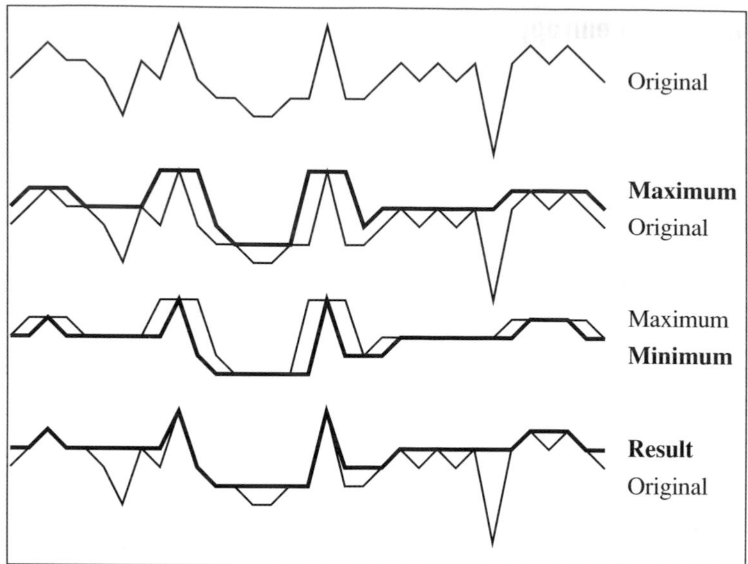

file back down to those points which were large enough to survive the first pass, giving a new profile that ignores the noise spikes in the original.

Profile plots sometimes offer a better tool for visualizing the reduction of noise in images than do grey scale representations. **Figure 23** shows the brightness values along the same line in several of the previous images obtained by processing **Figure 3.** Although these are only one-dimensional traverses across a two-dimensional image and therefore cannot show all of the data used in the transformations based on two-dimensional neighborhoods, the presence of noise and its removal by various operations is evident, as is the blurring of edges.

Figure 23. *Profile plots on several original and smoothed images from the preceding figures, showing the variation of brightness along the same horizontal line. Except for the profile for the averaged image, all of the brightness scales are identical.*

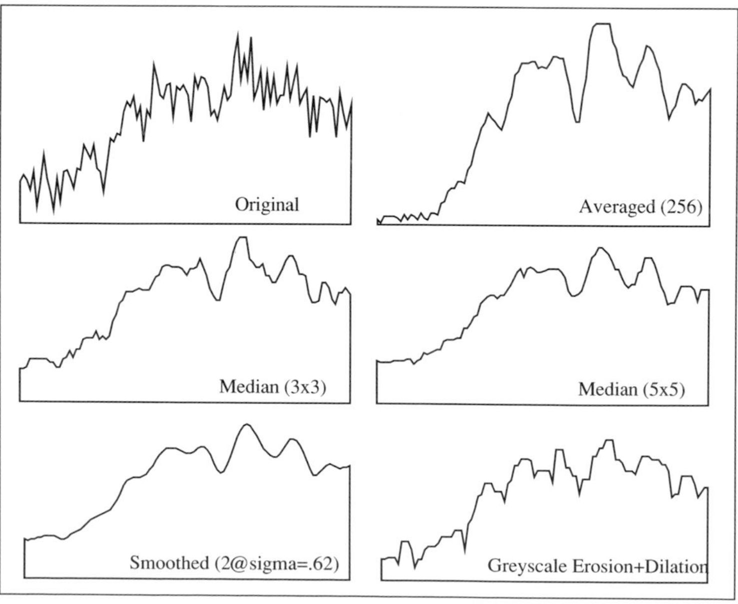

Maximum entropy

In addition to noise, images may contain other defects, such as blur due to motion or out-of-focus optics. The inverse filtering methods described in Chapter 4 are quite noise sensitive. When noise that is present can itself be characterized, it may be possible to use a maximum entropy approach to remove the artefacts.

Maximum entropy methods are a computer-intensive approach to removing artefacts, such as noise or blur, from images. It is based on some foreknowledge about the image contents and some assumptions about the nature of the degradation to be removed and the image to be restored (Skilling, 1986; Frieden, 1988). A conventional description of the method is to imagine an image containing N pixels, which has been formed by a total of M photons (where usually $M>N$). The number of photons in any single pixel (i.e., the pixel's brightness value) is P_i, where i is the pixel identification or location. This is usually written for convenience as a single subscript, but we understand that it really refers to a pixel at a given X, Y location.

The measured image has normalized pixel brightness values $p_i = P_i / M$ which only approximate the true image that would be collected if there were no artefacts. The method used to approach this ideal image is to alter pixel brightness values to maximize the entropy in the image, subject to some constraints. The justification for this method is given in terms of statistical probability and Bayes' theorem, and will not be derived here. In some cases, it produces dramatic improvements in image quality.

The entropy of the brightness pattern is given in a formal sense by calculating the number of ways that the pattern could have been formed by rearrangement, or $S = M!/p_1!\, p_2!, \ldots p_N!$ where ! indicates factorial. For large values of M, this reduces by Stirling's approximation to the more familiar $S = -\sum p_i \log p_i$. This is the same calculation of entropy used in statistical mechanics. In the particular case of taking the log to the base 2, the entropy of the image is the number of bits per pixel needed to represent the image, according to information theory.

The entropy in the image would be maximized in an absolute sense simply by setting the brightness of each pixel to the average brightness, M/N. Clearly, this is not the "proper" solution. It is the application of constraints that produces usable results. The most common constraint for images containing noise is based on a chi-squared statistic, calculated as $\chi^2 = 1/\sigma^2 \sum (p_i - p_i')^2$. In this expression, the p_i values are the original pixel values, the p_i' are the altered brightness values, and σ is the standard deviation of the values. An upper limit can be set on the value of χ^2 allowed in the calculation of a new set of p_i' values to maximize the entropy. A typical (but essentially arbitrary) limit for χ^2 is N, the number of pixels in the array.

Note that this constraint is not the only possible choice. A sum of the absolute value of differences or some other weighting rule could also be chosen. This is not quite enough information to produce an optimal image, so other constraints may be added. One is that the totals of the p_i and p_i' values be equal. Bryan and Skilling (1980) also require, for instance, that the distribution of the $p_i - p_i'$ values corresponds to the expected noise characteristics of the imaging source (e.g., a Poisson distribution for simple counting statistics). And, of course, we must be careful to include such seemingly obvious constraints as non-negativity (no pixel can collect fewer than zero photons). Jaynes (1985) makes the point that there is practically always a significant amount of real knowledge about the image that can be used as a constraint, but it is assumed to be so obvious that it is ignored.

An iterative solution for the values of p_i' produces a new image with the desired smoothness and noise characteristics which is often an improvement of the original image. Other formulations of the maximum entropy approach may compare one iteration of the image to the next, by calculating not the total entropy but the cross entropy, $-\sum p_i \log (p_i / q_i)$ where q_i is the previous image brightness value for the same pixel, or the modeled brightness for a theoretical image. In this formulation, the cross entropy is to be minimized. The basic principle remains the same.

Contrast expansion

Acquiring a noise-free image, or processing one to reduce noise, does not by itself ensure that the resulting image can be viewed or interpreted well by an observer or a program. If the brightness range within the image is very small, there may not be enough contrast to assure visibility. Typical digitizers, as discussed in Chapter 1, convert the analog voltage range from the camera or other sensor to numbers from 0 to 255 (8 bits). For a common video camera, this corresponds to a total voltage range of 0.7 volts and (depending on the camera design) to a variation in brightness covering several orders of magnitude in numbers of photons.

If the inherent range of variation in image brightness is much smaller than the dynamic range of the camera, subsequent electronics, and digitizer, then the actual range of numbers will be much less than the full range of 0 through 255. **Figure 24a** shows an example. The specimen is a thin section through tissue, with a blood vessel shown in cross section in a bright field microscope. Illumination in the microscope and very light staining of the section produce very little total contrast. The histogram shown next to the image is a plot of the number of pixels at each of the 256 possible brightness levels. The narrow peak indicates that only a few of the levels are represented.

Visibility of the structures present can be improved by stretching the contrast so that the values of pixels are reassigned to cover the entire available range, as in **Figure 24b.** The mapping is lin-

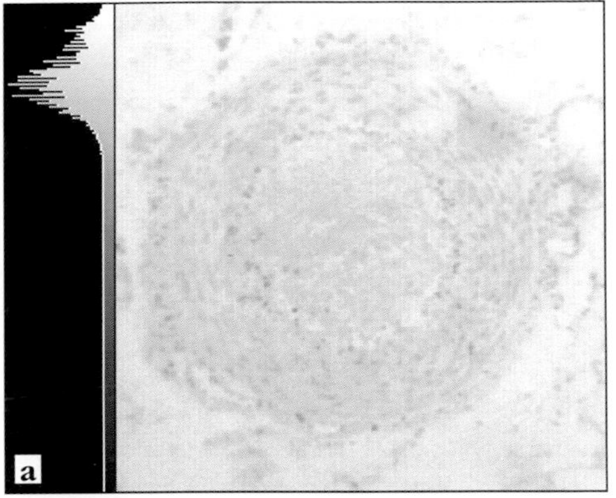
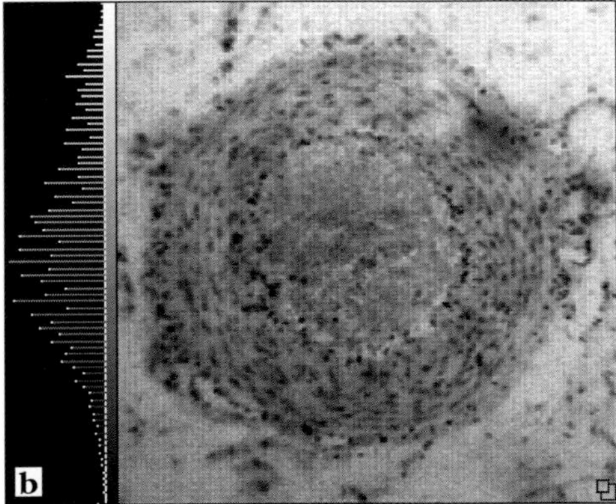
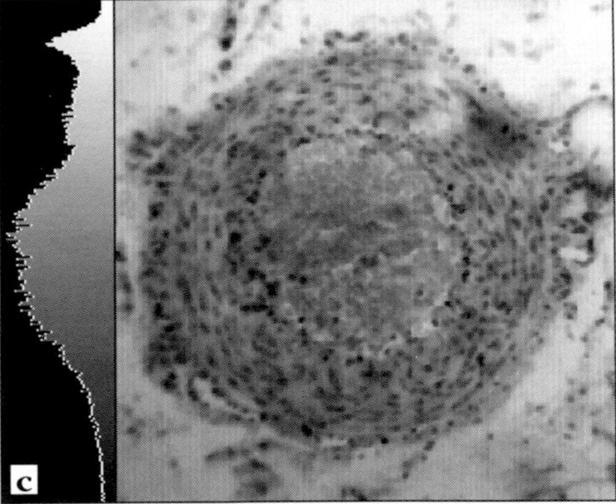

Figure 24. Contrast expansion:
a) *this light microscope image of a blood vessel has very low initial contrast, as shown by its brightness histogram;*
b) *linear expansion of the brightness range by manipulating the display shows a full range of black to white values but causes gaps in the histogram;*
c) *averaging multiple frames produces an image with more than 8 bits, which can be scaled to the full 8 bit range of the display without gaps. It also averages image noise to produce a smoother image.*

ear and one-to-one. This means that the darkest pixels in the original image are assigned to black, the lightest images are assigned to white, and intermediate grey values in the original image are given new values which are linearly interpolated between black and white. All of the pixels in the original image that had one particular grey value will also have the same relative grey shade in the resulting image, but it will be a different value.

This histogram plotted with the image in the figure now shows pixel counts for grey levels that are spread out across the available brightness scale. However, notice that most of the grey values still show no pixels in the histogram, indicating that no pixels have those values. The reassignment of grey values has increased the visual contrast for the pixels present, but has not increased the ability to discriminate subtle variations in grey scale that were not recorded in the original image. It has also magnified the brightness difference associated with noise in the original image.

Figure 24c shows the same field of view recorded to utilize the entire range of the camera and digitizer. This was actually done by averaging together many video frames. The mean brightness of various structures is similar to that shown in **Figure 24b,** after linear expansion of the contrast range. However, all of the 256 possible grey values are now present in the image, and very small variations in sample density can now be distinguished or measured in the specimen.

This is a rather extreme case. It is not always practical to adjust the illumination, camera gain, etc. to exactly fill the available pixel depth (number of grey levels that can be digitized or stored). Furthermore, increasing the brightness range too much can cause pixel values at the dark and/or light ends of the range to exceed the digitization and storage capacity and to be clipped to the limiting values, which also causes a loss of information. Consequently, it is common to acquire images that do not completely cover the available brightness range.

If these images still have enough different grey levels to reveal the specimen's important features, then linear contrast expansion may be a useful and acceptable method to increase the viewer's visual discrimination. More important, it may make it possible to more directly compare images acquired with slightly different brightness ranges by adjusting them all to the same expanded contrast scale. Of course, this only works if the brightest and darkest classes of features are present in all of the images and fields of view.

Other manipulations of pixel brightness values can also be performed. Operations that are one to one (i.e., all pixels that originally had a single grey scale value are assigned to another single value) need not be linear. An example would be one that converted brightness to density, which involves a logarithmic relationship. For color images, a transfer function can be used to correct colors for distortion due to the color temperature of the light source or for atmospheric scattering and absorption in satellite images. These functions may be implemented using either a mathematical function or a LUT and for color images is most easily performed when the image is represented as hue, saturation, and intensity (as opposed to red, green, and blue) values for each pixel. Discussion of the general use of transfer functions, and their implementation using LUTS, is presented in Chapter 3 on image processing.

Nonuniform illumination

The most straightforward strategy for image analysis uses the brightness of regions in the image as a means of identification: It is assumed that the same type of feature will have the same brightness (or color, in a color image) wherever it appears in the field of view. If this brightness is different from that of other features, or can be made so by appropriate image processing as discussed in Chapter 3, then it can be used to discriminate the features for counting, measurement, etc. Even if there are a few other types of objects that cannot be distinguished on the basis of brightness or color alone, subsequent measurements may suffice to select the ones of interest.

This approach is not without pitfalls, which are discussed further in Chapter 5 in conjunction with converting grey scale images to binary (black and white) images. Additionally, other approaches are available, such as region growing or split-and-merge, which do not have such stringent requirements for uniformity of illumination. Since simple brightness thresholding is by far the simplest and fastest method to isolate features in an image (when it can be used), it is important to consider the problems of image shading.

When irregular surfaces are viewed, the amount of light scattered to the viewer or camera from each region is a function of the orientation of the surface with respect to the source of light and the viewer, even if the surface material and finish is uniform. In fact, this principle can be used to estimate the surface orientation, using a technique known as shape-from-shading. Human vision seems to apply these rules very easily and rapidly, since we are not generally confused by images of real-world objects. We will not pursue those methods here, however.

Most of the images we really want to process are essentially two-dimensional. Whether they come from light or electron microscopes or satellite images, the variation in surface elevation is usually small compared to the lateral dimensions, giving rise to what is often called "two-and-one-half D." This is not always the case of course (consider a metal fracture surface examined in the SEM), but we will treat such problems as exceptions to the general rule and recognize that more elaborate processing may be needed.

Even surfaces of low relief need not be flat. A simple example is the curvature of the earth as viewed from a weather satellite, which produces a shading across the field of view. Shading also occurs in a macroscopic or microscopic surface that is illuminated from one side. Even elaborate collections of lights and ring lights can only approximate uniform illumination of the scene.

For transmission imaging, a condenser lens system produces a fairly uniform light source, but it is easy for these systems to get out of perfect alignment and produce shading as well. Finally, it was mentioned in Chapter 1 that lenses or cameras themselves (especially ones with glass envelopes) may cause vignetting, in which the corners of the image are darker than the center, because the light is partially absorbed.

Most of these defects can be minimized by carefully setting up the imaging conditions. Even if defects cannot be eliminated altogether, they can be assumed to be constant over some period of time. This allows correction through image processing. In most instances, it is possible to acquire a background image in which a uniform reference surface or specimen is inserted in place of the actual sample to be viewed, and the light intensity recorded. This image can then be used to level the subsequent images. The process is often called background subtraction, but in many cases this is a misnomer. If the image acquisition device is logarithmic with a gamma of 1.0, then the background image is subtracted point by point from each acquired image. If the camera or sensor is linear, then the correct procedure is to divide the acquired image by the background. For other sensor response functions, there is no simple correct arithmetic method and the calibrated response must first be determined and applied to convert the measured signal to a linear space.

Notice that in the process of subtracting (or dividing) one image by another, some of the dynamic range of the original data will be lost. The greater the variation in background brightness, the less the remaining variation from that level can be recorded in the image and will be left after the leveling process. These factors, along with the inevitable increase in statistical noise that results from subtracting one signal from another, argue that all practical steps should be taken to make illumination uniform while acquiring images, before resorting to processing methods.

Figure 50 in Chapter 1 showed an example of leveling in which the background illumination function could be acquired separately. This is most commonly done by removing the specimen (for instance, a slide) from the light path and storing an image representing the variation. This can then be used for leveling. However, in many cases it is not practical to remove the specimen, or its presence contributes to the brightness variation. This includes situations in which the specimen thickness varies, affecting the overall absorption of light. Another case occurs when the surface being examined is not perfectly flat, causing incident light or SEM images to show a varying background.

Figure 25 shows an example of the latter effect. The SEM image shows particles on a substrate, which because of the geometry of the surface and of the SEM chamber cause a portion of the image to appear darker than the rest. Furthermore, moving the specimen or changing the magnification alters the pattern of light

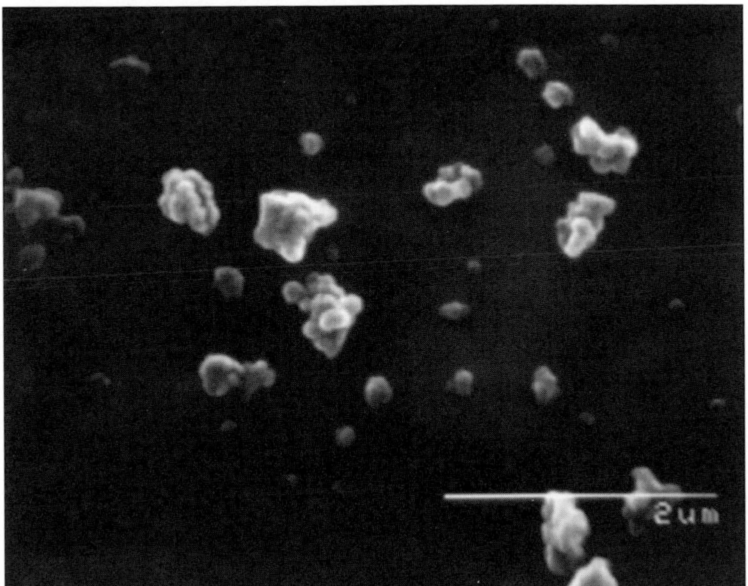

Figure 25. *SEM image of particles on a substrate showing nonuniform brightness.*

and dark. In this case, it is necessary to perform the correction using the image itself. Fortunately, in many of these situations the variation of background brightness is a smooth and well-behaved function of location and can be approximated by simple functions, such as polynomials.

Fitting a background function

By selecting a number of points in the image, a list of brightness values and locations can be acquired. The list is then used to perform least-squares fitting of a function $B(x,y)$ that approximates the background and can be subtracted (or divided) just as a physically acquired background image. When the user marks these points, for instance by using a pointing device such as a mouse, trackball, or light pen, it is important to select locations that all have the same brightness and are well distributed across the image. Locating many points in one small region and few or none in other parts of the image requires the function to extrapolate the polynomial and can introduce significant errors. For a second-order polynomial, the functional form of the fitted background is

$$B(x,y) = a_0 + a_1 \cdot x + a_2 \cdot y + a_3 \cdot x^2 + a_4 \cdot y^2 + a_5 \cdot xy \quad (2$$

This equation has six fitted constants and so in principle could be fitted with only that number of marked points. Likewise, a third-order polynomial would have ten coefficients. However, in order to get a good fit and diminish sensitivity to minor fluctuations in individual pixels and to have enough points to properly sample the entire image area, it is usual to require several times this minimum number of points.

Figure 26. Automatic leveling of nonuniform illumination:
a) *reflection light microscope image of ceramic specimen, with nonuniform background brightness due to a non-planar surface;*
b) *background function calculated as a polynomial fit to the brightest point in each of 81 squares (a 9×9 grid);*
c) *leveled image after subtracting b from a.*

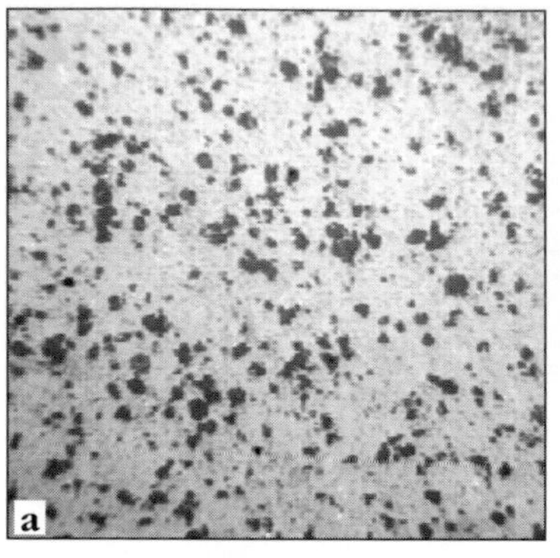

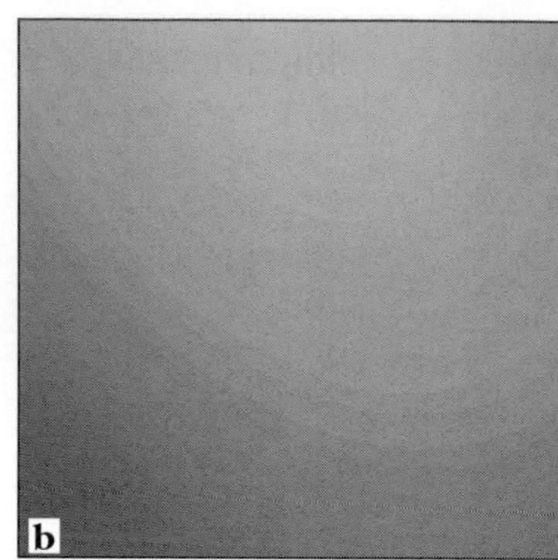

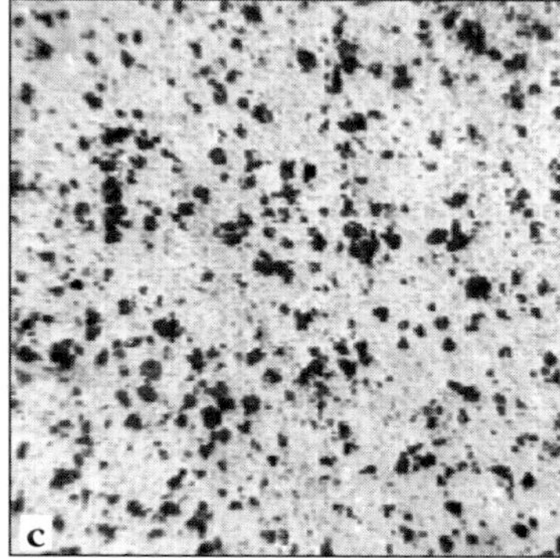

In some cases, it is practical to locate the points automatically for background fitting. This is easiest when there is a distinct structure or phase present that is well distributed throughout the image area and contains the darkest (or lightest) pixels present. In that case, the image can be subdivided into a grid of smaller squares or rectangles, the darkest (or lightest) pixels in each subregion region located, and these points used for the fitting.

Figure 26 shows an example of this approach, in which the specimen (a polished ceramic) has an overall variation in brightness due to the curvature of its surface. The brightest pixels in each region of the specimen represent the matrix, so they should all be the same. Subdividing the image into a 9×9 grid and locating the brightest pixel in each square gives a total of 81 points, which are then used to calculate a second-order polynomial (six coefficients) by least-squares. The fitting routine in this case reported a fitting error (rms value) of less than 2 brightness values out of the total 0 to 255 range for pixels in the image.

Figure 26b shows the calculated brightness using the $B(x,y)$ function and **Figure 26c** shows the result after subtracting the background from the original, pixel by pixel, to level the image. This removes the variation in background brightness and permits setting brightness thresholds to delineate the pores for measurement, as discussed in Chapter 5.

Another approach sometimes used to remove gradual variation in overall brightness employs the frequency transforms discussed

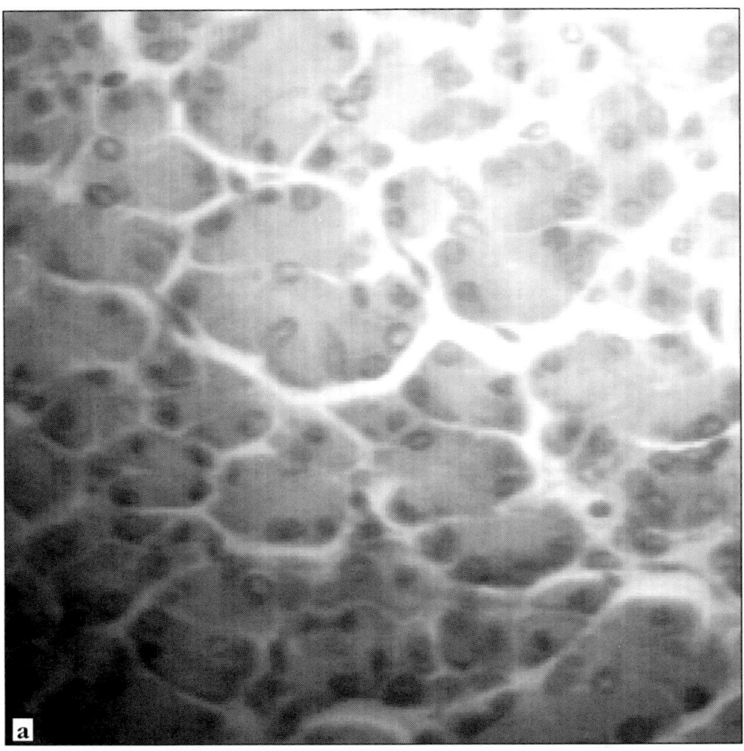

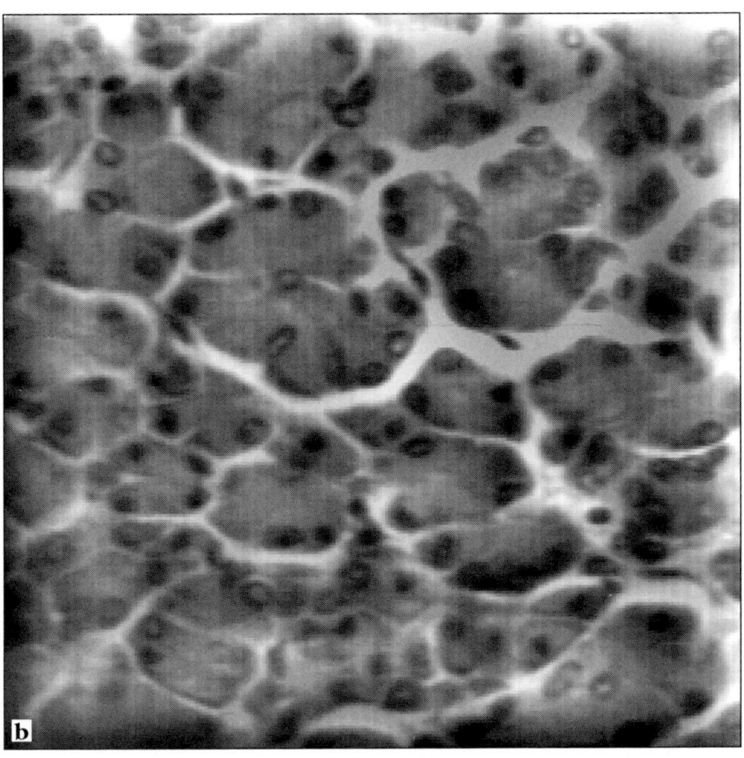

Figure 27. Leveling of image brightness and contrast by removal of low-frequency terms in 2D FFT:

a) *original image, showing nonuniform illumination;*

b) *attempt to level the brightness by reducing the magnitude to zero of the lowest four frequency components. Notice that in addition to the variations near the edge, the brightness of similar structures is not constant throughout the image.*

in Chapter 4. Background variation in the image is assumed to be a low-frequency signal that can be separated in frequency space from the higher frequencies defining the features present. If this assumption is justified and the frequencies corresponding to the background can be identified, then they can be removed by a simple filter in the frequency space representation.

Figure 27 shows an example of this approach. The brightness variation in the original image is due to off-centered illumination in the microscope. Transforming the image into frequency space with a two-dimensional FFT (as discussed in Chapter 4), reducing the magnitude of the first four frequency components by filtering the frequency space image, and finally retransforming produces the image in **Figure 27b.**

This transform method is not entirely successful for the image in the example. The edges of the image show significant variations, which are present because the frequency transform attempts to match the left and right and the top and bottom edges. In addition, the brightness of dark and light regions throughout the image that have the same appearance and would therefore be expected to properly have the same brightness show considerable local variations. This is because the brightness variation is a function of the local details, including the actual brightness values and the shapes of the features. There are few practical situations in which leveling can be satisfactorily performed by this method.

Rank leveling

Another approach can be used when the background variation is more irregular than can be fit to simple functions. It is particularly useful when the surface is irregular, such as when examining details on a fracture surface in the SEM. The assumption behind this method is that features of interest are limited in size and smaller than the scale of background variations and that the background is everywhere either lighter or darker than the features. It happens that both requirements are often met in practical situations.

Rank neighborhood operations are discussed in detail elsewhere in this chapter and in Chapter 3. The basic idea behind neighborhood operations is to compare each pixel to its neighbors or combine the pixel values in some small region, minimally the 8 touching pixels in a 3×3 square. This operation is performed for each pixel in the image, resulting in a new image. In many practical implementations, the new image replaces the original image with only a temporary requirement for additional storage; these implementation considerations are discussed in Chapter 3.

For our present purposes, the neighborhood comparison works as follows: examine the pixels in a 3×3 or other similar small region. If the background is known to be *darker* than the features, find the darkest pixel in each neighborhood and replace the value of the original pixel with that darker brightness value. For

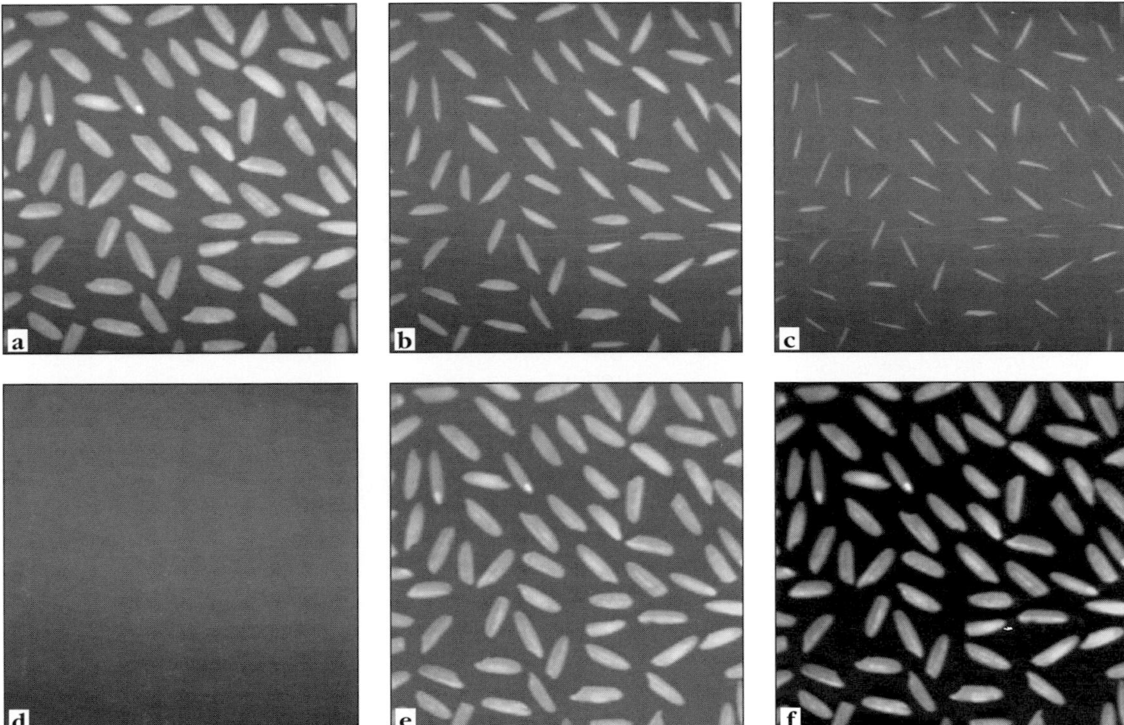

Figure 28. Constructing a background image with a rank operation:
a) *an image of rice grains with nonuniform illumination;*
b) *each pixel replaced with the darkest neighboring pixel in an octagonal 5×5 neighborhood;*
c) *another repetition of the "darkest neighbor" or grey scale erosion operation;*
d) *after four repetitions only the background remains;*
e) *result of subtracting d from a;*
f) *the leveled result with contrast expanded.*

the case of a background *lighter* than the features, the brightest pixel in the neighborhood is used instead. The result of applying this operation to the entire image is to shrink the features by the radius of the neighborhood region and to extend the local background brightness values into the area previously covered by features.

Figure 28 illustrates this method used on an image of rice grains on a dark and uneven background. A neighborhood is used consisting of 21 pixels in an octagonal 5×5 pattern centered on each pixel in the image. The darkest pixel value in that region replaces the original central pixel. This operation is repeated for every pixel in the image, always using the original image pixels and not the new ones from applying the procedure to other pixels. After this procedure is complete, the rice grains are reduced in size, as shown in **Figure 28b.** Repeating the operation continues to shrink the grains and extends the background based on the local background brightness.

After four repetitions **(Figure 28d),** the rice grains have been removed. This is possible because the maximum width of any

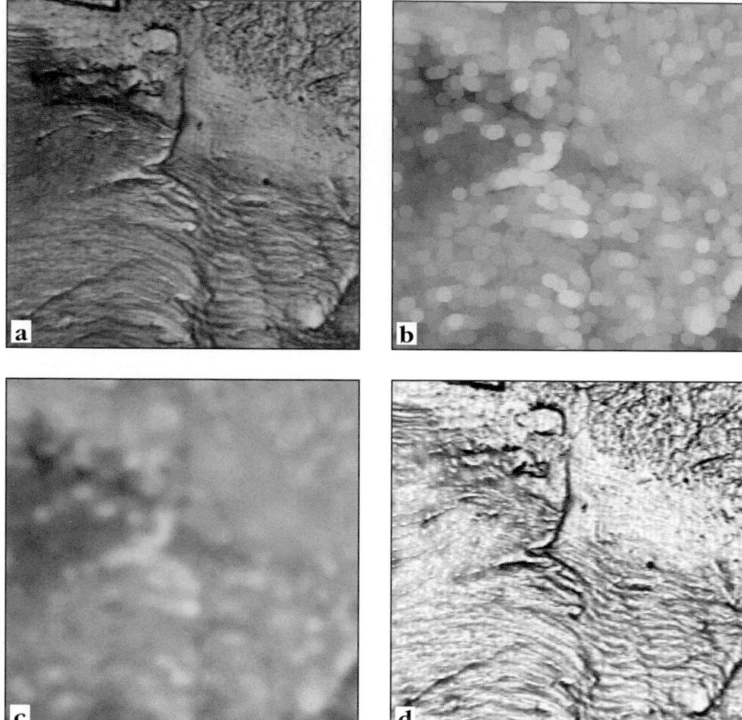

Figure 29. Leveling an uneven fracture surface image (TEM replica):
a) *original image shows brightness variations due to local variations in surface orientation;*
b) *two applications of a brightest rank operation using a 5×5 octagonal neighborhood around each pixel;*
c) *image b smoothed using a Gaussian kernel with sigma = 1.6 pixels;*
d) *subtraction of image c from image a, showing the leveled background and more visible fatigue striations.*

grain is not larger than four times the width of the 5-pixel-wide neighborhood used for the ranking. Knowing how many times to apply this operation depends upon knowing the width (smallest dimension) of the largest features present or simply watching the progress of the operation and repeating until the features are removed. In some cases, this can be judged from the disappearance of a peak from the image histogram. The background produced by this method has the large-scale variation present in the original image; subtracting it produces a leveled image **(Figure 28f)** that clearly defines the features and allows them to be separated from the background by thresholding.

This method is particularly suitable for the irregular background brightness variations that occur in details on fracture surfaces. **Figure 29** shows an example. The original TEM image of this fatigue fracture has facets at different orientations having differing overall brightnesses. Applying a ranking operation to select the brightest pixel in a 5-pixel-wide octagonal neighborhood produces the result shown in **Figure 29.** This was blurred using a Gaussian smoothing kernel with a standard deviation of 1.6 pixels (these neighborhood smoothing operations are discussed earlier in this chapter) and then subtracted from the original image to produce the result in **Figure 29d.** The leveled background improves the visibility of the fatigue striations on the fracture.

It is interesting in this example to note that the fatigue marks in

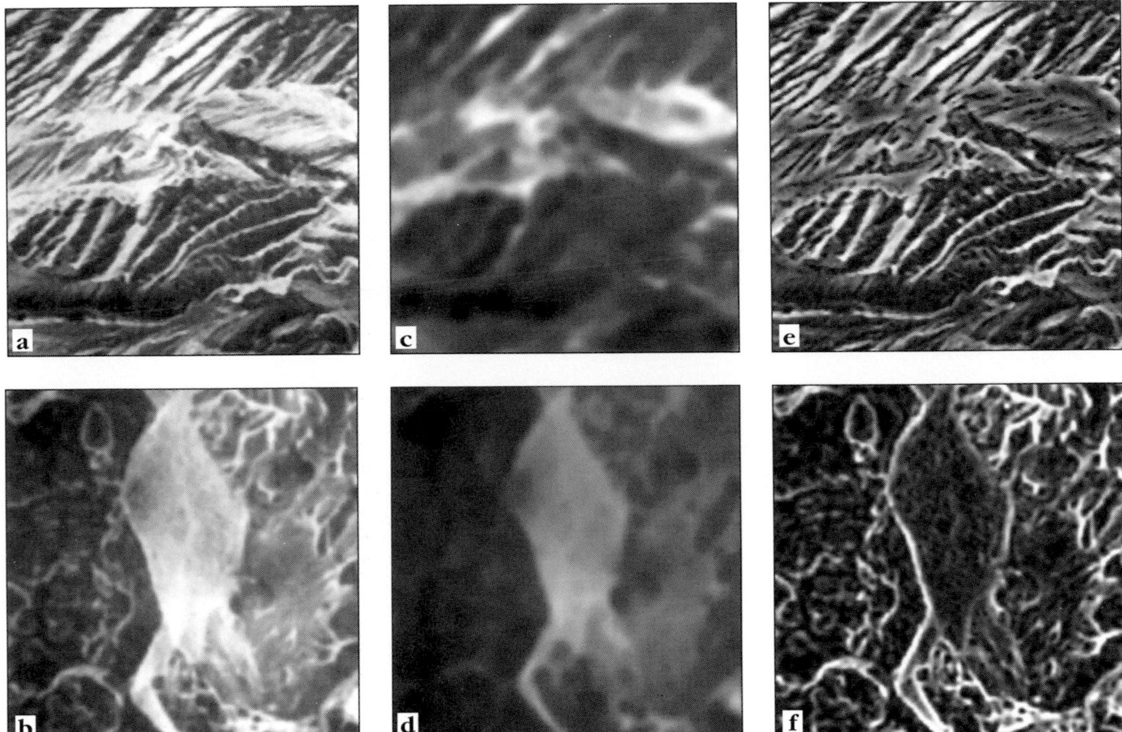

Figure 30. Application of rank leveling to SEM images:
a, b) *original images of metal fractures showing local brightness variations due to surface orientation;*
c, d) *background image produced by two applications of a 5-pixel-wide rank filter keeping the darkest pixel in each neighborhood followed by smoothing with a Gaussian filter having a standard deviation of 1.0 pixels;*
e, f) *leveled result after subtraction of the background from the original.*

the original image are not simply the darkest pixels in the image. The original image was produced by shadowing a TEM replica with carbon, causing each line to have a white and dark line. This influences the result; the background rank leveling method provides only an approximate correction for this type of image.

Better results are often possible with SEM images, in which local ridges and variations produce bright lines on a dark background. **Figure 30** shows two images of fracture surfaces in metals. The background in each case was produced by two applications of the ranking operation keeping the darkest pixel in a 5-pixel-wide octagonal neighborhood, followed by smoothing with a Gaussian kernel having a standard deviation of 1.0 pixels. Subtracting this background from the original makes the markings–fatigue striations in one image and brittle quasi-cleavage marks in the other–more visible by removing the overall variation caused by surface orientation.

This method is also useful for examining particles and other surface decorations on freeze-fractured cell walls in biological specimens; examination of surface roughness on irregular particles, pollen, etc.; and other similar problems. In some cases, it can be

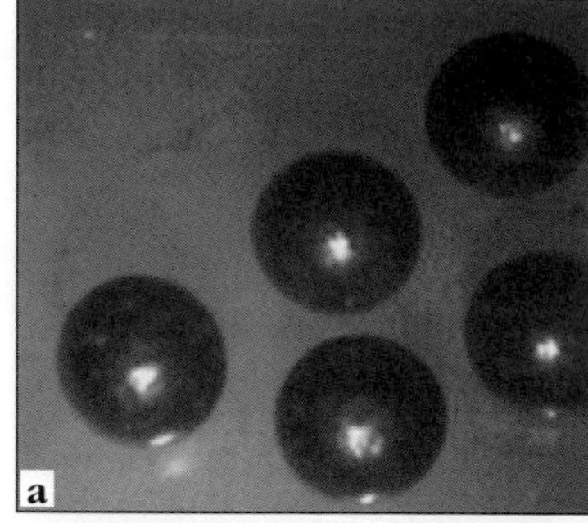

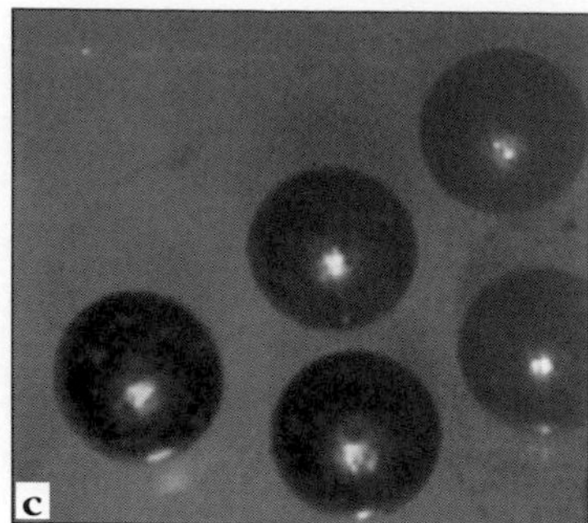

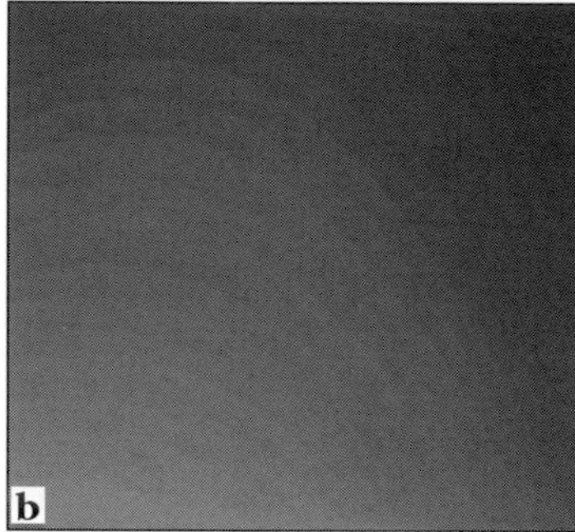

Figure 31. Effect of leveling on an image with limited grey scale range:
a) *original image;*
b) *fitted polynomial background;*
c) *subtracting image b from a–the background is not uniform, but the dark features are not because the original pixels were fully black in the original image.*

used to enhance the visibility of dislocations in TEM images of materials, which appear as dark lines in different grains, whose overall brightness varies due to lattice orientation.

However, the ability to level brightness variations by subtracting a background image, whether it is obtained by measurement, mathematical fitting, or image processing, is not a cost-free process. It uses up part of the dynamic range, or grey scale, of the image. **Figure 31** shows an example. The original image has a shading variation that can be fit rather well by a quadratic function, but this has a range of about half of the total 256 grey levels. After it has been subtracted, the leveled image does not have enough remaining brightness range to show detail in the dark areas of some features. This clipping may interfere with further analysis of the image.

Non-planar views

Computer graphics is much concerned with methods for displaying the surfaces of three-dimensional objects. Some of these methods will be used in Chapter 8 to display representations of three-dimensional structures obtained from a series of two-dimensional image slices or from direct three-dimensional imaging methods such as tomography.

One particular use of computer graphics that most of us take for granted can be seen each evening on the local news. Most TV stations in the US have a weather forecast that uses satellite images from the GOES satellite. These pictures show the US as it appears from latitude 0, longitude 108 W (the satellite is shifted to 98 W in summertime to get a better view of hurricanes developing in the south Atlantic) at an elevation of about 22,000 miles.

The satellite image shows cloud patterns and the movement of storms and other weather systems. The coastline, Great Lakes, and a few other topographic features are evident, but may be partially obscured by clouds. Given the average citizen's geographical knowledge, that picture would not help most viewers to recognize their location. Therefore, computer graphics are used to superimpose political outlines, such as the state borders, and perhaps other information, such as cities, to assist the viewer. Most US TV stations have heavy investments in computer graphics for advertising, news, etc., but they rarely generate these weather lines themselves, instead obtaining them from a company specializing in the niche market.

How are these lines generated? It is not simply a matter of overlaying a conventional map, say a Mercator projection (as used in school classrooms), over the satellite image. The earth's curvature and the foreshortening of the image need to be taken into account. **Figure 32** shows an example of the broadcast use of these images. **Figure 33** shows a GOES image of North America that is clearly foreshortened at the top and shows noticeable curvature from west to east across the width of the region.

The coordinates, in latitude and longitude, of points on the earth's surface are used to calculate a perspective view of the roughly spherical globe as it is seen from the satellite. Since the viewpoint is constant, this is a one-time calculation, which nevertheless needs to be done for a great many points to construct good outline maps for superimposition. The calculation can be visualized as shown in the diagram of **Figure 34.**

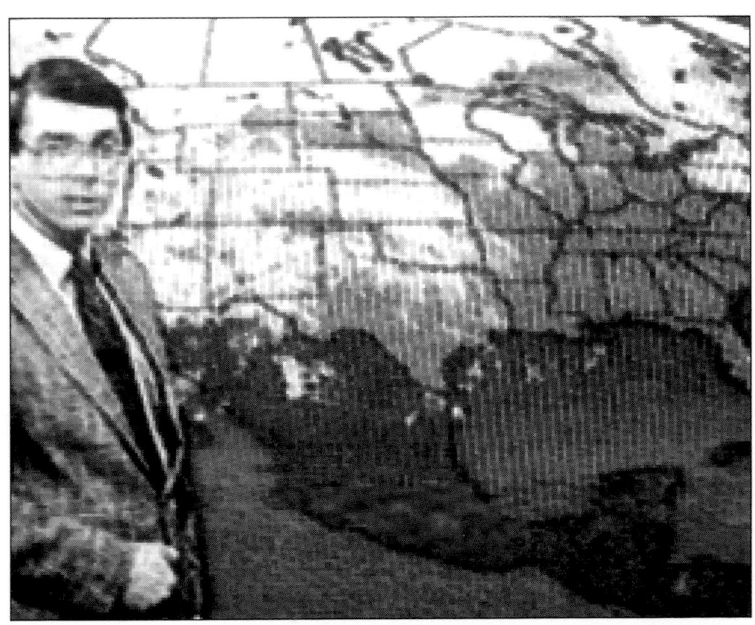

Figure 32. *Television weather forecast using the GOES weather satellite image. The satellite is located on the equator and therefore shows the US in a foreshortened view. There is also curvature evident from west to east. The political boundary lines are superimposed by computer graphics, as discussed in the text. (WRAL-TV, Channel 5, Raleigh, NC.)*

Figure 33. GOES-7 image of North America with political boundary lines superimposed. The dark area just west of Baja California is the shadow of the moon, during the eclipse of 11 June, 1991. (Image courtesy National Environmental Satellite, Data and Information Service.)

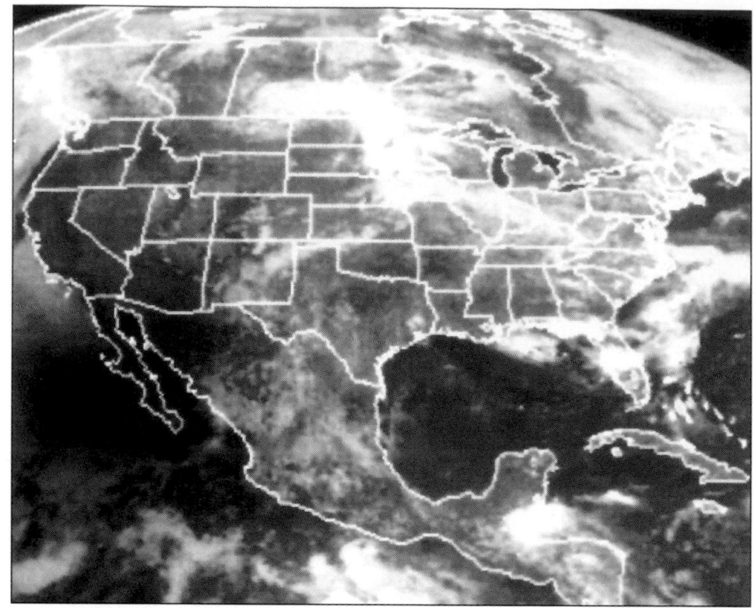

The location of a point on the spherical earth (specified by its latitude and longitude) is used to determine the intersection of a view line to the satellite with a flat image plane, inserted in front of the sphere. This requires only simple trigonometry, as indicated in **Figure 35.** The coordinates of the points in that plane are the location of the point in the viewed image. As shown, a square on the ground is viewed as a skewed trapezoid, and if the square is large enough, its sides are noticeably curved.

Figure 34. Diagram of satellite imaging. As in any perspective geometry, the "flat" image is formed by projecting view lines from the three-dimensional object to the viewpoint and constructing the image from the points at which they intersect the image plane.

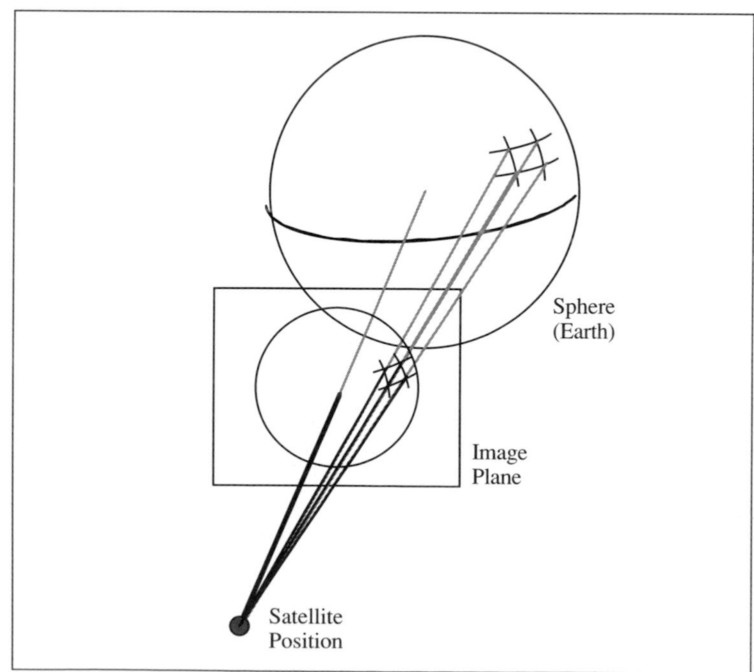

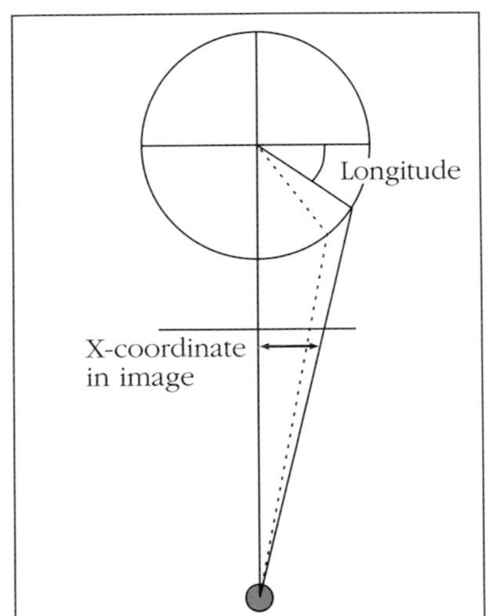

Figure 35. *Simple trigonometry can be used to calculate the location of points in the image plane from the longitude of the point on the earth, and the location of the satellite. This is the view from the North Pole; a similar view from the equator gives the y-coordinate.*

Computer graphics

Computer graphics is similarly used to construct perspective drawings of three-dimensional objects so that they can be viewed on the computer screen, for instance in CAD (computer-aided design) programs. The subject goes far beyond our needs here; the interested reader should refer to standard texts, such as Foley and Van Dam (1984) or Hearn and Baker (1986). The display process is the same as that just described, with the addition of perspective control that allows the user to adjust the apparent distance of the camera or viewpoint to control the degree of foreshortening that occurs (equivalent to choosing a long or short focal-length lens for a camera–the short focal-length lens produces more distortion in the image).

Neglecting perspective distortion for the moment (i.e., using a telephoto lens), we can represent the translation of a point in three dimensions by matrix multiplication of its x, y, z coordinates by a set of values that describes rotation and translation. This is simpler to examine in more detail in two dimensions, since our main interest here is with two-dimensional images. Consider a point with Cartesian X,Y coordinates and how it moves when we shift or rotate it and the other points in the object with respect to the coordinate system.

From simple geometry, we know that a translation of an object simply adds offsets to X and Y, to produce

$$\begin{aligned} X' &= X + \Delta X \\ Y' &= Y + \Delta Y \end{aligned} \qquad (3$$

while stretching the object requires multiplicative coefficients which may not be the same

$$\begin{aligned} X' &= a\,X \\ Y' &= b\,Y \end{aligned} \qquad (4$$

and rotation of an object by the angle ϑ introduces an interdependence between the original X and Y coordinates of the form

$$X' = X + Y \sin \vartheta \qquad (5$$
$$Y' = Y - X \cos \vartheta$$

In general, the notation for two-dimensional translations is most commonly written using so-called homogeneous coordinates and matrix notation. The coordinates X, Y are combined in a vector along with an arbitrary constant 1 to allow the translation values to be incorporated into the matrix math, producing the result

$$[X' \; Y' \; 1] = [X \; Y \; 1] \cdot \begin{vmatrix} a & b & 0 \\ c & d & 0 \\ e & f & 1 \end{vmatrix} \qquad (6$$

which multiplies out to

$$X' = aX + cY + e \qquad (7$$
$$Y' = bX + dY + f$$

By comparing this matrix form to the examples above, we see that the e and f terms are the translational shift values. The diagonal values a and d are the stretching coefficients, while b and c are the sine and cosine terms involved in rotation. When a series of transformations is combined, including rotation, translation, and stretching, it produces a series of matrices that can be multiplied together. When this happens, for instance to produce rotation about some point other than the origin or to combine nonuniform stretching with rotation, the individual terms are combined in ways that complicate their simple interpretation. However, only the same six coefficients are needed.

If only these terms are used, we cannot produce curvature or twisting of the objects. By introducing higher-order terms, more complex stretching, twisting, etc. of figures is possible. This creates a more complex equation of the form

$$X' = a_1 + a_2X + a_3Y + a_4XY + a_5X^2 + a_6Y^2 + \ldots \qquad (8$$

and a similar relationship for Y'. There is no fundamental reason to limit this polynomial expansion to any particular maximum power, except that as the complexity grows, the number of coefficients needed rises (and so does the difficulty of obtaining them) and the mathematical precision needed to apply the transformation increases. It is unusual to have terms beyond second power, which can handle most commonly encountered cases of distortion and can even approximate the curvature produced by looking at a spherical surface–at least over small ranges of angles.

Of course, some surface mappings are better handled by other functions. The standard Mercator projection of the spherical earth onto a cylinder **(Figure 36)** sends the poles to infinity and greatly magnifies areas at high latitudes. It would require many polynomial terms to approximate it, but since the actual geometry of the mapping is known, it is easy to use the cosecant function to efficiently perform the transformation.

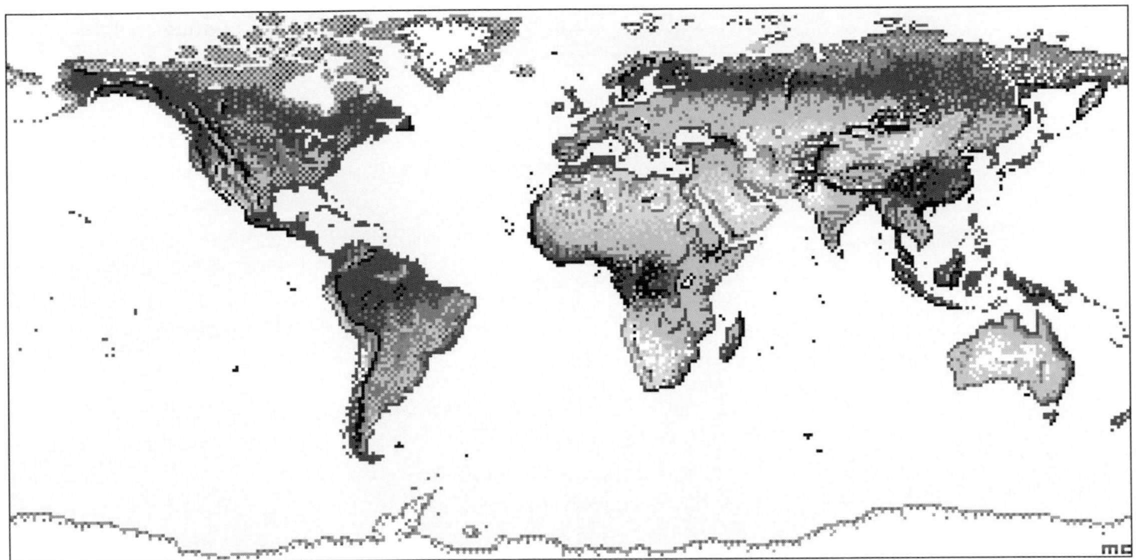

Figure 36. *The standard Mercator projection of the earth used in maps projects the points on the sphere onto a cylinder, producing distortion at high latitudes.*

Geometrical distortion

Now we must examine what to do with these mathematical operations. Images are frequently obtained that are not of flat surfaces viewed normally. The example of the satellite image used above is an obvious case. The same is true for viewing surfaces in the SEM, in which the specimen surface is often tilted to increase the contrast in the detected image. If the surface is not flat, different regions may be tilted at arbitrary angles, or continuous curvature may be present. This becomes important if we want to measure comparisons within or between images. Many airborne cameras and radars introduce a predictable distortion (which is therefore correctable) due to the use of a moving or sideways scan pattern or by imaging a single line onto continuously moving film. In all of these cases, knowing the distortion is the key to correcting it.

This situation does not commonly arise with light microscopy, because the depth of field of the optics is so low that surfaces must be flat and normal to the optical axis to remain in focus. There are other imaging technologies, however, that do frequently encounter non-ideal surfaces or viewing conditions.

Making maps from aerial or satellite images is one application (Thompson, 1966). Of course, there is no perfect projection of a spherical surface onto a flat one, so various approximations and useful conventions are employed. In each case, however, there is a known relationship between the coordinates on the globe and those on the map which can be expressed mathematically. But what about the image? If the viewpoint is exactly known (as in the case of the weather satellite), or can be calculated for the moment of exposure (as in the case of a space probe passing by a planet), then the same kind of mathematical relationship can be determined.

This is usually impractical for aerial photographs, since the position of the airplane is not precisely controlled. The alternative is to locate a few known reference points in the image whose locations on the globe or on the map are known and use them to determine the equations relating image position to map location. This technique is generally known as image warping, or rubber sheeting, and while the equations are the same as those used in computer graphics, the techniques for determining the coefficients are quite different.

We have seen that a pair of equations calculating X', Y' coordinates for a transformed view from original coordinates X, Y may include constants, linear terms in X and Y, plus higher-order terms, such as XY, X^2, etc. Adding more terms of a higher order makes it possible to introduce more complex distortions in the transformation. If the problem is simply one of rotation, only linear terms are needed, and a constraint on the coefficients can be introduced to preserve angles. In terms of the simple matrix shown above, this would require that the two stretching coefficients a and d must be equal. That means that only a few constants are needed; they can be determined by locating a few known reference points and setting up simultaneous equations.

More elaborate stretching to align images with each other or with a map requires correspondingly more terms and more points. In SEM pictures of surfaces that are locally flat but oriented at an angle to the point of view, the distortion is essentially trapezoidal, as shown in **Figure 37.** The portion of the surface that is closest to the lens is magnified more than regions farther away and distances are foreshortened in the direction of tilt. In order to measure and compare features on these surfaces, or even to properly apply image processing methods (which generally assume that neighboring pixels in various directions are at equal distances from the center), it may be necessary to transform this image to correct the distortion. Since the exact tilt angle and working distance may not be known, a method that uses only reference points within the image itself is required.

All that is necessary is the ability to identify four points whose real X, Y coordinates on the surface are known and whose image coordinates X', Y' can be measured. Then the following equations are written

$$\begin{aligned} X &= a_1 + a_2X' + a_3Y' + a_4X'Y' \\ Y &= b_1 + b_2X' + b_3Y' + b_4X'Y' \end{aligned} \quad (9$$

for each of the four sets of coordinates. This allows solving for the constants a_i and b_i. Of course, if more points are available, they can be used to obtain a least-squares solution which minimizes the effect of the inevitable small errors in measuring image coordinates.

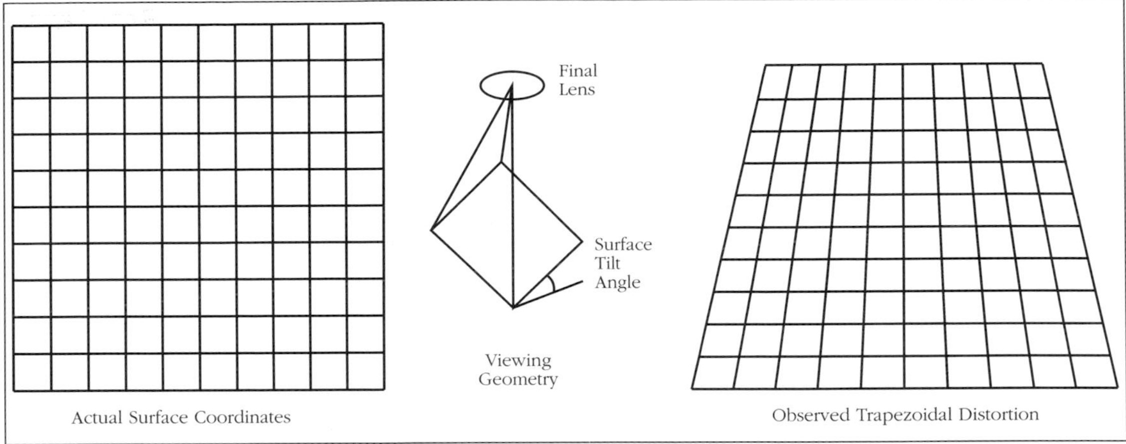

Figure 37. *Trapezoidal distortion commonly encountered in the SEM, due to observing a tilted surface with a short focal length lens.*

Note that by limiting the equation to those terms needed to accomplish the rotation and stretching involved in the trapezoidal distortion which we expect to be present, we minimize the number of points needed for the fit. More than the three terms shown above are required, because angles are not preserved in this kind of foreshortening. Using the fewest terms possible, though, is preferred to a general equation involving many higher order terms, both in terms of the efficiency of the calculation (number of reference points) and the precision of the coefficients.

Likewise, if we know that the distortion in the image is produced by viewing a globe, the appropriate sine and cosine terms can be used in the fitting equations. Of course, if we have no independent knowledge about the shape of the surface or the kind of imaging distortion, then arbitrary polynomials often represent the only practical approach.

Alignment

Another very common situation is the alignment of serial section images. In this case there is no "ground truth", only relative alignment between the successive slices. By using features within the image that can be recognized in two successive slices, or by introducing fiducial marks, such as holes drilled through the specimen block before the sections are cut, alignment can be performed. Points may be located manually by the user or automatically by the imaging system, although the latter method works best for artificial markings (such as holes) and somewhat poorly when trying to use image details that match only imperfectly from one section to the next. This is discussed in more detail in Chapter 7.

Serial sections cut with a microtome from a block of embedded biological material are commonly foreshortened in the cutting

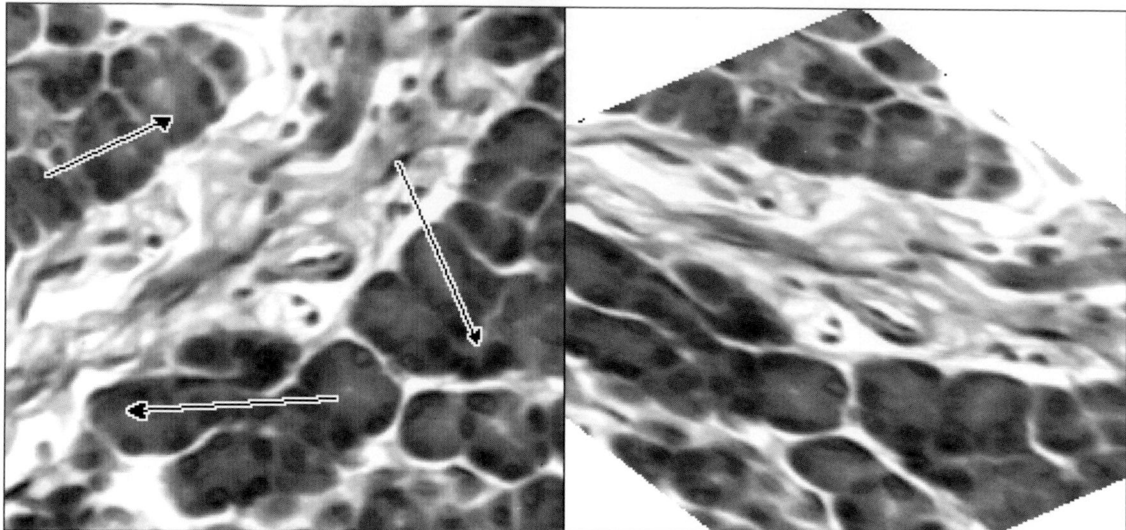

Figure 38. *An image with three displacement vectors (left), and the rotation and stretching transformation which they produce (right). Notice that portions of the original image are lost and some areas of the transformed image have no information.*

direction by 5 to 15 percent, due to compression of the block by the knife. Then the sections are rotated arbitrarily before they are viewed. The result is a need for an alignment equation of the form

$$X = a_1 + a_2X' + a_3Y' \qquad (10$$

with only three constants (and a similar equation for Y). Hence, locating three reference points that are common to two sequential images allows one to be rotated and stretched to align with the other. **Figure 38** shows an image in which three points have been marked with vectors to indicate their movement to perform this alignment, and the resulting transformation of the image by stretching.

This kind of warping can be performed to align images with other images, as in serial section reconstruction, or to align images along their edges to permit assembling them as a mosaic (Milgram, 1975). Aligning side-by-side sections of a mosaic is often attempted with SEM images, but fails because of the trapezoidal distortion discussed above. Features along the image boundaries do not quite line up, causing the mosaic to be imperfect. Using rubber sheeting can correct this problem.

Such corrections are routinely performed for satellite and space probe pictures. **Figure 39** shows an example of a mosaic image constructed from multiple images taken of the surface of Mars from orbit. Boundaries between images are visible because of brightness differences, due to variations in illumination or exposure, but the features line up well across the seams. When images are being aligned, it is possible to write the equations either in

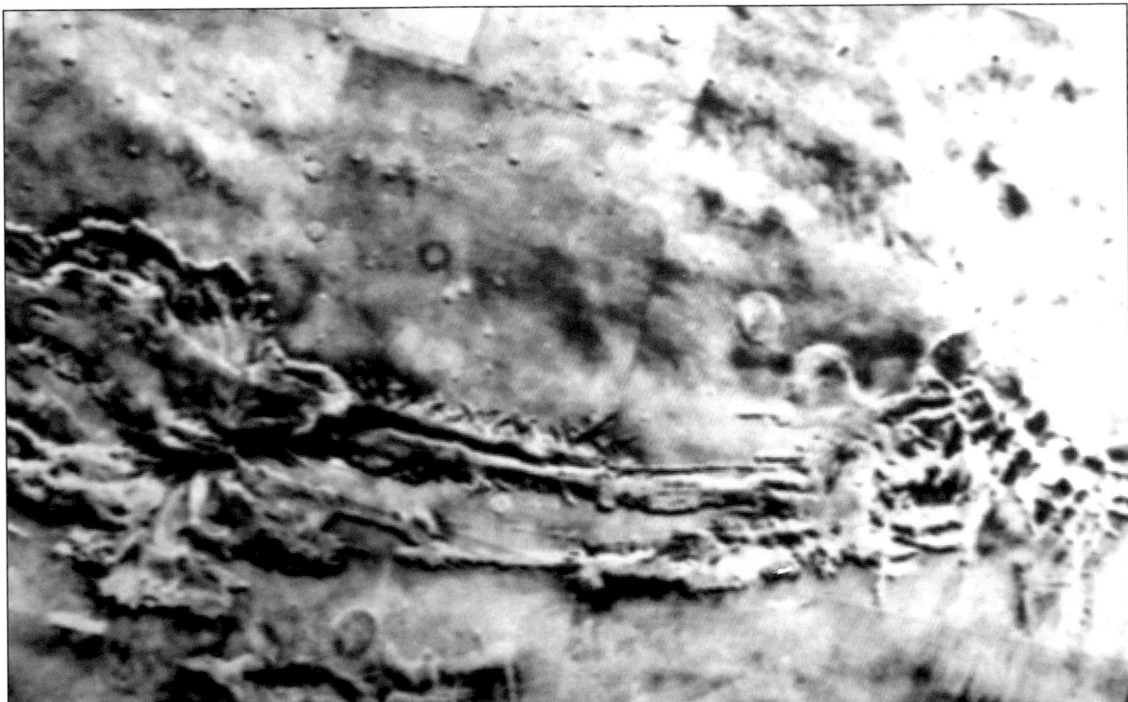

Figure 39. *Mosaic image of the Valles Marineris on Mars, assembled from satellite images.*

terms of the coordinates in the original image as a function of the geometrically corrected one, or vice versa. In practice, it is usually preferable to use the grid of x,y coordinates in the corrected image to calculate for each of the coordinates in the original image and to perform the calculation in terms of actual pixel addresses.

Unfortunately, these calculated coordinates for the original location will only rarely be integers. This means that the location generally lies "between" the pixels in the original image. Several methods are used to deal with this problem. The simplest is to truncate the calculated values, discarding the fractional part of the address and using the pixel lying toward the origin of the coordinate system. Slightly better results are obtained by rounding the address values to select the nearest pixel, whose brightness is then copied to the transformed image array.

Either method introduces some error in location that can cause distortion of the transformed image. **Figure 40** shows examples using a test pattern, in which the biasing of the lines and apparent variations in their width is evident.

When this distortion is unacceptable, another method requiring more calculation may be used. The brightness value for the transformed pixel may be calculated by interpolating between the four pixels surrounding the calculated address. This is called bilinear interpolation, and is calculated simply from the fractional part of the X and Y coordinates. First the interpolation is done in one di-

__Figure 40. Rotation and stretching of a test image:__
__a)__ original;
__b)__ rotation only, no change in scale;
__c)__ rotation and uniform stretching while maintaining angles;
__d)__ general rotation and stretching in which angles may vary.

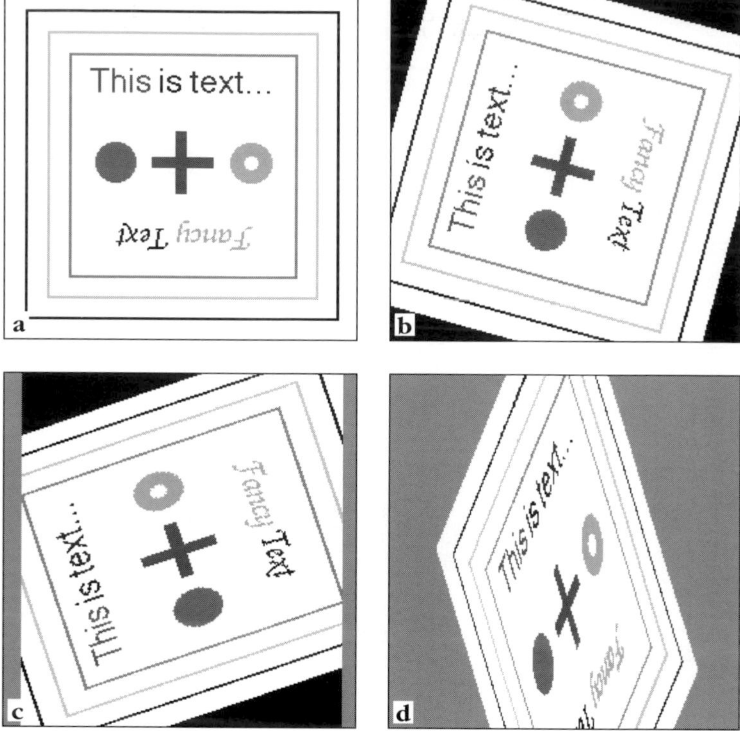

rection and then in the other, as indicated in **Figure 41.** For a location with coordinates $j+x$, $k+y$ where x and y are the fractional part of the address, the equations for the first interpolation are

Figure 41. *Diagram of pixel interpolation. The brightness values of the neighbors are first interpolated horizontally, and then these two values are interpolated vertically, using the fractional part of the pixel addresses.*

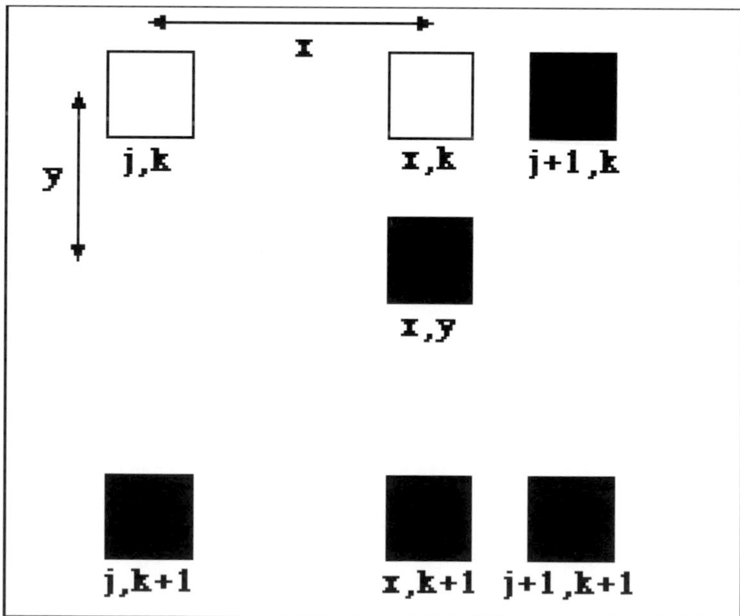

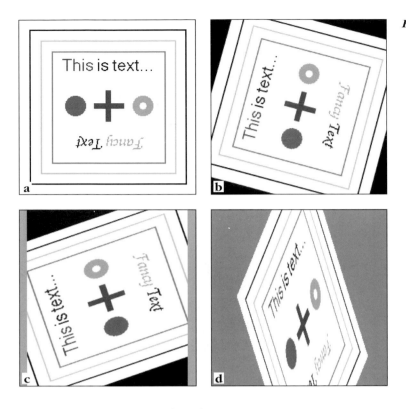

Figure 42. *Same generalized rotation and stretching as in Figure 40, but with bilinear interpolation. Note the smoothing of the lines and boundaries.*

$$B_{x,k} = (1 - x) \cdot B_{j,k} + x \cdot B_{j+1,k}$$
$$B_{x,k+1} = (1 - x) \cdot B_{j,k+1} + x \cdot B_{j+1,\,k+1} \qquad (11$$

and then the second interpolation, in the y direction, gives the final value

$$B_{x,y} = (1 - y) \cdot B_{x,k} + y \cdot B_{x,k+1} \qquad (12$$

Weighted interpolations over larger regions are also used in some cases. The advantage of interpolation is that dimensions are altered as little as possible in the transformation, and in particular boundaries and other lines are not biased or distorted. **Figure 42** shows the same examples as **Figure 40,** using bilinear interpolation. Careful examination of the figure shows that the lines appear straight, not "aliased" or stair-stepped, because some of the pixels along the sides of the lines have intermediate grey values resulting from the interpolation. In fact, computer graphics sometimes uses this same method to draw lines on CRT displays, so that the stair-stepping inherent in drawing lines on a discrete pixel array is avoided. The technique is called anti-aliasing and produces lines whose pixels have grey values according to how close they lie to the mathematical location of the line. This fools the viewer into perceiving a smooth line.

For image warping or rubber-sheeting, interpolation has the advantage of preserving dimensions, but not brightness values. The nearest-pixel method, which rounds pixel addresses, distorts dimensions but preserves the brightness values. Choosing the

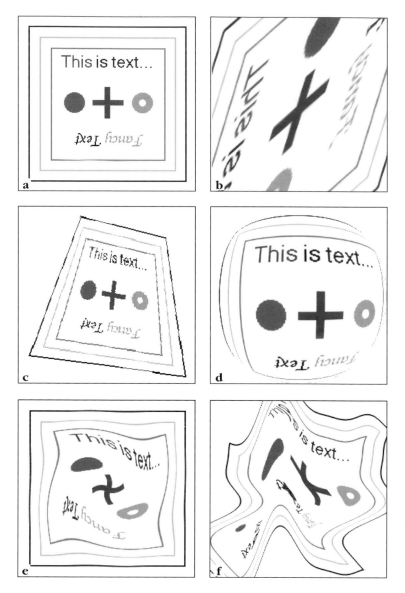

***Figure 43.* Some additional examples of image warping:**
a) *original test image;*
b) *linear warping with reversal;*
c) *quadratic warping showing trapezoidal foreshortening (no interpolation);*
d) *cubic warping in which lines are curved (approximation here is to a spherical surface);*
e) *twisting the center of the field while holding the edges fixed (also cubic warping);*
f) *arbitrary warping in which higher order and trigonometric terms are required.*

method appropriate to a particular imaging task depends primarily on which kind of information is more important, and secondarily on the additional computational effort required for the interpolation.

Figure 43 illustrates the effect of adding higher-order terms to the warping equations. With quadratic terms, the trapezoidal distortion of a short focal-length lens or SEM can be corrected. It is also possible to closely model the distortion of a spherical surface over modest distances. With higher-order terms, arbitrary distortion is possible. However, this is rarely useful in an image processing situation, since the reference points to determine such a distortion are not likely to be available.

3

Image Enhancement

The preceding chapter discussed methods for correcting or alleviating the principal defects in as-acquired images. There is a grey area between simply correcting these defects and going beyond to enhance the images. Enhancement is the subject of this chapter. Methods are available that increase the visibility of one component or aspect of an image, though generally at the expense of others, whose visibility is diminished. In this regard, image processing is a bit like word processing or food processing. It is possible to rearrange things to make a product that is more pleasing or interpretable, but the total amount of data does not change. In the case of images, this generally means that the number of bytes (or pixels) is not reduced. On the other hand, most image analysis procedures attempt to extract only the "important" information from the image. An example would be to identify and count features in an image, reducing the amount of data from perhaps a million bytes to a few dozen, or even a single "Yes" or "No" answer in certain quality control, medical, or forensic applications.

Image processing for purposes of enhancement can be performed in either the spatial domain (the array of pixels comprising our conventional view of the image) or other domains, such as the Fourier domain discussed in Chapter 4. In the spatial domain, pixel values may be modified according to rules that depend on the original pixel value (local or point processes). Alternatively, pixel values may be combined with or compared to others in their immediate neighborhood in a variety of ways. Examples of each of these approaches were used in Chapter 2, to replace brightness values to expand image contrast, for in-

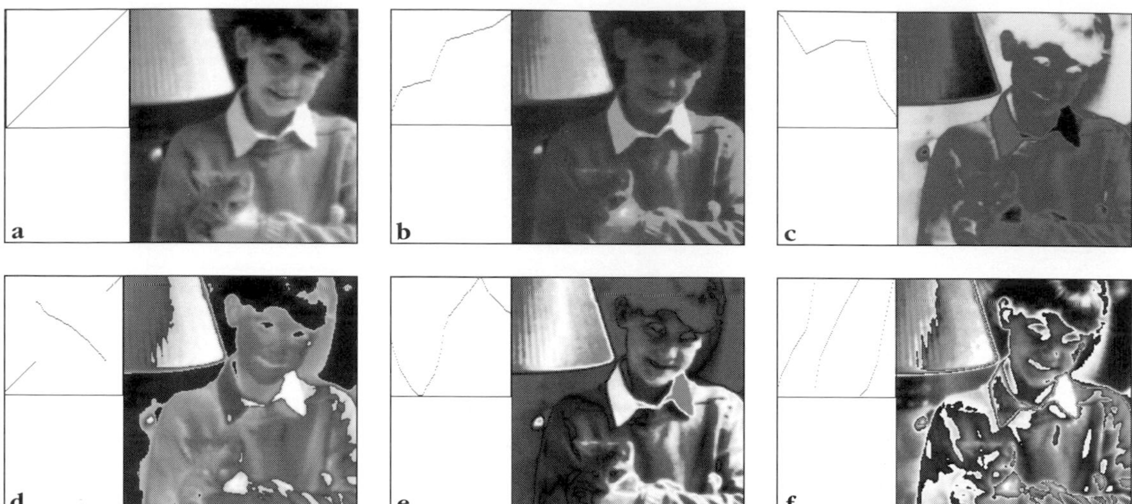

Figure 1. *An original image with a full range of brightness values and several examples of arbitrary hand-drawn display transfer functions which expand or alter the contrast in various parts of the range. The plot with each image shows the stored pixel brightness values on the horizontal axis and the displayed brightness on the vertical axis.*

Image a) *has a transfer function that is the identity function, so that actual stored brightnesses are displayed.*

Images b) *through* ***f)*** *illustrate various possibilities, including reversal and increased or decreased slope over parts of the brightness range.*

stance, or to smooth noise by kernel averaging or median filtering. Related techniques used in this chapter perform further enhancements.

Contrast manipulation

In Chapter 2, Figure 24 showed the example of expanding the contrast of a dim image by reassigning pixel brightness levels. In most systems, this can be done almost instantaneously by writing a table of values into the display hardware. This LUT substitutes a display brightness value for each stored value and thus does not require actually modifying any of the values stored in memory for the image. Linearly expanding the contrast range by assigning the darkest pixel value to black, the brightest value to white, and each of the others to linearly interpolated shades of grey makes the best use of the display and enhances the visibility of features in the image.

It was also shown, in Chapter 1, that the same LUT approach can be used with colors by assigning a triplet of red, green, and blue values to each stored grey scale value. This pseudo-color also increases the visible difference between similar pixels; sometimes it is an aid to the user who wishes to see small or gradual changes in image brightness.

A typical computer display can show 2^8 or 256 different shades of grey, and many can produce colors with the same 2^8 brightness values for each of the red, green, and blue components to produce a total of 2^{24} or 16 million different colors. This is often described as "true color," since the gamut of colors that can be displayed is adequate to reproduce most natural scenes. It does not imply, of course, that the colors displayed are photometrically accurate or identical to the original color in the displayed scene. Indeed, that kind of control is very difficult and requires special hardware and calibration.

More important, the 16 million different colors that such a system is capable of displaying, and even the 256 shades of grey, are far more than the human eye can distinguish. Under good viewing conditions, we can typically see only a few tens of different grey levels and hundreds of distinguishable colors. That means the display hardware of an image processing system is not being used very well to communicate the image information to the user. If many of the pixels in the image are quite bright, for example, they cannot be distinguished. If there are also some dark pixels present, we cannot simply expand the contrast. Instead, a more complicated relationship between stored and displayed values is needed.

In general, we can describe the manipulation of the grey scale LUT in terms of a transfer function relating the stored brightness value for each pixel to a displayed value. If this relationship is one-to-one, then for each stored value there will be a unique (though not necessarily visually discernible) displayed value. In some cases, it is advantageous to use transfer functions that are not one-to-one: several stored values are displayed with the same brightness value, so that other stored values can be spread further apart to increase their visual difference.

Figure 1 shows an image in which the 256 distinct pixel brightness values cannot all be discerned even on the display CRT; the printed version of the image is necessarily much worse. As discussed in Chapter 1, the number of distinct printed grey levels in a halftone image is determined by the variation in dot size of the printer. For a simple 300-dot-per-inch laser writer, this requires a tradeoff between grey scale resolution (number of shades) and lateral resolution (number of halftone cells per inch). A typical compromise is 50 cells per inch and more than 30 grey levels, or 75 cells per inch and 17 grey levels. The Lino used for this book is capable of much higher resolution and more grey levels.

For comparison purposes, a good-quality photographic print can reproduce 20 to 30 grey levels (the negative can do much better). An instant print such as the Polaroid film commonly used with laboratory microscopes can show 10 to 15. However, both have much higher spatial resolution, and so the images appear sharper to the eye.

Figure 2. *Examples of display transfer functions.*

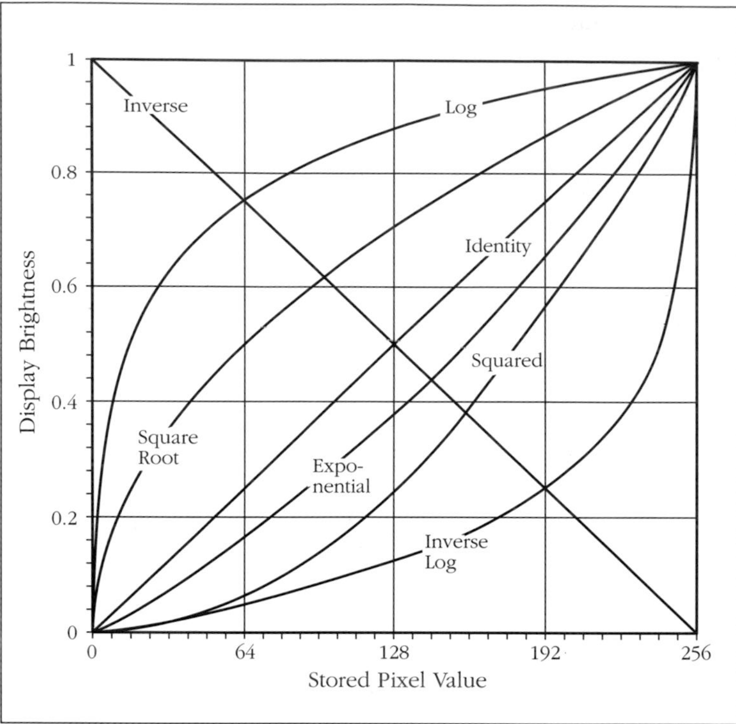

Even so, looking at the original image in **Figure 1,** the viewer cannot see the detail in the bright and dark regions of the image, even on the video screen (and certainly not on the print). Modifying the LUT can increase the visibility in one or both regions, provided something else is given up in exchange. **Figure 1** shows several modifications to the original image that were produced simply by manipulating the transfer function and the LUTs by drawing a new relationship between stored and displayed brightness. In this case, a freehand drawing was made that became the transfer function; it was adjusted purely for visual effect.

Note some of the imaging possibilities. A nonlinear relationship can expand one portion of the grey scale range while compressing another. In photographic processing and also in analog display electronics, this is called varying the gamma (the slope of the exposure-density curve). Using a computer, however, we can draw in transfer functions that are far more complicated, nonlinear, and arbitrary than can be achieved in the darkroom.

Reversing all of the contrast range produces the equivalent of a photographic negative, which sometimes improves the visibility of details (especially in dark regions of the original image). Reversing only a portion of the brightness range produces a visually strange effect, called solarization by photographers, that can also be used to show detail in shadowed or saturated areas.

Increasing the slope of the transfer function so that it "wraps around" produces an image in which several quite different stored brightness values may have the same display brightness. If the overall organization of the image is familiar to the viewer, though, this contouring may not be too disruptive, and it actually increases visibility for small differences. However, like the use of pseudo-color, this kind of treatment is easily overdone and may confuse rather than enhance most images.

Certainly, experimentally modifying the transfer function until the image "looks good" and best shows the features of most interest to the viewer provides an ultimately flexible (if dangerous) tool. In most cases, it is desirable to have more reproducible and meaningful transfer functions available which can be applied equally to a series of images, so that proper comparison is possible.

The most common kinds of transfer functions are shown in **Figure 2**. These are curves of displayed vs. stored brightness following simple mathematical relationships, such as logarithmic or power law curves. A logarithmic or square root curve will compress the displayed brightnesses at the bright end of the scale, while expanding those at the dark end. Additionally, this kind of relationship can convert an image from a camera with a linear response to the more common logarithmic response. An inverse log or squared curve will do the opposite. The bell curve compresses middle grey values and spreads the scale at both the bright and dark extremes. An inverse curve simply produces a negative image.

Any of these functions may be used in addition to contrast expansion, which stretches the original scale to the full range of the display. Curves or tables of values for these transfer functions are typically precalculated and stored, so that they can be loaded quickly to modify the display LUT. Many systems allow quite a few different tables to be kept on hand for use when an image requires it, just as a series of color LUTs may be available on disk for pseudo-color displays. **Figure 3** illustrates the use of several transfer functions to enhance the visibility of structures in an image.

Histogram equalization

In addition to pre-calculated and stored tables, it is sometimes advantageous to construct a transfer function for a specific image. Unlike the arbitrary, hand-drawn functions shown above, however, we would like to have a specific algorithm that gives reproducible and (hopefully) optimal results. The most popular of these methods is called histogram equalization. To understand it, we must begin by understanding the image brightness histogram.

Figure 4 shows an example of an image with its histogram. The plot shows the number of pixels in the image having each of the

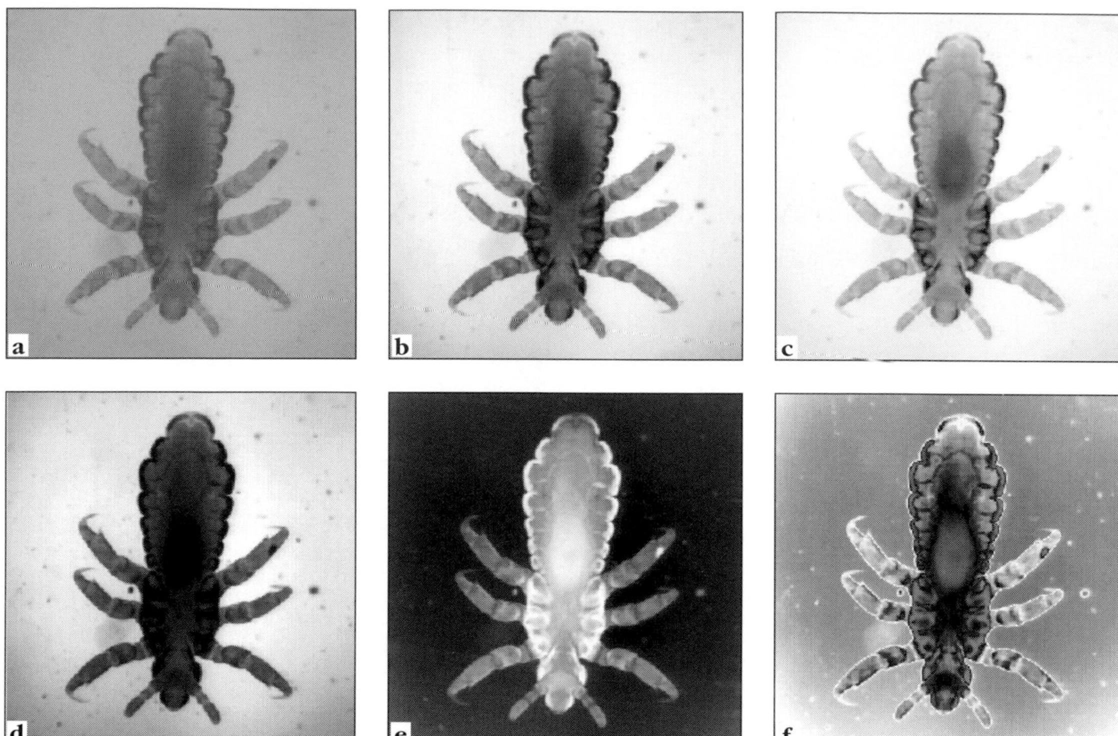

Figure 3. Manipulation of the grey scale transfer function:

a) *an original, moderately low-contrast transmission light microscope image (prepared slide of a head louse);*

b) *expanded linear transfer function adjusted to the minimum and maximum brightness values in the image;*

c) *positive gamma (log) function;*

d) *negative gamma (log) function;*

e) *negative linear transfer function;*

f) *nonlinear transfer function (high slope linear contrast over central portion of brightness range, with negative slope or solarization for dark and bright portions).*

256 possible values of stored brightness. Peaks in the histogram correspond to the more common brightness values, which often identify particular structures that are present. Valleys between the peaks indicate brightness values that are less common in the image. The flat regions at the two ends of the histogram show that no pixels have those values, indicating that the image brightness range does not cover the full 0–255 range available.

Generally, images have unique brightness histograms. Even images of different areas of the same sample or scene, in which the various structures present have consistent brightness levels wherever they occur, will have different histograms, depending on the area fraction of each structure. Changing the overall illumination will shift the peaks in the histogram. In addition, most real images exhibit some variation in brightness within features (e.g., from the edge to the center) or in different regions.

From the standpoint of efficiently using available grey levels on

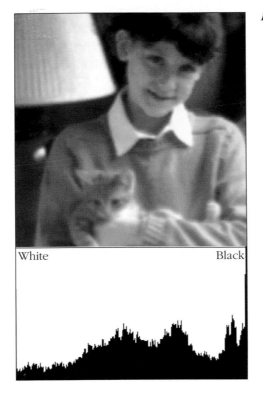

__Figure 4.__ An image with its brightness histogram. The plot shows the number of pixels with each of the 256 possible brightness values.

the display, some grey scale values are under-utilized. It might be better to selectively spread out the displayed grey levels in the peak areas, compressing them in the valleys so that the same number of pixels in the display show each of the possible brightness levels. This is called histogram equalization. The transfer function is simply the original brightness histogram of the image, replotted as a cumulative plot as shown in **Figure 5**.

Histogram equalization reassigns the brightness values of pixels based on the image histogram. Individual pixels retain their brightness order–that is, they remain brighter or darker than other pixels–but the values are shifted, so that an equal number of pixels have each possible brightness value. In many cases, this spreads out the values in regions where different regions meet, showing detail in areas with a high brightness gradient.

An image having a few regions with very similar brightness values presents a histogram with peaks. The sizes of these peaks give the relative area of the different phase regions and are useful for image analysis. Performing a histogram equalization on the image spreads the peaks out, compressing other parts of the histogram by assigning the same or very close brightness values to those pixels that are few in number and have intermediate brightnesses. This makes it possible to see minor variations within regions that appeared nearly uniform in the original image.

Figure 5. The original and cumulative histogram from Figure 4. The cumulative plot gives the transfer function for histogram equalization. The image shows the result of applying this function.

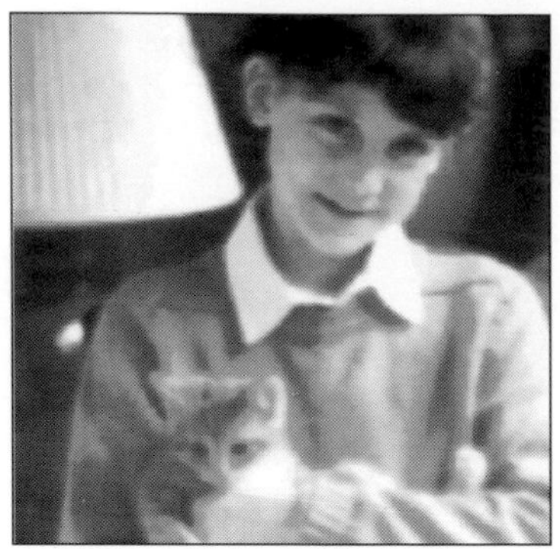

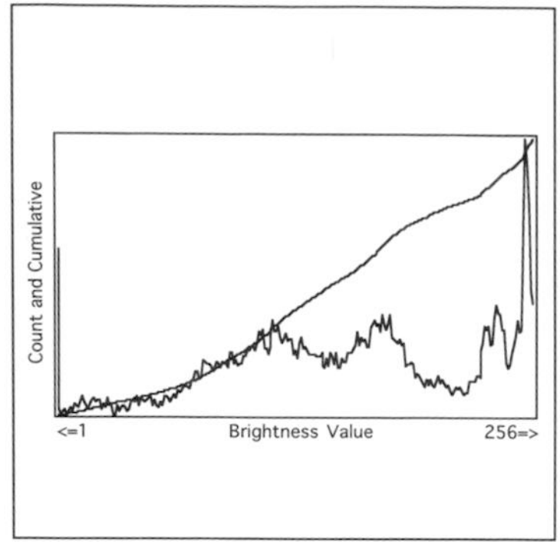

The process is quite simple. For each brightness level j in the original image (and its histogram), the new assigned value k is calculated as

$$k = \sum_{i=0}^{j} N_i / T$$

where the sum counts the number of pixels in the image (by integrating the histogram) with brightness equal to or less than j, and T is the total number of pixels (or the total area of the histogram).

Figure 6 shows an example. The original metallographic specimen has three phase regions with dark, intermediate, and light grey values. These peaks are separated in the histogram **(Figure 7)** by much lower regions having pixels with intermediate brightness values, often because they happen to fall on the boundary between lighter and darker phase regions. Histogram equalization shows the shading within phase regions, indiscernable in the original image. It also spreads out the brightness values in the histogram, as shown.

Some pixels that originally had different values are now assigned the same value, which represents a loss of information, while other values that were once very close together have been spread out, leaving gaps in the histogram. This image of a pol-

Figure 6. Metallographic light microscope image of a three-phase metal alloy. In the original image (a), phase regions are characterized by fairly uniform brightness values. After histogram equalization (b) the shading in these regions is evident because the brightness values for the pixels have been spread apart.

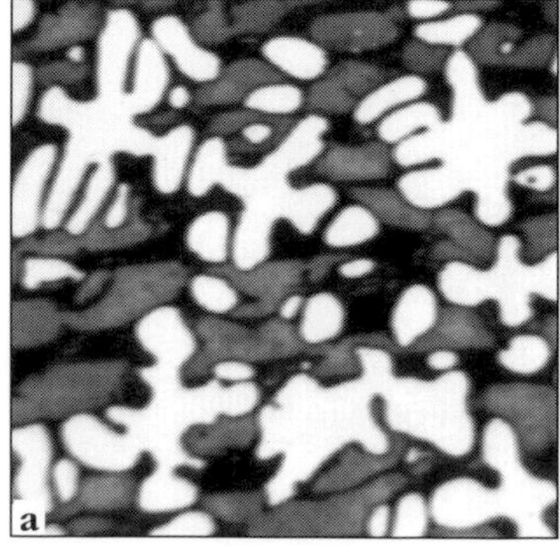

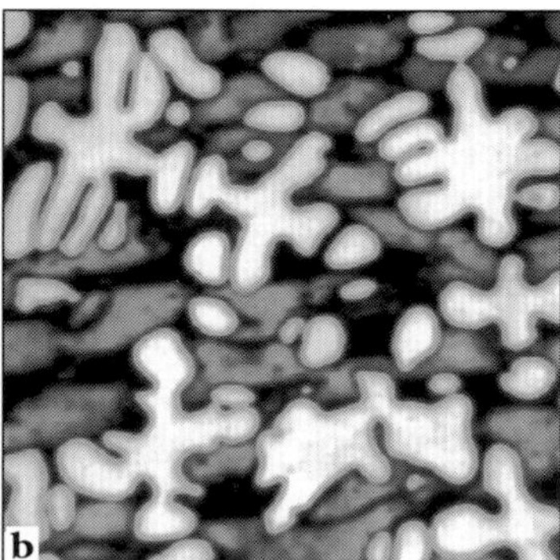

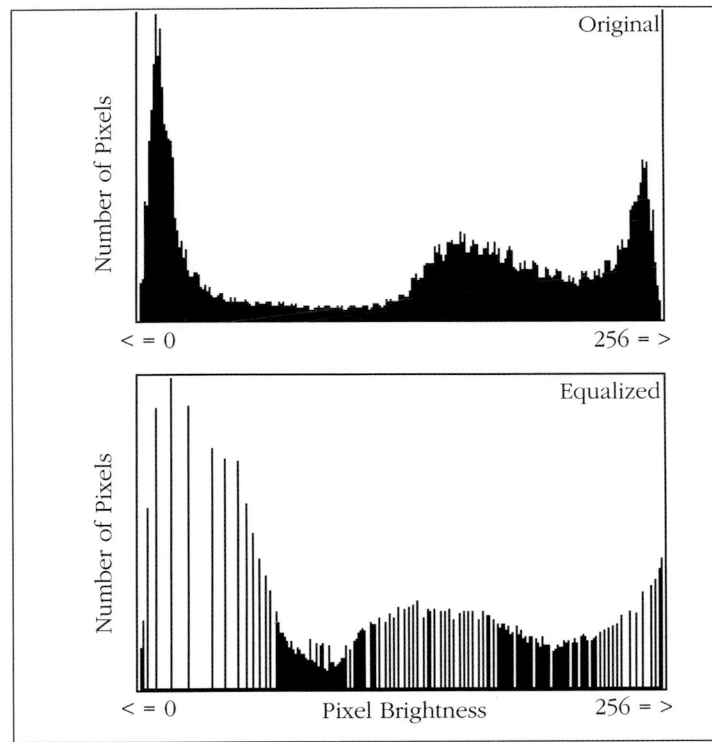

Figure 7. *Brightness histograms from the images in Figure 6. The horizonal scale is brightness, from zero (white) to 255 (black). The vertical scale is the number of pixels in the image with that brightness value. The original image shows three major peaks corresponding to the three phase regions in the original specimen, with few pixels having intermediate values. After equalization, the brightness values are reassigned to cover the brightness range uniformly. This causes some pixels with initially different brightness values to be assigned the same value, and other values to be missing altogether.*

ished metal shows well-defined peaks corresponding to different phases present. The histogram-equalized image is less satisfying in terms of showing the distinction between the phases, but much better at showing the gradation in the white phase, which was not visible in the original.

The equalization process need not be performed on an entire image. Enhancing a portion of the original image, rather than the entire area, is also useful in many situations. This is particularly true when large regions of the image correspond to different types of structures or scenes and are generally brighter or darker than the rest of the image. When portions of an image can be selected, either manually or by some algorithm based on the variation in the brightness histogram, a selective equalization can be used to bring out local detail.

Figure 8 shows regions of the same test image used previously, with three regions separately selected and equalized. Two of these regions are arbitrary rectangular and elliptical shapes, drawn by hand. In many cases, this kind of manual selection is the most straightforward way to specify a region. The third area is the lampshade, which can be isolated from the rest of the image because locally the boundary is a sharp transition from white to black. Methods for locating boundary edges are discussed later in the chapter.

Each of the three regions shown was used to construct a brightness histogram, which was then equalized. The resulting re-

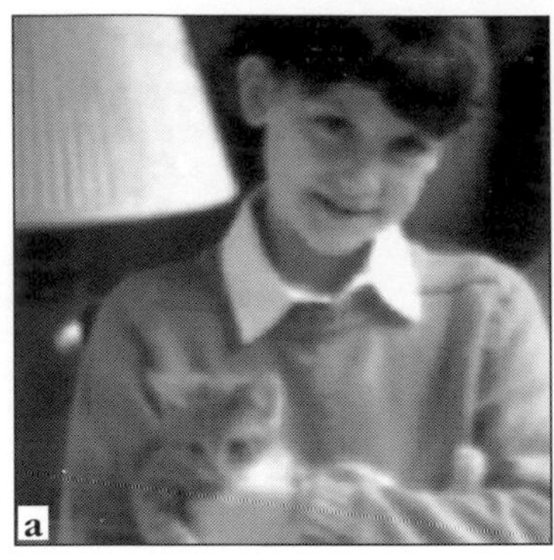

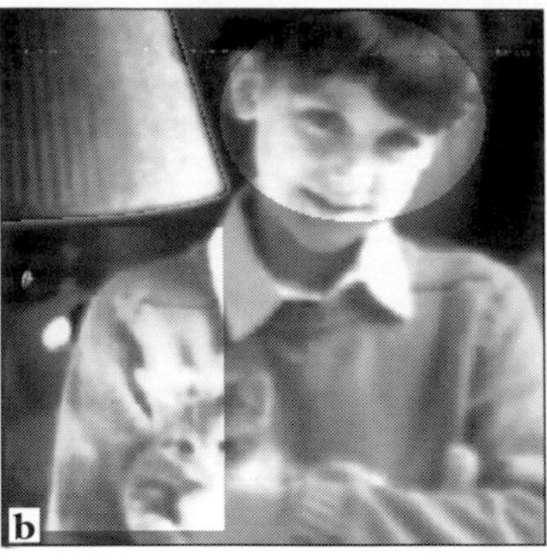

Figure 8. *Selective equalization can be performed in any designated region of an image. In this example, three regions have been selected and histogram equalization performed within each one separately. In the dark regions (the girl's face and the area behind her shoulder), this lightens the image and shows some of the detail that is otherwise not visible. In the light region (the lampshade), this results in an overall average darkening and expansion of the contrast to show shading. In both cases, the process is ultimately limited by the number of discrete grey levels which were actually present in those regions in the original image.*

assigned brightness values were then substituted only for the pixels within the region. In the two dark regions (the girl's face and the region near her shoulder), equalization produces an overall brightening and spreads out the brightness values so that the small variations are more evident. In the bright area (the lampshade), the overall brightness is reduced; again, more variation is evident.

In all cases, the brightness values in the equalized regions show some contouring–visible steps in brightness produced by the small number of different values present in these regions in the original image. Contouring is usually considered to be an image defect, since it distorts the actual smooth variation in values present in the image. When it is introduced specifically for effect, it may be called posterization.

It should be noted, of course, that once a region has been selected, either manually or automatically, the contrast can be modified in any way desired: by loading a pre-stored LUT, calculating a histogram equalization function, or simply stretching the grey scale linearly to maximize contrast. However, when these operations are applied to only a portion of the entire image, it is not possible to manipulate only the display LUT. Since the stored grey values in other regions of the image are to be shown with their original corresponding display values, it is necessary to actually modify the contents of the stored image to alter the display. It is a very fast operation, since this is performed using a transfer function that is loaded or precalculated from the histogram.

Histogram equalization of image regions can dramatically improve the local visibility of details, but it usually alters the relationship between brightness and structure. In most cases, it is desirable for the brightness level of pixels associated with a particular type of feature in the image to be the same, wherever in the field of view it may occur. This allows rapid classification of the features for counting or measurement. Locally modifying the grey scale relationship voids this assumption, making the display brightness of features dependent on other features that happen to be nearby or in the selected region.

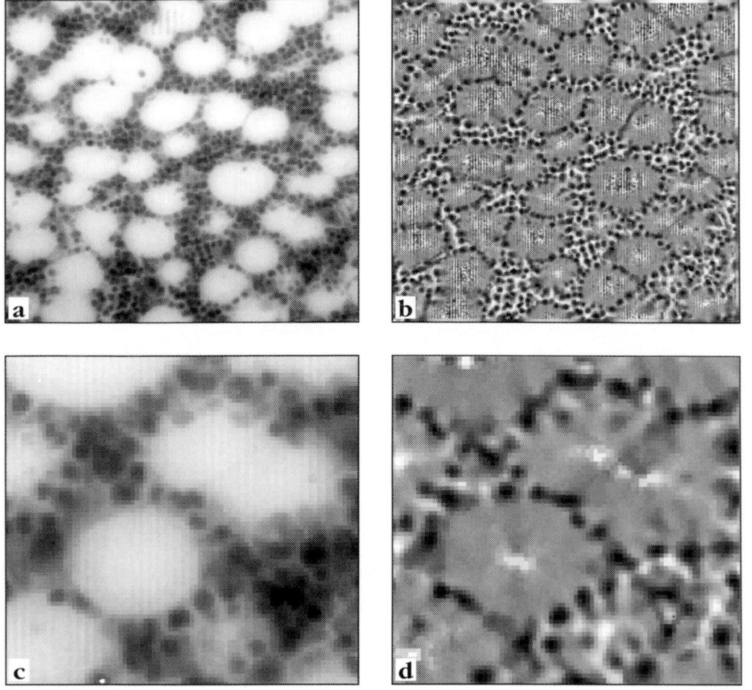

Figure 9. *Local equalization applied to every pixel in an image. This is a transmission light micrograph of bone marrow. For each pixel in the original image (a), a 9×9 neighborhood has been used to construct a histogram. Equalization of that histogram produces a new brightness value for each pixel, but this is only saved for the central pixel. The process is repeated to apply to each pixel in the original image except those too near the edge, producing the result (b). Enlargements to show individual pixels are shown in (c) and (d). The effect of this local equalization is to enhance edges and reveal detail in light and dark regions. However, in the center of uniform regions it can produce artefacts and noise.*

Histogram equalization in Figure 6 assigns the same new grey value to each pixel having a given original grey value, everywhere in the region. The result is that regions often have very noticeable and abrupt boundaries, which may or may not follow feature boundaries in the original image. Another approach performs the equalization in a region around each pixel in the image, with the result applied separately to each individual pixel. This is normally done by specifying a neighborhood size (typically round or square). All of the pixels in that region are counted into a histogram, but the equalization procedure is applied only to the central pixel. This process is then repeated for each pixel in the image, always using the original brightness values to construct the histogram.

Figure 9 shows an example in which the neighborhood size is a 9×9 pixel square. The process is not applied within a distance of four pixels of the edges of the image, where the region cannot be centered on a pixel. Special rules can be made for these points, if required. The calculation is quite simple in this method, since for each pixel the equalized brightness value is just the number of darker pixels in the neighborhood. For the case of a 9×9 region, the maximum number of pixels is 81, so the procedure produces an image in which the maximum number of distinct brightness values is 81, instead of the original 256.

The process of local equalization enhances contrast near edges, revealing details in both light and dark regions. However, it can be seen in the example that in the center of large, nominally uniform regions, this can produce artificial contrast variations that in-

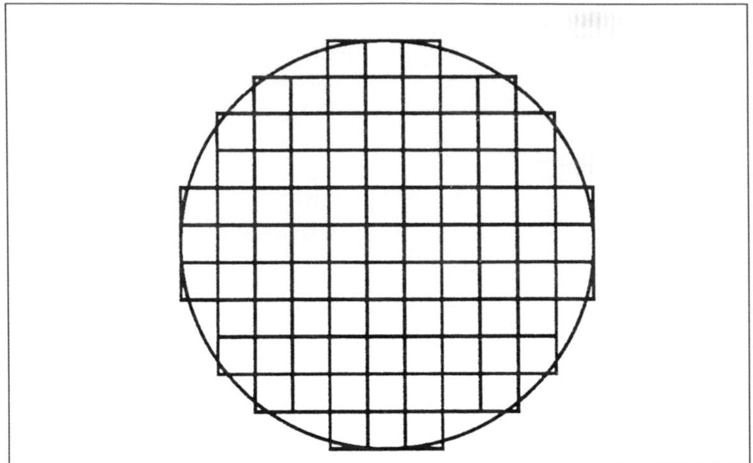

Figure 10. *Approximation to a circle 11 pixels wide contains a total of 89 pixels. Using a round neighborhood minimizes directional distortion and artefacts in the image due to local equalization.*

troduce artefacts into the image. The solution is to increase the size of the region so that it is larger than any uniform area in the image. However, this slows down the process and loses some of the ability to locally increase contrast at boundaries.

Somewhat more uniform results can be obtained with a circular region 11 pixels wide, as shown in **Figure 10.** It contains 89 pixels, including the central one. If a brightness histogram is formed from just those 89 pixels, a transfer function can be constructed that would assign a new brightness value to each pixel, but the assignment will be performed only for the one central pixel. Then the process can be repeated for the next pixel, using a slightly shifted neighborhood region of 89 pixels. Of course, it is necessary to construct a new image so that only the original values of the neighboring pixels are used to perform the equalization.

Since it is not necessary to build the entire table of substitute brightness values, an efficient way to perform this calculation is to simply count the number of pixels in the neighborhood region that are darker than or equal to the central pixel. The ratio of this number to 89 (the total number of pixels in the neighborhood), multiplied by 255 (the maximum grey value in the image, if it is a conventional 8-bit image), gives the new pixel brightness value.

Clever use of logic, to add in the brightness of each new row or column of pixel values and remove the old ones as the process is repeated for each pixel in the image, can make this operation moderately fast. The resulting image can only have a total of 89 possible different pixel values with this size of neighborhood. Of course, larger neighborhoods can also be used with correspondingly more pixels and possible grey levels.

Figure 11 shows an example of the application of local or neighborhood equalization using the 11-pixel-wide circular region de-

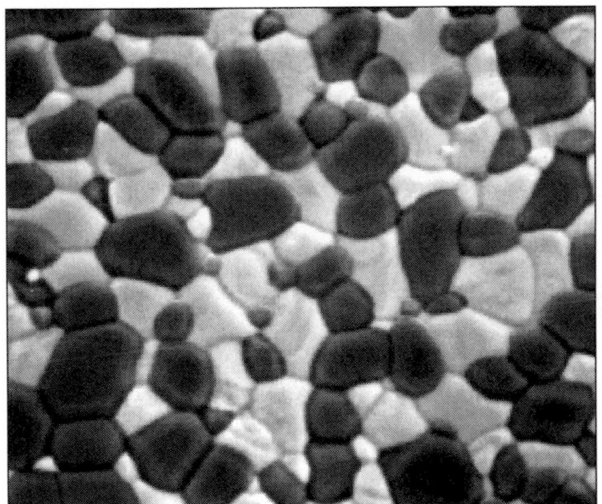
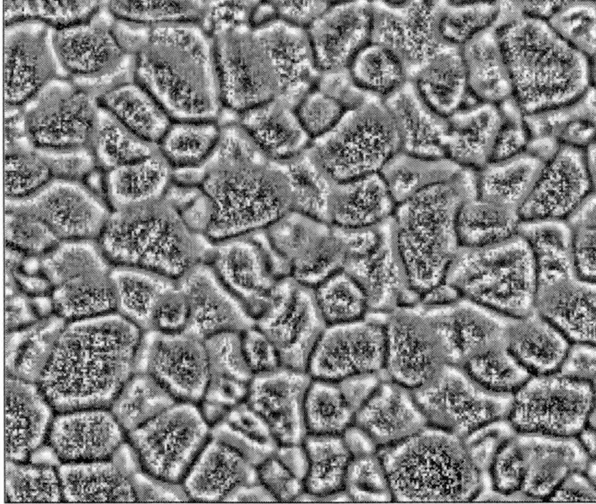

Figure 11. *Local equalization of a two-phase material (alumina-zirconia) using an 11-pixel diameter circle. Note the increased contrast at boundaries, and the gradients within the grains producing noise artefacts within the grains.*

scribed. Notice that the gradient within each of the uniform grey or white grain areas is an artefact of the method, because the regions overlap more of the adjacent areas when they are near the edges. This method tends to highlight edges and boundaries and shows separations and detail in nearly uniform regions (note the improved separation between dark features).

Laplacian

Local, or neighborhood, equalization of image contrast produces an increase in local contrast at boundaries. This has the effect of making edges easier for the viewer to see, consequently making the image appear sharper. This section will discuss several different approaches to edge enhancement that are less sensitive to overall brightness levels and feature sizes than the equalization discussed above.

The first set of operations uses neighborhoods with multiplicative kernels of integer weights identical in principle to those used in Chapter 2 for noise smoothing. In the section on smoothing, kernels were written as an array of integers. For example,

1	2	1
2	4	2
1	2	1

This 3×3 kernel is understood to mean that the central pixel brightness value is multiplied by 4, the values of the 4 touching neighbors to the sides and above and below are multiplied by 2, and the 4 diagonally touching neighbors by 1. The total value is added up and then divided by 16 (the sum of the 9 weights) to produce a new brightness value for the pixel. Other arrays of weights were also shown, some involving much larger arrays than this simple 3×3. For smoothing, all of the kernels were symmetrical about the center, and most of the examples had only positive weight values.

A very simple kernel that is still symmetrical, but does not have exclusively positive values, is the 3×3 Laplacian operator

–1	–1	–1
–1	+8	–1
–1	–1	–1

This subtracts the brightness values of each of the neighboring pixels from the central pixel. Consequently, in a region of the image that is uniform in brightness or has a uniform gradient of brightness, the result of applying this kernel is to reduce the grey level to zero. When a discontinuity is present within the neighborhood in the form of a point, line, or edge, the result of the Laplacian is a non-zero value. It may be either positive or negative, depending on where the central point lies with respect to the edge, etc.

In order to display the result when both positive and negative pixel values arise, it is common to add a medium grey value (128 for the case of a single-byte-per-pixel image with grey values in the range from 0 to 255) so that the zero points are middle grey and the brighter and darker values produced by the Laplacian can be seen. Some systems plot the absolute value of the result, but this tends to produce double lines along edges that are confusing both to the viewer and to subsequent processing and measurement operations.

As the name of the Laplacian operator implies, it is an approximation to the linear second derivative of brightness B in directions x and y

$$\nabla^2 B \equiv \frac{\partial^2 B}{\partial x^2} + \frac{\partial^2 B}{\partial y^2}$$

which is invariant to rotation, and hence insensitive to the direction in which the discontinuity runs. This highlights the points, lines, and edges in the image and suppresses uniform and smoothly varying regions, with the result shown in **Figure 12**. By itself, this Laplacian image is not very easy to interpret. Subtracting the Laplacian enhancement of the edges from the original image restores the overall grey scale variation which the human viewer can comfortably interpret. It also sharpens the image by locally increasing the contrast at discontinuities **(Figure 12).** This can be done simply by changing the central weight in the kernel, so that it becomes

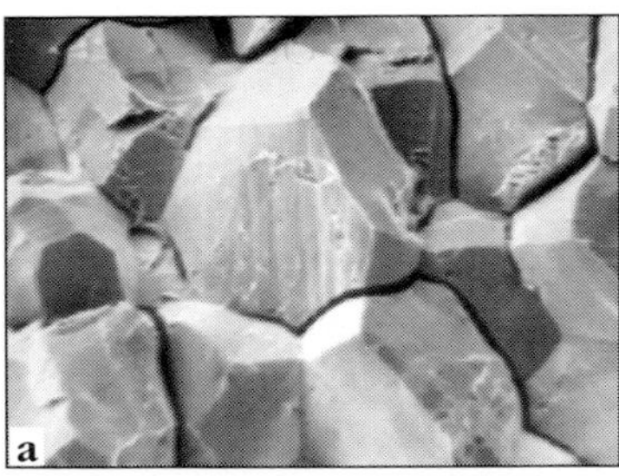

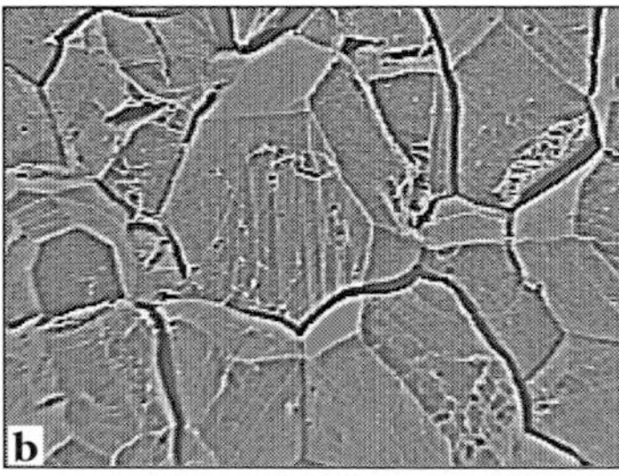

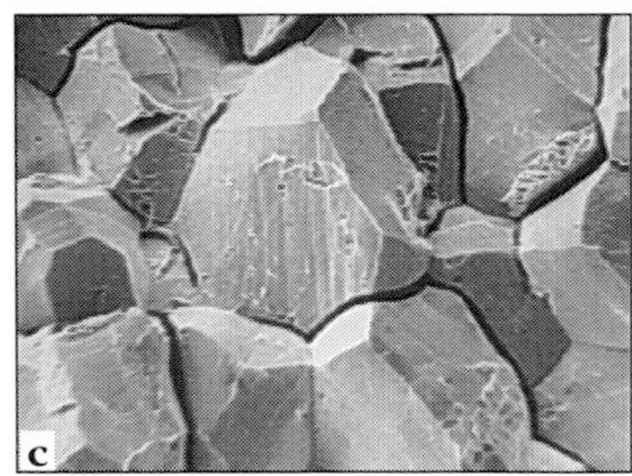

Figure 12. Enhancement of contrast at edges, lines, and points using a Laplacian:
a) *original SEM image of ceramic fracture;*
b) *application of Laplacian operator;*
c) *subtraction of the Laplacian from the original image.*

+1	+1	+1
+1	−7	+1
+1	+1	+1

This kernel is often described as a sharpening operator, because of the improved image contrast that it produces at edges. Justification for the procedure can be found in two different explanations. First, consider blur in an image to be modeled by a diffusion process, which would obey the partial differential equation

$$\frac{\partial f}{\partial t} = k\nabla^2 f$$

where the blur function is $f(x,y,t)$, and t is time. If this is expanded into a Taylor series around time τ, we can express the unblurred image as

$$B(x,y) = f(x,y,\tau) - \tau\frac{\partial f}{\partial t} + \frac{\tau^2}{2}\frac{\partial^2 f}{\partial t^2} - \ldots$$

If the higher-order terms are ignored, this is just

$$B = f - k\tau\nabla^2 f$$

In other words, the unblurred image B can be restored by subtracting the Laplacian (times a constant) from the blurred image. While the modeling of image blur as a diffusion process is at best approximate and the scaling constant is unknown or arbitrary, this at least gives some plausibility to the approach.

At least equally important is the simple fact that the processed image "looks good." **Figure 13** illustrates this with an astronomical photograph of Saturn. The visibility of the fine detail in the rings and atmosphere is enhanced by processing. The human visual system itself concentrates on edges and ignores uniform re-

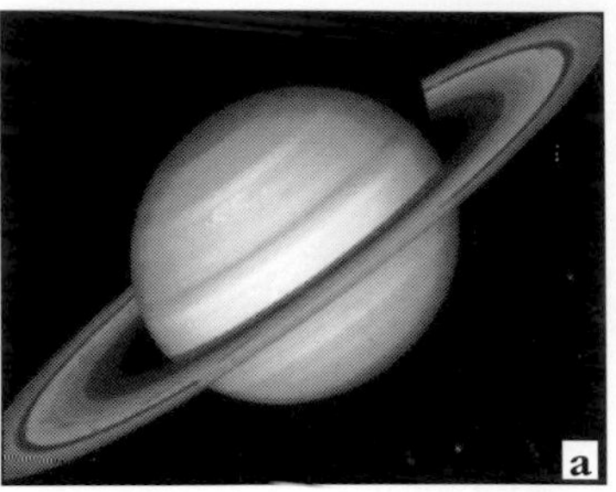

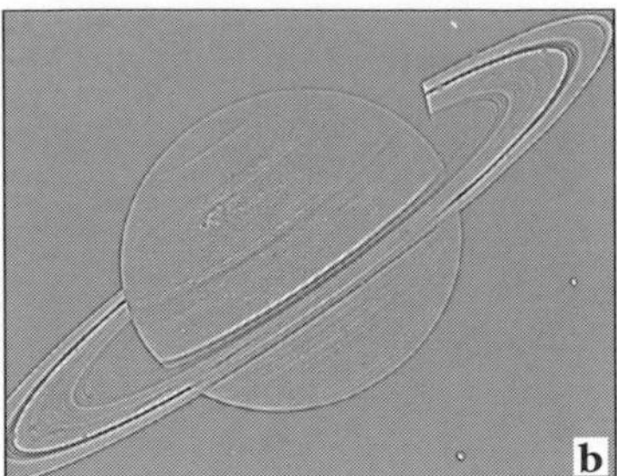

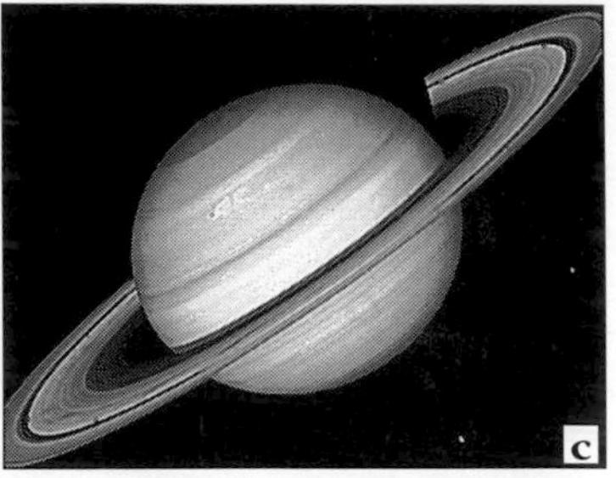

Figure 13. Application of a Laplacian operator to enhance the visibility of band structures in the rings and atmosphere of Saturn:
a) *original image;*
b) *application of Laplacian operator (notice the haloes around the tiny moons);*
c) *subtraction of the Laplacian from the original image.*

gions (Marr & Hildreth, 1980; Marr, 1982; Hildreth, 1983). This capability is hard-wired into our retinas. Connected directly to the rods and cones of the retina are two layers of processing neurons, which perform an operation very similar to the Laplacian. The horizontal cells in the second layer average together the signals from several neighboring sensors in the first layer, and the bipolar cells in the third layer subtract that signal from the original sensor output. This is called local inhibition and helps us to extract boundaries and edges.

At a more practical level, consider the ability of the eye to respond to cartoons and line drawings. These are highly abstracted bits of information about the original scene, yet they are entirely recognizable and interpretable. The cartoon provides the eye with exactly the minimum information it would otherwise have to extract from the scene itself to transmit up to higher levels of processing in the brain. (Similar inhibition in the time domain, using the next two layers of retinal neurons, helps us detect motion.)

One characteristic of human vision that confirms this behavior is the presence of Mach bands, a common illusion resulting from local brightness inhibition (Mach, 1906; Cornsweet, 1970). **Figure 14** shows a series of vertical bands of uniform intensity. The human viewer does not perceive them as uniform, instead seeing an undershoot and overshoot on each side of the steps, as shown in the plot. This increases the contrast at the step, and hence its visibility.

To see how this works using the Laplacian, we will use a one-dimensional kernel of the form

$$-1 \qquad +2 \qquad -1$$

and apply it to a series of brightness values along a line profile, across a step of moderate steepness

2 2 2 2 2 4 6 6 6 6 6

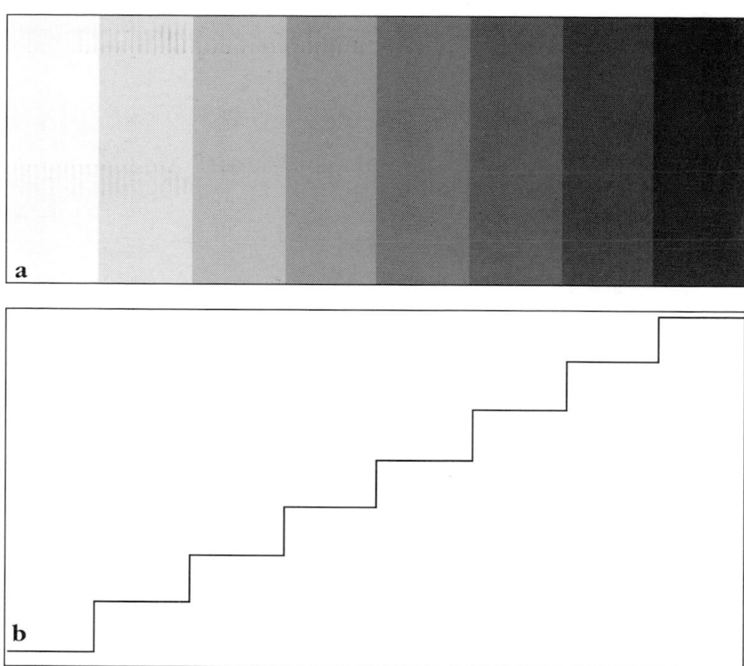

Figure 14. Illustration of Mach bands:
a) *uniform grey bands;*
b) *brightness profile of the bands;*
c) *application of a Laplacian to the bands in image a, showing increased contrast at the boundaries (this is the way the human eye perceives the uniform bands in image a);*
d) *brightness profile of image c.*

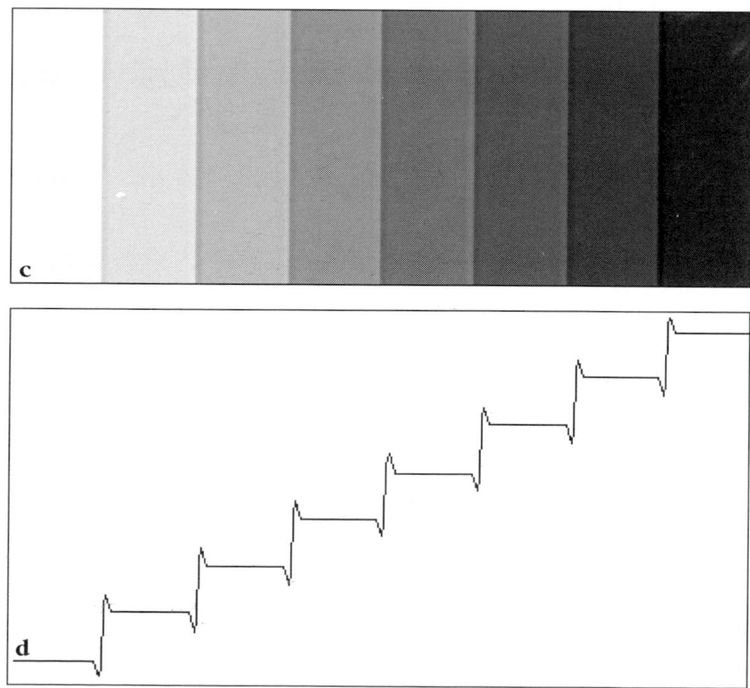

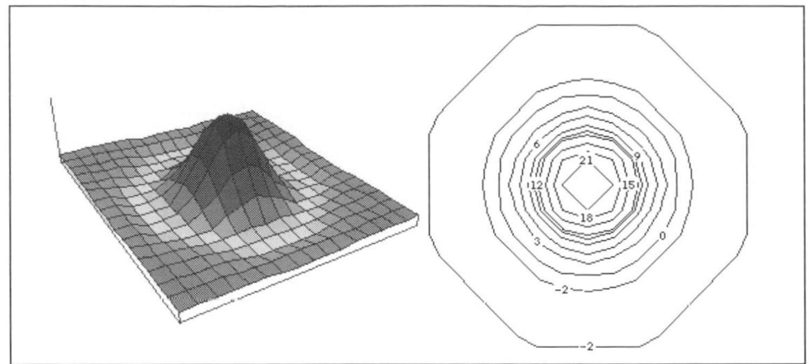

Figure 15. Isometric and contour plot views of the 17×17 Mexican hat kernel.

Shifting the kernel to each position, multiplying the kernel values times the brightness values, then adding, gives the result

0 0 0 0 –2 0 +2 0 0 0 0

which can be subtracted from the original to give

2 2 2 2 0 4 8 6 6 6 6

The undershoot and overshoot in brightness on either side of the step correspond to the Mach band effect.

Another way to describe the operation of the Laplacian is as a high-pass filter. In Chapter 4, image processing in the Fourier domain is discussed in terms of the high- and low-frequency components of the image brightness. A low-pass filter, such as the smoothing kernels discussed above and in Chapter 2, removes the high-frequency variability associated with noise, which can cause nearby pixels to vary in brightness. Conversely, a high-pass filter allows these high frequencies to remain (pass through the filter), while removing the low frequencies forming the gradual overall variation in brightness.

As with smoothing kernels, there are many different sets of integers and different-size kernels that can be used to apply a Laplacian to an image. The simplest just uses the four immediately touching pixels that share a side with the central pixel

	–1	
–1	+4	–1
	–1	

Larger kernels may combine a certain amount of smoothing by having positive weights for pixels in a small region near the central pixel, surrounded by negative weights for pixels farther away. Several examples are shown below. Because of the shape of these kernels when they are plotted as isometric views **(Figure 15),** they are sometimes described as a Mexican hat or sombrero filter; this name is usually reserved for kernels with more than one positive-weighted pixel at the center.

5 × 5 Laplacian kernel

0	0	-1	0	0
0	-1	-2	-1	0
-1	-2	16	-2	-1
0	-1	-2	-1	0
0	0	-1	0	0

7 × 7 Mexican hat kernel

0	0	-1	-1	-1	0	0
0	-1	-3	-3	-3	-1	0
-1	-3	0	7	0	-3	-1
-1	-3	7	24	7	-3	-1
-1	-3	0	7	0	-3	-1
0	-1	-3	-3	-3	-1	0
0	0	-1	-1	-1	0	0

13 × 13 Mexican hat kernel

0	0	0	0	0	-1	-1	-1	0	0	0	0	0
0	0	0	-1	-1	-2	-2	-2	-1	-1	0	0	0
0	0	-2	-2	-3	-3	-4	-3	-3	-2	-2	0	0
0	-1	-2	-3	-3	-3	-2	-3	-3	-3	-2	-1	0
0	-1	-3	-3	-1	4	6	4	-1	-3	-3	-1	0
-1	-2	-3	-3	4	14	19	14	4	-3	-3	-2	-1
-1	-2	-4	-2	6	19	24	19	6	-2	-4	-2	-1
-1	-2	-3	-3	4	14	19	14	4	-3	-3	-2	-1
0	-1	-3	-3	-1	4	6	4	-1	-3	-3	-1	0
0	-1	-2	-3	-3	-3	-2	-3	-3	-3	-2	-1	0
0	0	-2	-2	-3	-3	-4	-3	-3	-2	-2	0	0
0	0	0	-1	-1	-2	-2	-2	-1	-1	0	0	0
0	0	0	0	0	-1	-1	-1	0	0	0	0	0

17 × 17 Mexican hat kernel

0	0	0	0	0	0	-1	-1	-1	-1	-1	0	0	0	0	0	0
0	0	0	0	-1	-1	-1	-1	-1	-1	-1	-1	-1	0	0	0	0
0	0	-1	-1	-1	-2	-3	-3	-3	-3	-3	-2	-1	-1	-1	0	0
0	0	-1	-1	-2	-3	-3	-3	-3	-3	-3	-3	-2	-1	-1	0	0
0	-1	-1	-2	-3	-3	-3	-2	-3	-2	-3	-3	-3	-2	-1	-1	0
0	-1	-2	-3	-3	-3	0	2	4	2	0	-3	-3	-3	-2	-1	0
-1	-1	-3	-3	-3	0	4	10	12	10	4	0	-3	-3	-3	-1	-1
-1	-1	-3	-3	-2	2	10	18	21	18	10	2	-2	-3	-3	-1	-1
-1	-1	-3	-3	-3	4	12	21	24	21	12	4	-3	-3	-3	-1	-1
-1	-1	-3	-3	-2	2	10	18	21	18	10	2	-2	-3	-3	-1	-1
-1	-1	-3	-3	-3	0	4	10	12	10	4	0	-3	-3	-3	-1	-1
0	-1	-2	-3	-3	-3	0	2	4	2	0	-3	-3	-3	-2	-1	0
0	-1	-1	-2	-3	-3	-3	-2	-3	-2	-3	-3	-3	-2	-1	-1	0
0	0	-1	-1	-2	-3	-3	-3	-3	-3	-3	-3	-2	-1	-1	0	0
0	0	-1	-1	-1	-2	-3	-3	-3	-3	-3	-2	-1	-1	-1	0	0
0	0	0	0	-1	-1	-1	-1	-1	-1	-1	-1	-1	0	0	0	0
0	0	0	0	0	0	-1	-1	-1	-1	-1	0	0	0	0	0	0

Derivatives

The Laplacian is a good high-pass filter, but not a particularly good tool for demarcating edges (Berzins, 1984). In most cases, boundaries or edges of features or regions appear at least locally as a step in brightness, sometimes spread over several pixels. The Laplacian gives a larger response to a line than to a step, and to a point than to a line. In an image that contains noise, typically present as points varying in brightness due to counting statistics, detector characteristics, etc., the Laplacian will show such points more strongly than the edges or boundaries that are of interest.

Another approach to locating edges uses first derivatives in two or more directions. It will be helpful to first examine simple, one-dimensional first derivatives. Some images are essentially one-dimensional, such as chromatography preparations in which proteins are spread along lanes in an electrical field **(Figure 16)** or tree ring patterns from drill cores **(Figure 17).** Applying a first derivative to such an image, in the direction of important variation, demarcates the boundaries and enhances the visibility of small steps and other details, as shown in **Figures 16** and **17.**

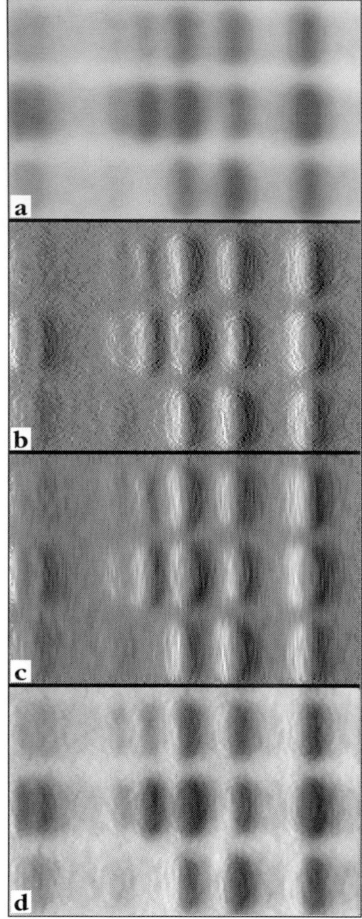

Figure 16. Image of a protein separation gel:
a) *original;*
b) *difference between each pixel and its neighbor to the left;*
c) *vertical averaging of image b to reduce noise;*
d) *horizontal derivative using a 3×3 kernel as discussed in the text.*

Of course, for an image with digitized finite pixels, a continuous derivative cannot be performed. Instead, the difference value between adjacent pixels can be calculated as a finite derivative. This difference is also somewhat noisy, but averaging in the direction perpendicular to the derivative can smooth the result, as shown in **Figures 16** and **17.**

A derivative image with smoother appearance can be produced with fewer steps by applying an asymmetrical kernel. Consider a set of kernels of the form shown below. There are 8 possible rotational orientations of this kernel about the center.

$$\begin{matrix} 1 & 0 & -1 \\ 2 & 0 & -2 \\ 1 & 0 & -1 \end{matrix} \qquad \begin{matrix} 2 & 1 & 0 \\ 1 & 0 & -1 \\ 0 & -1 & -2 \end{matrix} \qquad \begin{matrix} 1 & 2 & 1 \\ 0 & 0 & 0 \\ -1 & -2 & -1 \end{matrix}$$

Applying the first pattern of values shown to the tree ring and protein separation images is shown in **Figures 16** and **17.**

One improvement comes from averaging together the adjacent pixels in each vertical column before taking the difference; this reduces noise in the image. A second, more subtle effect is that

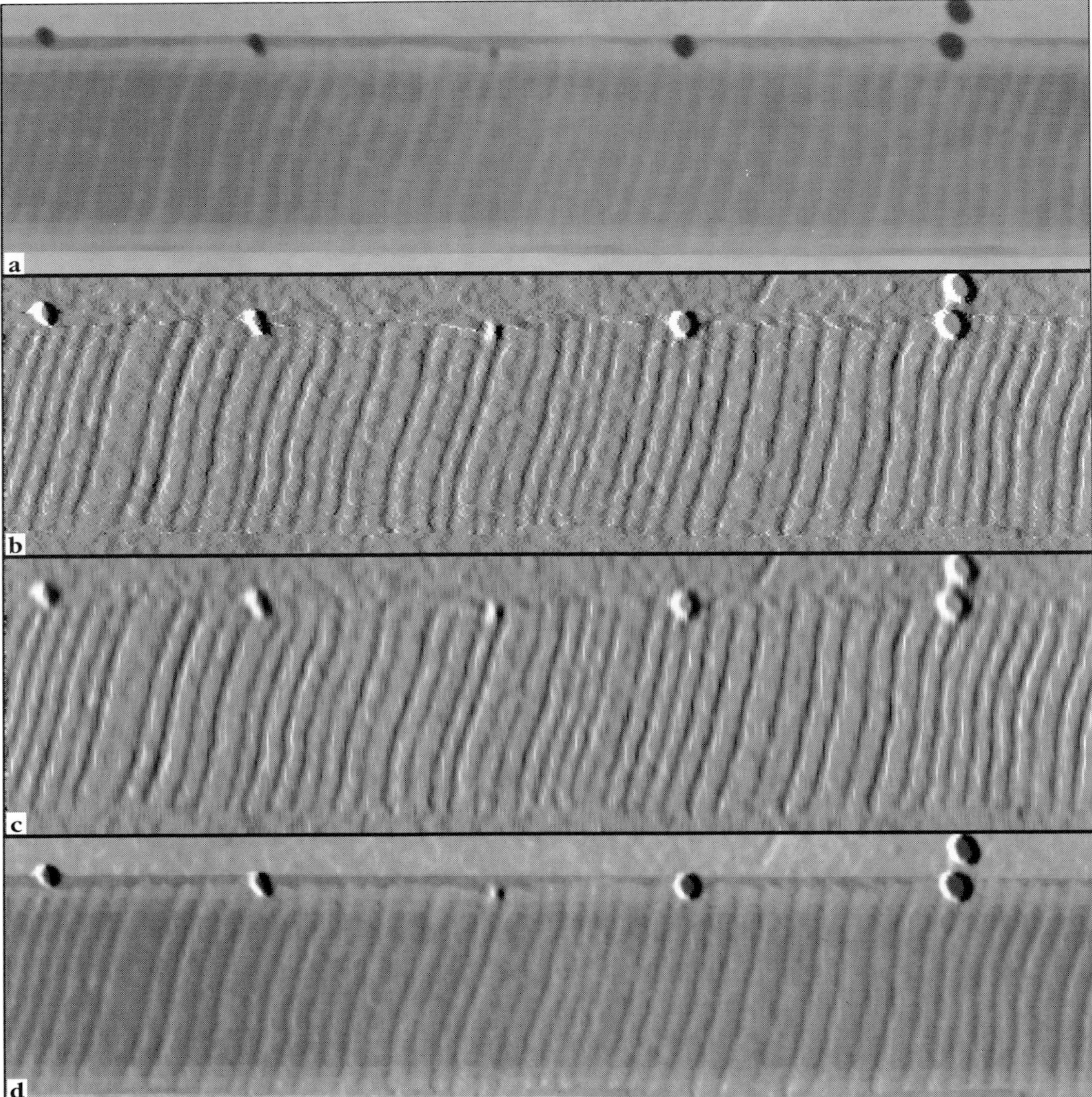

Figure 17. Image of tree rings in a drill core:
a) *original;*
b) *difference between each pixel and its neighbor to the left;*
c) *vertical averaging of image b to reduce noise;*
d) *horizontal derivative using a 3 × 3 kernel as discussed in the text.*

these kernels are 3 pixels wide and thus replace the central pixel with the difference value. The simple subtraction described above causes a half-pixel shift in the image, which is absent with this kernel. Finally, the method shown here is faster, since it requires only a single pass through the image.

Obviously, other kernel values can be devised that will also produce derivatives. As the kernel size increases, more directions are possible. Since this is fundamentally a one-dimensional derivative, it is possible to directly use the coefficients of Savitsky and Golay (1964), which were originally published for use with such one-dimensional data as spectrograms or other strip-chart recorder output. These coefficients, like the smoothing weights shown in Chapter 2, are equivalent to least-squares fitting a high-order polynomial to the data. In this case, though, the first derivative of the polynomial is evaluated at the central point. Both second degree (quadratic) and fourth degree (quartic) polynomials are shown.

Table of Coefficients for First Derivative Quadratic Fit

#	5	7	9	11	13	15	17	19	21	23	25
−12											−.0092
−11										−.0109	−.0085
−10									−.0130	−.0099	−.0077
−9								−.0158	−.0117	−.0089	−.0069
−8							−.0196	−.0140	−.0104	−.0079	−.0062
−7						−.0250	−.0172	−.0123	−.0091	−.0069	−.0054
−6					−.0330	−.0214	−.0147	−.0105	−.0078	−.0059	−.0046
−5				−.0455	−.0275	−.0179	−.0123	−.0088	−.0065	−.0049	−.0038
−4			−.0667	−.0364	−.0220	−.0143	−.0098	−.0070	−.0052	−.0040	−.0031
−3		−.1071	−.0500	−.0273	−.0165	−.0107	−.0074	−.0053	−.0039	−.0030	−.0023
−2	−.2000	−.0714	−.0333	−.0182	−.0110	−.0071	−.0049	−.0035	−.0026	−.0020	−.0015
−1	−.1000	−.0357	−.0250	−.0091	−.0055	−.0036	−.0025	−.0018	−.0013	−.0010	−.0008
0	0	0	0	0	0	0	0	0	0	0	0
+1	+.1000	+.0357	+.0250	+.0091	+.0055	+.0036	+.0025	+.0018	+.0013	+.0010	+.0008
+2	+.2000	+.0714	+.0333	+.0182	+.0110	+.0071	+.0049	+.0035	+.0026	+.0020	+.0015
+3		+.1071	+.0500	+.0273	+.0165	+.0107	+.0074	+.0053	+.0039	+.0030	+.0023
+4			+.0667	+.0364	+.0220	+.0143	+.0098	+.0070	+.0052	+.0040	+.0031
+5				+.0455	+.0275	+.0179	+.0123	+.0088	+.0065	+.0049	+.0038
+6					+.0330	+.0214	+.0147	+.0105	+.0078	+.0059	+.0046
+7						+.0250	+.0172	+.0123	+.0091	+.0069	+.0054
+8							+.0196	+.0140	+.0104	+.0079	+.0062
+9								+.0158	+.0117	+.0089	+.0069
+10									+.0130	+.0099	+.0077
+11										+.0109	+.0085
+12											+.0092

Table of Coefficients for First Derivative Quartic Fit

#	5	7	9	11	13	15	17	19	21	23	25
−12											+.0174
−11										+.0200	+.0048
−10									+.0231	+.0041	−.0048
−9								+.0271	+.0028	−.0077	−.0118
−8							+.0322	−.0003	−.0119	−.0159	−.0165
−7						+.0387	−.0042	−.0182	−.0215	−.0209	−.0190
−6					+.0472	−.0123	−.0276	−.0292	−.0267	−.0231	−.0197
−5				+.0583	−.0275	−.0423	−.0400	−.0340	−.0280	−.0230	−.0189
−4			+.0724	−.0571	−.0657	−.0549	−.0431	−.0335	−.0262	−.0208	−.0166
−3		+.0873	−.1195	−.1033	−.0748	−.0534	−.0388	−.0320	−.0219	−.0170	−.0134
−2	+.0833	−.2659	−.1625	−.0977	−.0620	−.0414	−.0289	−.0210	−.0157	−.0120	−.0094
−1	−.6667	−.2302	−.1061	−.0575	−.0346	−.0225	−.0154	−.0110	−.0081	−.0062	−.0048
0	0	0	0	0	0	0	0	0	0	0	0
+1	+.6667	+.2302	+.1061	+.0575	+.0346	+.0225	+.0154	+.0110	+.0081	+.0062	+.0048
+2	−.0833	+.2659	+.1625	+.0977	+.0620	+.0414	+.0289	+.0210	+.0157	+.0120	+.0094
+3		−.0873	+.1195	+.1033	+.0748	+.0534	+.0388	+.0320	+.0219	+.0170	+.0134
+4			−.0724	+.0571	+.0657	+.0549	+.0431	+.0335	+.0262	+.0208	+.0166
+5				−.0583	+.0275	+.0423	+.0400	+.0340	+.0280	+.0230	+.0189
+6					−.0472	+.0123	+.0276	+.0292	+.0267	+.0231	+.0197
+7						−.0387	+.0042	+.0182	+.0215	+.0209	+.0190
+8							−.0322	+.0003	+.0119	+.0159	+.0165
+9								−.0271	−.0028	+.0077	+.0118
+10									−.0231	−.0041	+.0048
+11										−.0200	−.0048
+12											−.0174

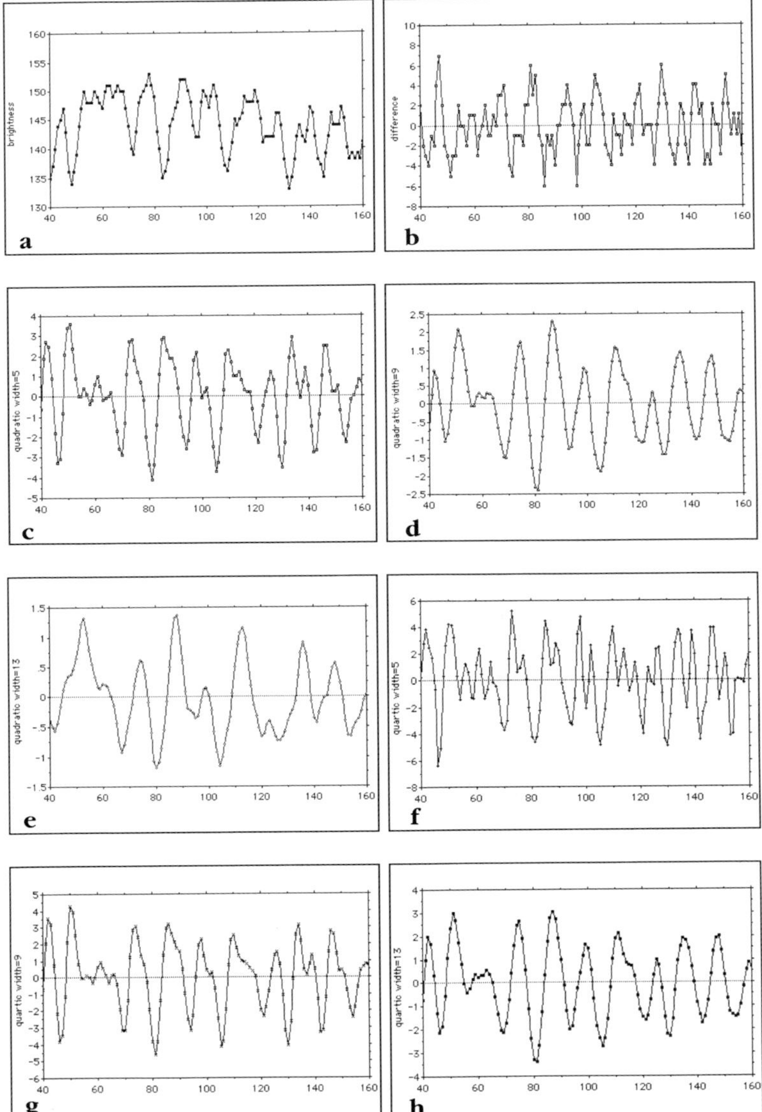

Figure 18. Horizontal brightness profile for a line in the center of the tree ring image (Figure 17) and its derivatives:

a) *original brightness plotted for each pixel along a fragment of the line;*

b) *finite difference plot showing the difference between adjacent pixels;*

c) *derivative calculated using the weights for a quadratic polynomial fit to 5 points;*

d) *a quadratic fit to 9 points;*

e) *a quadratic fit to 13 points;*

f) *derivative calculated using the weights for a quartic polynomial fit to 5 points;*

g) *a quartic fit to 9 points;*

h) *a quartic fit to 13 points.*

Figure 18 shows a fragment of the brightness profile along the center of the tree ring image in **Figure 17.** The first derivative plots shown were obtained by using the pixel difference approximation, and by using these weights to fit quadratic and quartic polynomials over widths of 5, 9, and 13 pixels around each point. The fits produce much smoother results and suppress noise. However, by increasing the fitting width, the small-scale real variations in the data are suppressed. It is generally necessary, as in any fitting or smoothing operation, to keep the kernel size smaller than the features of interest.

Using one-dimensional derivatives to extract one-dimensional data from two-dimensional images is a relatively unusual and specialized operation. However, extending the same principles to locating boundaries with arbitrary orientations in two-dimen-

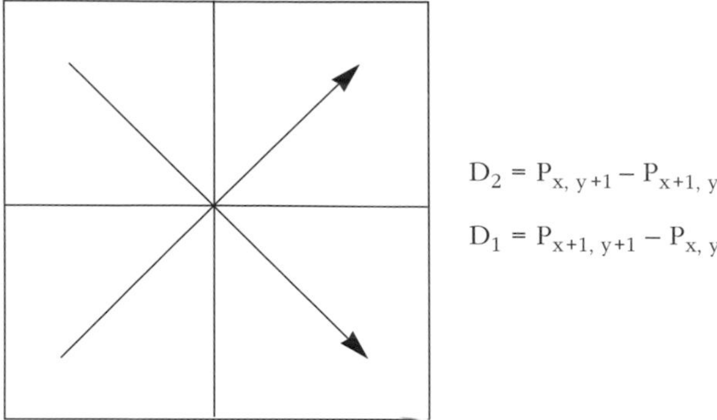

Figure 19. *Robert's Cross Operator uses the differences between four neighboring pixels.*

sional images is one of the most common of all image enhancement operations. The problem, of course, is finding a method that is insensitive to the (local) orientation of the edge.

One of the earliest approaches to this task was the Roberts' Cross operator (Roberts, 1965). It uses the same difference technique shown above for the one-dimensional case, but with two pixel differences at right angles to each other, as diagrammed in **Figure 19.** These two differences represent a finite approximation to the derivative of brightness. Two-directional derivatives can be combined to obtain a magnitude value that is insensitive to the orientation of the edge: by squaring, adding, and taking the square root of the total.

This method has the same problems as the difference method used in one dimension. Noise in the image is magnified by the single-pixel differences, and the result is shifted by one-half of a pixel in both the x and y directions. In addition, the result may not be invariant with respect to edge orientation. As a practical matter, the computers in common use when this model was first proposed were not very fast, nor were they equipped with separate, floating-point math coprocessors. This made the square root of the sum of the squares impractical to calculate. Two alternatives were used: adding the absolute values of the two directional differences, or comparing the two absolute values of the differences, keeping the larger one. Both of these methods make the result quite sensitive to direction. In addition, even if the square root method is used, the magnitude of the result will vary, because the pixel spacing is not the same in all directions, and edges in the vertical and horizontal directions spread the change in brightness over more pixels than edges in the diagonal directions.

In several of the comparison sequences that follow, the Roberts' Cross image will be shown **(Figures 22b and 32c).** In all cases, the square root of the sum of squares of the differences was used. Even so, the images are characterized by varying sensitivity with respect to edge orientation, as well as a high noise level.

The Sobel and Kirsch operators

Just as for the example of the horizontal derivative above, the use of a larger kernel offers reduced sensitivity to noise by averaging several pixels and eliminating image shift. In fact, the derivative kernels shown above, or other similar patterns using different sets of integers, are widely used. Some common examples of these coefficients are shown in the table below.

+1	0	−1	+1	0	−1	+1	−1	−1	+5	−3	−3
+1	0	−1	+2	0	−2	+2	+1	−1	+5	0	−3
+1	0	−1	+1	0	−1	+1	−1	−1	+5	−3	−3
+1	+1	0	+2	+1	0	+2	+1	−1	+5	+5	−3
+1	0	−1	+1	0	−1	+1	+1	−1	+5	0	−3
0	−1	−1	0	−1	−2	−1	−1	−1	−3	−3	−3
+1	+1	+1	+1	+2	+1	+1	+2	+1	+5	+5	+5
0	0	0	0	0	0	−1	+1	−1	−3	0	−3
−1	−1	−1	−1	−2	−1	−1	−1	−1	−3	−3	−3

and so forth for eight rotations…

It actually makes little difference which of these patterns of values is used, as long as the magnitude of the result does not exceed the storage capacity of the computer being used. This is often a single byte per pixel, which, since the result of the above operation may be either negative or positive, can handle only values between −127 and +128. If large steps in brightness are present, this may result in the clipping of calculated values, so that major boundaries are broadened or distorted in order to see smaller ones. The alternative is to employ automatic scaling, using the maximum and minimum values in the derivative image to set the white and dark values. To avoid a loss of precision, though, this requires two passes through the image: one to perform the calculations and find the extreme values and the second to actually compute the values and scale the results for storage.

As for the Roberts' Cross method, if the derivatives in two orthogonal directions are computed, they can be combined as the square root of the sums of their squares to obtain a result independent of orientation.

$$\text{Magnitude} = \sqrt{\frac{\partial B^2}{\partial x} + \frac{\partial B^2}{\partial y}}$$

This is the Sobel (1970) method. It is one of the most commonly used techniques, even though it requires a fair amount of computation to perform correctly. (As for the Roberts' Cross, some computer programs attempt to compensate for hardware limitations by adding or comparing the two values, instead of squaring, adding, and taking the square root.)

With appropriate hardware, such as a shift register or array processor, the Sobel operation can be performed in essentially

Figure 20. *A metallographic image (a) with two directional derivatives (b and c), and the Kirsch image (d) produced by keeping the maximum value from each of 8 directions.*

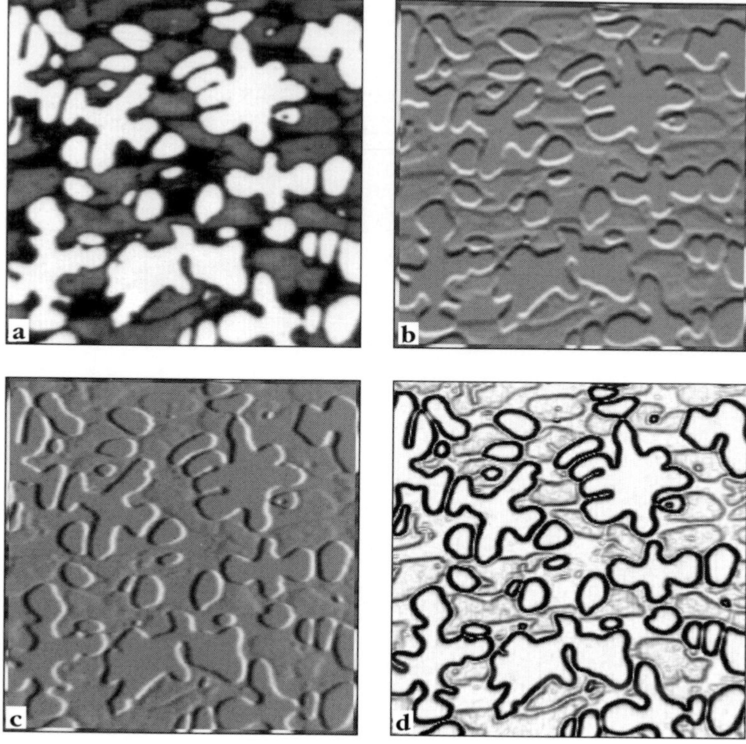

real time. This usually means 1/30th of a second per image, so that conventional video images can be processed and viewed. It often means viewing one frame while the following one is digitized, but in the case of the Sobel, it is even possible to view the image live, delayed only by two video scan lines. Two lines of data can be buffered and used to calculate the derivative values using the 3×3 kernels shown above. Specialized hardware to perform this real-time edge enhancement is used in some military applications, making it possible to locate edges in images needed for tracking, alignment of hardware in midair refueling, and other purposes.

At the other extreme, some general-purpose image analysis systems that do not have hardware for fast math operations perform the Sobel operation using a series of operations. First, two derivative images are formed, one using a horizontal and one a vertical orientation of the kernel. Then each of these is modified using a LUT to replace the value of each pixel with its square. The two resulting images are added together, and another LUT is used to convert each pixel value to its square root. No multiplication or square roots are needed. However, if this method is applied in a typical system with 8 bits per pixel, the loss of precision is severe, reducing the final image to no more than 4 bits of useful information.

A more useful method, when the mathematical operations

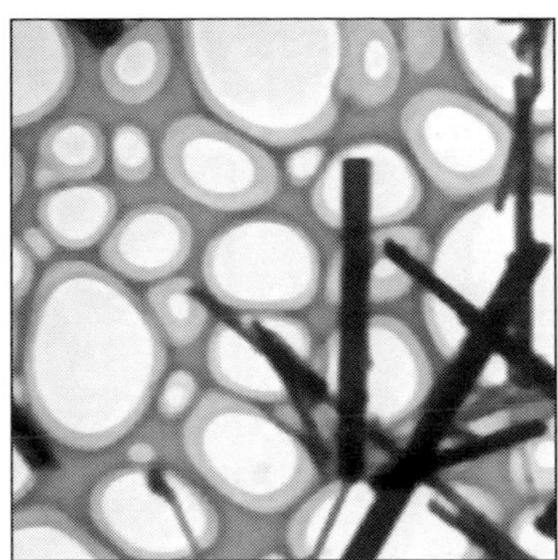

Figure 21. Original image (asbestos fibers on a holey carbon film), imaged in a TEM. This image is the basis for the processing shown in Figure 22.

needed to calculate the square root of the sum of squares for the Sobel must be avoided, is the Kirsch operator (1971). This method applies each of the eight orientations of the derivative kernel and keeps the maximum value. It requires only integer multiplication and comparisons. For many images, the results for the magnitude of edges are very similar to the Sobel. **Figure 20** shows an example. Vertical and horizontal derivatives of the image, and the maximum derivative values in each of eight directions, are shown.

Figures 21 and **22** illustrate the formation of the Sobel edge-finding image and compare it to the Laplacian, Roberts' Cross, and Kirsch operators. The example image contains many continuous edges running in all directions around the holes in the carbon film, as well as some straight edges at various orientations along the asbestos fibers. The Laplacian image is quite noisy, and the Roberts' Cross does not show all of the edges equally well. The individual vertical and horizontal derivatives are shown with the zero value shifted to an intermediate grey, so that both the negative and positive values can be seen. The absolute values are also shown.

Combining the two directional derivatives by a sum, or maximum operator, produces quite noisy and incomplete boundary enhancement. The square root of the sum of squares produces a good image, with little noise and continuous edge markings. The result from the Kirsch operator is very similar to the Sobel for this image.

In addition to the magnitude of the Sobel operator, it is also possible to calculate a direction value for each pixel as

$$\text{Direction} = \text{Arc Tan}\left(\frac{\partial B/\partial y}{\partial B/\partial x}\right)$$

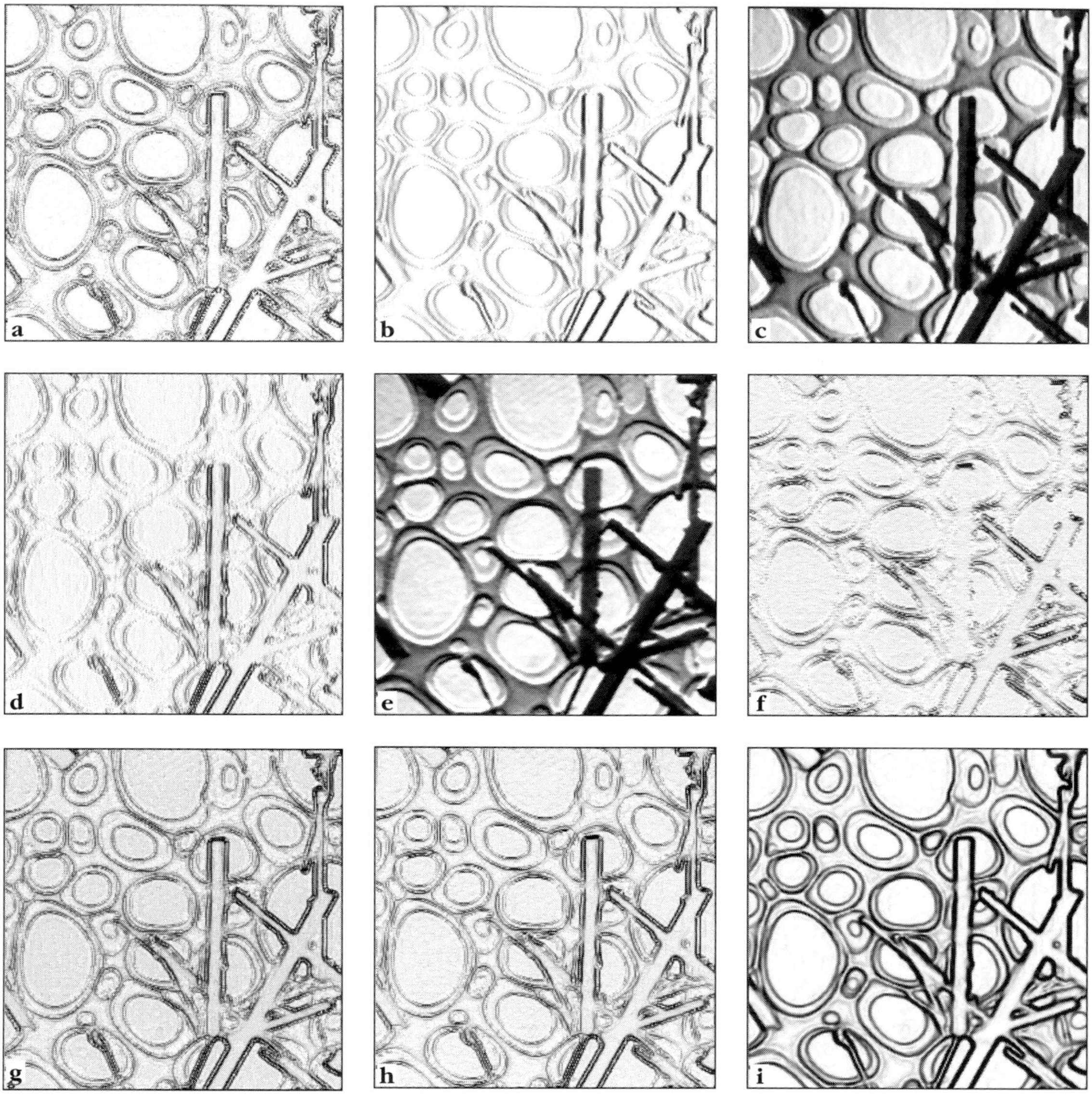

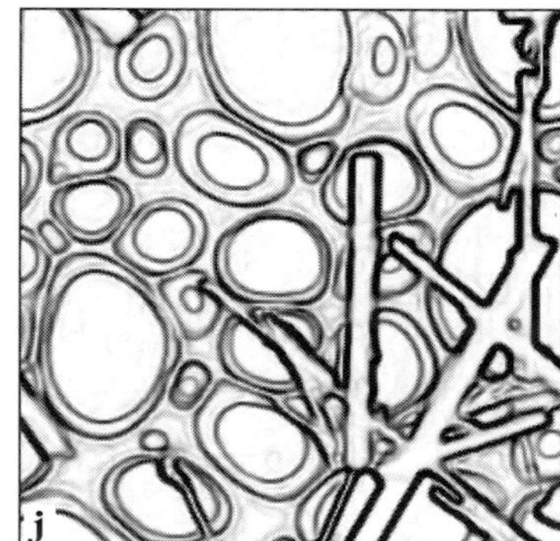

Figure 22. Edge enhancement of the image in Figure 20:
a) *Laplacian operator;*
b) *Roberts' Cross operator;*
c) *horizontal derivative, scaled to full grey scale range;*
d) *absolute value of image c;*
e) *vertical derivative, scaled to full grey scale range;*
f) *absolute value of image e;*
g) *sum of absolute values from images d and f;*
h) *maximum of values in images d and f, pixel by pixel;*
i) *Sobel operator (square root of sum of squares of values);*
j) *Kirsch operator.*

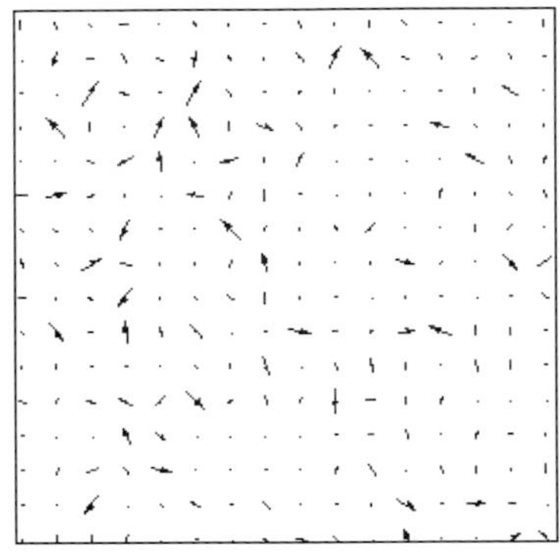
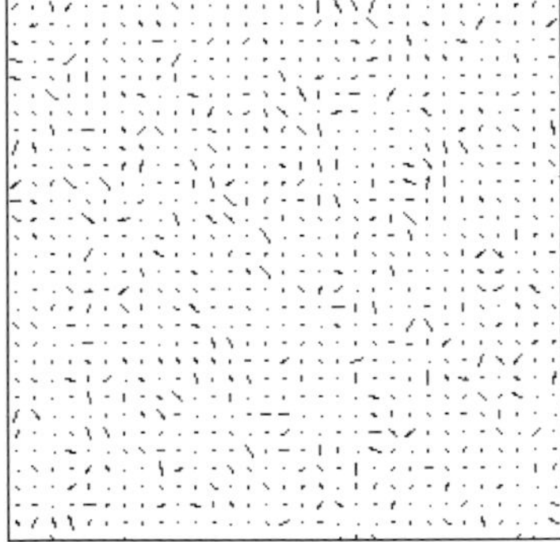

Figure 23. Applying a Sobel operator to the image in Figure 20. Each vector has the direction and magnitude given by the operator, but even the fine vector field is too sparse to show any details of the image.

This assigns a value to each pixel for the gradient direction, which can be scaled to the grey scale of the image. **Figure 23** shows the vector results from applying the Sobel operator to the image of Figure 19. The magnitude and direction are encoded, but the vector field is too sparse to show any image details.

Figure 24 shows only the direction information for the image in **Figure 21,** using grey values to represent the angles. The progression of values around each more-or-less circular hole is evident. The use of a pseudo-color scale for this display is particularly suitable, since a rainbow of hues can show the progression without the arbitrary discontinuity required by the grey scale (in this example, at an angle of zero degrees).

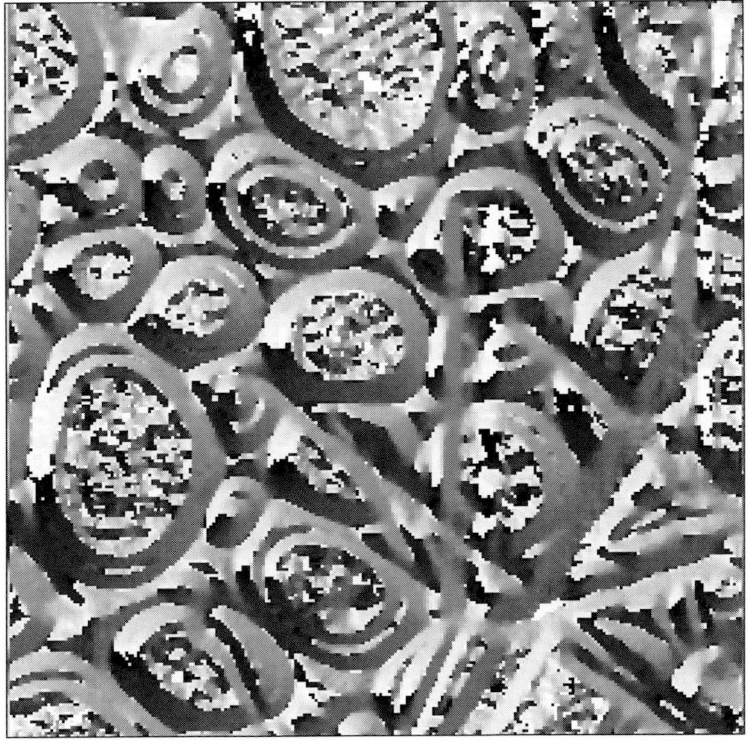

Figure 24. Direction of the Sobel operator for the image in Figure 21.

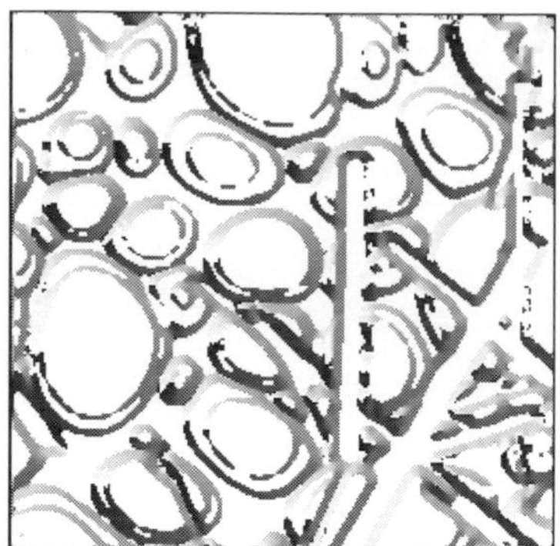

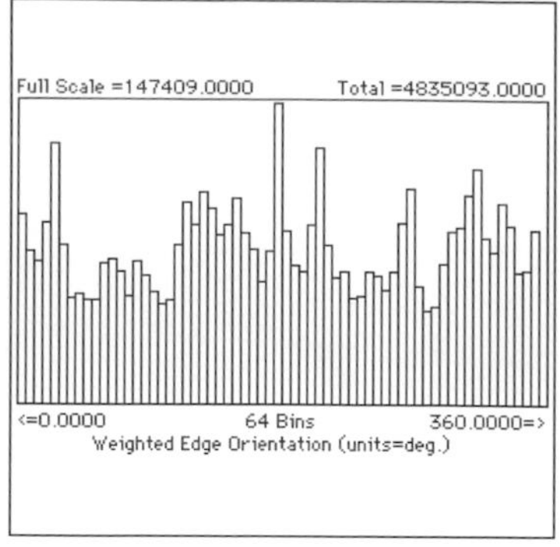

Figure 25. Uses of the edge orientation image in Figure 24:
left) *masking only those pixels whose edge magnitude is large (the 40% of the pixels with the largest magnitude);*
right) *generating a histogram of weighted orientation, where each pixel is classified according to the local Sobel direction (horizontal axis) and the bins sum the Sobel magnitude (vertical axis).*

The use of the direction image to reveal image texture will be discussed below. It is evident from **Figure 24** that the pixels in rather homogeneous regions of the image do not show a strong orientation; the edge direction image is simply noisy there. One way to improve the result is to show the direction information only for those pixels also having a strong magnitude for the brightness gradient. In **Figure 25,** this is done by using the magnitude image as a mask, selecting (by thresholding, discussed in Chapter 5) the 40% of the pixels with the largest gradient magnitude, and showing the direction only for those pixels.

Figure 25 also shows a histogram plot of the preferred orientation in the image. This is constructed by sorting each pixel in **Figure 24** into one of 64 bins based on orientation, then summing up for all of the pixels in each bin the total of the gradient magnitude values. This kind of weighted plot is particularly common for interpreting the orientation of lines, such as dislocations in metals and the traces of faults in geographic maps. Further examples will be discussed below.

The use of an edge-enhancing operator to modify images is useful in many situations. We have already seen examples of sharpening using the Laplacian, to increase the contrast at edges and make images appear sharper to the viewer. Gradient, or edge-finding, methods also do this, but they also modify the image, so that its interpretation becomes somewhat different. Since this contrast increase is selective, it responds to local information in the image in a way that manipulating the brightness histogram cannot.

For example, **Figure 26** shows several views of galaxy M51. In the original image, it is quite impossible to see the full range of brightness, even on a high-quality photographic negative. It is even less possible to print it. The extremely light and dark areas simply cover too great a range. Compressing the range nonlinearly, using a logarithmic transfer function, can make it possible to see both ends of the scale at the same time. However, this is accomplished by reducing small variations, especially at the bright end of the scale, so that they are not visible.

A rather common approach to dealing with this type of image is

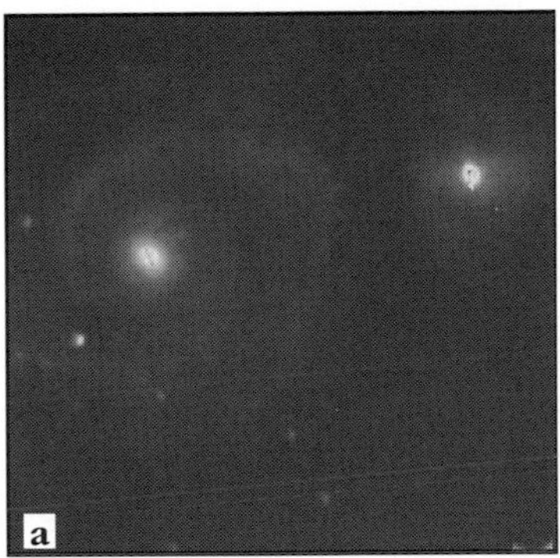

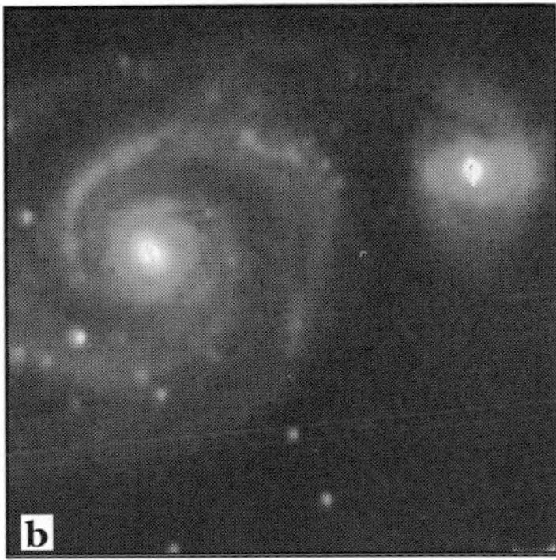

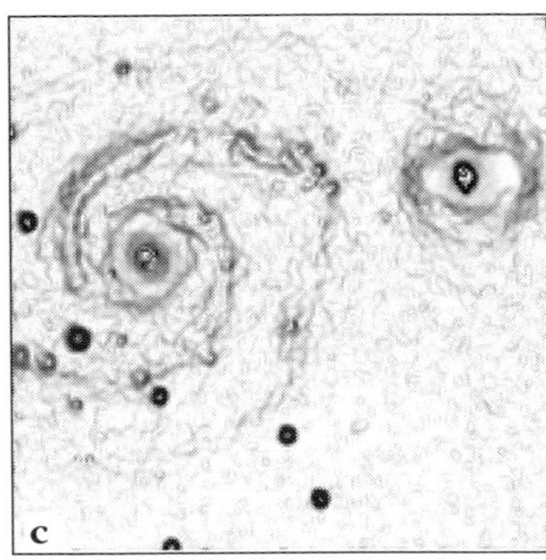

Figure 26. Enhancing an astronomical image (M51):
a) *original telescope image, with brightness range too great for printing;*
b) *application of "unsharp masking" by subtracting a smoothed image to reduce contrast selectively and show detail;*
c) *gradient of original image using a Sobel operator, which also shows the fine structure of the galaxy.*

called unsharp masking. Traditionally, it has been applied using photographic darkroom techniques. First, a contact print is made from the original negative onto film, leaving a small gap between the emulsions so that the image is blurred. After the film is developed, a new print is made with the two negatives clamped together. The light areas on the original negative are covered by dark areas on the printed negative, allowing little light to come through. Only regions where the slightly out-of-focus negative does not match the original are printed. This is functionally equivalent to the Laplacian, which subtracts a smoothed (out of focus) image from the original to suppress gradual changes and pass high frequencies or edges.

Closely related to unsharp masking is the subtraction of one smoothed version of the image from another having a different degree of smoothing. This is called the difference of Gaussians (DOG) method and is believed to be similar to the way the human visual system locates boundaries (Marr, 1982) and other features (the effect of inhibition increasing contrast at boundaries was shown in Chapter 1). Smoothing an image using Gaussian kernels with different standard deviations suppresses high-frequency information, which corresponds to small details and spacing that are present. Large structures are not affected. The difference between the two images keeps only those structures (lines, points, etc.) that are in the intermediate size range between the two operators. Examples of this operation will be shown below in **Figure 32.** **Figure 27** shows a plot of two Gaussian curves with different standard deviations, and their difference, which is very similar to a cross section of the Laplacian. This edge extractor is also sometimes called a Marr-Hildreth operator.

The gradient enhancement shown in **Figure 26** uses a Sobel operator to mark edges. This shows the structure within the galaxy in a very different way, by emphasizing local spatial variations re-

Figure 27. *The difference of Gaussian ("DOG") operator in one dimension. Two Gaussian curves with different standard deviations are shown, with their difference. The result is a sharpening operation much like the Laplacian.*

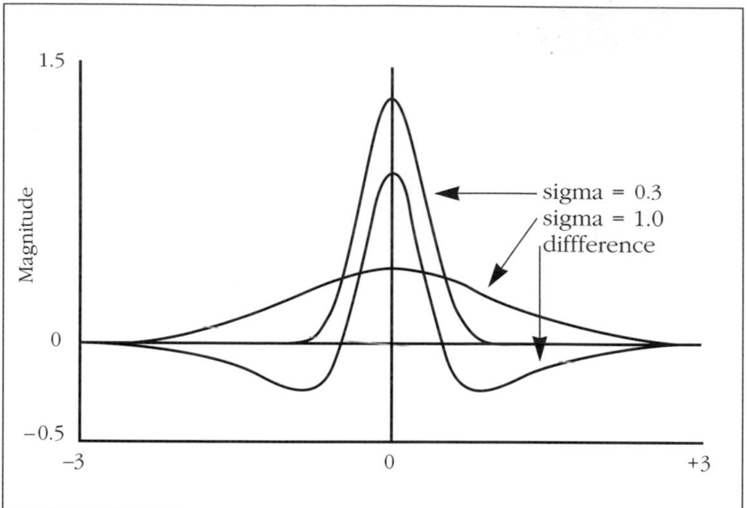

gardless of the absolute value of the brightness. This produces a distinctly different result than the Laplacian or unsharp masking.

Figure 28 shows an example at a very different scale. The specimen is a polished aluminum metal. The individual grains exhibit different brightnesses because their crystallographic lattices are randomly oriented in space. Also, the etching procedure used darkens some grains more than others. It is the grain boundaries that are usually important in studying metal structures, since the configuration of grain boundaries results from prior heat treatment and controls many mechanical properties. The human visual process detects the grain boundaries using its sensitivity to boundaries and edges. Most image analysis systems use a gradient operation, such as a Sobel, to perform a similar enhancement prior to measuring the grain boundaries.

In the example in **Figure 28,** another method has been employed. This is a variance operator, which calculates the sum of squares of the brightness differences for the 8 pixels surrounding each pixel in the original image. This value, like the other edge-enhancement operators, is very small in uniform regions of the image and becomes large whenever a step is present. In this example, the dark lines (large magnitudes of the variance) are further processed by thinning, to obtain single pixel lines before they are superimposed on the original image. This thinning or ridge finding method is discussed further below.

Performing derivative operations using kernels can be considered a template matching, or cross-correlation, process. The pattern of weights in the kernel is a template that gives the maximum response when it matches the pattern of brightness values in the image pixels. The number of different kernels used for derivative calculations indicates that there is no single best definition of what constitutes a boundary. Also, it might be helpful at

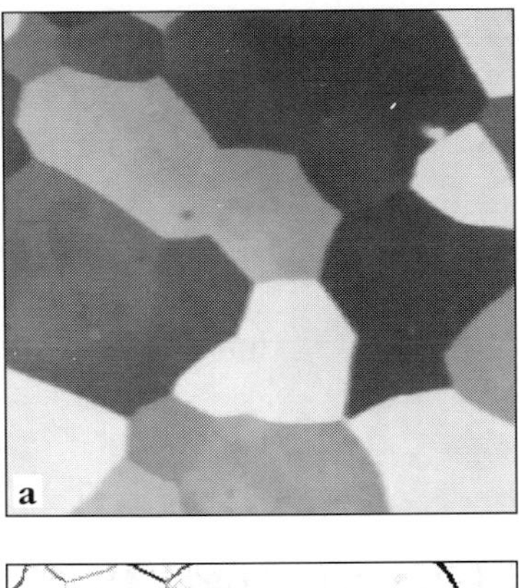

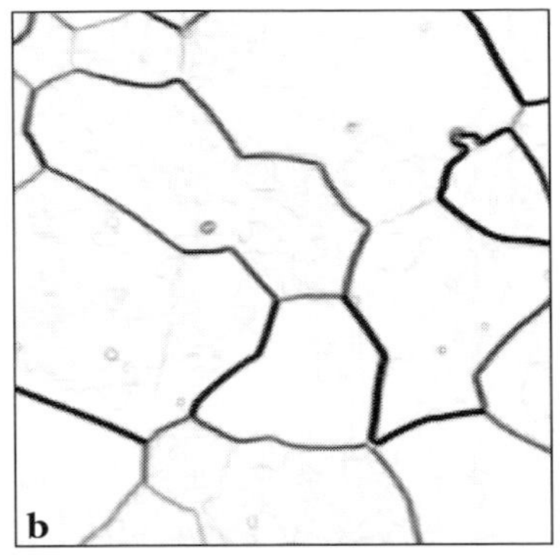

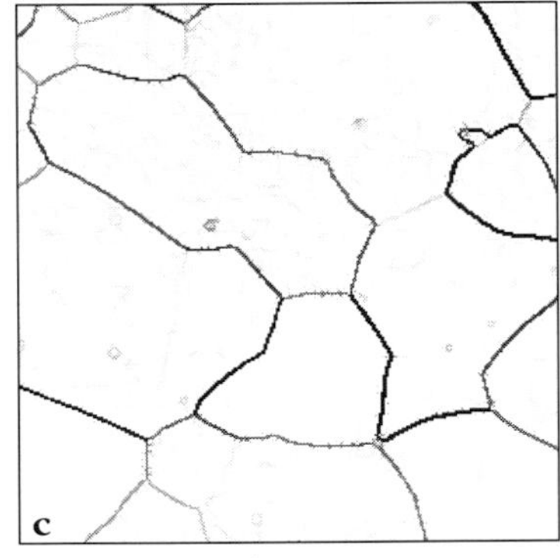

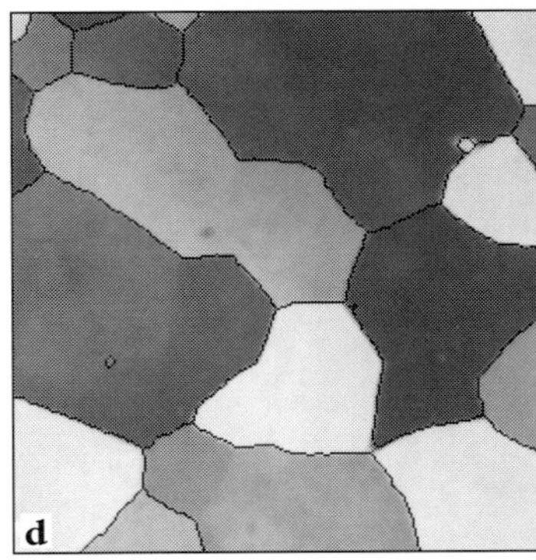

Figure 28. Delineating boundaries between grains:
a) *aluminum metal, polished and etched to show different grains (contrast arises from different crystallographic orientation of each grain, so that some boundaries have less contrast than others);*
b) *variance edge-finding algorithm applied to image a;*
c) *grey scale skeletonization (ridge finding) applied to image b (points not on a ridge are suppressed);*
d) *thresholding and skeletonization of the boundaries to a single line of pixels produces the grain boundaries, shown superimposed on the original image.*

the same time to look for other patterns that are not representative of an edge.

These ideas are combined in the Frei and Chen algorithm (1977), which applies a set of kernels to each point in the image. Each kernel extracts one kind of behavior in the image, only a few of which are indicative of the presence of an edge. For a 3×3 neighborhood region, the kernels, which are described as orthogonal or independent basis functions, are shown below.

number	kernel			number	kernel		
0	1	1	1	4	$\sqrt{2}$	−1	0
	1	1	1		−1	0	1
	1	1	1		0	1	$-\sqrt{2}$
1	−1	$-\sqrt{2}$	−1	5	0	1	0
	0	0	0		−1	0	1
	1	$\sqrt{2}$	1		0	−1	0
2	−1	0	1	6	−1	0	1
	$-\sqrt{2}$	0	$\sqrt{2}$		0	0	0
	−1	0	1		1	0	−1
3	0	−1	$\sqrt{2}$	7	1	−2	1
	1	0	−1		−2	4	−2
	$-\sqrt{2}$	1	0		1	−2	1
				8	−2	1	−2
					1	4	1
					−2	1	−2

Figure 29. ***Application of the Frei and Chen edge detector:***
a) *original (light microscope image of head louse);*
b) *result of Frei and Chen operator.*

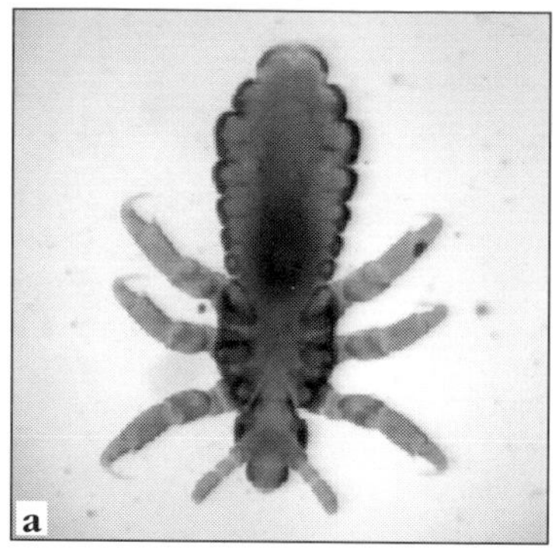

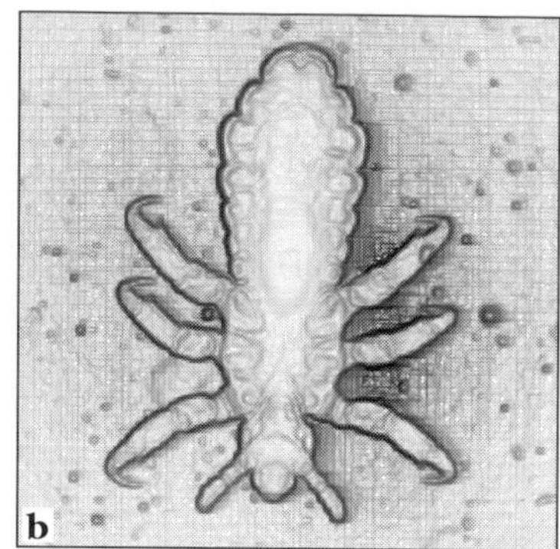

Only kernels 1 and 2 are considered to indicate the presence of an edge. The results of applying each kernel to each pixel are therefore summed to produce a ratio. The cosine of the square root of this value is effectively the vector projection of the information from the neighborhood in the direction of "edgeness," and is assigned to the pixel location in the derived image.

The advantage compared to more conventional edge detectors, such as the Sobel, is sensitivity to a configuration of relative pixel values independent of the magnitude of the brightness, which may vary from place to place in the image. **Figure 29** shows an example of the Frei and Chen operator. This may be compared to other edge-finding processing, shown in **Figures 30** through **31,** which apply some of the other operations discussed in this chapter to the same image.

The noise or blurring introduced by the other operations is evident, as is the ability of the Frei and Chen to reveal even the rather subtle edge information present in the original. **Figure 30** shows the application of a Laplacian operator, or high-pass filter, using different-sized kernels; **Figure 31** shows the difference of Gaussians, which is fundamentally similar. **Figure 32** shows the use of derivatives, including the Roberts' Cross and Sobel methods.

Rank operations

The neighborhood operations discussed in the preceding section use linear arithmetic operations to combine the values of various pixels. Another class of operators also using a neighborhood instead performs comparisons. In Chapter 2, the median filter was introduced. This sorts the pixels in a region into brightness order, finds the median value, and replaces the central pixel with that value. Used to remove noise from images, this operation completely eliminates extreme values from the image.

Rank operations also include the maximum and minimum operators, which find the brightest or darkest pixels in each neigh-

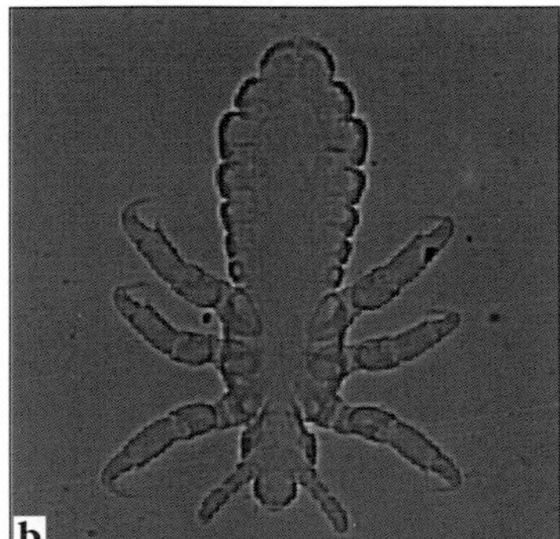
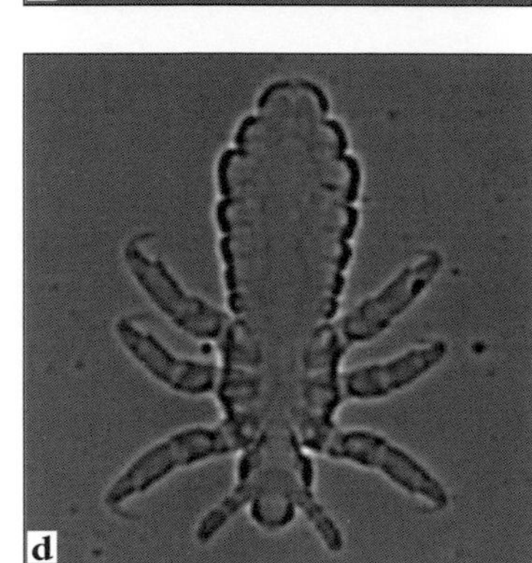

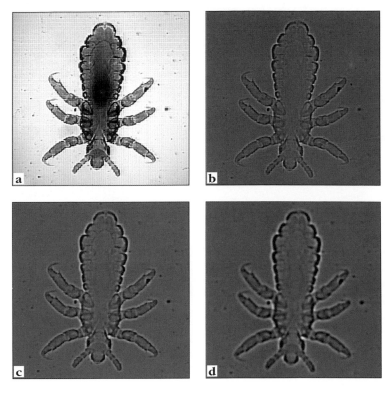

Figure 30. Application of Laplacian difference operations to the same image as in Figure 29:
a) *sharpening (addition of the 3×3 Laplacian to the original grey scale image);*
b) *5×5 Laplacian;*
c) *7×7 Laplacian;*
d) *9×9 Laplacian.*

borhood and place that value into the central pixel. By loose analogy to the erosion and dilation operations on binary images, which are discussed in Chapter 6, these are sometimes called grey scale erosion and dilation. The erosion effect of this ranking operation was demonstrated in Chapter 2, in the context of removing features from an image to produce a background for leveling.

One of the important variables in the use of a rank operator is the size of the neighborhood. Generally, shapes that are squares (for convenience of computation) or approximations to a circle (to minimize directional effects) are used. As the size of the neighborhood is increased, however, the computational effort in performing the ranking increases rapidly. Also, these ranking operations cannot be easily programmed into specialized hardware, such as array processors. In consequence, it is not common to use regions larger than those shown in **Figure 33.**

Several uses of rank operators are appropriate for image enhancement and the selection of one portion of the information present in an image. For example, the top hat operator (Bright & Steel, 1987) has been implemented in various ways, but can be described using two different-sized regions, as shown in **Figure 34.** If we assume that the goal of the operator is to find bright points, then the algorithm compares the maximum brightness value in a small central region to the maximum brightness value

Figure 31. Difference of Gaussians applied to the same image as Figure 29:
a) original image minus 3×3 Gaussian smooth;
b) difference between smoothing with σ = 0.625 and σ = 1.0 pixels;
c) difference between smoothing with σ = 1.6 and σ = 1.0 pixels;
d) difference between smoothing with σ = 4.1 and σ = 2.6 pixels.

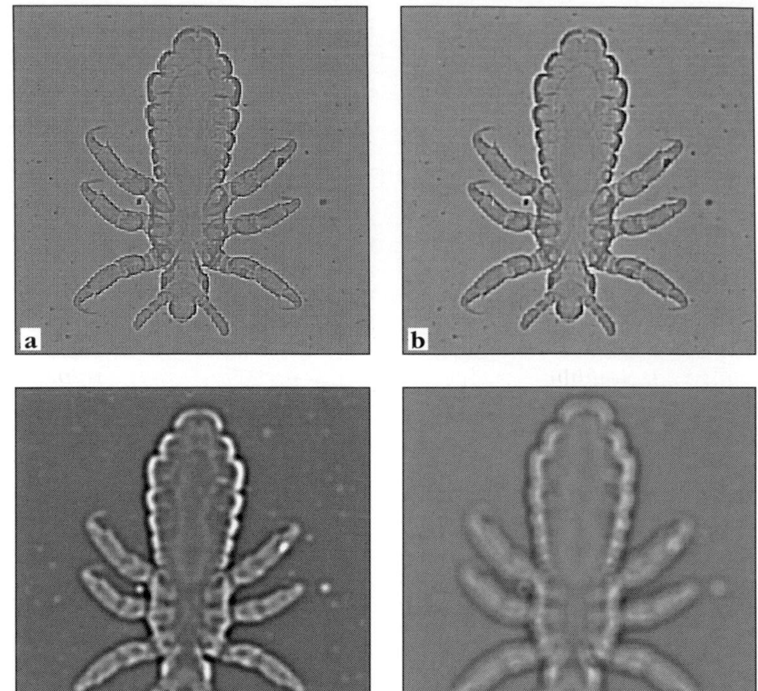

Figure 32. Derivative edge finding applied to the image from Figure 29:
a) single derivative (from the upper left);
b) brightest value at each point after applying two crossed derivatives;
c) Roberts' Cross operator;
d) Sobel operator.

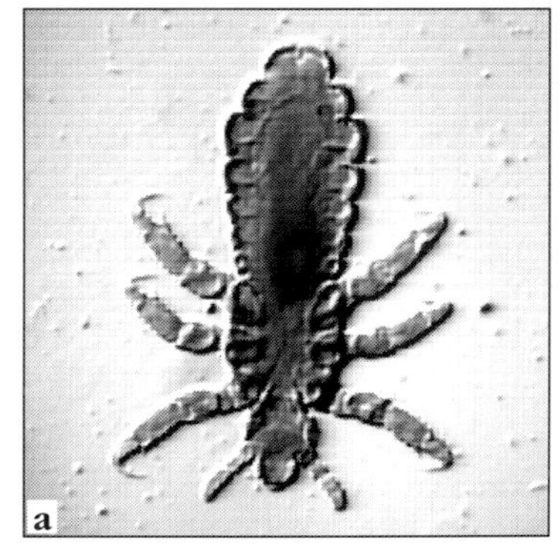

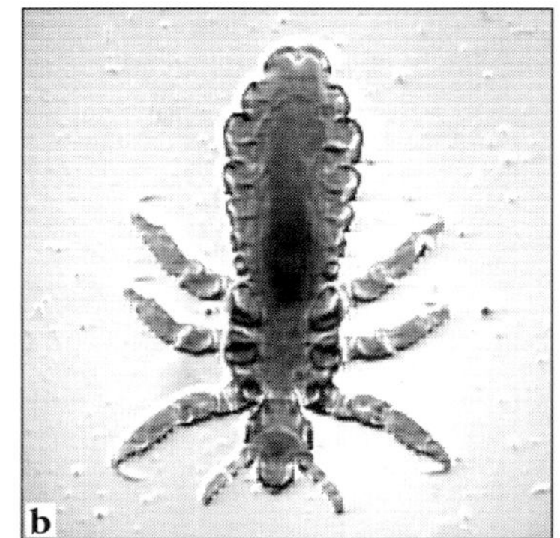

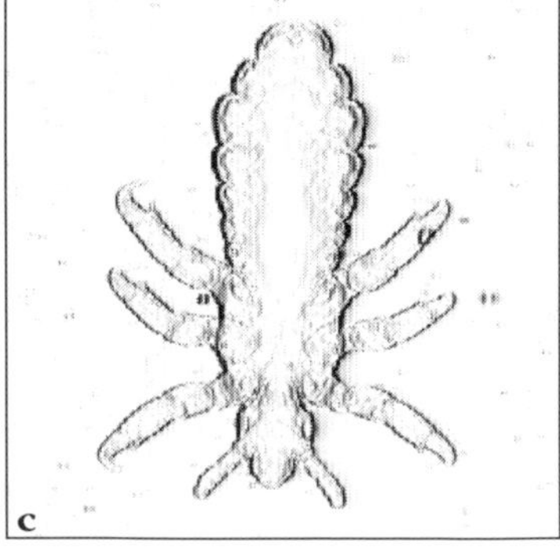

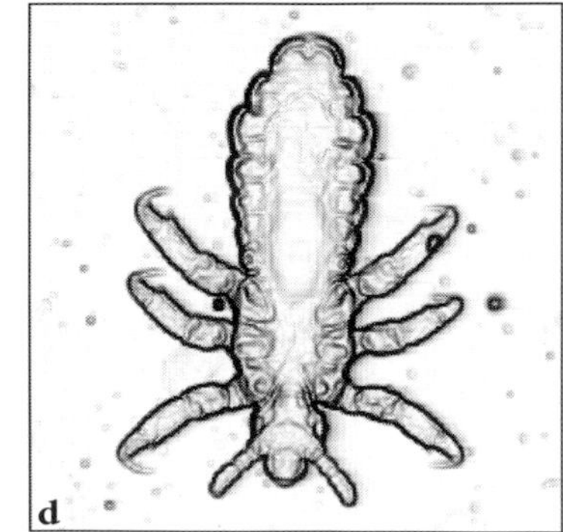

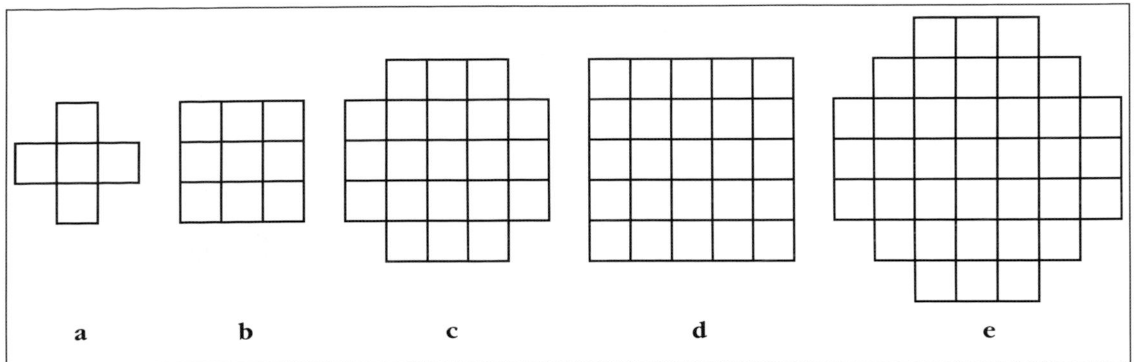

Figure 33. Neighborhood patterns used for ranking operations:
a) *4 nearest-neighbor cross;* ***b)*** *3×3 square containing nine pixels;*
c) *5×5 octagonal region with 21 pixels;* ***d)*** *5×5 square containing 25 pixels;*
e) *7×7 octagonal region containing 37 pixels.*

in a larger one. If the difference between these two values exceeds some arbitrary threshold, then the value of the central pixel is retained. Otherwise, it is removed.

Some systems contain specific programs to execute this algorithm, while others provide general-purpose ranking operations which can be combined to achieve this result. **Figure 35** shows the application of a top hat filter, in which the bright points in the diffraction pattern (calculated using a fast Fourier transform as discussed in Chapter 4) are retained and the overall variation in background brightness is suppressed. Performing the inverse transform on only the major points provides an averaged image, combining the repetitive information from many individually noisy atom images.

An equivalent result could be obtained by calculating two images from the original: one retaining the maximum brightness value in a 5-pixel-wide octagonal region and the second doing the same for just the central pixel and its 4 edge-touching neighbors. Subtracting one from the other gives the difference between the maxima in the two regions. Next, thresholding to select only those points with a value greater than 12 would apply the same arbitrary threshold used in **Figure 35.**

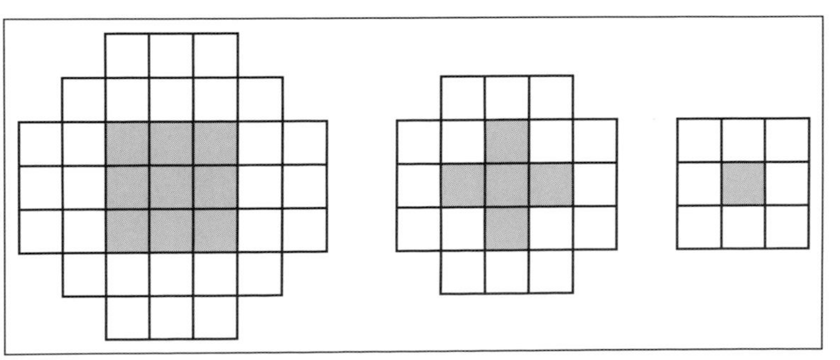

Figure 34. *Neighborhood patterns used for a top hat filter. The brightest value in the outer (white) region is subtracted from the brightest value in the inner (shaded) region. If the difference exceeds a threshold, then the central pixel is kept. Otherwise it is erased.*

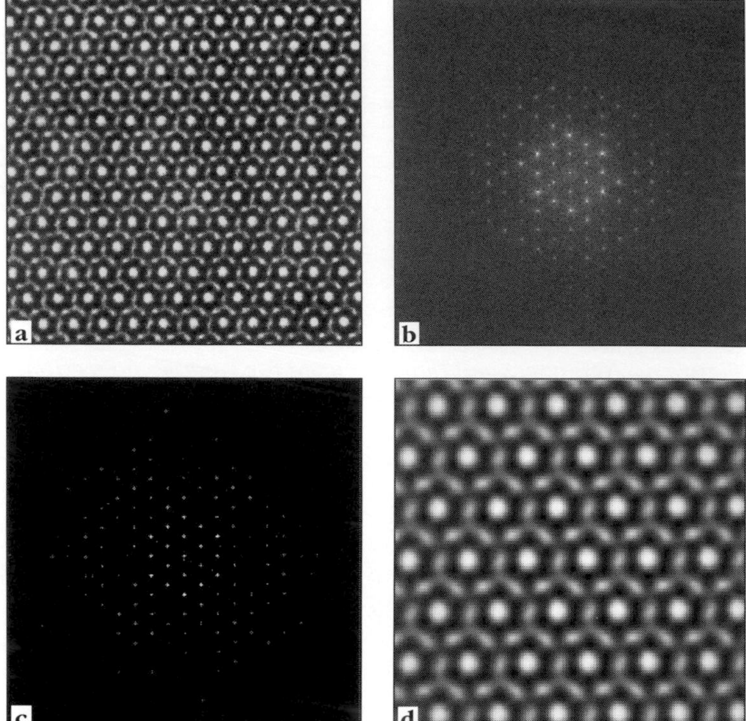

Figure 35. Application of a top hat filter to select points in a diffraction pattern:
a) *high-resolution TEM image of silicon nitride, showing atomic positions;*
b) *FFT magnitude image calculated from image a;*
c) *application of a top hat filter to image b, selecting the locally bright points on a nonuniform background;*
d) *inverse transform using only the points selected in image c, enlarged to show detail.*

The top hat filter is basically a point finder. The size of the point is defined by the smaller of the two neighborhood regions and may be as small as a single pixel in some cases. The larger region defines the local background, which the points of interest must exceed in brightness. Unlike the Laplacian, though, which subtracts the average value of the surrounding background from the central point, the top hat method finds the maximum brightness in the larger region (the "brim" of the hat) and subtracts that from the brightest point in the interior region. If the difference exceeds some arbitrary threshold (the "height" of the hat's crown), then the central pixel is kept.

In a sketch depicting the operation of the algorithm, the brim rests on the data and the point that pokes through the top of the hat is kept. If the central region is larger than a single pixel, though, this depiction is not quite accurate. When any of the points in the central region exceeds the brim value, the central pixel value (which may not be the bright one) is kept. This may produce small haloes around single bright points that are smaller than the central neighborhood region. However, any bright point that is part of a feature larger than the central region will not be found by the top hat filter.

Of course, it should be noted that some images have features of interest that are darker, rather than lighter, than their surroundings. The logic of the top hat filter works just as well when it is

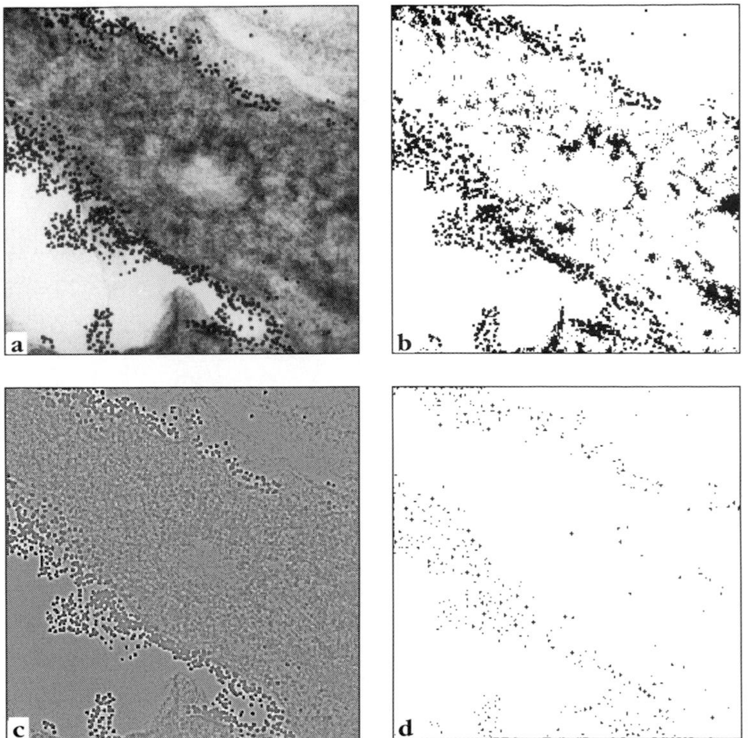

Figure 36. Application of a top hat filter:

a) *TEM image of Golgi stained rat skeletal muscles, with gold particles (dark) on variable background;*

b) *thresholding of image a selects dark pixels, but cannot isolate the particles;*

c) *unsharp masking, produced by subtracting a smoothed version of the image from the original;*

d) *the top hat filter finds (most of) the particles in spite of the variation in the background.*

inverted and darkness, rather than lightness, is the test criterion. **Figure 36** shows such a case, in which the small (and quite uniformly sized) dark features are gold particles in Golgi stained muscle tissue. In this example, simply thresholding the dark particles does not work, because other parts of the image are just as dark. Similarly, a method such as unsharp masking, accomplished in the example by subtracting the average value (using a Gaussian smoothing filter with a standard deviation of 0.6 pixels) from the original, produces an image in which the particles are quite visible to a human viewer, but are still not distinguishable to a computer program.

It is possible to apply a top hat filter to one-dimensional data. The method is sometimes used, for instance, to select peaks in spectra. **Figure 37** shows an example. The brim of the hat rests on the profile and in only a few places does the plot poke through the crown. Peaks that are too low, too broad, or adjacent to others are not detected.

It is also possible, in principle, to design a top hat filter that is not circularly symmetrical, but has regions shaped to select particular features of interest–even lines. Of course, the orientation of the feature must match that of the filter, so this is not a very general operation. When features with a well-defined shape and orientation are sought, cross-correlation in either the spatial or frequency domain is generally more appropriate.

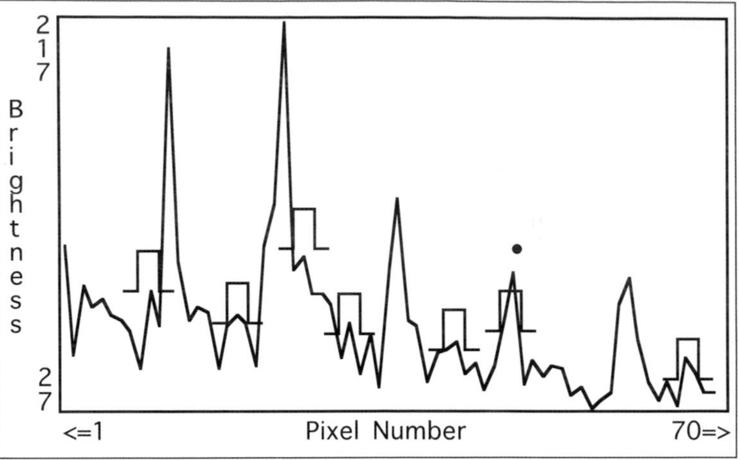

Figure 37. *Diagram of application of the top hat filter to one-dimensional data (a brightness profile from the diffraction pattern in Figure 34). Several placements of the filter are shown. In only one (marked •) does the central value exceed the threshold.*

A close relative of the top hat filter is the rolling ball filter. Instead of selecting points that exceed the local background, this filter eliminates them, replacing those pixel values with the neighborhood value. This is most easily described for an image in whose noise pixels are dark. The filter's name suggests an analogy to placing a ball on the image, again visualized as a surface in which elevation at each point is the brightness of the pixel.

As the ball rolls on the surface, it is in contact with several pixels. An outer, large neighborhood and an inner, smaller one, both approximately circular, define the contact points by their minimum (darkest) values. The permitted difference value is a function of the radius of the ball. Any point that is darker and corresponds to points that the ball cannot touch is considered to be a noise point; its value is replaced with the darkest value in the inner region. Again, while the description here uses dark points as the targets to be removed, it is straightforward to reverse the logic and remove bright noise points.

The top hat filter is an example of a suppression operator. It removes pixels from the image if they do not meet some criteria of being "interesting" and leaves alone those pixels that do. Another operator of this type, which locates lines rather than points, is variously known as ridge-finding or grey scale skeletonization (by analogy to skeletonization of binary images, discussed in Chapter 6). We have already seen a number of edge-finding and gradient operators that produce bright or dark lines along boundaries. These lines are often wider than a single pixel and it may be desirable to reduce them to a minimum width.

The ridge-finding algorithm suppresses pixels (by reducing their value to zero) if they are not part of the center ridge of the line. This is defined as any pixel whose value is less than all of its 8 neighbors, or whose 8 touching neighbors have a single maxi-

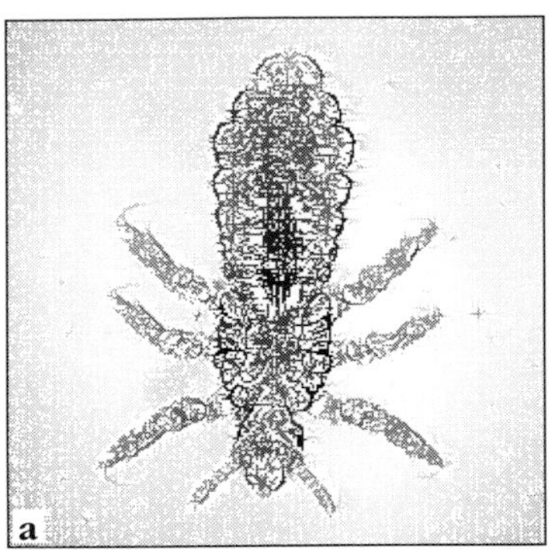

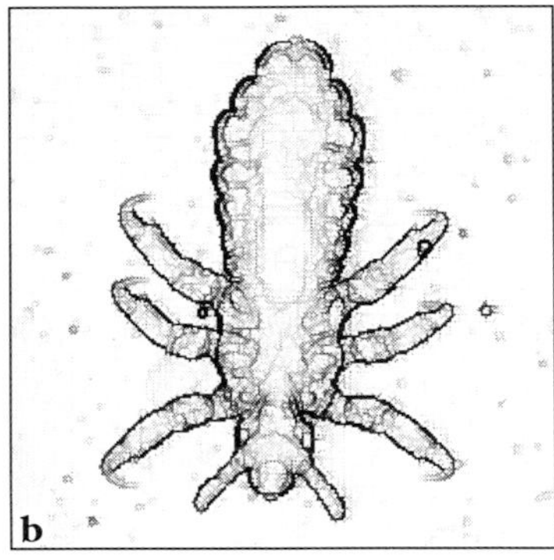

Figure 38. Grey scale skeletonization (ridge finding):
a) *applied to the original image in Figure 29;*
b) *applied to the edge image produced by the Sobel operator shown in Figure 3.*

mum that is greater than the pixel. **Figure 38** shows an example of the application of this operator to the image of the head louse in **Figure 29** and to the edges derived from that image in **Figure 32.** In both cases, the reduction of lines to single pixel width is accompanied by many smaller lines radiating from the principal ridge.

Figure 39 shows the direct application of ridge finding to an image of axons, which appear in the light microscope as dark outlines. Here, the grey scale skeleton of the outlines is converted to a binary image by thresholding (Chapter 5) and then reduced to a single line by binary image skeletonization (Chapter 6). The resulting image is then suitable for feature measurement, shown in **Figure 39d** by grey scale labeling of each feature.

Many structures are best characterized by a continuous network, or tesselation, of boundaries. **Figure 40** shows an example, a ceramic containing grains of two different compositions (the dark grains are alumina and the light ones zirconia). The grains are easily distinguishable by the viewer, but it is the grain boundaries that are important for measurement to characterize the structure–and not just the boundaries between light and dark grains, but also those between light and light or dark and dark grains.

Figure 41 shows the applicaton of various edge-finding operators to this image. In this case, the variance produces the best boundary demarcation, without including too many extraneous lines due to the texture within the grains. Thresholding this image (as discussed in Chapter 5) and processing the binary image (as discussed in Chapter 6) to thin the lines to single pixel width produces an image of only the boundaries, as shown in **Figure 42.** It is then possible to use the brightness of the pixels in the original image to classify each grain as either *a* or *b*. Images of only those boundaries lying between *a* and *a*, *b* and *b*, or *a* and *b* can then be obtained (as shown in the figure and discussed in Chapter 6). It is also possible to count the number of neighbors

Figure 39. Converting boundaries to features:
a) *axons seen in cross section in a light microscope section;*
b) *grey scale skeletonization of image a;*
c) *binary skeletonization and pruning of image b;*
d) *features within closed outlines of image c.*

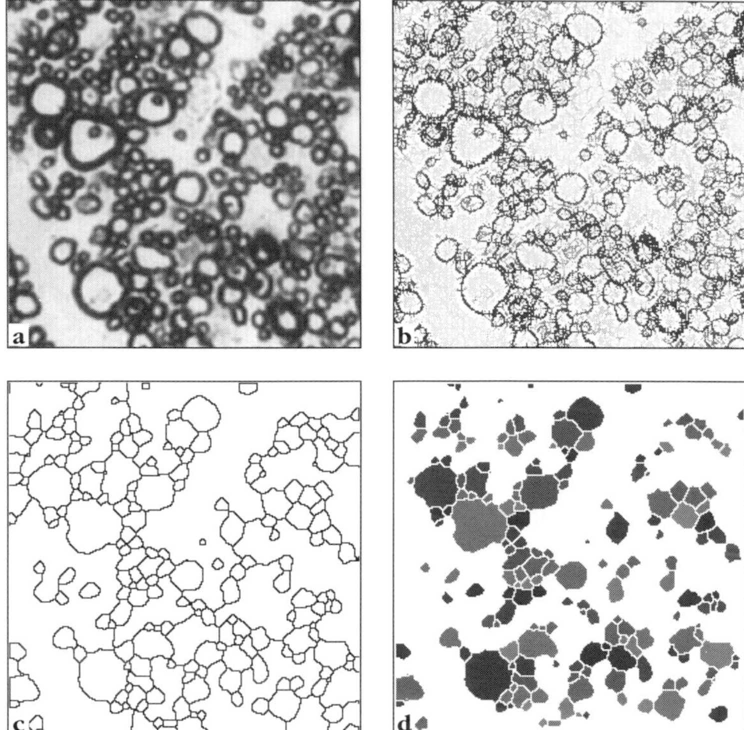

around each grain and use a color or grey scale to code them, as shown in **Figure 43.** This goes beyond the usual scope of image processing, however, and into the realm of image measurement and analysis.

Figure 40. *SEM image of thermally etched alumina-zirconia multiphase ceramic. The two phases are easily distinguished by brightness, but the boundaries between two light or two dark regions are not. (Image courtesy of Dr. K. B. Alexander, Oak Ridge National Labs, Oak Ridge, TN.)*

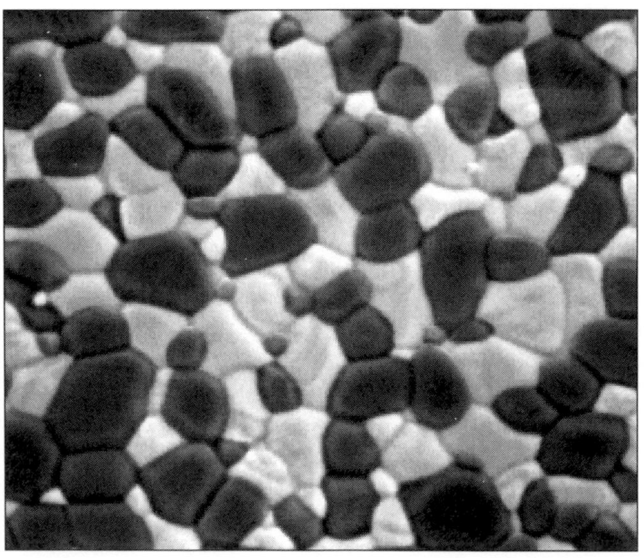

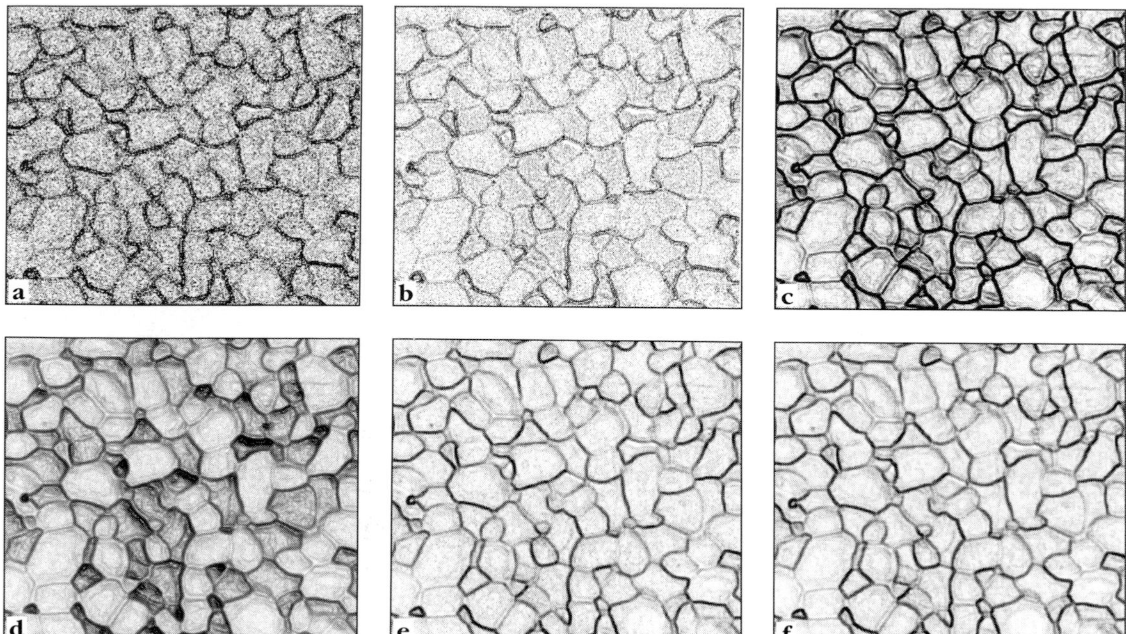

Figure 41. Processing of Figure 39 to enhance edges (all operations performed on 3×3 neighborhood regions):
a) *absolute value of the Laplacian;*
b) *absolute value of the difference between original and Gaussian smooth;*
c) *Sobel gradient operator;*
d) *Frei and Chen edge operator;*
e) *variance operator;*
f) *range operator.*

Texture

Many images contain regions characterized not so much by a unique value of brightness, but by a variation in brightness, often called texture. This is a somewhat loosely defined term that refers to the local variation in brightness from one pixel to the next or within a small region. If the brightness is interpreted as elevation in a representation of the image as a surface, then the texture is a measure of the surface roughness, another term without an accepted or universal quantitative meaning.

Rank operations are also used to detect this texture in images. One of the simplest (but least versatile) of the texture operators is simply the range or difference between maximum and minimum brightness values in the neighborhood. For a flat or uniform region, the range is small. Larger values of the range correspond to surfaces with a larger roughness. The size of the neighborhood region must be large enough to include dark and light pixels, which generally means being larger than any small uniform details that may be present. **Figure 44** shows an example.

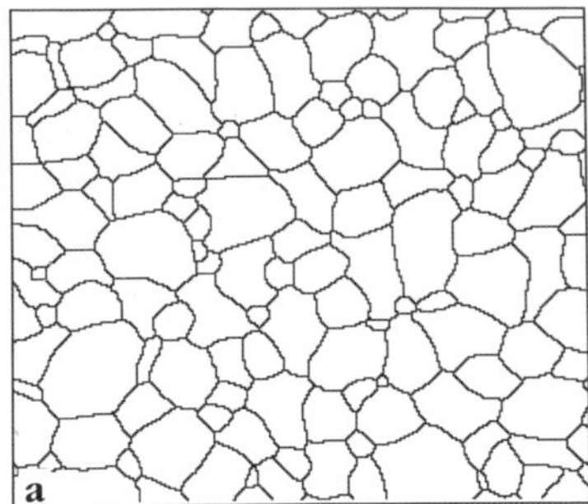

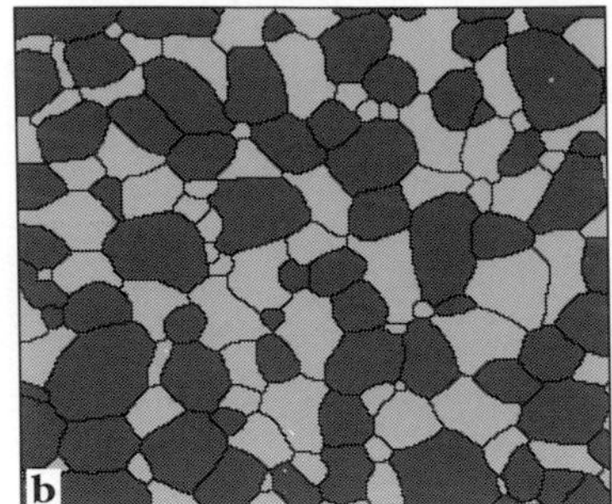

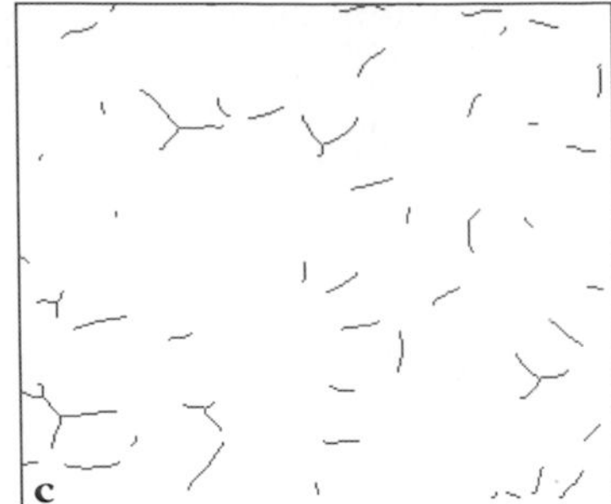

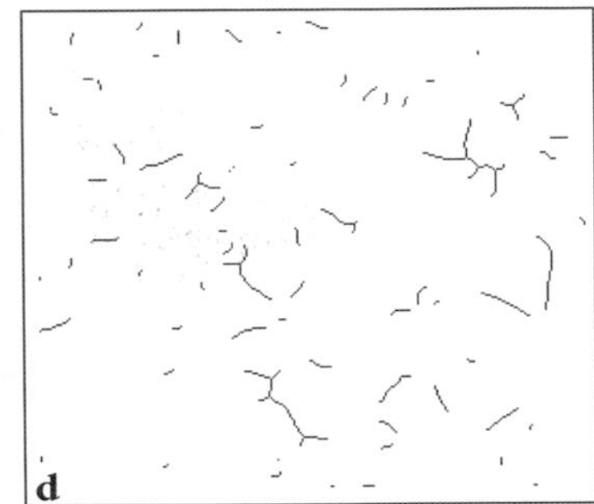

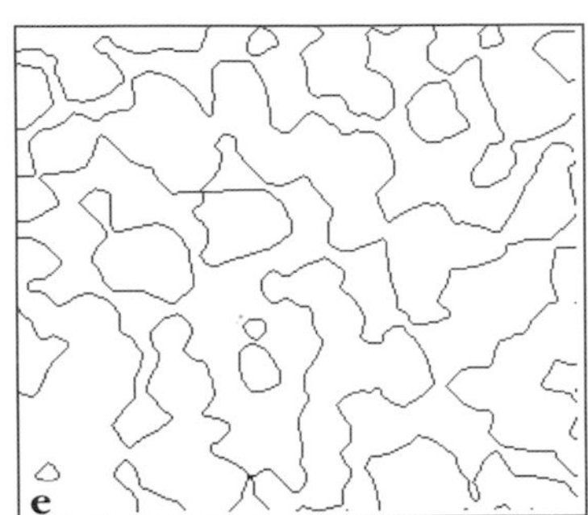

Figure 42. Grain boundary images derived from the variance image in Figure 40e by thresholding and skeletonization:

a) *boundaries between the grains;*

b) *grains grey scale coded to show phase identification;*

c) *only those boundaries between two dark (alumina) grains, making up 16.2% of the total;*

d) *only those boundaries between two light (zirconia) grains, making up 15.2% of the total;*

e) *only those boundaries between a light and dark grain, making up 68.6% of the total boundary.*

The range operator converts the original image to one in which brightness represents the texture, the original feature brightness is gone, and different structural regions may be distinguished by the range brightness. As shown in **Figure 45,** the range operator also responds to the boundaries between regions that are of different average brightness and is sometimes used as an edge-defining algorithm. Comparison to other edge-finding methods discussed in this chapter shows that the Sobel and Frei and Chen are superior, but the range operation requires no arithmetic and is very fast.

Another estimator of texture is the variance in neighborhood regions. This is the sum of the squares of the differences between the brightness of the central pixel and its neighbors. Because the value can become quite large, the result is sometimes displayed as the square root of this difference. If the sum of squares is first normalized by dividing by the number of pixels in the neigh-

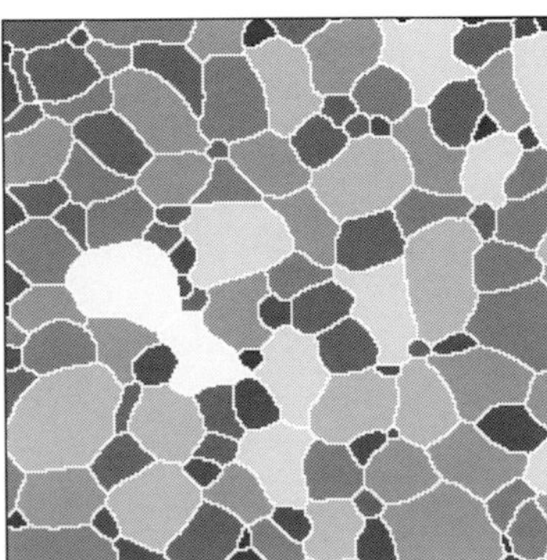

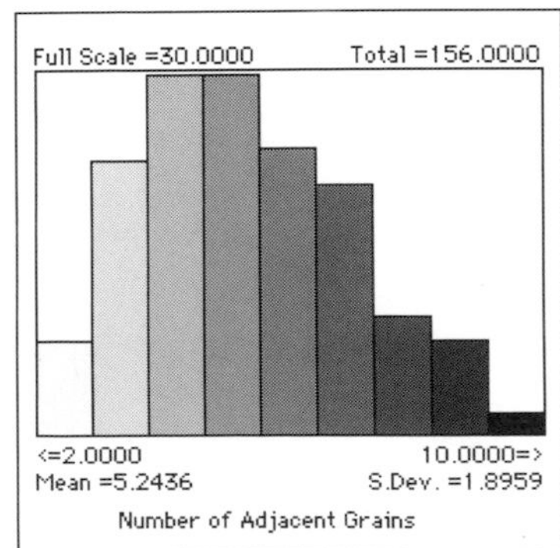

Figure 43. *The grains from Figure 42 grey scale coded to show the number of neighbors touching each, and a plot of the frequency of each number of neighbors. Further analysis shows that both the size and the number of neighbor plots are different for the two different phases.*

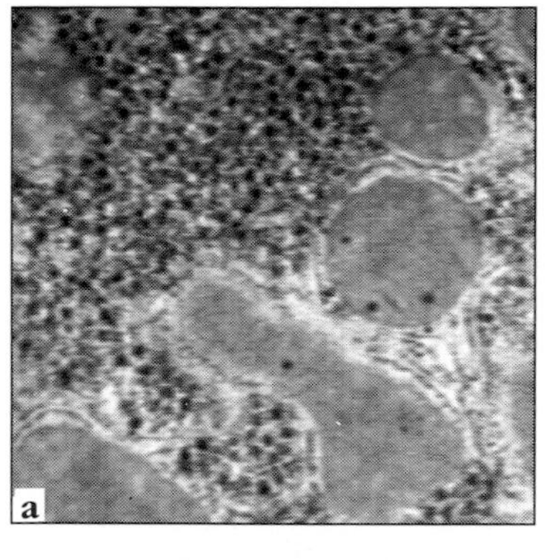

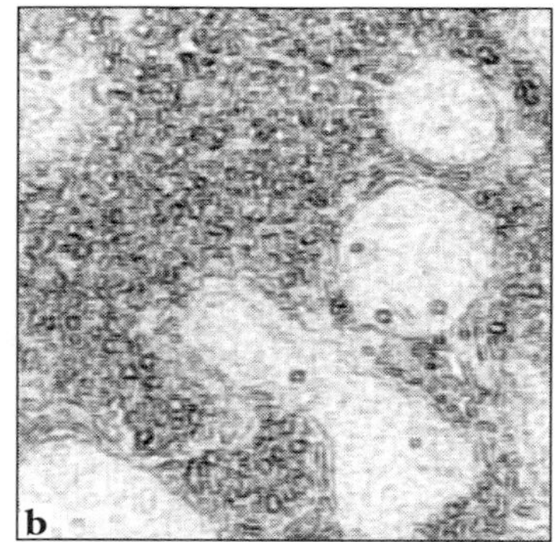

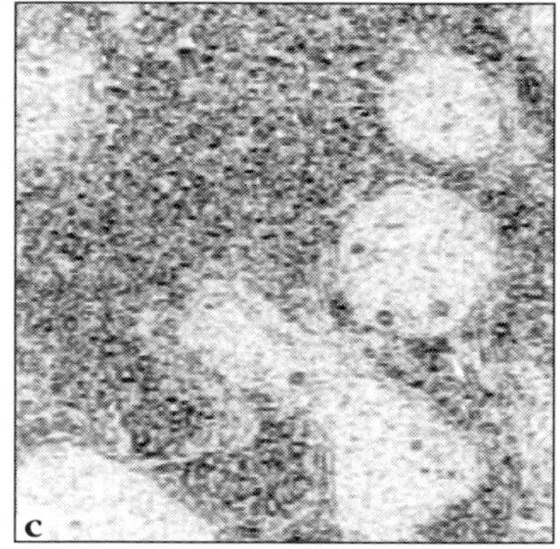

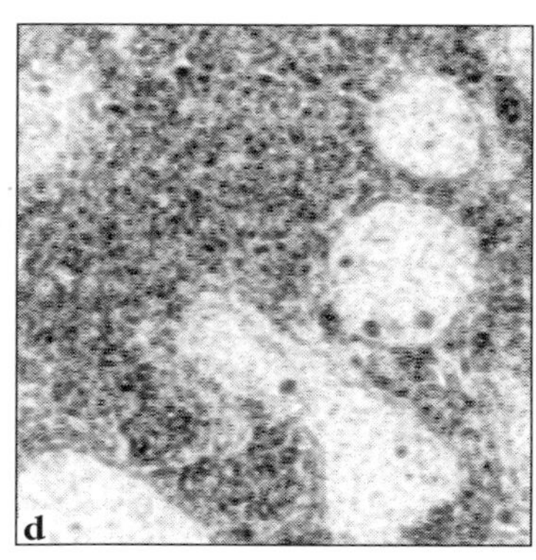

Figure 44. Enhancement of texture:

a) *transmission electron microscope image of liver thin section;*

b) *range image (difference between maximum and minimum brightness values in a 3×3 neighborhood);*

c) *root-mean-square (RMS) image (square root of the sum of squares of differences between the central pixel and its neighbors in a 3×3 neighborhood);*

d) *RMS image using a 5-pixel-wide octagonal neighborhood.*

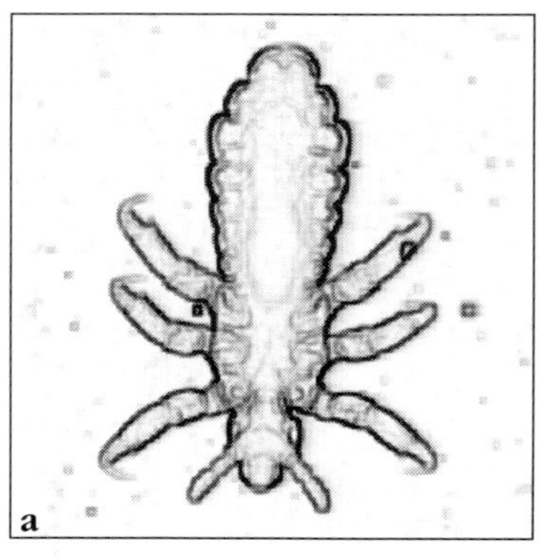

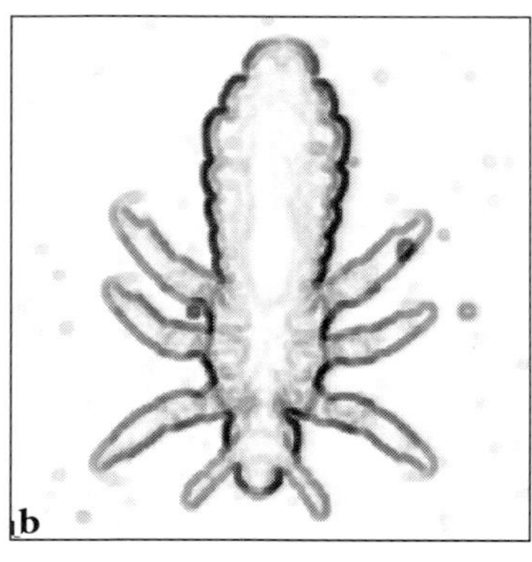

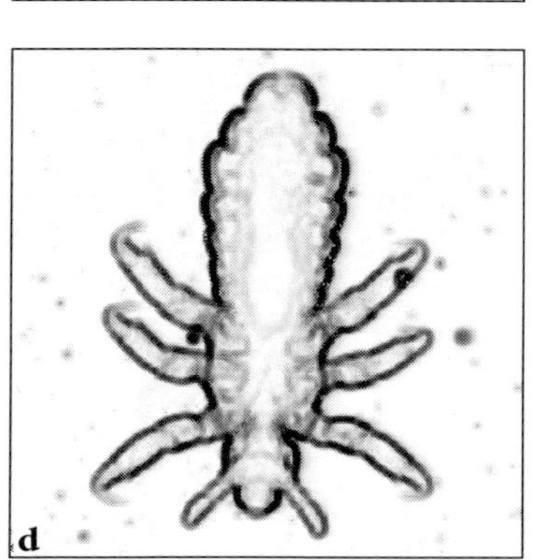

Figure 45. Application of range and variance operators to the same image as in Figure 29:

a) *range (3×3 neighborhood);*

b) *range (5-pixel-wide octagonal neighborhood);*

c) *variance (3×3 neighborhood);*

d) *variance (5-pixel-wide octagonal neighborhood).*

Figure 46. ***Application of Haralick texture operators to the image in Figure 44:***
a) *3×3 neighborhood;*
b) *5×5 neighborhood.*

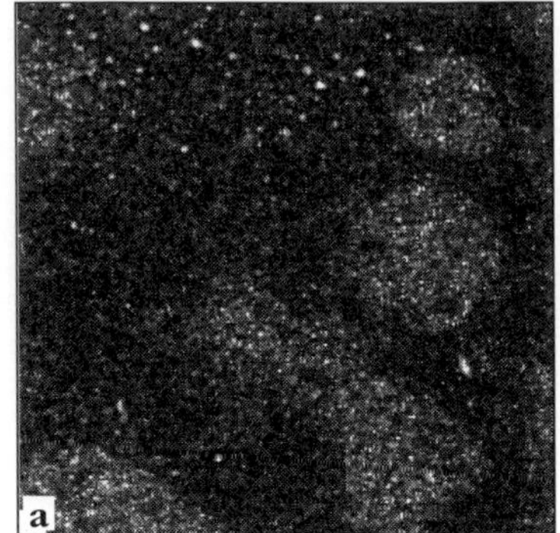

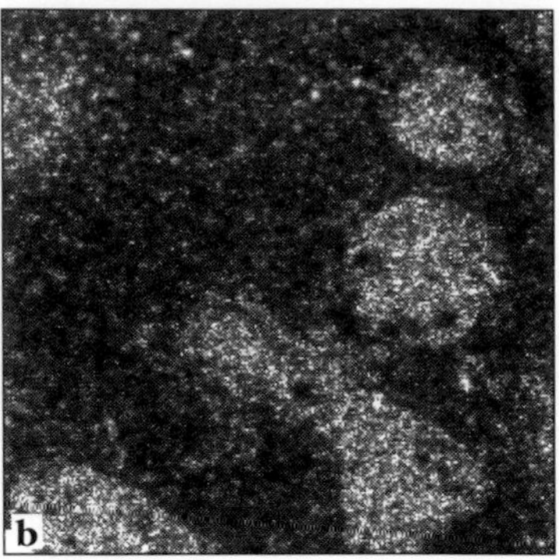

borhood, this is just the root-mean-square (RMS) difference of values and corresponds to a similar RMS measure of roughness for surfaces.

Like the range, the variance also responds to the variation of pixels in the region. It is less sensitive to the individual extreme pixel values and produces an image with less noise than the range operator. **Figures 41** and **45** show the comparison between applying the RMS operator with a 3×3 pixel neighborhood and the range operator with a 5-pixel-wide octagonal neighborhood. Like the range operator, the variance also responds to boundaries between regions of different brightnesses and is sometimes used as an edge detector.

Satellite images are especially appropriate for characterization by texture operators. Categorization of crops, construction, and other land uses produce distinctive textures that humans can recognize. Therefore, methods have been sought that duplicate this capability in software algorithms. In a classic paper on the subject, Haralick listed 14 such texture operators that utilize pixels within a region and assess their brightness differences (Haralick et al., 1973). This region is not a neighborhood around each pixel, but comprises all of the pixels within a contiguous block delineated by some boundary or other identifying brightness, etc. A table is constructed with the number of adjacent pixel pairs within the region as a function of their brightnesses. This pixel table is then used to calculate the texture parameters.

In the expressions below, the array $P(i,j)$ contains the number of nearest-neighbor pixel pairs (in 90-degree directions only) whose brightnesses are i and j, respectively. R is a renormalizing constant equal to the total number of pixel pairs in the image or any rectangular portion used for the calculation. In principle, this can be extended to pixel pairs that are separated by a distance d and to pairs aligned in the 45-degree direction (whose separation distance is greater than ones in the 90-degree directions). The summations are carried out for all pixel pairs in the region. Haralick applied this to rectangular regions, but it is equally applicable to pixels within irregular outlines.

The first parameter shown is a measure of homogeneity using a second moment. Since the terms are squared, a few large differences will contribute more than many small ones. The second one shown is a difference moment, which is a measure of the contrast in the image. The third is a measure of the linear dependency of brightness in the image, obtained by correlation.

$$f_1 = \sum_{i=1}^{N} \sum_{j=1}^{N} \left(\frac{P(i,j)}{R} \right)^2$$

$$f_2 = \sum_{n=0}^{N-1} n^2 \left\{ \sum_{|i-j|=n} \left(\frac{P(i,j)}{R} \right) \right\}$$

$$f_3 = \frac{\sum_{i=1}^{N} \sum_{j=1}^{N} \{ i \cdot j \cdot P(i,j) / R \} - \mu_x \cdot \mu_y}{\sigma_x \cdot \sigma_y}$$

In these expressions, N is the number of grey levels, and μ and σ are the mean and standard deviation, respectively, of the distributions of brightness values accumulated in the x and y directions. Additional parameters describe the variance, entropy, and information measure of brightness value correlation. Haralick has shown that when applied to large rectangular areas in satellite photos, these parameters can distinguish water from grassland, different sandstones from each other, and woodland from marsh or urban regions.

Some of these operators are obviously easier than others to calculate for all of the pixels in an image. The resulting values can be scaled to create a useful derived image that can be discriminated with thresholds. In any given instance, it sometimes requires experimentation with several texture operators to find the one that gives the best separation between the features of interest and their surroundings.

Some of these same operations can be applied to individual pixels to produce a new image, in which the brightness is proportional to the local texture. **Figure 46** illustrates the use of the Haralick angular second moment operator (f_2 above) applied to 3×3 and 5×5 pixel neighborhoods centered on each pixel to calculate a texture value, which is then assigned to the pixel. This result can be compared to **Figure 44.**

Fractal analysis

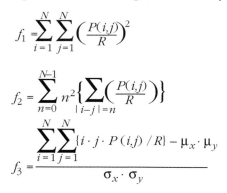

The characterization of surface roughness by a fractal dimension has been applied to fracture surfaces, wear and erosion, corrosion, etc. (Mandelbrot et al., 1984; Underwood & Banerji, 1986; Mecholsky & Passoja, 1985; Mecholsky et al., 1986, 1989; Srinivasan et al., 1991; Fahmy et al., 1991). It has also been shown (Pentland, 1983; Peleg et al., 1984) that the brightness pattern in images of fractal surfaces is also mathematically a fractal and that this also holds for SEM images (Russ, 1990a). A particularly effi-

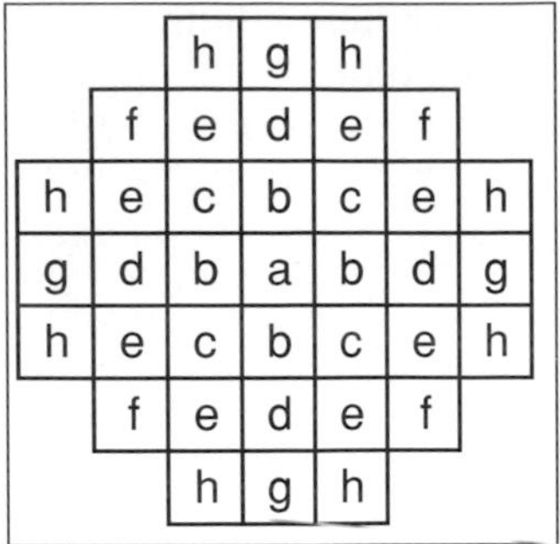

Figure 47. *Octagonal 7-pixel-wide neighborhood (37 pixels total) used for local rescaled-range (Hurst coefficient) calculation. Pixel labels identify groups with the same distance from the central pixel.*

cient method for computing the fractal dimension of surfaces from elevation images is the Hurst coefficient, or rescaled range analysis (Hurst et al., 1965; Feder, 1988; Russ, 1990c). This procedure plots the greatest difference in brightness (or elevation, etc.) between points along a linear traverse of the image or surface as a function of the search distance, on log-log axes. When the range is scaled by dividing by the standard deviation of the data, the slope of the resulting line is directly related to the fractal dimension of the profile.

Performing such an operation at the pixel level is interesting, because it may permit local classification that can be of use for image segmentation. Processing an image so that each pixel value is converted to a new brightness scale indicating local roughness (in the sense of a Hurst coefficient) permits segmentation by simple brightness thresholding. It uses two-dimensional information on the brightness variation, compared to the one-dimensional comparison used in measuring brightness profiles.

Figure 47 shows a neighborhood region consisting of 37 pixels in a 7-pixel-wide octagonal shape. The size is a compromise between the desire to include many pixel values (for accurate results) and the need for fast calculation. Qualitatively similar results are obtained with 5-, 9-, and 11-pixel-wide regions. Unlike some neighborhood operators, such as smoothing kernels, the use of progressively larger neighborhood regions for the Hurst operator does not select information with different dimensions or scales in the image. Instead, it increases the precision of the fit and reduces the noise introduced by individual light or dark pixels–at least up to a region size as large as the defined structures in the image.

Each of the pixels in the diagram of **Figure 47** is labeled to indicate its distance from the center of the octagon. The distances (in pixel units) and the number of pixels at each distance are listed in **Table 1.** The distances range from 1 pixel (the 4 touching neighbors sharing a side with the central pixel) to 3.162 pixels ($\sqrt{10} = \sqrt{(3 \cdot 3 + 1 \cdot 1}$).

Application of the operator proceeds by examining the pixels in the neighborhood around each pixel in the original image. The brightest and darkest pixel values in each of the distance classes are found and their difference used to construct a Hurst plot.

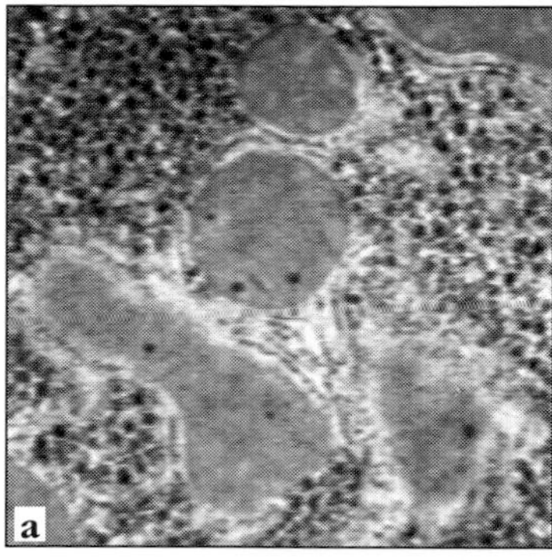
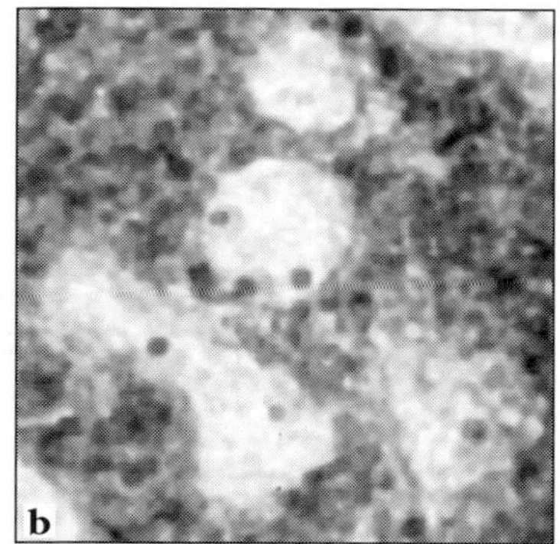
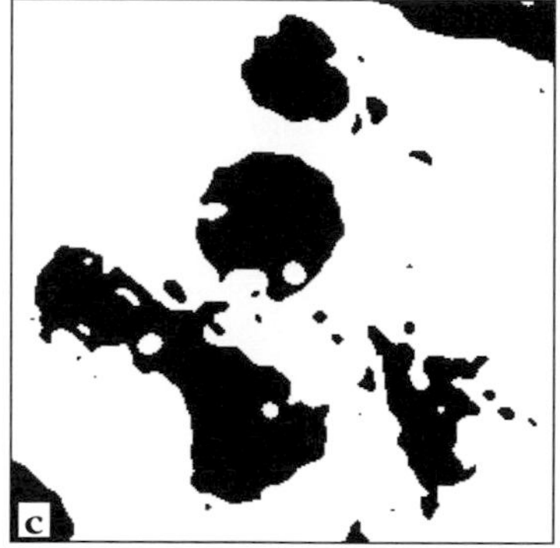
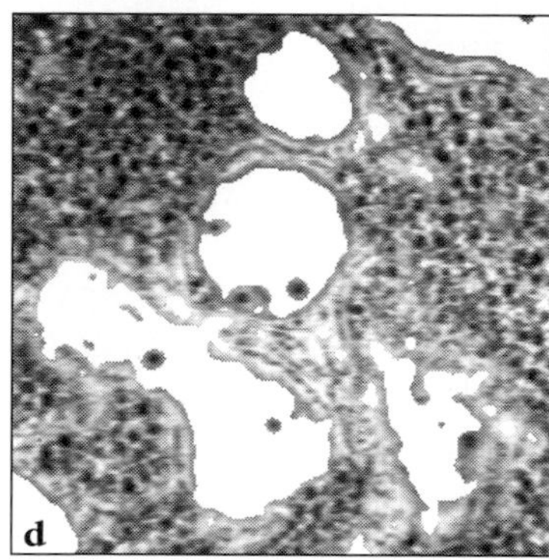

Figure 48. Segmentation based on texture using a Hurst operator:
a) *liver (transmission electron micrograph of thin section);*
b) *Hurst transform image;*
c) *thresholded binary from image b;*
d) *high-texture regions in original using image c as a mask.*

Table 1. Distance of pixels labeled in Figure 47 from the center of the neighborhood.

Pixel class	Number	Distance from center
a	1	0
b	4	1
c	4	1.414 (√2)
d	4	2
e	8	2.236 (√5)
f	4	2.828 (√8)
g	4	3
h	8	3.162 (√10)

Performing a least-squares fit of the slope of the log (brightness difference) vs. log (distance) relationship is simplified because the distance values (and their logarithms) are unvarying and can be stored beforehand in a short table. It is also unnecessary to divide by the standard deviation of pixel brightnesses in the image, since this is a constant for each pixel in the image and the slope of the Hurst plot will be arbitrarily scaled to fit the brightness range of the display anyway.

Building the sums for the least-squares fit and performing the necessary calculations is moderately complex. Hence, it is time consuming compared to simple neighborhood operations such as smoothing, etc., but still well within the capability of typical desktop computer systems. Unfortunately, the comparison operations involved in this operator do not lend themselves to array processors or other specific hardware solutions.

Figure 48a shows a portion of a TEM of a thin section of liver tissue, used in **Figures 44** and **46.** The image contains many dif-

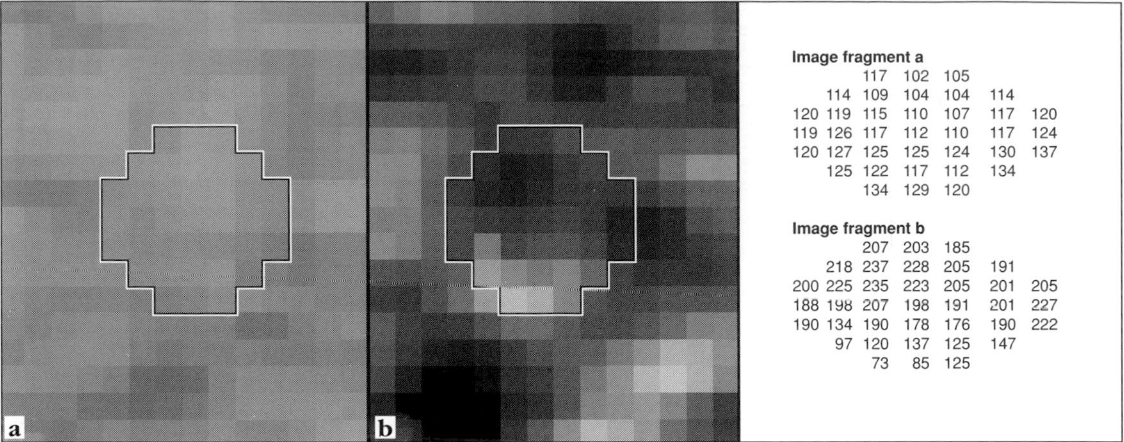

Figure 49. *Enlarged portions of smooth (a) and rough (b) areas of Figure 46a, showing individual pixels in representative 7-pixel-wide octagonal neighborhoods with the numerical values of the pixels (0 = white, 255 = black).*

ferent structures at the organelle level, but for classification purposes the large, relatively uniform grey regions and the much more highly textured regions containing many small dark particles can be distinguished visually. Unfortunately, the average brightness level of the two areas is not sufficiently different to permit direct thresholding (discussed in Chapter 5). There are many pixels in the highly textured region that are brighter, the same, or darker than the average grey level of the smooth region. The conversion of the original image to one whose texture information permits thresholding of the regions is shown in the figure.

Figure 49 shows highly magnified images of two representative locations in each of these regions, with outlines showing specific locations of the octagonal neighborhood of **Figure 47** and the brightness values of those pixels. The convention for pixel values in these 8-bit monochrome images is white = 0, black = 255. Sorting through the pixels in each distance class, finding the brightest and darkest and their difference, and constructing a plot of log (brightness range) vs. log (distance) is shown for these two specific pixel locations in **Table 2** and **Figure 50.** Notice that the slopes of the Hurst plots are quite different and that the lines fit the points rather well as shown by the r-squared values.

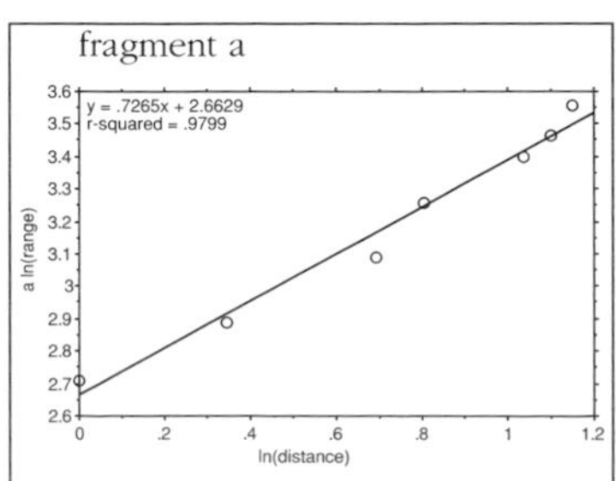

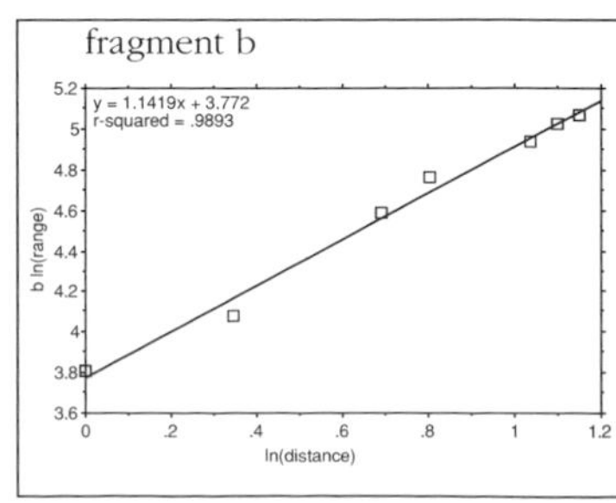

Figure 50. *Hurst plots of the logarithm of the maximum brightness range vs. log of distance for the two neighborhoods shown in Figure 48.*

Table 2. Distance and brightness data for the neighborhoods in Figure 49.

Distance (pixels)	1	√2	2	√5	√8	3	√10
Image fragment a							
brightest	110	107	104	104	104	102	102
darkest	125	125	126	130	134	134	137
range	15	18	21	26	30	32	35
Image fragment b							
brightest	178	176	137	120	97	85	73
darkest	223	235	235	237	237	237	237
range	45	59	98	117	140	152	159

Scaling the Hurst values to the brightness range of an image (in this example by multiplying arbitrarily by 64) and applying the operation to each pixel in the image produces the result shown in **Figure 48b. Figures 48c** and **48d** show the use of the processed image for segmentation by thresholding (Chapter 5).

Figure 51 shows an image of the broken end of a steel test specimen. Part of the surface was produced by fatigue and part by the terminal tearing failure. Visual examination easily distinguishes the two regions, based on texture. Measuring the area of the fatigue crack is important for determining the mechanical properties of the steel. However, the boundary is quite difficult to locate by computer processing.

Figure 52 shows the brightness histograms of two regions of the image, each 100 pixels square. The brightness values overlap extensively, although the variation of brightness values in the rough

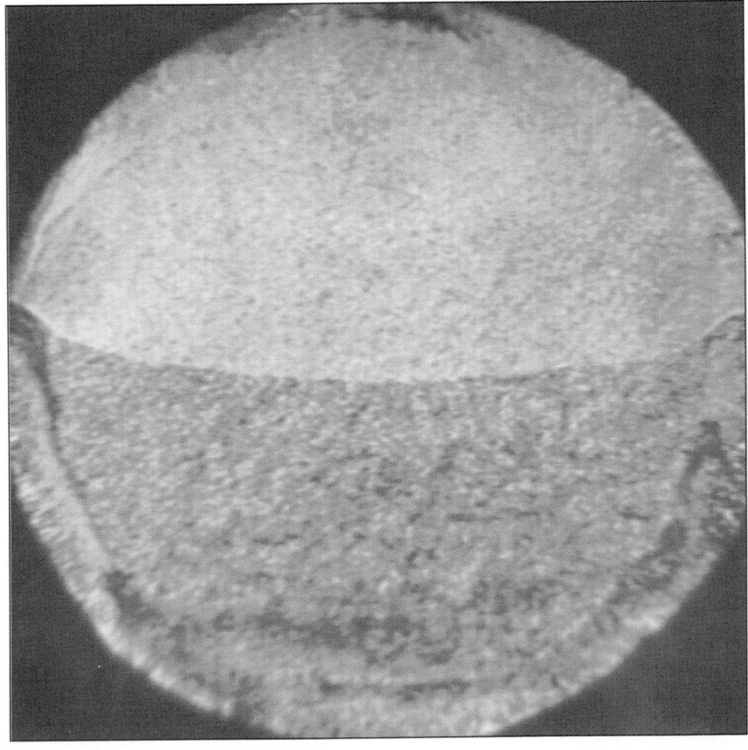

Figure 51. *Fracture surface of a steel test specimen. The smooth portion of the fracture occurred by fatigue, and the rougher portion by tearing.*

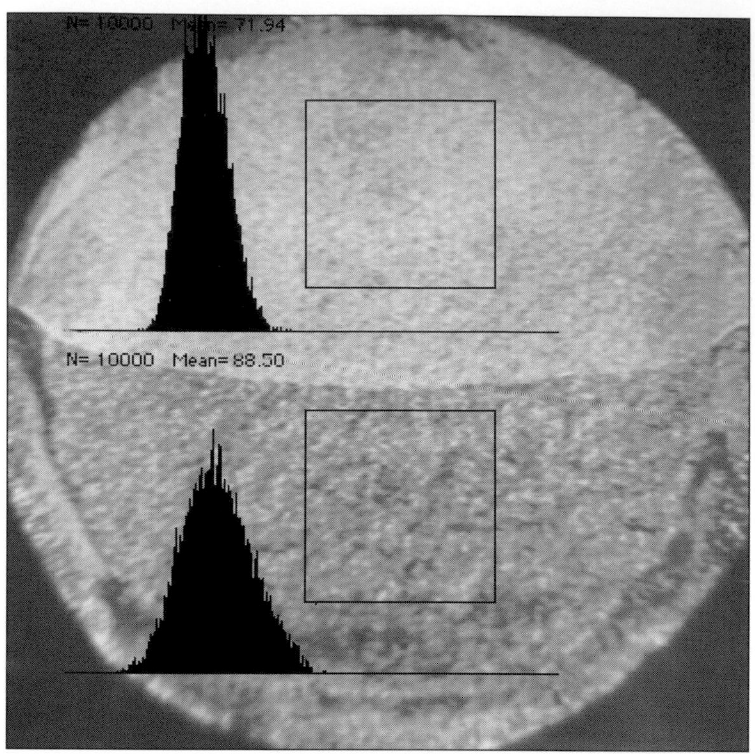

Figure 52. *Brightness histograms of two 100 × 100 pixel regions (marked) in Figure 51, showing greater variation in the rough area, but extensive overlap of brightness values with the smooth region.*

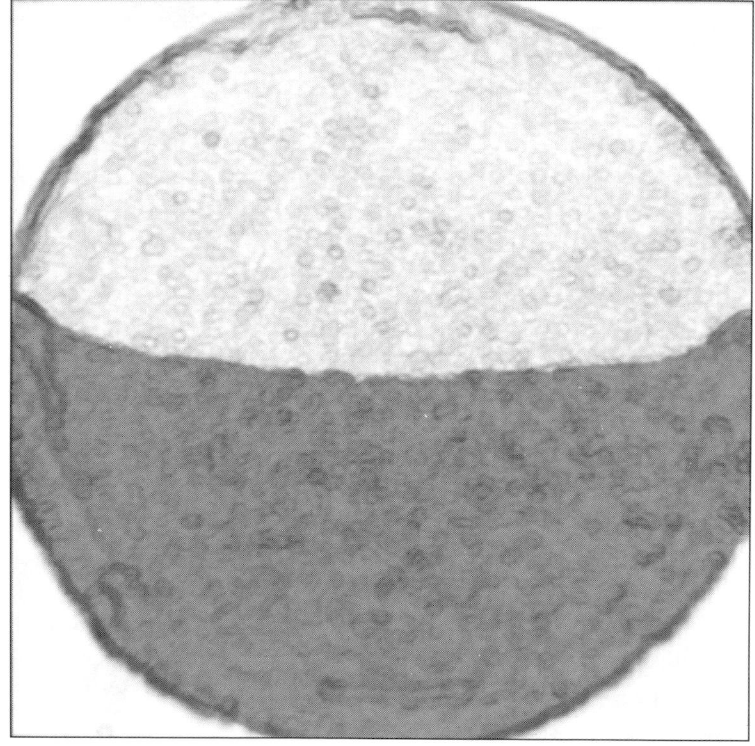

Figure 53. *Application of the local Hurst operator to the image in Figure 51, showing the larger values (darker pixels) for the rough portion of the fracture surface.*

region is greater than in the smooth region. This means that simple thresholding is not useful. Applying the local Hurst operator

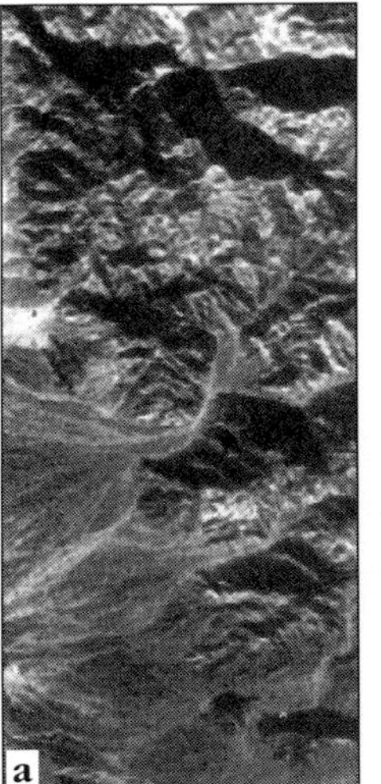

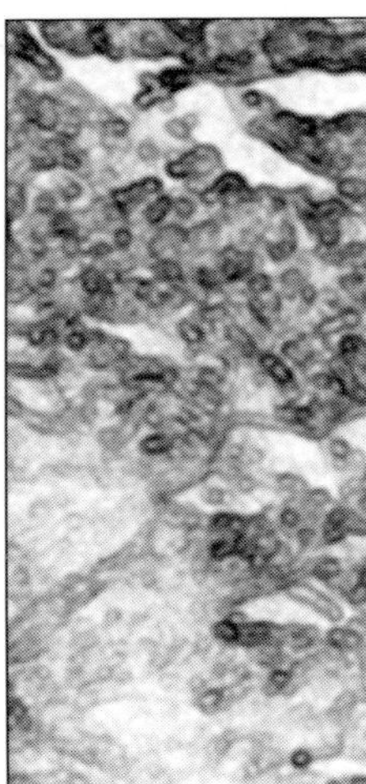

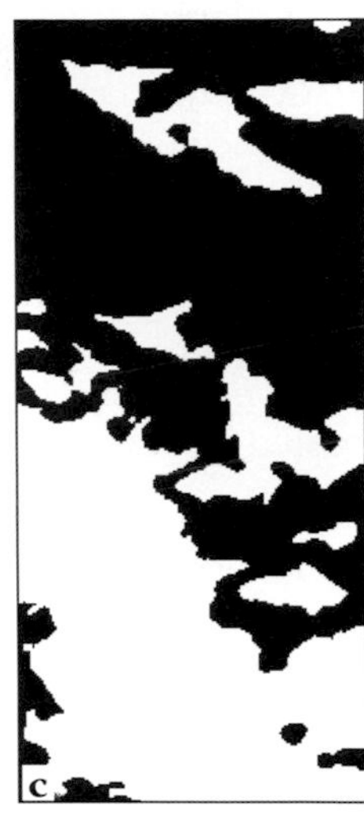

Figure 54. Aerial photograph (Death Valley, California):
a) *original, showing differences in local texture;*
b) *application of the Hurst operator;*
c) *binary image formed by thresholding image b to select high values of roughness.*

to this image produces the result shown in **Figure 53.** The two regions are clearly delineated, in spite of some local variations within each.

On an even larger scale, **Figure 54a** shows an aerial photograph of part of Death Valley, California. The terrain consists of comparatively smooth regions of desert and alluvial fans from the mountains, as well as much rougher terrain produced by weathering. Applying the same local Hurst operator to this image produces the result shown in **Figure 54b,** which can be directly thresholded to distinguish the two regions shown in **Figure 54c.**

Figure 55 shows several other processing operations applied to the same image as **Figure 54,** for comparison. Both the range and variance operators are sometimes used to characterize texture in images, but in this case, they perform as well as the Hurst operator. The Sobel operator highlights the edges and outlines the discontinuities in the image, but does not distinguish the smooth and rough regions.

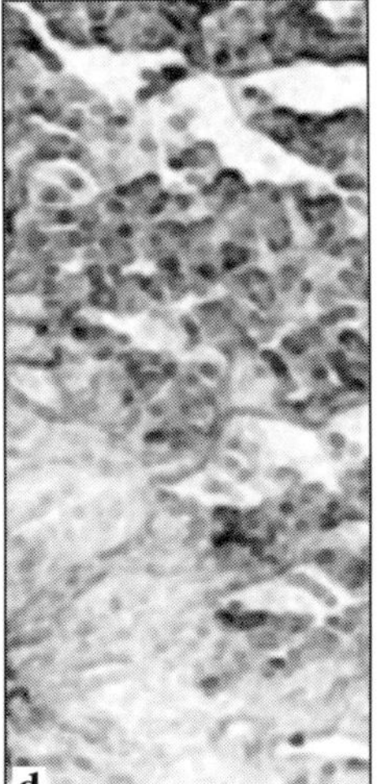

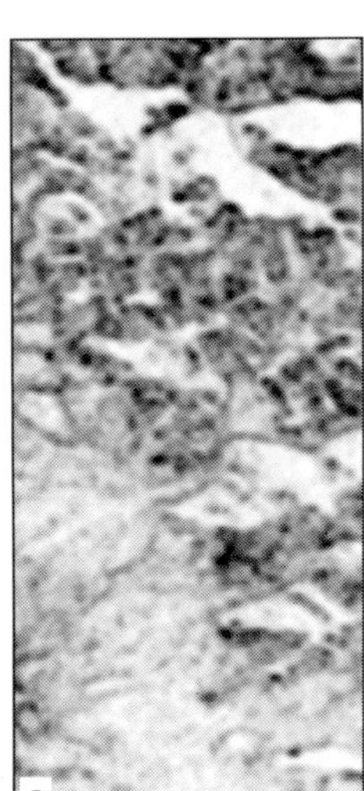

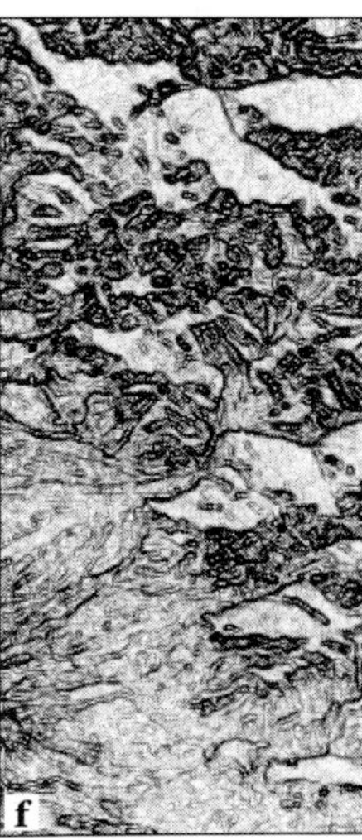

Figure 55. Other neighborhood operations applied to the image in Figure 54:
d) *range;*
e) *variance;*
f) *Sobel.*

Implementation notes

Many of the techniques discussed in this chapter and in Chapter 2 are neighborhood operators, which access pixels in a small area around each central pixel, perform some calculation or comparison with those values, and then derive a new value for the central pixel. In all cases, this new value is used to produce a new image, and it is the original values of pixels which are used in the neighborhood around the next pixel as the operation is repeated throughout the image.

Most image analysis systems, particularly those operating in mini or desktop computers, have limited memory (particularly when the large size of images is considered). Creating a new image for every image processing operation is an inefficient use of this limited resource. Consequently, the strategy generally used is to perform the operation "in place", to process one image and replace it with the result.

This requires only enough temporary memory to hold a few lines of the image. The operations are generally performed left to right along each scan line and top to bottom through the image. Duplicating the line that is being modified, and keeping copies of the preceding lines whose pixels are used, allows the new (modified) values to be written back into the original image memory. The number of lines is simply $(n + 1)/2$, where n is the neighborhood dimension (e.g., 3×3, 5×5, etc.). Usually, the time required to duplicate a line from the image is small and by shuffling through a series of pointers, it is only necessary to copy each line once when the moving process reaches it, then re-use the array for subsequent vertical positions.

Some of the image processing methods described above create two or more intermediate results. For example, the Roberts' Cross or Sobel filters apply two directional derivatives whose magnitudes are subsequently combined. It is possible to do this pixel by pixel, so that no additional storage is required. However, in some implementations, particularly those that can be efficiently programmed into an array processor (which acts on an entire line through the image at one time), it is faster to obtain the intermediate results for each operator applied to each line and then combine them for the whole line. This requires additional storage for the intermediate results.

Another consideration in implementing neighborhood operations is how to best treat pixels near the edges of the image. Many of the example images shown here are taken from the center of larger original images, so edge effects are avoided. In others, a band around the edge of the image is skipped, which is one of the most common ways to respond to the problem. With this approach, the programs skip pixels within a distance of $(n - 1)/2$ pixels from any edge, where n is the total width of the neighborhood.

Other possibilities include having special neighborhood rules near edges to sort through a smaller set of pixels, duplicating rows of pixels at edges (i.e., assuming each edge is a mirror), or using warp-around addressing (i.e., assuming that the left and right edges and the top and bottom edges of the image are contiguous). None of these methods is particularly attractive, in general. Since the largest and smallest brightness values are used to find the maximum range, the duplication of rows of pixels would not provide any extra information for range operations. In all cases, the use of fewer pixels for calculations would degrade the precision of the results. There is no reason whatsoever to assume that the image edges should be matched, and indeed, quite different structures and regions will normally occur there. The most conservative approach is to accept a small shrinkage in useful image size after processing, by ignoring near-edge pixels.

Image math

The image processing operations discussed so far in this chapter operate on one image and produce a modified result, which may be stored in the same image memory. Another class of operations uses two images to produce a new image (which may replace one of the originals). These operations are usually described as image arithmetic, since operators such as addition, subtraction, division, and multiplication are included. They are performed pixel by pixel, so that the sum of two images simply contains pixels whose brightness values are the sums of the corresponding pixels in the original images. There are some additional operators used, as well, such as comparing two images to keep the brighter (or darker) pixel. Other operations, such as Boolean OR or AND logic, are generally applied to binary images; they will be discussed in that context in Chapter 6.

Actually, image addition has already been used in a method described previously. In Chapter 2, the averaging of images to reduce noise was discussed. The addition operation is straightforward, but a decision is required about how to deal with the result. If two 8-bit images (with brightness values from 0 to 255 at each pixel) are added together, the resulting value can range from 0 to 510. This exceeds the capacity of the image memory. One possibility is simply to divide the result by two, obtaining a resulting image that is correctly scaled to the 0 to 255 range. This is what is usually applied in image averaging, in which the N images added together produce a total, which is then divided by N to rescale the data.

Another possibility is to find the largest and smallest actual values in the sum image, and then dynamically rescale the result to this maximum and minimum, so that each pixel is assigned a new value B = range · (sum – minimum) / (maximum – minimum), where range is the capacity of the image memory, typically 255. This is superior to performing the division by two and

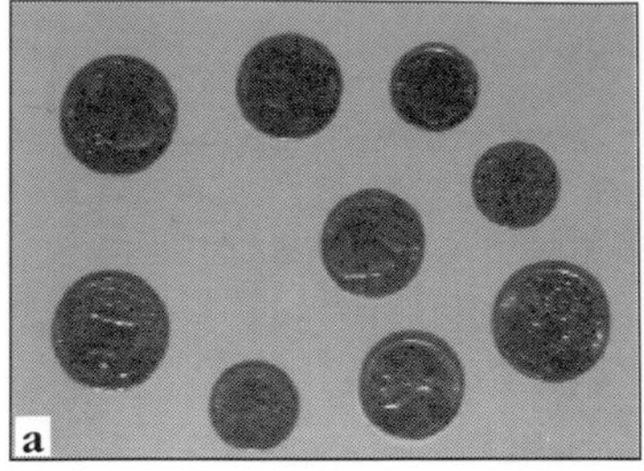

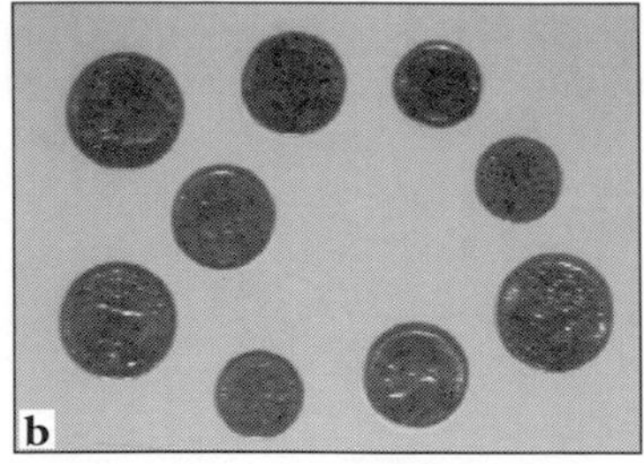

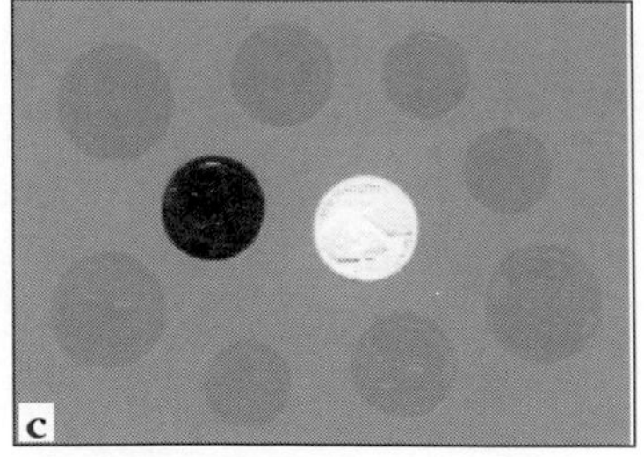

Figure 56. Showing image differences by subtraction:
***a)** original image; **b)** image after moving one coin; **c)** difference image after pixel by pixel subtraction.*

then subsequently performing a linear expansion of contrast, as discussed in Chapter 2, because the precision of the resulting values is higher. When the integer division by two is performed, fractional values are truncated and some information may be lost.

On the other hand, when dynamic ranging or automatic scaling is performed, it becomes more difficult to perform direct comparison of images after processing, since the brightness scales may not be the same. In addition, autoscaling takes longer, since two complete passes through the image are required: one to determine the maximum and minimum and one to apply the autoscaling calculation. Many of the images printed in this book have been autoscaled in order to maximize printed contrast. Whenever possible, this operation has been performed as part of the processing operation to maintain precision.

Adding together images superimposes information and can in some cases be useful to create composites, which help to communicate complex spatial relationships. We have already seen that adding the Laplacian or a derivative image to the original can help provide some spatial guidelines to interpret the information from the filter. Usually, this kind of addition is handled directly in the processing by changing the central value of the kernel. For the Laplacian, this modification is called a sharpening filter, as noted above.

Subtracting images

Subtraction is widely used and more interesting than the addition operation. In Chapter 2, subtraction was used to level images by removing background. This chapter has already mentioned uses of subtraction, such as that employed in unsharp masking, where the smoothed image is subtracted, pixel by pixel, from the original. In such an operation, the possible range of values for images whose initial range is 0 to 255 becomes –255 to +255. The data can be rescaled to fit into a single byte, replacing the original image, by adding 255 and dividing by two, or the same autoscaling method described above for addition may be employed. The same advantages and penalties for fixed and flexible scaling are encountered.

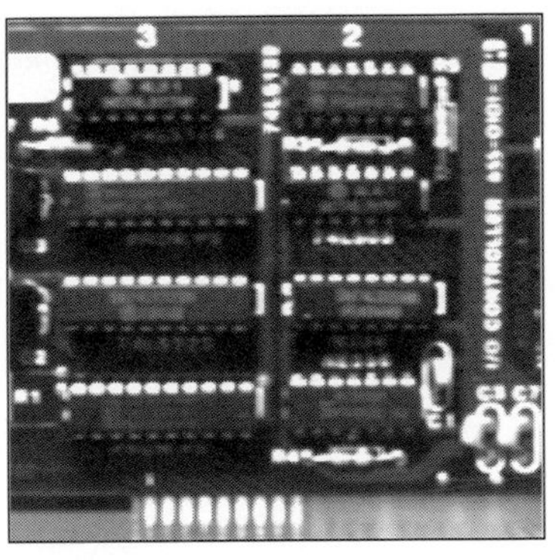

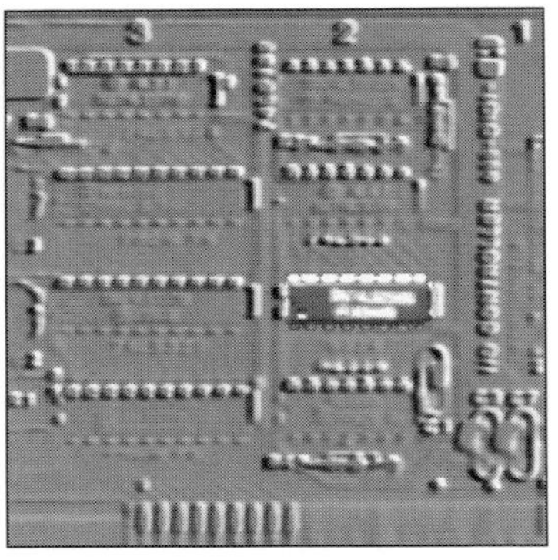

Figure 57. *Difference images for quality control. A master image is subtracted from images of each subsequent part. In this example, the missing chip in a printed circuit board is evident in the difference image.*

Subtraction is primarily a way to discover differences between images. **Figure 56** shows two images of coins and their difference. The parts of the picture that are essentially unchanged in the two images cancel out, except for minor variations, appearing as a uniform medium grey due to the precision of digitization, changes in illumination, etc. The coin that has been moved between the two image acquisitions is clearly shown. The dark image shows where the image was; the bright one shows where it has gone.

Subtracting one image from another effectively removes from the difference image all features that do not change, while highlighting those that do. If the lighting and geometry of view is consistent, the only differences in pixel values where no changes occur are statistical variations in the brightness, due to camera or electronic noise. The bright and dark images show features that have been added or removed from the field of view.

A major use of image subtraction is quality control. A master image is acquired and stored that shows the correct placement of parts on circuit boards **(Figure 57),** the alignment of labels on packaging, etc. When the image is subtracted from a series of images acquired from subsequent objects, the differences are strongly highlighted, revealing errors in production. This subtraction is often carried out at video frame rates using dedicated hardware. Since it is unrealistic to expect parts to be exactly aligned, a tolerance can be specified by the area of bright and dark (mismatched) pixels present after the subtraction. **Figure 58** shows this schematically.

The same technique is used in reconnaissance photos to watch for the appearance or disappearance of targets in a complex scene. Image warping, as discussed in Chapter 2, may be required to align images taken from different points of view before the subtraction can be performed. A similar method is used in astronomy. "Blinking" images taken of the same area of the sky at different times is the traditional way to search for moving planets or asteroids. This technique alternately presents each image to a human viewer, who notices the apparent motion of the point of light that is different in the two images. Some use of

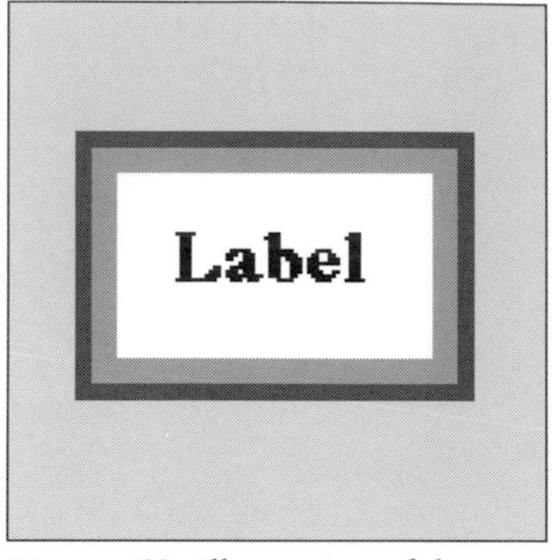

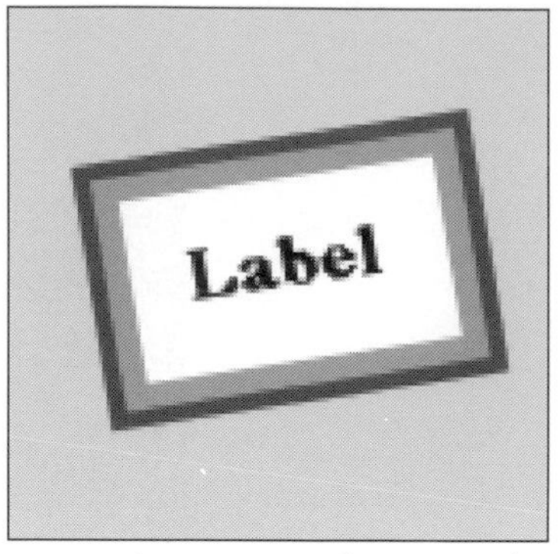

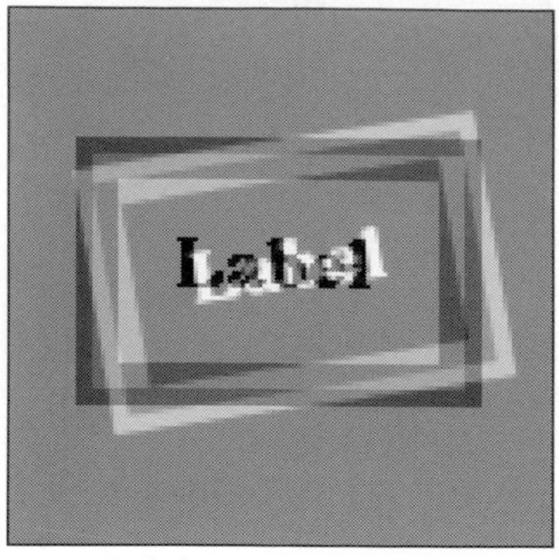

Figure 58. *Illustration of the use of image subtraction to detect misalignment in label positioning. The area of white and dark pixels measures the extent of positioning error.*

computer searching using subtraction has been used, but for dim objects in the presence of background noise has not proved as sensitive as a human observer.

Object motion can be measured using subtraction, if the features are large enough and the sequential images are acquired fast enough that they overlap in successive frames. In this case, the subtraction shows a bright area of mismatch, which can be measured. The length of the unmatched region divided by the elapsed time gives the velocity; direction can be determined by the orientation of the region. This technique is used at microscopic scales to track the motion of cells on slides **(Figure 59)** in response to chemical cues.

At the other extreme, subtraction is used with satellite photos to track ice floes in the north Atlantic. For motion between two successive images that is too large for this method, it may be possible to identify the same objects in successive images based on size, shape, etc. and thus track motion. Or, one can assume that where paths cross, the points causing the least deviation of the path give the correct match **(Figure 60).** However, the direct subtraction technique is much simpler and more direct.

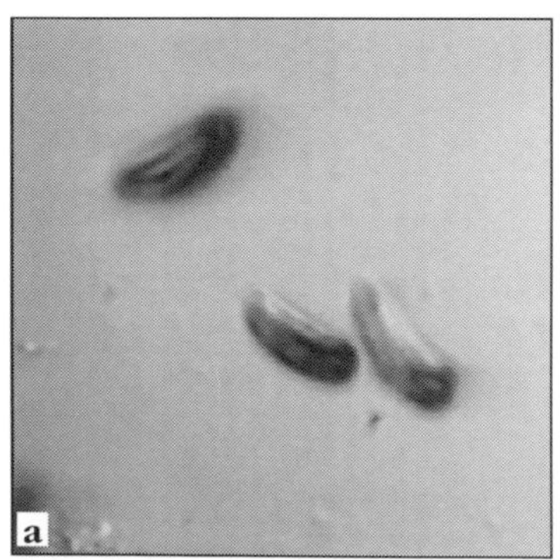

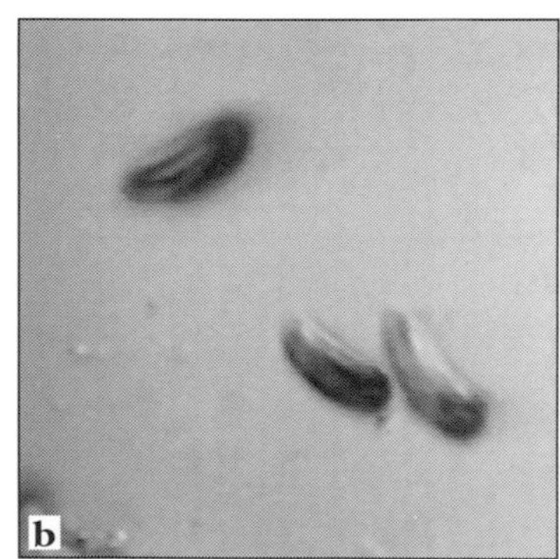

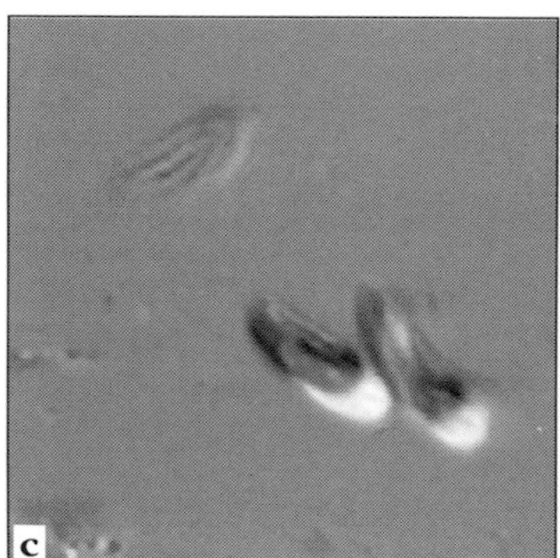

Figure 59. *Two frames from a videotape sequence of free swimming single-celled animals in a drop of pond water, and the difference image. The length of the white region divided by the time interval gives the velocity.*

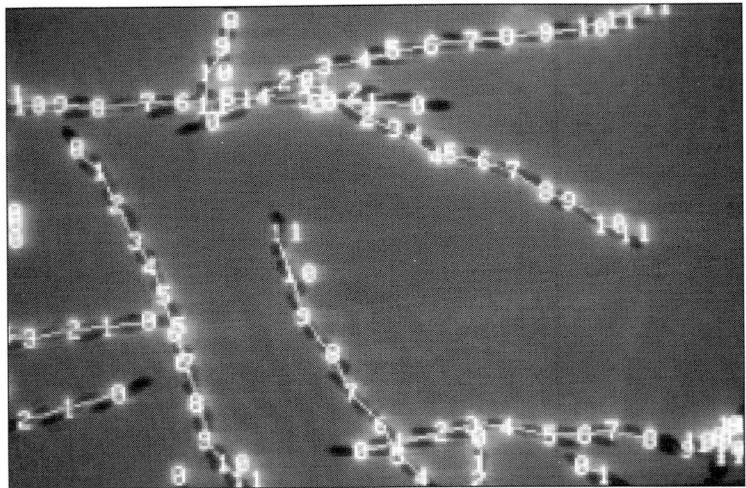

Figure 60. *Analysis of motion in a more complex situation than shown in Figure 59. Where the paths of the swimming microorganisms cross, they are sorted out by assuming that the path continues in a nearly straight direction. (Gualtieri & Coltelli, 1991)*

Multiplication and division

Image multiplication is perhaps the least used of the mathematics modes, but it is generally included for the sake of completeness in systems offering the other arithmetic operations. One possible use is superimposing one image on another in the particular case when the superimposed data is proportional to the absolute brightness of the original image. An example is texture; **Figure 61** shows an illustration. A Gaussian random brightness pattern is superimposed on the smooth polygonal approximation of a shaded sphere in order to provide an impression of roughness. Similar multiplicative superimposition may be used to add fluorescence or other emission images to a reflection or transmission image.

One of the difficulties with multiplication is the extreme range of values that may be generated. With 8-bit images whose pixels can have a range between 0 and 255, the possible products can range from 0 to more than 65,000. This is a 2-byte product, only

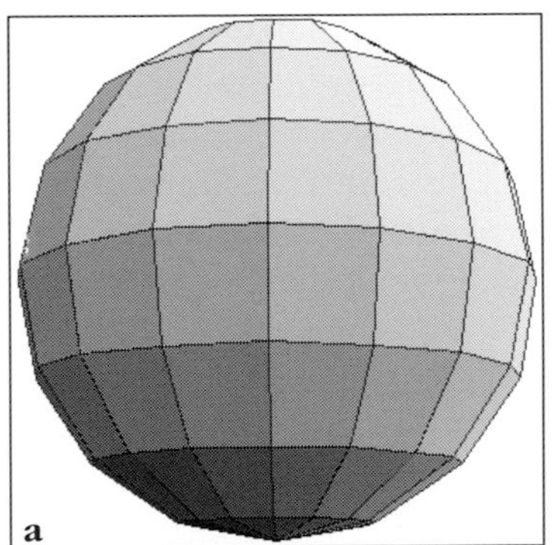

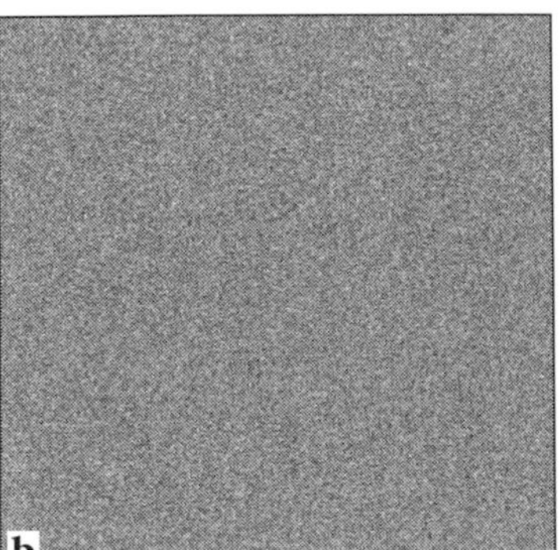

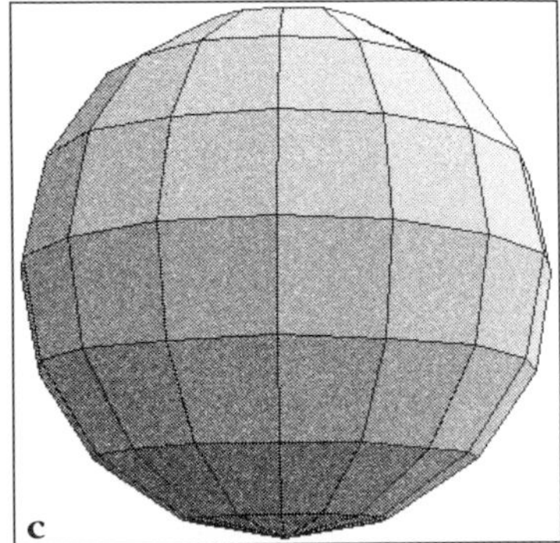

Figure 61. Multiplication of images can be used to superimpose texture on an image:
a) *smooth faceted globe;*
b) *Gaussian random values;*
c) *product of a times b.*

the high byte of which can be stored back into the same image memory, unless automatic scaling is used. A significant loss of precision may result for values in the resulting image.

The magnitude of the numbers also creates problems with division. First, division by 0 must be avoided. This is usually done by adding 1 to all brightness values, so that the values are interpreted as 1 to 256 instead of 0 to 255. Then it is necessary to first multiply each pixel in the numerator by some factor that will produce quotients covering the 0 to 255 range, while maintaining some useful precision for the ends of the range. Automatic scaling is particularly useful for these situations, but it cannot be used in applications requiring comparison of results to each other or to a calibration curve.

An example of division in which automatic scaling is useful is the removal of background (as discussed in Chapter 2) when linear detectors or cameras are used. An example of division when absolute values are required is calculating ratios of brightness from two or more Landsat bands (an example is shown in Chapter 1) or two or more filter images when examining fluorescent probes in the light microscope. In fluorescence microscopy, the time variation of emitted light intensity is normalized by alternately collecting images through two or more filters at different wavelengths above and below the line of interest, and calibrating the ratio against the activity of the element(s) of interest. In satellite imagery, ratios of intensities (particularly Band 4 = 0.5 to 0.6 μm, Band 5 = 0.6 to 0.7 μm, Band 6 = 0.7 to 0.8 μm, and Band 7 = 0.8 to 1.1 μm) are used for terrain classification and the identification of some rock types. The thermal inertia of different rock formations may also be determined by ratioing images obtained at different local times of day, as the formations heat or cool.

As an example of mineral identification, silicates exhibit a wavelength shift in the absorption band with composition. Granites, diorites, gabbros, and olivene peridotes have progressively decreasing silicon content. The absorption band shifts to progressively longer wavelengths in the 8- to 12-μm thermal infrared band as the bond-stretching vibrations between Si and O atoms in the silicate lattice change. The Thermal Infrared Multispectral Mapper satellite records six bands of image data in this range, which are combined and normalized to locate the absorption band and identify rock formations. Carbonate rocks (dolomite and limestone) have a similar absorption response in the 6- to 8-μm range, but this is difficult to measure in satellite imagery because of atmospheric absorption. At radar wavelengths, different surface roughnesses produce variations in reflected intensity in the Ka, X, and L bands and can be combined in the same ways to perform measurements and distinguish the coarseness of sands, gravels, cobbles, and boulders (Sabins, 1987).

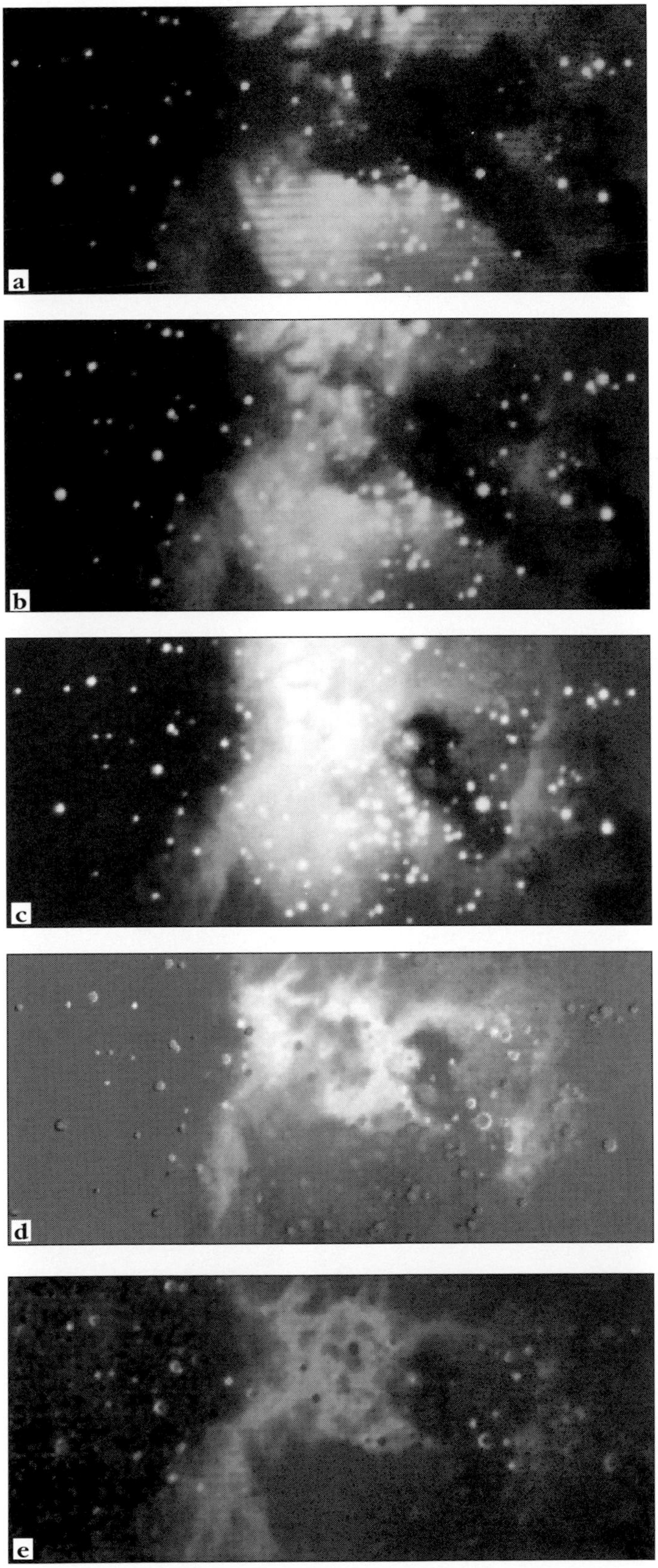

Figure 62. Combining views of NGC-2024 to show star-forming regions and dust.

a) *1.2-µm infrared image;*

b) *1.6-µm infrared image;*

c) *2.2-µm infrared image;*

d) *2.2-µm image minus 1.6-µm image;*

e) *1.6-µm image divided by 1.2-µm image.*

a

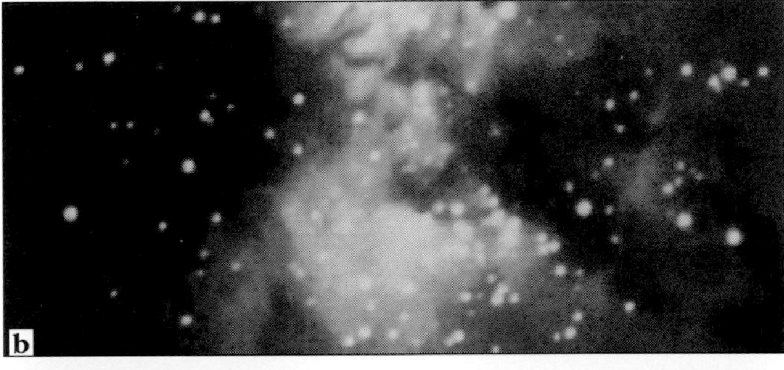

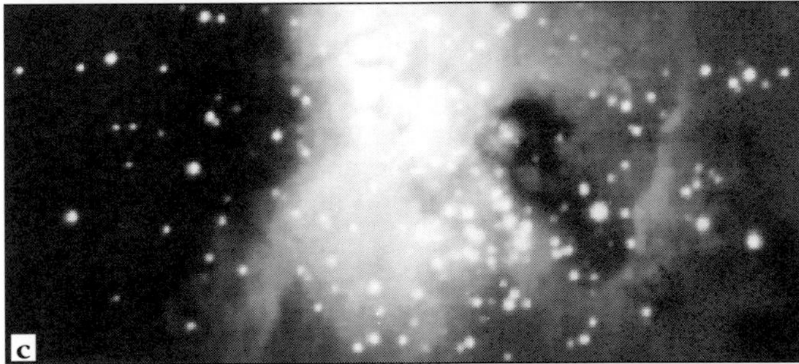

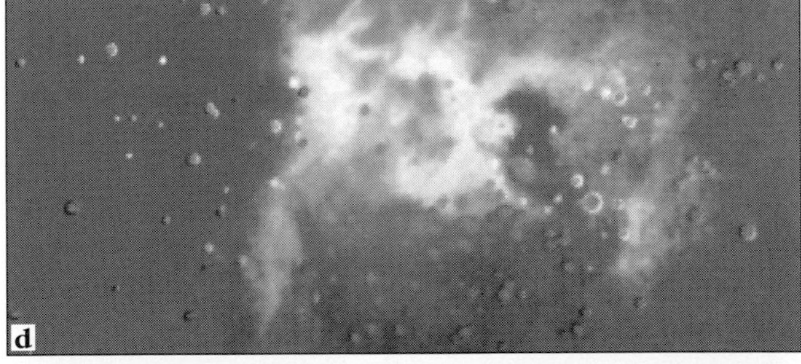

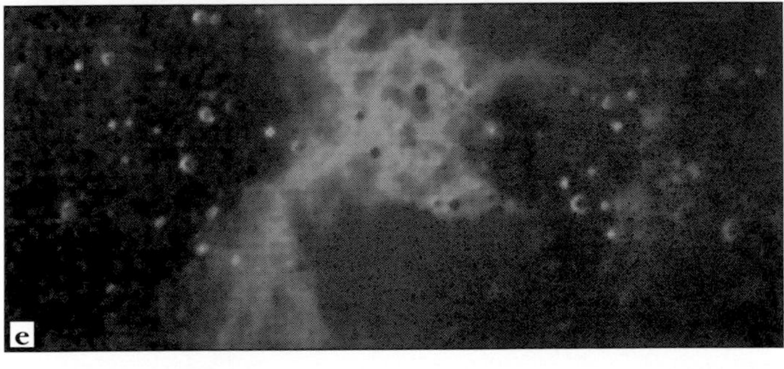

Figure 63. Principle of the confocal scanning light microscope. Light reflected from out-of-focus planes or points does not reach the detector.

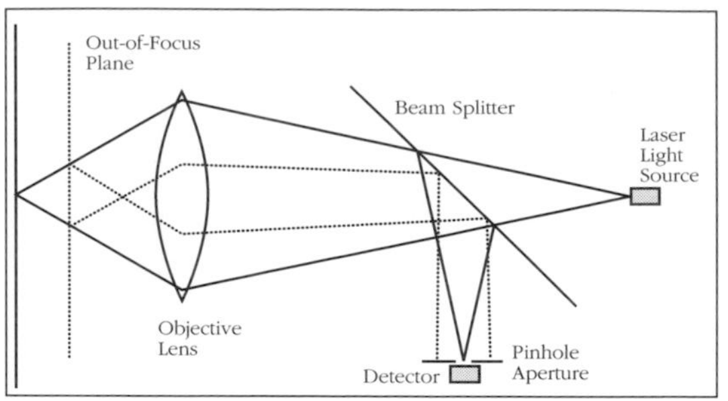

In the same way, Bands 1 (0.55 to 0.68 µm, or visible red) and 2 (0.72 to 1.10 µm, or reflected infrared) from multispectral satellite imagery are used to recognize vegetation. Band 1 records the chlorophyll absorption and Band 2 gives the reflection from the cell structure of the leaves. The ratio $(B_2 - B_1) / (B_2 + B_1)$ eliminates variations due to differences in solar elevation (illumination angle) and is used to measure the distribution of vegetation in images. Typically, this approach also combines data from successive scans to obtain the spectral vegetation index as a function of time. Other ratios have been used to image and to measure chlorophyll concentrations due to phytoplankton in the ocean (Sabins, 1987).

Ratios are also used in astronomical images. **Figure 62** shows infrared images of the star-forming region in NGC-2024. Infrared light penetrates dust, which blocks most visible light. Ratios or differences of the different wavelength images show details in the dust and enhance the visibility of the young stars.

Image math also includes the logical comparison of pixel values. For instance, two images may be combined by keeping the brighter (or darker) of the corresponding pixels at each location. This is used, for instance, to build up a CSLM image with great depth of field. Normal light microscope images have limited depth of field because of the high numerical aperture of the lenses. In the CSLM, the scanning light beam and aperture on the detector reduce this depth of field even more by eliminating

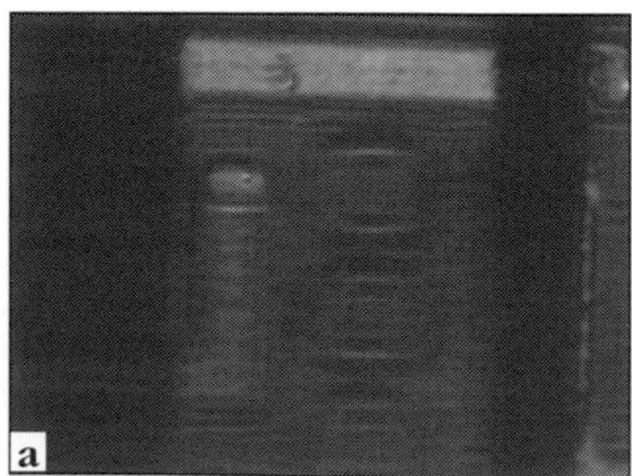

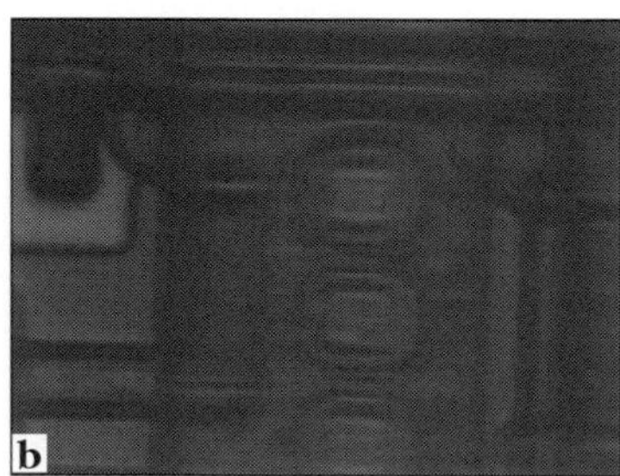

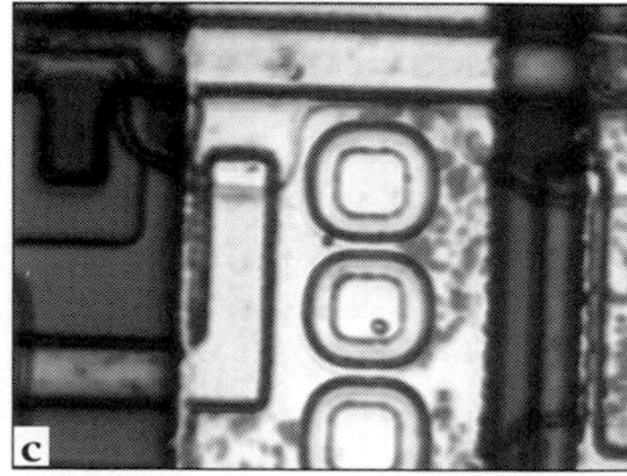

Figure 64. *Combining CSLM images by keeping the brightest value at each pixel location. Images a and b are two individual focal plane images from a series of 25 on an integrated circuit. Only the portion of the surface which is in focus is bright. Since the in-focus point is brightest, combining all of the individual planes produces image c, which shows the entire surface in focus.*

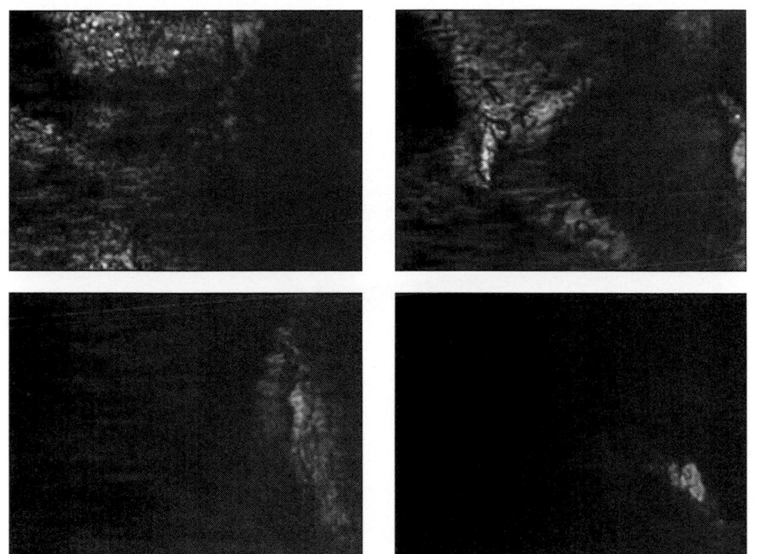

Figure 65. *Four individual focal ections from a confocal light microscope series on a ceramic fracture surface. The images are 40 μm wide, and the images in the stack of 26 images are spaced 1 μm apart in depth.*

light scattered from any point except the single point illuminated in the plane of focus, as indicated in **Figure 63.**

A single, two-dimensional image is formed by scanning the light over the sample (or, equivalently, by moving the sample itself with the light beam stationary). For a specimen with an irregular surface, this image is very dark, except at locations where the surface lies in the plane of focus. By moving the specimen vertically, many such planar images can be acquired. The display of a complete three-dimensional set of such images is discussed in Chapter 8. However, at each pixel location, the brightest value of light reflectance occurs at the in-focus point. Consequently, the images from many focal depths can be combined by keeping only the brightest value at each pixel location to form an image with an unlimited depth of field. **Figure 64** shows an example.

An additional effect can be produced by shifting each image slightly before performing the comparison and superimposition. **Figures 65** and **66** show an example. The 26 individual images, four of which are shown in **Figure 65,** are combined in this way to produce a perspective view of the surface.

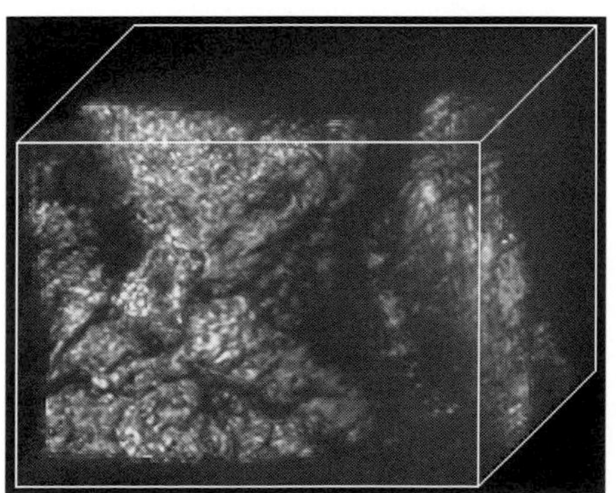

Figure 66. *Surface reconstruction from the images shown in Figure 63. Each image is shifted two pixels to the right and up, and combined by keeping the brightest value at each pixel location. The result is a perspective view of the entire surface.*

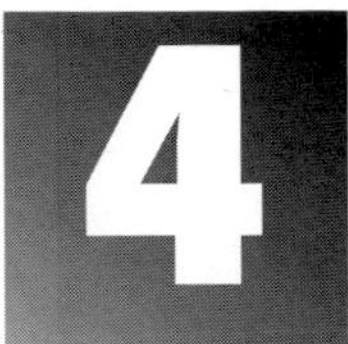

Processing Images in Frequency Space

Some necessary mathematical preliminaries

What frequency space is all about

It is unusual to pick up a book on image analysis without finding at least a portion of it devoted to a discussion of Fourier transforms (see especially Pratt, 1991; Gonzalez & Wintz, 1987; and Jain, 1989). In part, this is due to the utility of working in frequency space to perform certain image measurement and processing operations. Many of these same operations can be performed in the original (spatial domain) image only with significantly greater computational effort. Another reason for the lengthy sections on these methods is that the authors frequently come from a background in electrical engineering and signal processing and so are familiar with the mathematics and the use of these methods for other types of signals, particularly the one-dimensional (time varying) electrical signals that make up much of our modern electronics.

However, the typical image analyst interested in applying computer methods to images for purposes of enhancement or measurement is often not comfortable with the pages of mathematics (and intimidating notation) used in these discussions. Furthermore, he or she may not have the fortitude to relate these concepts to the operation of a dedicated image analysis computer. Unable to see the connection between the topics discussed and the typical image problems encountered in real life, the analyst might therefore find it easier to skip the subject. This is a loss, because the use of frequency space methods can offer benefits in many real-life applications, and it is not essential to deal deeply with the mathematics to arrive at a practical working knowledge of these techniques.

The Fourier transform and other frequency space transforms are applied to two-dimensional images for many different reasons. Some of these have little to do with the purposes of enhancing the visibility and selection of features or structures of interest. For instance, some of these transform methods are used as a means of image compression, in which less data than the original image must be transmitted or stored. In this type of application, it is necessary to reconstruct the image (bring it back from the frequency to the spatial domain) for viewing. It is desirable to be able to accomplish both the forward and reverse transform rapidly and with a minimum loss of image quality. This is a somewhat elusive concept that certainly includes the alteration of grey levels, definition of feature boundaries, and introduction or removal of fine-scale texture in the image. It is usual to find that the greater the degree of compression, the greater the loss of image fidelity.

Speed is usually a less important concern to image measurement applications, since the acquisition and subsequent analysis of the images are likely to require some time anyway, but the computational advances (both in hardware and software or algorithms) made to accommodate the requirements of the data compression application are of course directly useful for this task, as well. On the other hand, the amount of image degradation that can be tolerated by most visual uses of the compressed and restored images is far greater than is usually acceptable for image analysis purposes. Consequently, the amount of image compression that can be achieved with minimal loss of fidelity is rather small.

Since in most cases the transmission of an image from the point of acquisition to the computer used for analysis is not a major concern, we will ignore this entire subject here and assume that the transform retains all of the data, even if this means that there is no compression at all. Indeed, this is exactly true for most of these methods. The transform encodes the image information completely and it can be exactly reconstructed, at least to within the arithmetic precision of the computer being used–which is generally better than the precision of the original image sensor or analog-to-digital converter.

Although there are many different types of image transforms that can be used, the best known (at least, the one with the most recognizable name) is the Fourier transform. This is due in part to the availability of a powerful and very efficient algorithm for computing it, known as the Fast Fourier Transform, or FFT (Cooley & Tukey, 1965; Bracewell, 1989), which we will encounter in due course. Although most of the examples in this text were actually computed using a newer approach (the Fast Hartley Transform, or FHT, see Hartley, 1942; Bracewell, 1984, 1986; Reeves,

1990), the frequency space images are presented in the same form that the Fourier method would yield. For the sake of explanation, it is probably easiest to describe the better-known method.

The usual approach to developing the mathematical background of the Fourier transform begins with a one-dimensional waveform and then expands to two dimensions (an image). In principle, this can also be extended to three dimensions, although it becomes much more difficult to visualize or display. Three-dimensional transforms between the spatial domain (now a volume image constructed of voxels instead of pixels) and the three-dimensional frequency space are used, for example, in some tomographic reconstructions.

The mathematical development that follows has been kept as brief as possible, but if you suffer from "integral-o-phobia" then it is permitted to skip this section and go on to the examples and discussion, returning here only when (and if) a deeper understanding is desired.

The Fourier transform

Using a fairly standard nomenclature and symbology, let us begin with a function $f(x)$, where x is a real variable representing time or distance in one direction across an image. It is very common to refer to this function as the spatial or time domain function and the transform F introduced below as the frequency space function. The function f is a continuous and well-behaved function. Do not be disturbed by the fact that in a digitized image, the values of x are not continuous but discrete (based on pixel spacing), and the possible brightness values are quantized as well. These values are considered to sample the real or analog image, which exists outside the computer.

Fourier's theorem states that it is possible to form any one-dimensional function $f(x)$ as a summation of a series of sine and cosine terms of increasing frequency. The Fourier transform of the function $f(x)$ is written $F(u)$ and describes the amount of each frequency term that must be added together to make $f(x)$. It can be written as

$$F(u) = \int_{-\infty}^{+\infty} f(x)e^{-2\pi iux}\,dx$$

where i is (as usual) $\sqrt{-1}$. The use of the exponential notation relies on the mathematical identity (Euler's formula)

$$e^{-2\pi iux} = \cos(2\pi ux) - i\sin(2\pi ux)$$

One of the very important characteristics of this transform is that given $F(u)$, it is possible to recover the spatial domain function $f(x)$ in the same way.

$$f(x) = \int_{-\infty}^{+\infty} F(u) e^{2\pi iux} du$$

These two equations together comprise the forward and reverse Fourier transform. The function $f(x)$ is generally a real function, such as a time-varying voltage or a spatially varying image brightness. However, the transform function $F(u)$ is generally complex, the sum of a real part R and an imaginary part I.

$$F(u) = R(u) + i\,I(u)$$

It is usually more convenient to express this in polar rather than Cartesian form

$$F(u) = |F(u)|\; e^{i\,\phi(u)}$$

where $|F|$ is called the magnitude and ϕ is called the phase. The square of the magnitude $P(u) = |F(u)|^2$ is commonly referred to as the power spectrum, or spectral density of $f(x)$.

The integrals from minus to plus infinity will in practice be reduced to a summation of terms of increasing frequency, limited by the finite spacing of the sampled points in the image. The discrete Fourier transform is written as

$$F(u) = \frac{1}{N} \sum_{x=0}^{N-1} f(x) e^{-i2\pi ux/N}$$

where N is the number of sampled points along the function $f(x)$ which are assumed to be uniformly spaced. Again, the reverse transform is similar (but not identical–note the absence of the $1/N$ term and the change in sign for the exponent).

$$f(x) = \sum_{u=0}^{N-1} F(u) e^{i2\pi ux/N}$$

The values of u from 0 to $N-1$ represent the discrete frequency components added together to construct the function $f(x)$. As in the continuous case, $F(u)$ is complex and may be written as real and imaginary or as magnitude and phase components.

The summation is normally performed over terms up to one-half the dimension of the image (in pixels), since it requires a minimum of two pixel brightness values to define the highest frequency present. This limitation is described as the Nyquist frequency. Because the summation has half as many terms as the width of the original image, but each term has a real and imaginary part, the total number of values produced by the Fourier transform is the same as the number of pixels in the original image width, or the number of samples of a time-varying function.

In both the continuous and the discrete cases, a direct extension from one-dimensional functions to two- (or three-) dimensional ones can be made by substituting $f(x,y)$ for $f(x)$ and $F(u,v)$ for $F(u)$, and performing the summation or integration over two (or three) variables instead of one. Since the dimensions x,y,z are orthogonal, so are the u,v,w dimensions. This means that the transformation can be performed separately in each direction. For a two-dimensional image, for example, it would be possible to perform a one-dimensional transform on each horizontal line of the image, producing an intermediate result with complex values for each point. Then a second series of one-dimensional transforms can be performed on each vertical line, finally producing the desired two-dimensional transform.

The program fragment listed below shows how to compute the FFT of a function. It is written in Fortran, but can be translated into any other language (you may have to define a type to hold the complex numbers). On input to the subroutine, *F* is the array of values to be transformed (usually the imaginary part of these complex numbers will be 0) and *LN* is the power of 2 (up to 10 for the maximum 1,024 in this implementation). The transform is returned in the same array *F*. The first loop reorders the input data, the second performs the successive doubling that is the heart of the FFT method, and the final loop normalizes the results.

```
                        SUBROUTINE FFT(F,LN)
      COMPLEX F(1024),U,W,T,CMPLX
      PI=3.14159265
      N=2**LN
      NV2=N/2
      NM1=N-1
      J=1
      DO 3 I=1,NM1
            IF (I.GE.J) GOTO 1
            T=F(J)
            F(J)=F(I)
            F(I)=T
1           K=NV2
2           IF (K.GE.J) GOTO 3
            J=J-K
            K=K/2
            GOTO 2
3           J=J+K
      DO 5 L=1,LN
            LE=2**L
            LE1=LE/2
            U=(1.0,0.0)
            W=CMPLX(COS(PI/LE1),-SIN(PI/LE1))
            DO 5 J=1,LE1
                  DO 4 I=J,N,LE
                        IP=I+LE1
                        T=F(IP)*U
                        F(IP)=F(I)-T
4                       F(I)=F(I)+T
5                 U=U*W
      DO 6 I=1MN
6           F(I)=F(I)/FLOAT(N)
      RETURN
      END
```

Applying this one-dimensional transform to each row and then each column of a two-dimensional image is not the absolute fastest way to perform the calculation, but it is by far the simplest and is actually used in many programs. A somewhat faster ap-

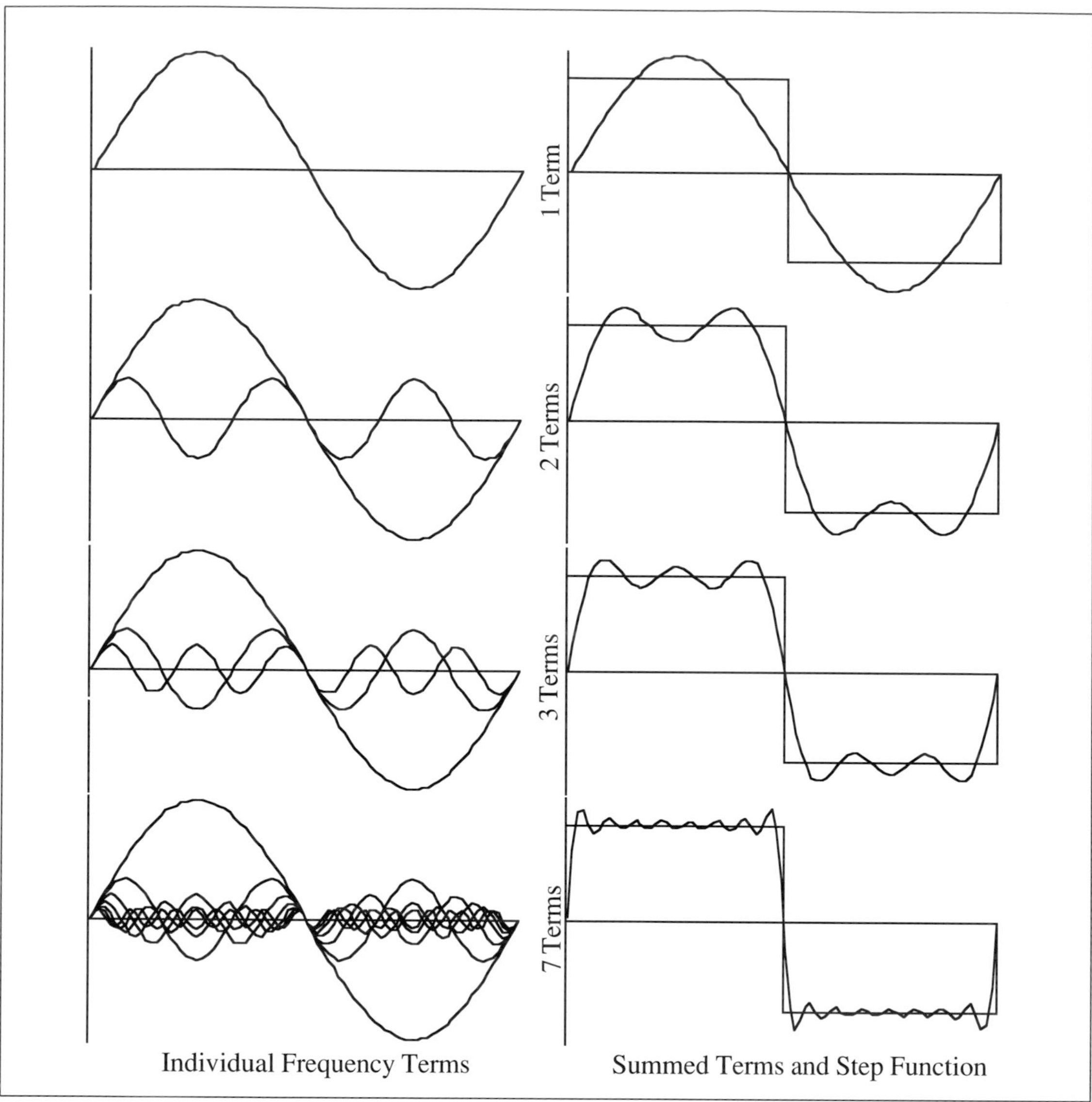

Figure 1. *Summation of Fourier frequency terms to fit a simple step function.*

proach, known as a butterfly because it uses various sets of pairs of pixel values throughout the two-dimensional image, produces identical results. Storing the array of *W* values can also provide a slight increase in speed.

The resulting transform of the original image into frequency space has complex values at each pixel. This is difficult to display in any meaningful way. In most cases, the display is based on only the magnitude of the value, ignoring the phase. If the square of the magnitude is used, this may be referred to as the image power spectrum, since different frequencies are represented at different distances from the origin, different directions represent different orientations in the original image, and the power at each location shows how much of that frequency and

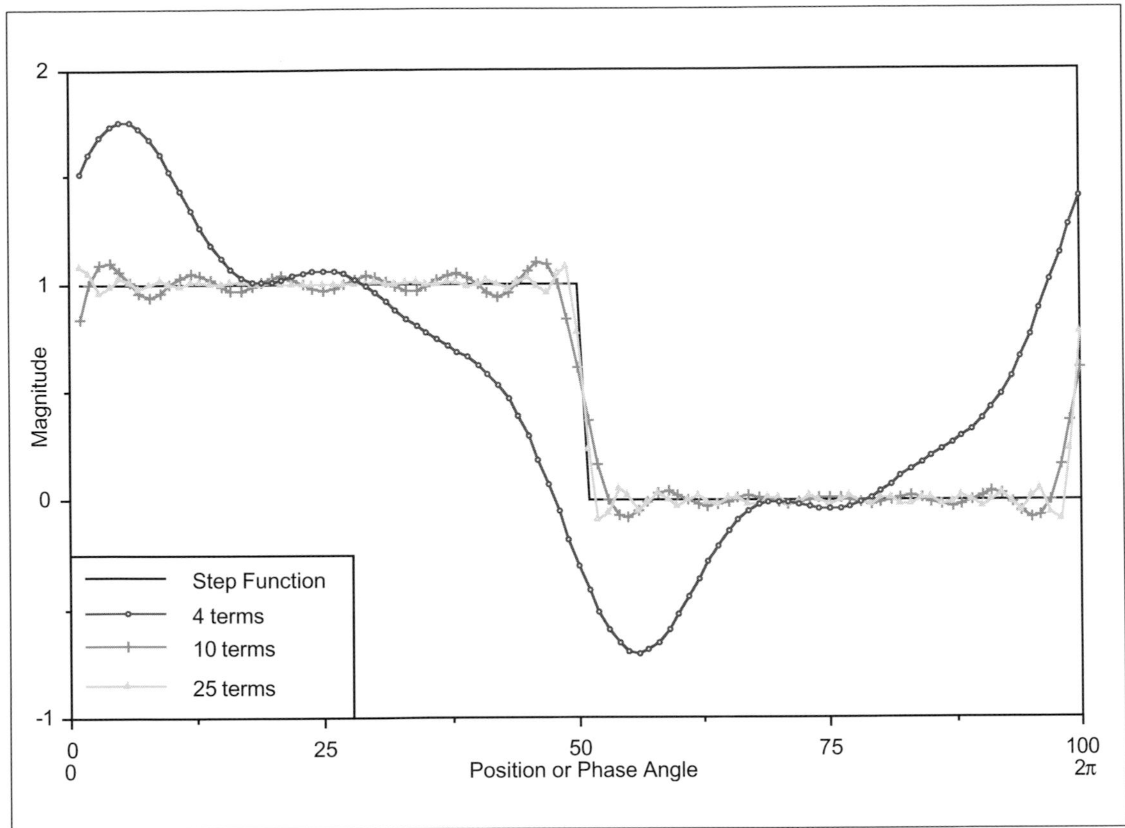

Figure 2. *Match between a step function and the first 4, 10, and 25 Fourier terms.*

orientation is present in the image. This display is particularly useful for isolating periodic structures or noise, which is discussed below. However, the power spectrum by itself cannot be used to restore the original image. The phase information is also needed, although it is rarely displayed and is usually difficult or impossible to interpret visually.

Fourier transforms of real functions

A common illustration in introductory-level math textbooks on the Fourier transform (which usually deal only with the one-dimensional case) is the quality of the fit to an arbitrary, but simple, function by the sum of a finite series of terms in the Fourier expansion. **Figure 1** shows the familiar case of a step function, illustrating the ability to add up a series of sine waves to produce the desired step. The coefficients in the Fourier series are the magnitudes of each increasing frequency needed to produce the fit. **Figure 2** shows the result of adding together the first 4, 10, and 25 terms. Obviously, the greater the number of terms included, the better the fit (especially at the sharp edge). **Figure 3** shows the same process for a ramp function.

Notice in both of these cases that the function is actually assumed to be repetitive or cyclical. The fit goes on at the right

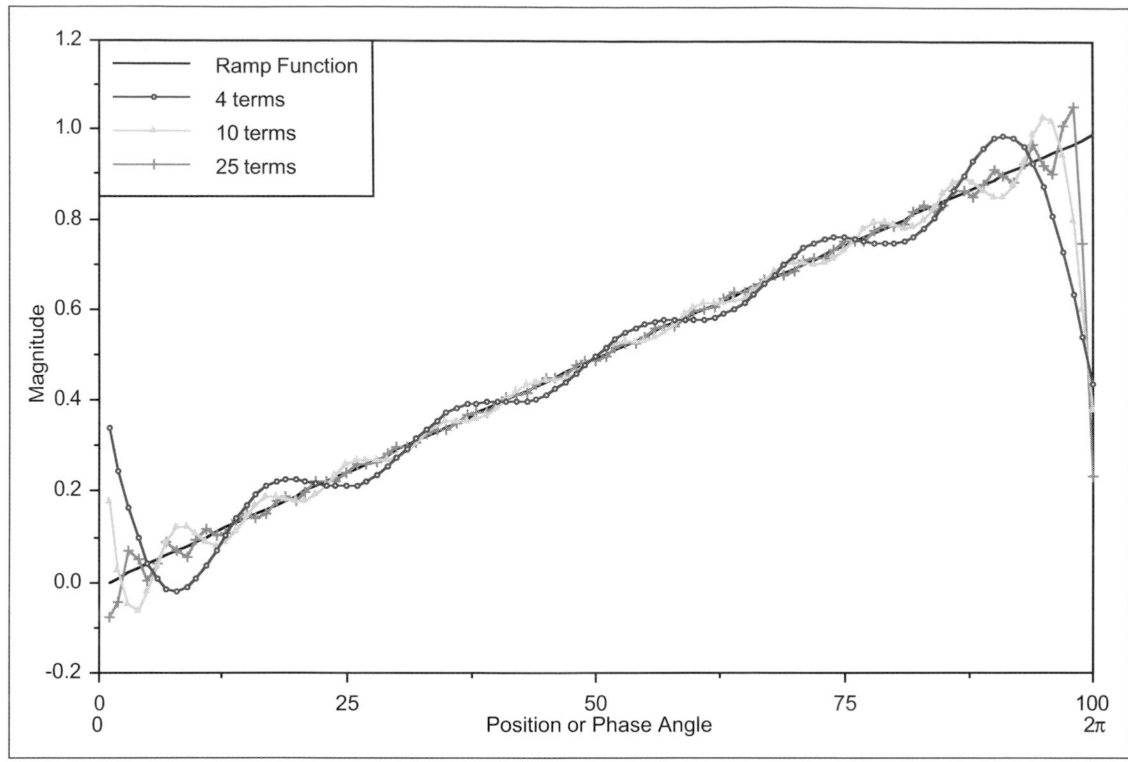

Figure 3. *Match between a ramp function and the first 4, 10, and 25 Fourier terms.*

and left ends of the interval as though the function were endlessly repeated there in both directions. This is also the case in two dimensions; the image in the spatial domain is essentially one tile in an endlessly repeating pattern. If the right and left edges or the top and bottom edges of the image are different, this can produce very noticeable effects in the resulting transform. One solution is to embed the image in a larger one consisting of either zeroes or the average brightness value of the pixels. This kind of padding makes the image twice as large in each direction, requiring four times as much storage and calculation. It is needed particularly when correlation is performed, as discussed below.

The magnitude of the Fourier coefficients from the fit shown in **Figures 2** and **3** is shown in **Figure 4,** plotted as amplitude vs. frequency. Notice that the step function consists only of odd terms, while the magnitudes for the ramp function transform decrease smoothly. Rather than the magnitudes, it is somewhat more common to plot the power spectrum of the transform, and to plot it as a symmetric function extending to both sides of the origin (zero frequency, or the DC level). As noted above, the power is simply the square of the magnitude. Because the range of values can be very large, the power spectrum is sometimes plotted with a logarithmic or other compressed vertical scale to show the smaller terms usually present at high frequencies, along with the lower frequency terms.

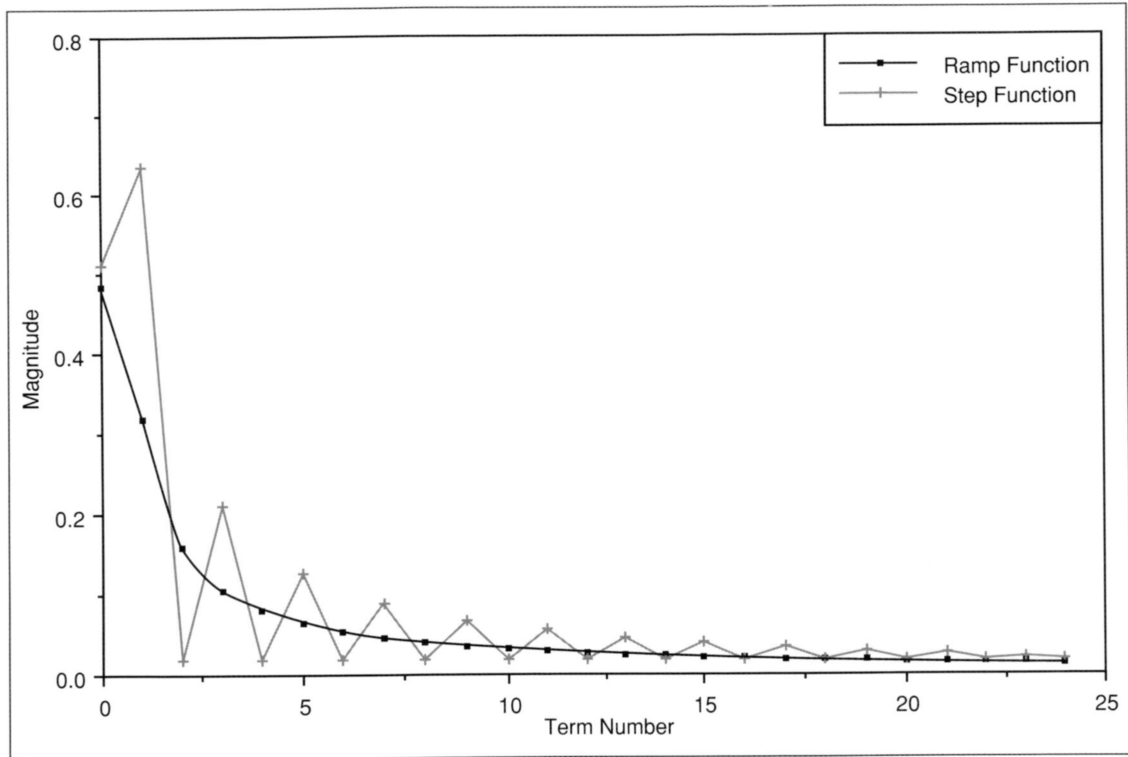

Figure 4. *Magnitude of the first 25 Fourier terms fit to the step and ramp in Figures 2 and 3.*

Figure 5 reiterates the duality of the Fourier transform process. The spatial and frequency domains show the information in very different ways, but the information is the same. Of course, the plot of amplitude in the frequency transform does not show the important phase information, but we understand that the values are actually complex.

It is important to recall, in examining these transforms, that the horizontal axis represents frequency. The low-frequency terms near the origin of the plot provide the overall shape of the function, while the high-frequency terms are needed to sharpen edges and provide fine detail. The second point to be kept in mind is that these terms are independent of each other (this is equivalent to the statement that the basis functions are orthogonal). Performing the transform to determine coefficients to higher and higher frequencies does not change the previous ones, and selecting any particular range of terms to reconstruct the function will do so to the greatest accuracy possible with those frequencies.

Proceeding to two dimensions, **Figure 6** shows the square wave simply extended uniformly in one direction. This produces a Fourier transform consisting of exactly the same frequency terms in the direction perpendicular to the step and nothing in any

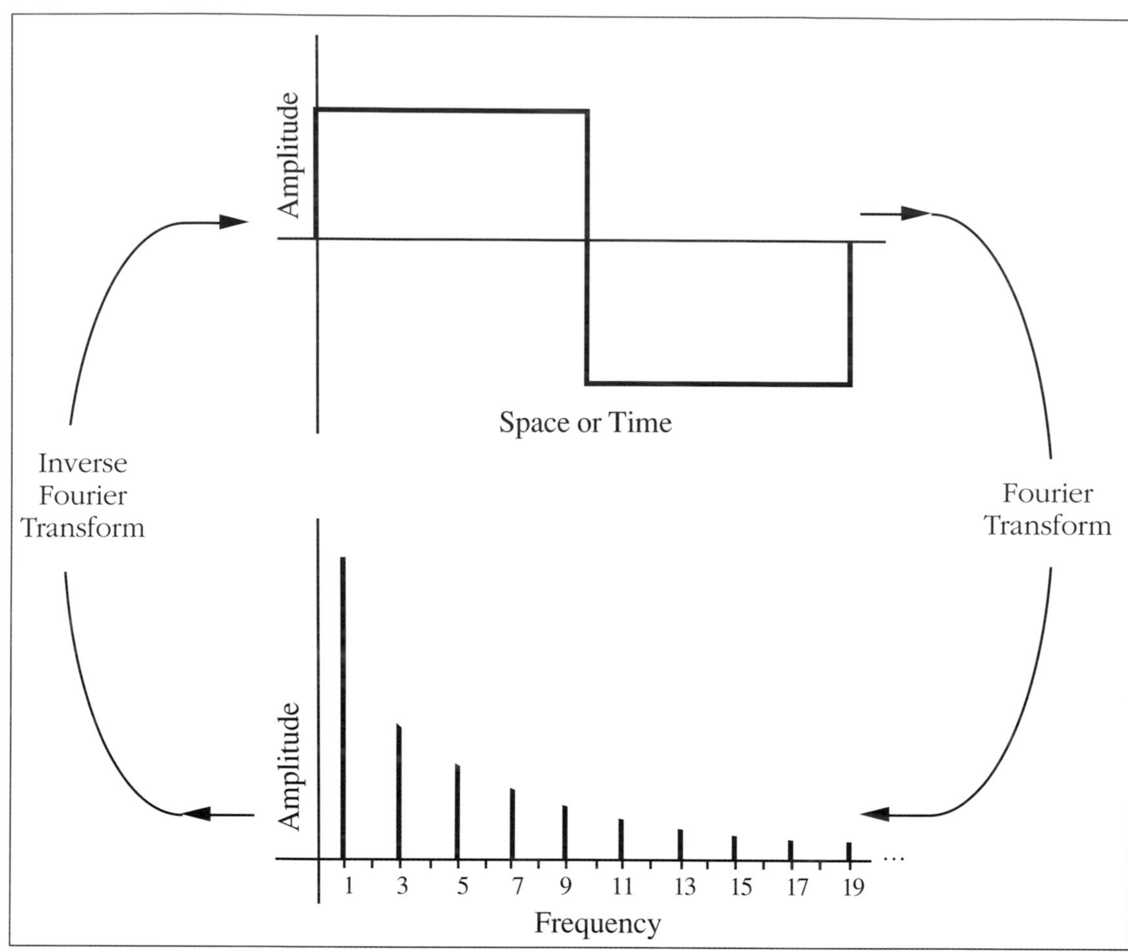

Figure 5. *Role of the forward and inverse transform and the spatial and frequency domain representations of a step function.*

other direction. **Figure 7** shows the transform of an image in which the brightness values vary in one direction as a linear ramp. Since the ramp varies in only one direction, the power spectrum consists of a single line of values whose brightness profile is the same as that for the one-dimensional function shown in **Figure 3.** The same power spectrum is obtained from the shifted ramp image shown in the figure (although the phase image is different). This image is 256 pixels wide, so a total of 128 terms are calculated. If only the first 25 of these terms are used in the reconstruction, the resulting ramp image, shown with grey scale coding in **Figure 8** and plotted isometrically in **Figure 9,** exhibits the same variation from the ideal ramp as shown in the one-dimensional case.

Figure 10 shows four images of perfectly sinusoidal variations in brightness. The first three vary in spacing (frequency) and orientation; the fourth is the superimposition of all three. For each, the two-dimensional frequency transform is particularly simple.

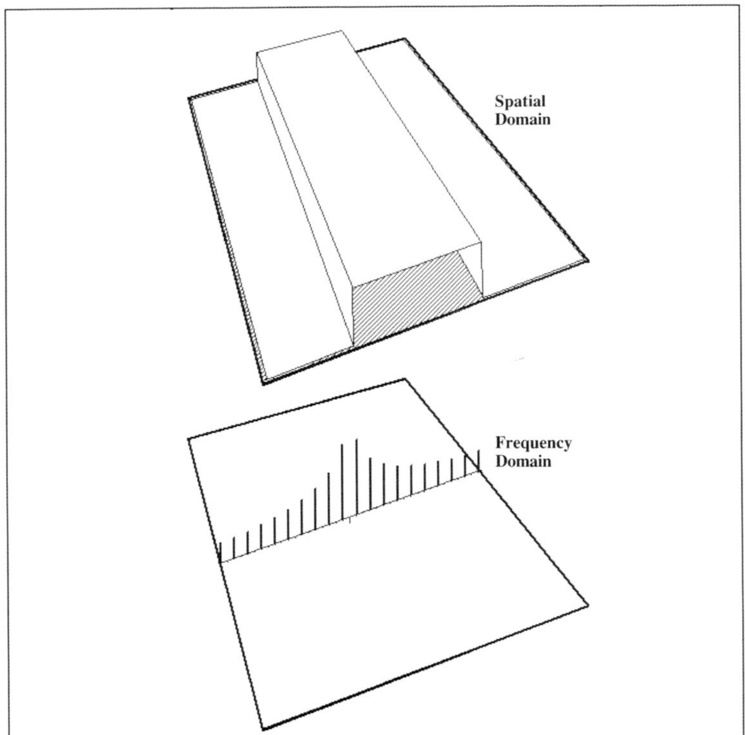

Figure 6. *Two-dimensional presentation of a step function and its frequency transform.*

Each of the pure tones has a transform consisting of a single point (identifying the frequency and orientation). Because of the redundancy of the plotting coordinates, the point is shown in two symmetrical locations around the origin. The superimposi-

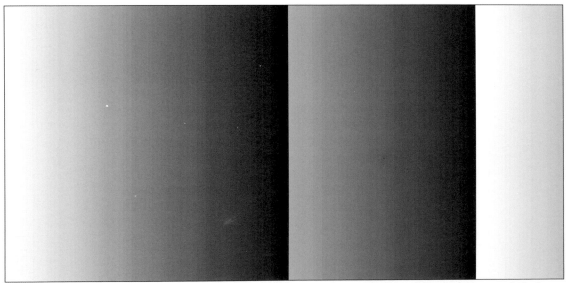

Figure 7. *Two-dimensional image of a simple one-dimensional ramp (left), and the same image shifted laterally (right).*

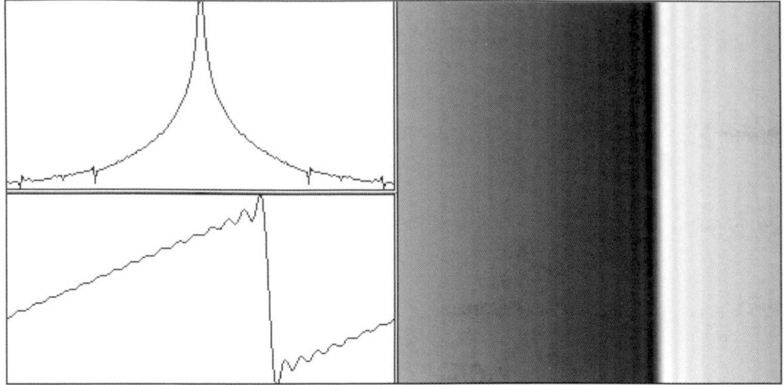

Figure 8. *The horizontal profile of the transform power spectrum from Figure 7 (top left), the retransformed image using the first 25 terms (right), and its horizontal brightness profile (bottom left).*

tion of the three sinusoids produces an image whose frequency transform is simply the sum of the three individual transforms. This principle of additivity will be important for much of the discussion below. Subtracting the information from a location in the frequency transform is equivalent to removing the corresponding information from every part of the spatial-domain image.

Figure 11 shows two images with the same shape in different orientations. The frequency transforms rotate with the feature. Two-dimensional power spectra are easiest to describe using polar coordinates, as indicated in **Figure 12** for the frequency transform of the step function. The frequency increases with radius ρ, and the orientation depends on the angle θ. It is common to display the two-dimensional transform with the frequencies plotted

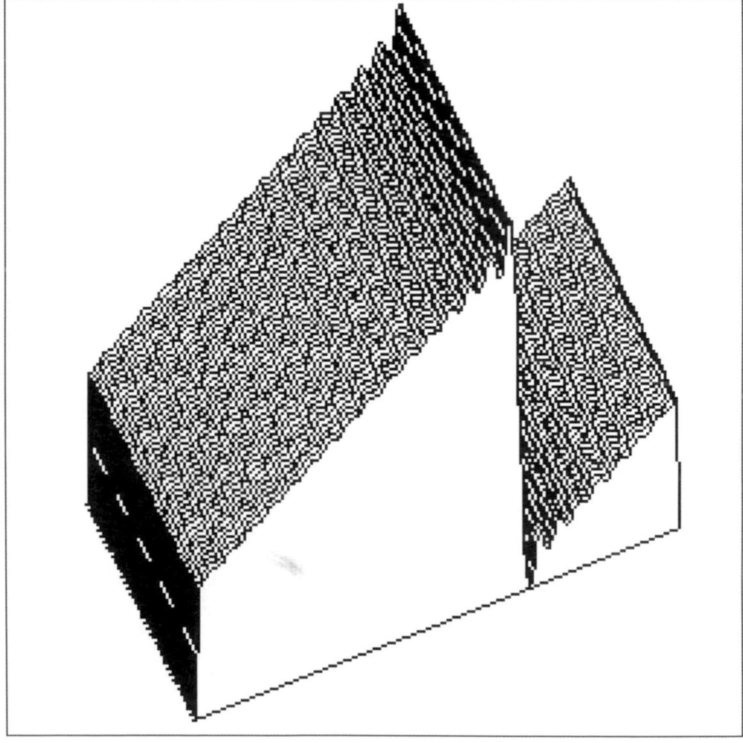

Figure 9. *Isometric plot of a reconstructed two-dimensional image of the results shown in Figure 8, based on the first 25 terms in the Fourier transform of the shifted linear ramp.*

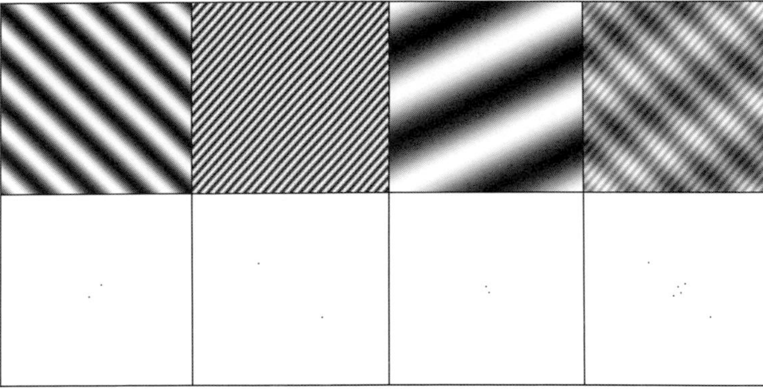

Figure 10. Three sinusoidal patterns, their frequency transforms, and their sum.

from the center of the image, which is consequently redundant (the top and bottom or left and right halves are simply duplicates, with symmetry about the origin). In some cases, this image is shifted so that the origin is at the corners of the image and the highest frequencies are in the center. One format can be converted to the other by swapping quadrants of the display. For most of the purposes of interest here (removing or selecting specific frequencies, etc.) the display with the origin centered will be simplest to use and has been adopted.

Figure 13 shows a two-dimensional step consisting of a rectangle. The two-dimensional frequency transform of this image produces the same series of diminishing peaks in the x and y axis directions as the one-dimensional step function. Limiting the

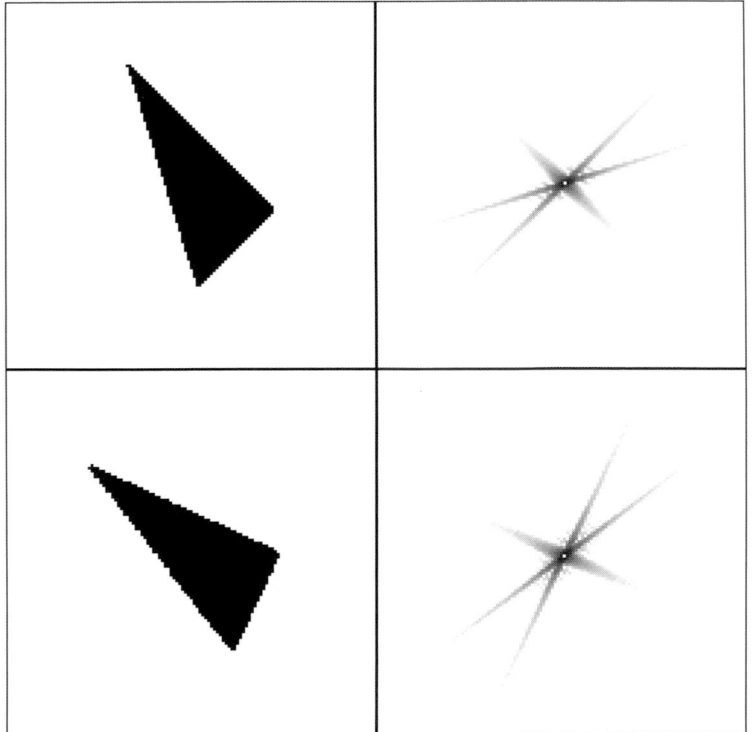

Figure 11. Rotation of a spatial-domain image (left), and the corresponding rotation of the frequency transform (right).

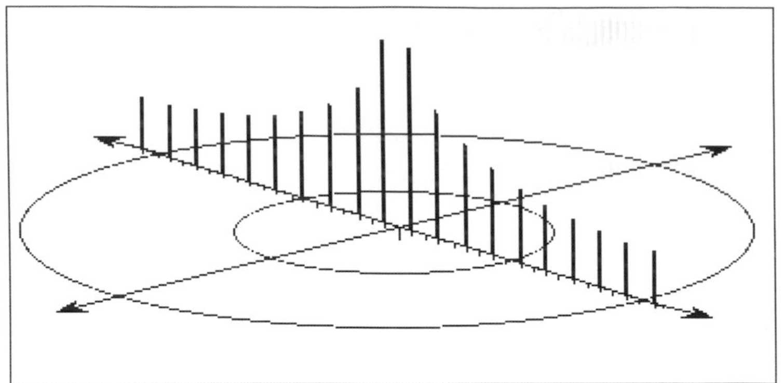

Figure 12. *Frequency transform of a step function rotates with orientation of the spatial image.*

reconstruction to only the central (low frequency) terms produces the reconstructions shown. Just as for the one-dimensional case, this limits the sharpness of the edge of the step and produces some ringing in the overall shape. The line profiles through the image show the same shape as previously discussed for the one-dimensional case. This can also be seen in **Figures 14** and **15,** where the magnitude, as well as the power spectrum with a logarithmic vertical scale, is showing. With a linear scale, the power spectrum would show only the central peak of this sinc function and the outer lobes would be virtually invisible. Notice also the different spacing of the lobes in the vertical and horizontal directions, resulting from the different dimensions of the original rectangle.

Frequencies and orientations

It is helpful to develop a little familiarity with the power spectrum display of the frequency-space transform of the image using simple images. **Figure 16** shows several shapes, more complex than the simple rectangular step function, with their two-dimensional frequency transforms. For each, the displayed power spectrum shows the orientation of the various edges and the various

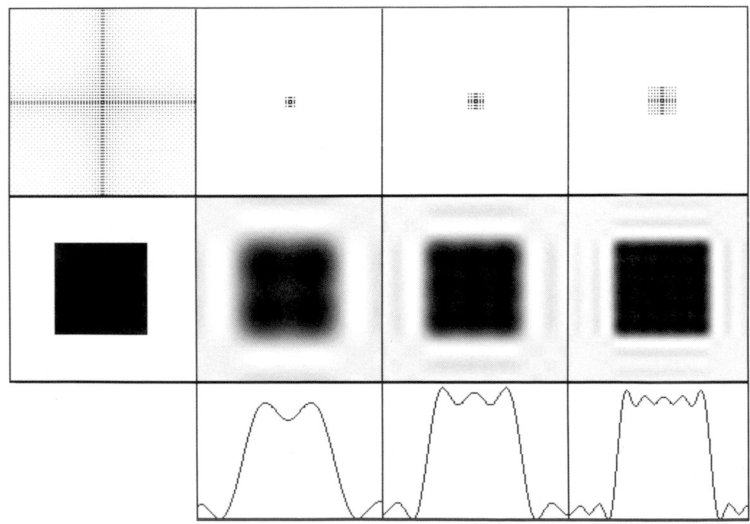

Figure 13. *A two-dimensional step function and its frequency transform (left), and reconstructions with different numbers of terms (shown as a portion of the frequency transform). Bottom row shows horizontal line profiles through the center of the reconstructed spatial image.*

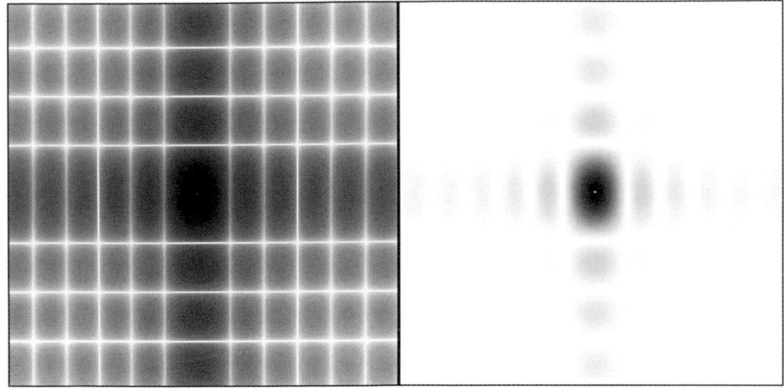

Figure 14. *The two-dimensional frequency transform of a rectangular step function shown as a logarithmic display of the power spectrum (left) and the magnitude (right).*

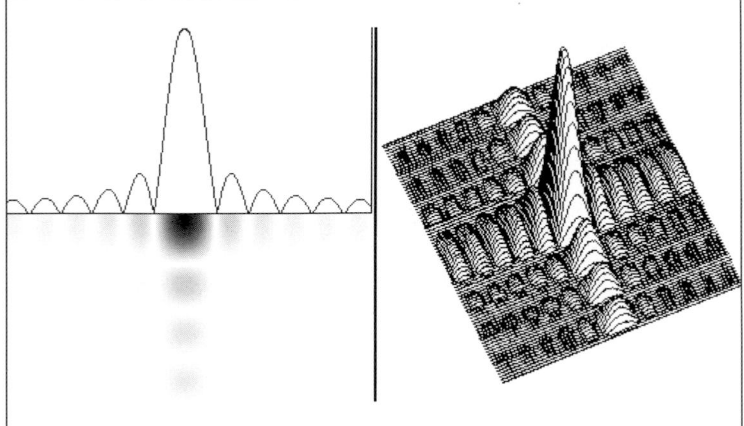

Figure 15. *The magnitude image from Figure 14 shown with cross section (left) and isometric display (right).*

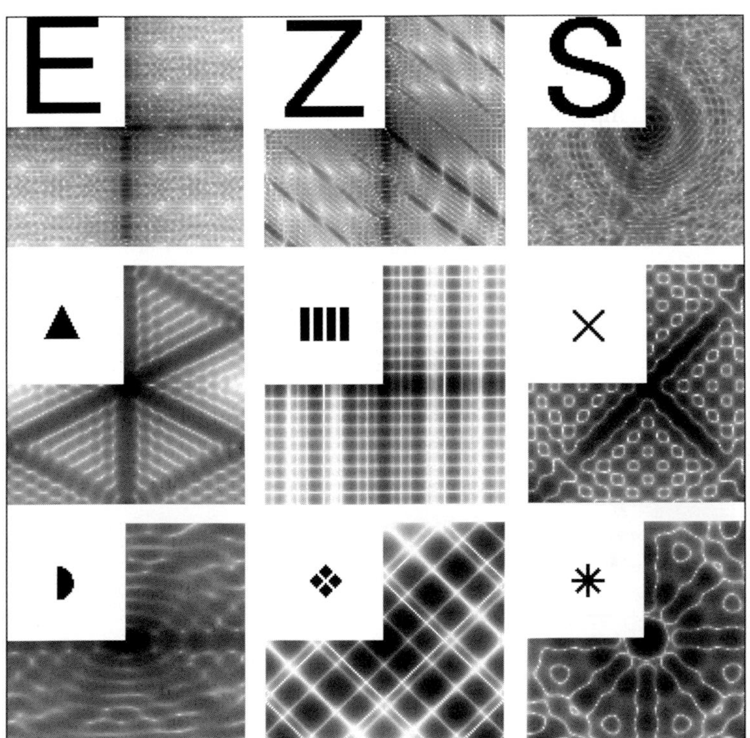

Figure 16. *Nine two-dimensional black and white shapes (insets) with their frequency transforms. (Image courtesy Arlo Reeves, Dartmouth Univ.)*

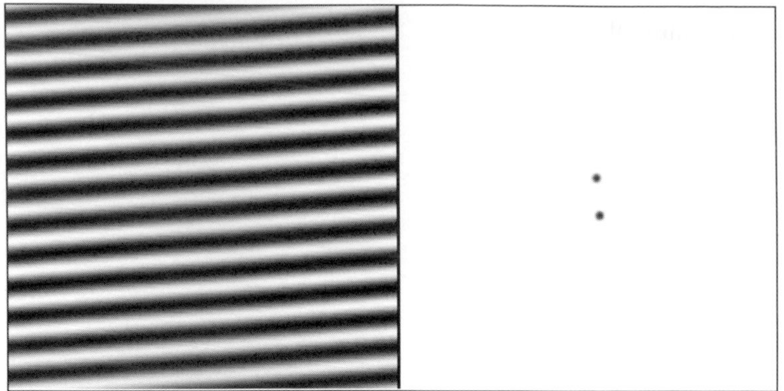

Figure 17. *A set of sinusoidal lines (left) and the frequency transform (right).*

frequencies show the terms needed to represent them. In only a few simple cases can a visual examination of the power spectrum identify the original generating shape.

In **Figure 17,** the lines can be represented by a single peak because their brightness profile is perfectly sinusoidal (as in **Figure 10** above); thus, only a single frequency is present. If the line profile is different, more terms are needed to represent the shape and consequently more peaks appear in the power spectrum. **Figure 18** shows an example in which the frequency transform consists of a series of peaks in the same orientation (perpendicular to the line angle).

In **Figure 19,** the lines have the aliasing common in computer displays (and in halftone printing technology), in which the lines at a shallow angle on the display are constructed from a series of steps corresponding to the rows of display pixels. This further complicates the frequency transform, which now has additional peaks representing the horizontal and vertical steps in the image that correspond to the aliasing, in addition to the main line of peaks seen in **Figure 18.**

It is possible to select only the peaks along the main row and eliminate the others with a mask or filter, as will be discussed below. After all, the frequency-domain image can be modified

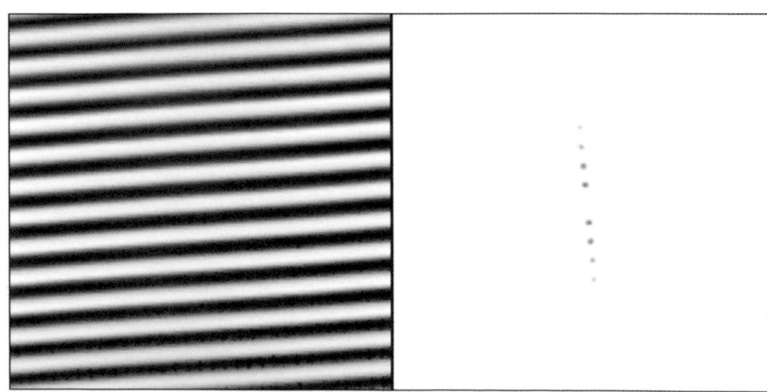

Figure 18. *The same lines as Figure 17 with a non-sinusoidal brightness profile.*

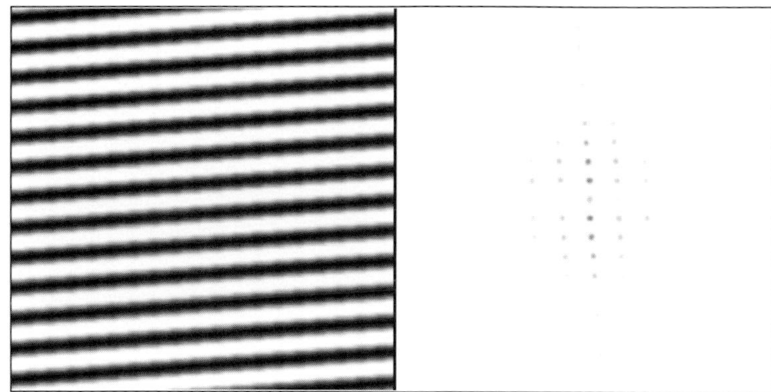

Figure 19. *The same lines as Figure 18 with aliasing.*

just like any other image. If this is done and only the peaks in the main row are used for the inverse transformation (back to the spatial domain), the aliasing of the lines is removed. In fact, that is how the images in **Figures 17** and **18** were produced. This will lead naturally to the subject of filtering (discussed in a later section): removing unwanted information from spatial-domain images by operating on the frequency transform.

Measuring images in the frequency domain

Orientation and spacing

The idealized examples shown in the preceding tutorial show that any periodic structure in the original spatial-domain image will be represented by a peak in the power spectrum image at a radius corresponding to the spacing and a direction corresponding to the orientation. In a real image, which also includes non-periodic information, these peaks will be superimposed on a broad, and sometimes noisy, background. However, finding the peaks is generally much easier than finding the original periodic structure. Also, measuring the peak locations is much easier and more accurate than trying to extract the same information from the original image, because all of the occurrences are effectively averaged together in the frequency domain.

Figure 20 shows an example of this peak measurement. The spatial-domain image is a very high-resolution TEM image of the lattice structure in pure silicon. The regular spacing of the bright spots represents the atomic structure of the lattice. Measuring all of the individual spacings of the spots would be very time-consuming and not particularly accurate. The frequency-domain representation of this image shows the periodicity clearly. The series of peaks indicates that the variation of brightness is not a simple sine wave, but contains many higher harmonics. The first-order peak gives the basic atomic spacing (and orientation), which can be measured by interpolating the peak position to a fraction of a pixel width, corresponding to an accuracy of a few parts in ten thousand.

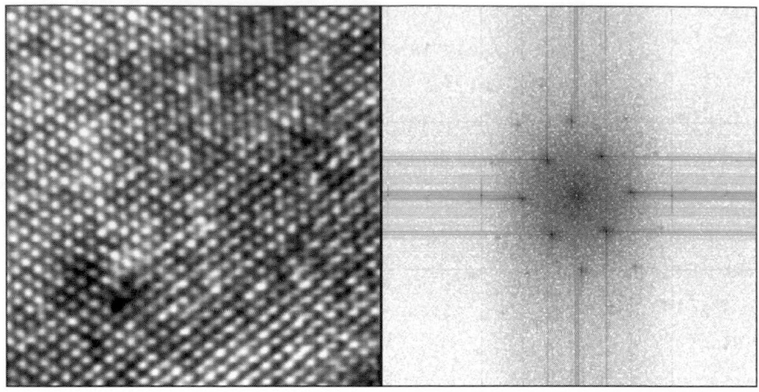

Figure 20. *High-resolution TEM image of atomic lattice in silicon (left), with the frequency transform (right). (Image courtesy Sopa Cehvacharoenkul, Microelectronics Center of North Carolina.)*

To the electron microscopist, the power spectrum image of the frequency-domain transform looks just like an electron diffraction pattern, which in fact it is. The use of microscope optics to form the diffraction pattern is an analog method of computing the frequency domain representation. This can be done with any image by setting up suitable optics. While it is a fast way to obtain the frequency-domain representation, however, it has two serious drawbacks for use in image processing.

First, the phase information is lost when the diffraction pattern is recorded, so it is not possible to reconstruct the spatial-domain image from a photograph of the diffraction pattern. It is possible to do so from the actual pattern by using suitable lenses (indeed, that is what happens in the microscope), so in principle it is possible to insert the various masks and filters discussed below. However, making these masks and filters is difficult and exacting work and must usually be performed individually for each image to be enhanced. Consequently, it is much easier (and more controllable) to use a computer to perform the transform and to apply any desired masks.

It is also easier to perform measurements on the frequency-domain representation using the computer. Locating the centers of peaks by curve fitting would require recording the diffraction pattern (typically with film, which may introduce nonlinearities or saturation over the extremely wide dynamic range of many patterns), followed by digitization to obtain numerical values. Considering the speed with which a spatial-domain image can be recorded, the frequency transform calculated, and interactive or automatic measurement performed, the computer is generally the tool of choice.

Figure 21 shows an electron microscope image of two adjacent grains in a ceramic (mullite) structure. The calculated diffraction patterns from each region can be analyzed to determine the orientation difference between the grains. This is made easier by the ability to adjust the display contrast so that both brighter and dimmer spots can be seen. Contrast adjustments can be made

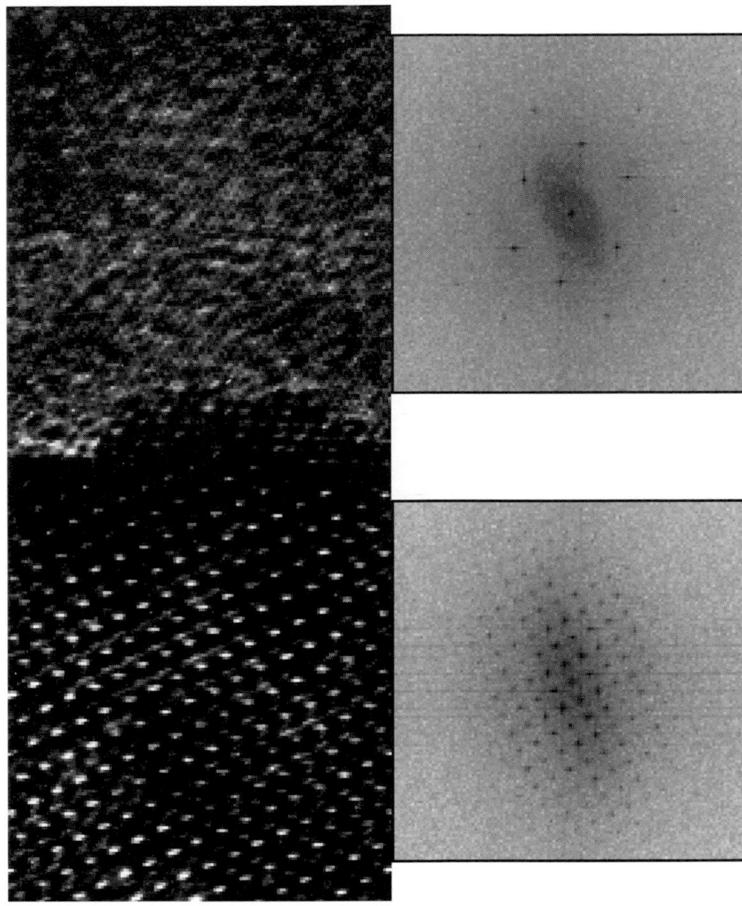

Figure 21. *High-resolution TEM image of two adjacent grains in mullite (left), with their frequency transforms (right). (Image courtesy Sopa Cehvacharoenkul, Microelectronics Center of North Carolina.)*

with much more flexibility than photographic film recording of the patterns can afford.

When spots from a periodic structure are superimposed on a general background, the total power in the spots expressed as a fraction of the total power in the entire frequency transform gives a useful quantitative measure of the degree of periodicity in the structure. This may also be used to compare different periodicities (different spacings or orientations) by comparing their summations of values in the power spectrum. For electron diffraction patterns, this is a function of the atomic density of various planes and the atomic scattering cross sections.

While the display of the power spectrum corresponds to a diffraction pattern and is the most familiar presentation of frequency-space information, it must not be forgotten that the phase information is also needed to reconstruct the original image. **Figure 22** shows a test image, consisting of a regular pattern of spots, and its corresponding power spectrum. If the phase information is erased (all phases set to zero), the reconstruction **(Figure 23)** shows some of the same periodicity, but the objects are no longer recognizable. The various sine waves have been shifted in phase, so the feature boundaries are not reconstructed.

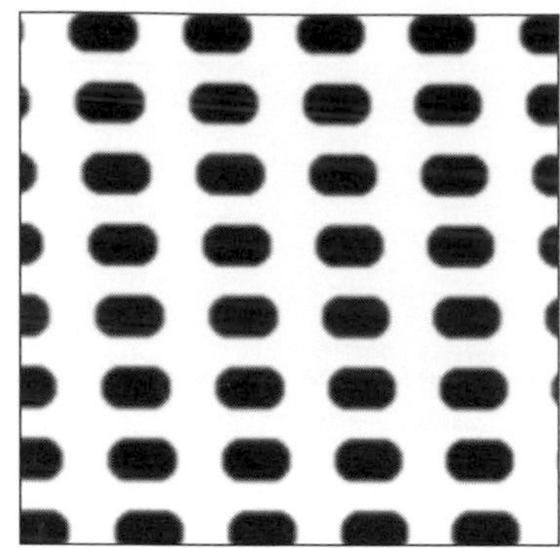

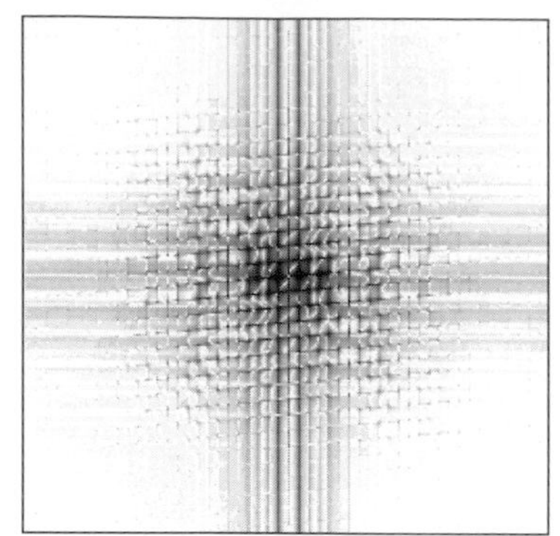

Figure 22. *Test image consisting of a regular pattern and its frequency transform power spectrum.*

The assumption that the image is one repetition of an endless sequence is also important. Most real images do not have perfectly matching left and right or top and bottom edges. This produces a large step function at the edge, which would be more apparent if the image were shifted by an arbitrary offset **(Figure 24).** As in the ramp example shown earlier, this does not alter the power spectrum image, although the phase image is shifted. The discontinuity requires high-frequency terms to fit, and since the edges are precisely horizontal and vertical, the power spectrum display shows a central cross superimposed on the rest of the data. For the test pattern of **Figure 22,** the result of eliminating these lines from the original frequency transform and then retransforming is shown in **Figure 25.** The central portion of the

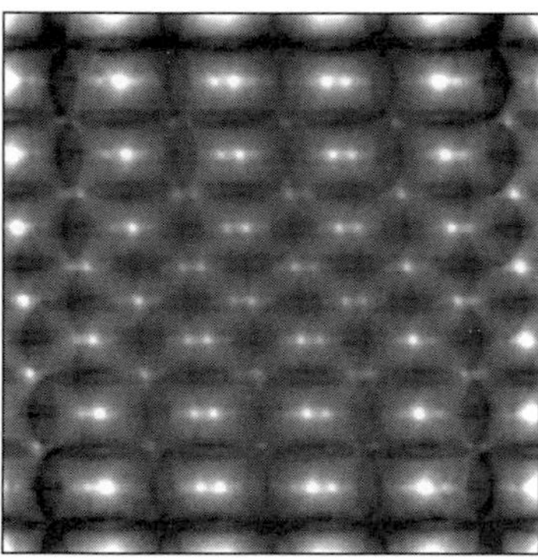

Figure 23. *Retransformation of Figure 22 with all phase information set to zero.*

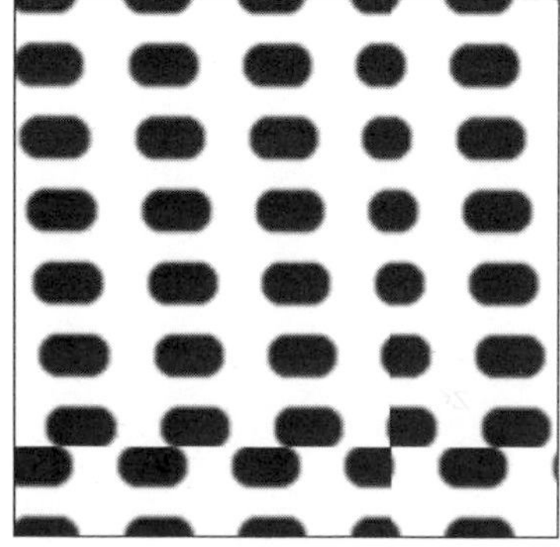

Figure 24. *The test image of Figure 22 with an arbitrary spatial shift, showing the discontinuities at the image boundaries*

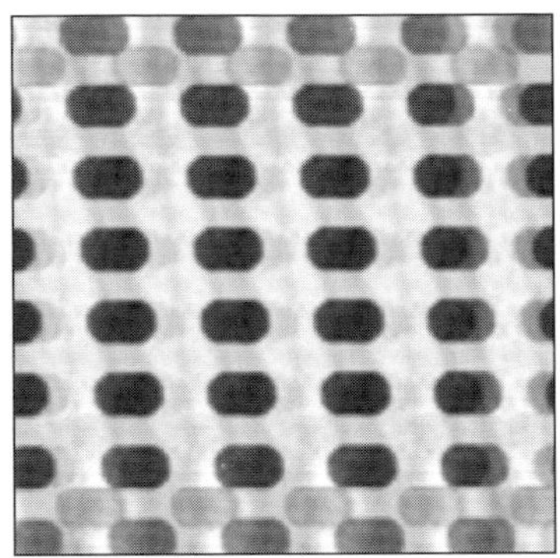

Figure 25. *Retransformation of Figure 22 with the central cross (horizontal and vertical lines) reduced to zero magnitude, so that the left and right edges of the image, and the top and bottom edges, are forced to match.*

image is unaffected, but at the edges the discontinuity is no longer fit. The pattern from each side has been reproduced on the other side of the boundary, superimposed on the correct data.

Preferred orientation

Figure 26 shows another example of a periodic structure, only much less perfect and larger in scale than the lattice images above. The specimen is a thin film of magnetic material viewed in polarized light. The stripes are oppositely oriented magnetic domains in the material that are used to store information in the film. The frequency transform of this image clearly shows the width and spacing of the domains. Instead of a single peak, there are arcs. They show the variation in stripe orientation, which is evident in the original image but difficult to quantify.

The length of the arcs and the variation of brightness (power) with angle along them can be easily measured to characterize the preferred orientation in the structure. Even for structures that are not perfectly periodic, the integrated power as a function of angle can be used to measure the preferred orientation. This is identical to the results of autocorrelation operations carried out in the spatial domain, in which a binary image is shifted and combined with itself in all possible displacements to obtain a matrix of fractional values, but it is much faster to perform with the fre-

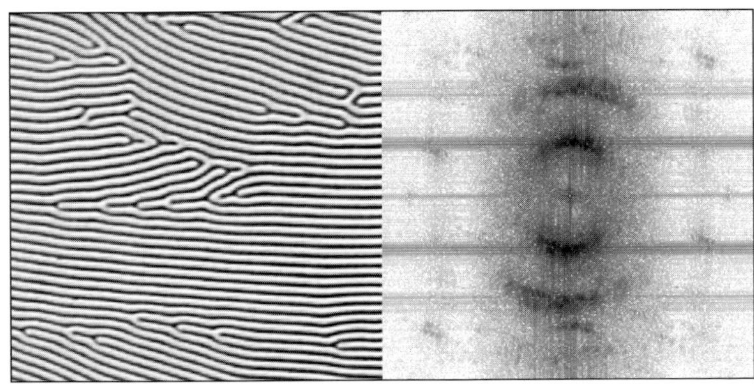

Figure 26. *Polarized light image of magnetic domains in thin film material (left), with the frequency transform (right).*

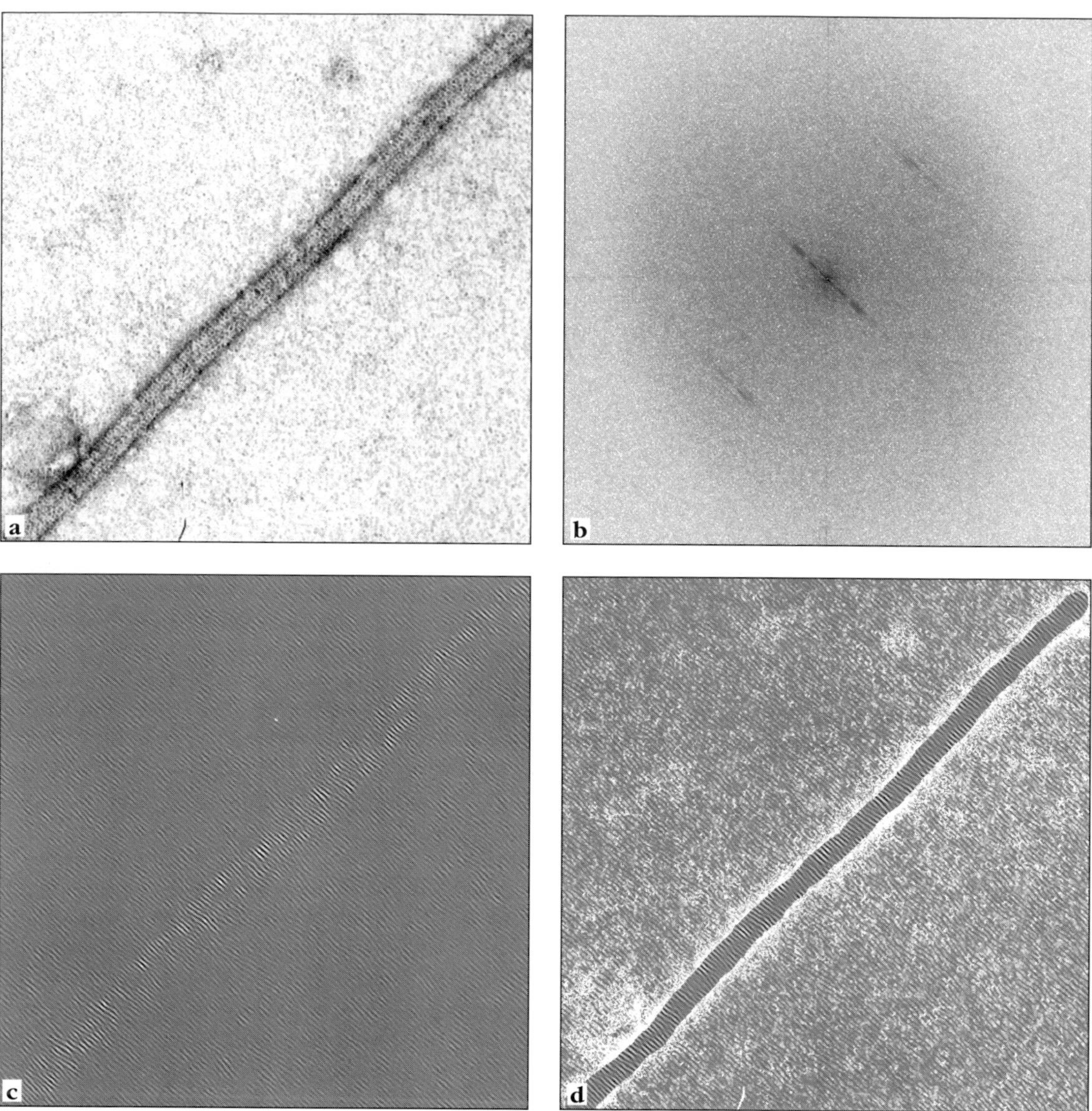

Figure 27. TEM image of a virus *(courtesy Dr. R. L. Grayson, Virginia Polytechnic Institute, Blacksburg, VA):* ***a)*** *original image, in which the internal helical structure is difficult to discern;* ***b)*** *frequency transform of image a, in which the regular repeating structure of the virus and its angular variation in orientation is evident;* ***c)*** *retransformation of just the peaks in the frequency transform, in which the periodic lines are not limited to the virus;* ***d)*** *using the virus particle as a mask, the helical pattern becomes evident.*

quency-domain representation. Also, this makes it easier to deal with grey scale values.

Reconstructing periodic structures that are not perfectly aligned can be performed by selecting the entire arc in the frequency transform. **Figure 27** illustrates this with a virus particle. The TEM image hints at the internal helical structure, but does not show it clearly. In the frequency transform, the periodic spacing and the variation in direction is evident. The spacing can be measured (2.41 nm) and the helix angle determined from the length of the arc. Retransforming only these arcs shows the periodicity but is not limited spatially to the virus particle. Using

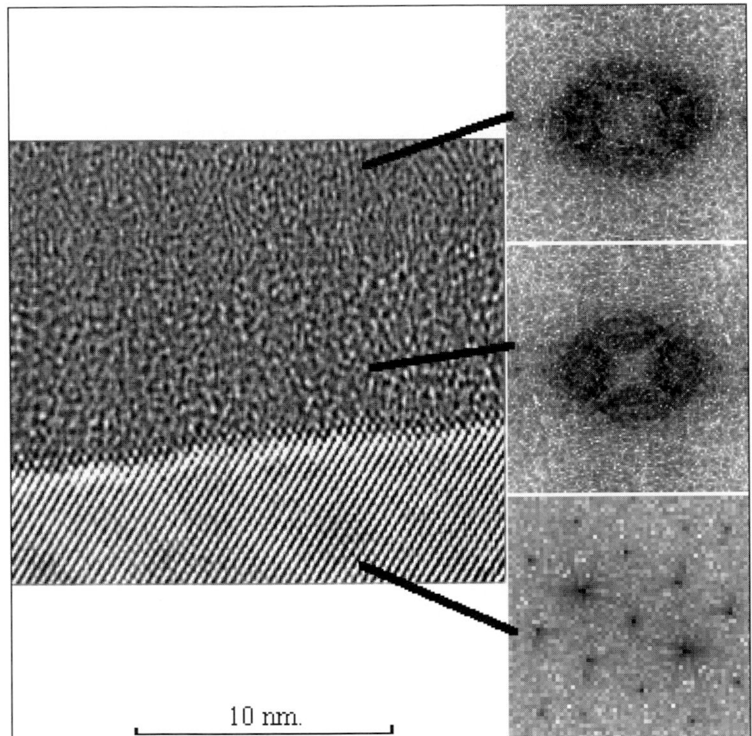

Figure 28. *TEM image of cross section of crystalline and amorphous silicon, and glue, with frequency transforms of each region shown at right. (Image courtesy Sopa Cehvacharoenkul, Microelectronics Center of North Carolina.)*

the spatial-domain image as a mask (as discussed in Chapter 6) makes the helical pattern evident.

One particular type of preferred orientation in images, which arises not from the specimen but rather from the imaging system itself, is astigmatism. This is a particular problem with electron microscopes because of the operating principles of electromagnetic lenses. Even skilled operators devote considerable time to making adjustments to minimize astigmatism and it is often very difficult to recognize it in images in order to correct it. Astigmatism results in the defocusing of the image and a consequent loss of sharpness in one direction, with an improvement in the perpendicular direction. This becomes immediately evident in the frequency transform, since the decrease in brightness or power falls off radially (at higher frequencies) and the asymmetry can be noted.

Figure 28 shows an example. The specimen is a cross section with three layers. The bottom is crystalline silicon, above which is a layer of amorphous (non-crystalline) silicon, followed by a layer of glue used to mount the sample for thinning and microscopy. The glue is difficult to distinguish by eye from the amorphous silicon. Frequency transforms for the three regions are shown. The bright spots in the pattern from the crystalline silicon give the expected diffraction pattern. While the two regions above do not show individual peaks from periodic structures, they are not the same. The amorphous silicon has short-range

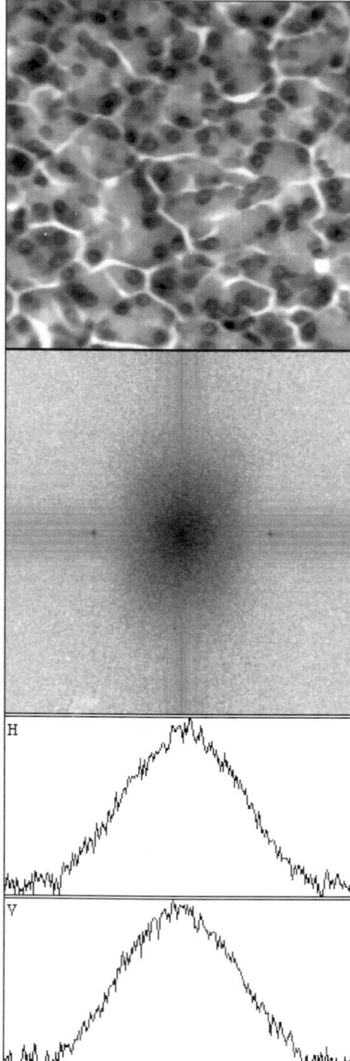

Figure 29. *Out-of-focus image with its power spectrum and horizontal and vertical line profiles, showing presence of high-frequency information as compared to Figure 30.*

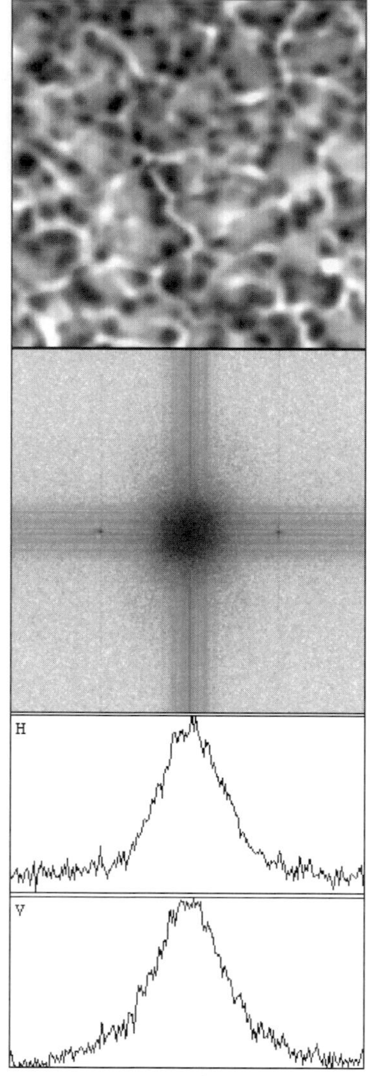

Figure 30. *Out-of-focus image with its power spectrum and horizontal and vertical line profiles, showing loss of high-frequency information as compared to Figure 29.*

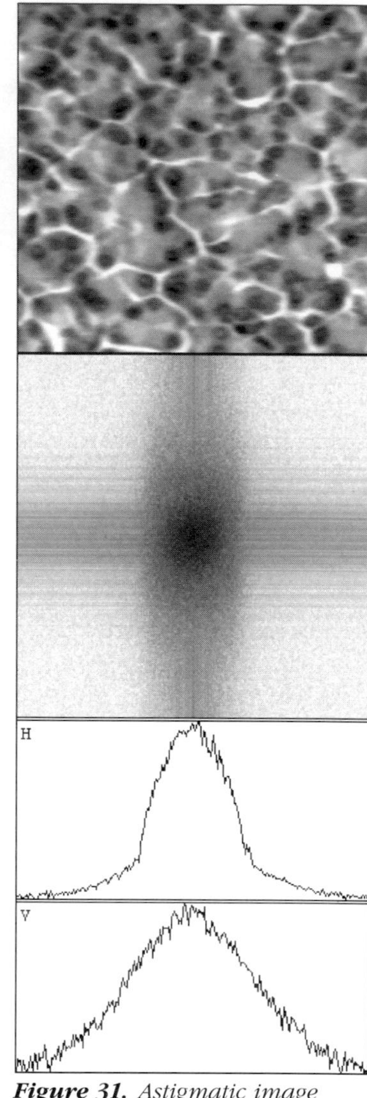

Figure 31. *Astigmatic image produced by misaligning lens, with its power spectrum and horizontal and vertical line profiles showing different high-frequency components.*

order in the atomic spacings, based on strong covalent atomic bonding. It is not visible to the human observer because of its chaotic overall pattern. This shows up in the frequency transform as a white cross in the dark ring, indicating that in the 45-degree directions there is a characteristic distance and direction to the next atom. This pattern is absent in the glue region, where there is no such structure.

In both regions, the dark circular pattern from the amorphous structure is not a perfect circle, but an ellipse. This indicates astigmatism. Adjusting the microscope optics to produce a uni-

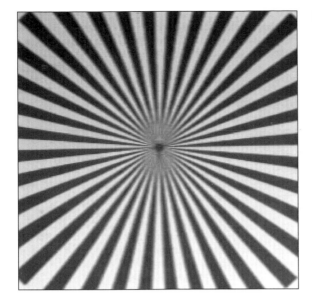

Figure 32. *Test pattern image.*

form circle will correct the astigmatism and provide uniform resolution in all directions in the original image. It is much easier to observe the effects of small changes in the frequency space display than in the spatial-domain image.

The frequency transform of an image can be used to optimize focus and astigmatism. When an image is in focus, the high-frequency information is maximized in order to sharply define the edges. This provides a convenient test for sharpest focus. **Figure 29** shows a light microscope image that is in focus. The line profiles of the power spectrum in both the vertical and horizontal directions show a more gradual dropoff at high frequencies than **Figure 30,** which is the same image out of focus. When astigmatism is present **(Figure 31),** the power spectrum is asymmetric, as shown by the profiles.

Figure 32 shows a test pattern of radial lines. Due to the finite spacing of detectors in the video camera used, as well as limitations in the electronics bandwidth which eliminate the very high frequencies required to resolve small details, these lines are incompletely resolved where they are close together. **Figure 33** shows the two-dimensional Fourier-transform power spectrum of this image, plotted isometrically to emphasize the magnitude values. The low-frequency information is at the center, as usual, and the frequencies increase radially.

It is evident that there is a well-defined boundary, different in the x and y directions, beyond which the magnitude drops abruptly. This corresponds to the spacing of the individual detectors in the camera, which is different in the horizontal and vertical directions. In many cases, it is not so obvious where the physical source of resolution limitation lies. However, the Fourier-transform power spectrum will still show the limit, permitting the resolution of any imaging system to be ascertained.

Figure 33. *Frequency transform of image in Figure 32, presented as an isometric view.*

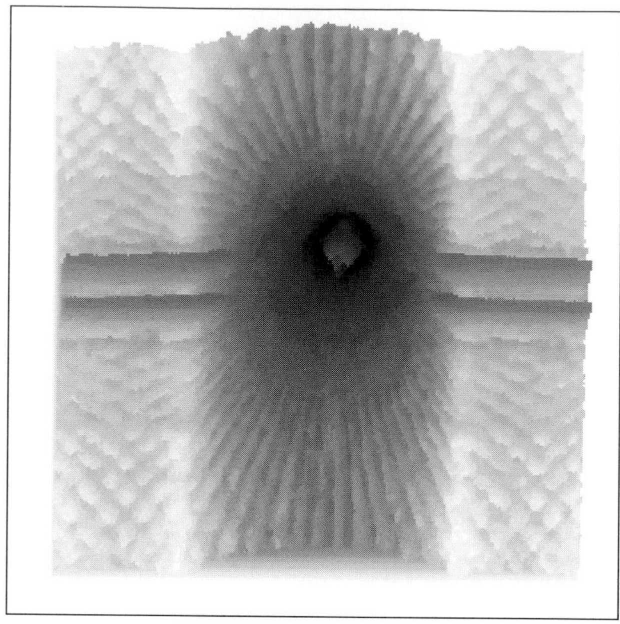

Texture and fractals

Besides the peaks in the power spectrum resulting from periodic structures that may be present and the ultimate limitation at high frequencies due to finite image resolution, it may seem as though there is only a noisy background containing little useful information. This is far from true. Many images represent the brightness of light scattered from surfaces or other data, such as surface elevation. In these images, the roughness or texture of the surface is revealed and may be measured from the power spectrum.

The concept of a fractal surface dimension will not be explained here in detail. Surfaces that are fractal have an area that is mathematically undefined. It is greater than the projected area covered by the irregular surface and increases as the measurement scale becomes finer. The fractal dimension is the slope of a line on a log-log plot of measured area vs. the size of the measuring tool. Many naturally occurring surfaces resulting from wear, erosion, agglomeration of particles, or fracture are observed to have this character. It has also been shown that images of these surfaces, whether produced by the scattering of diffuse light or the production of secondary electrons in an SEM, are also fractal. That is, the variation of brightness with position obeys the same mathematical relationship. The fractal dimension is an extremely powerful and compact representation of the surface roughness, which can often be related to the history of the surface and the properties that result.

Measuring surface fractals directly is rarely practical. The most common approach is to reduce the dimensionality and measure the fractal dimension of a boundary line produced by intersecting the surface with a sampling plane. This may either be pro-

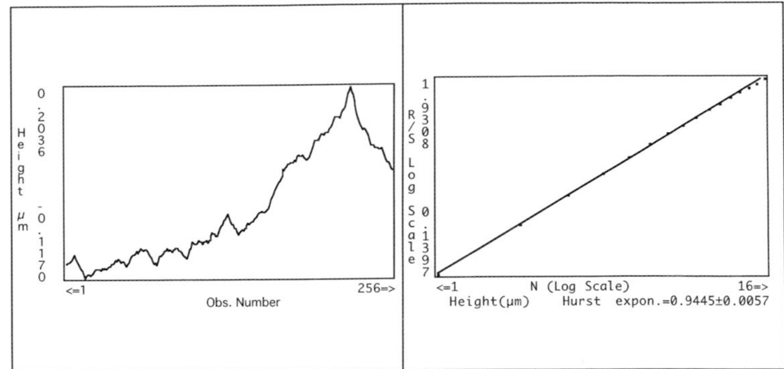

Figure 34. *A one-dimensional computer-generated line (left) with the rescaled range plot showing its Hurst coefficient (right).*

duced by cross sectioning or by polishing down into the surface to produce islands. In either case, the rougher the surface, the more irregular the line. This line also has a fractal dimension (the slope of a log-log plot relating the measured line length and the length of the measurement tool), which is just 1.0 less than that of the surface.

A closely related approach to measuring the fractal dimension of a line is the Hurst coefficient (also known as the rescaled range). First applied to time-series data, it plots the maximum difference between any two points in the sequence as a function of the temporal difference. The slope on a log-log scale is the coefficient K. If the values are elevation values along a traverse across a physical surface, then the fractal dimension is just $F = 2 - K$.

For many images, it is easy to perform this determination along a single line profile across the image. However, it is difficult to obtain a meaningful average value for the entire surface or to study systematically the variation in roughness with orientation that is often present, depending on the history of the surface.

Earlier figures showed the linear addition of frequency terms to construct a square or sawtooth wave. For a fractal profile, we expect that terms of increasingly higher frequency will continue to contribute to the summation, since by definition a fractal curve is self-similar and has detail extending to ever-finer scales (or higher frequencies). This also implies that the proportion of amplitudes of higher frequency terms must be self-similar. The curve that satisfies this criterion is exponential. The magnitudes of the coefficients in a Fourier-series fit to a fractal curve decrease exponentially with the log of frequency, while their phases are randomized.

Figure 34 shows a computer-generated fractal line and its rescaled range plot, whose slope gives the Hurst coefficient. The plot of Fourier magnitudes shown in **Figure 35** shows the expected exponential decrease. **Figure 36** shows a plot correlating the slope observed in the Fourier magnitude plot with the Hurst coefficient of ten such lines. This implies that there is a simple relationship between the fractal dimension of a profile and the ex-

Figure 35. Log-log plot of FFT magnitude vs. frequency for the line in Figure 34.

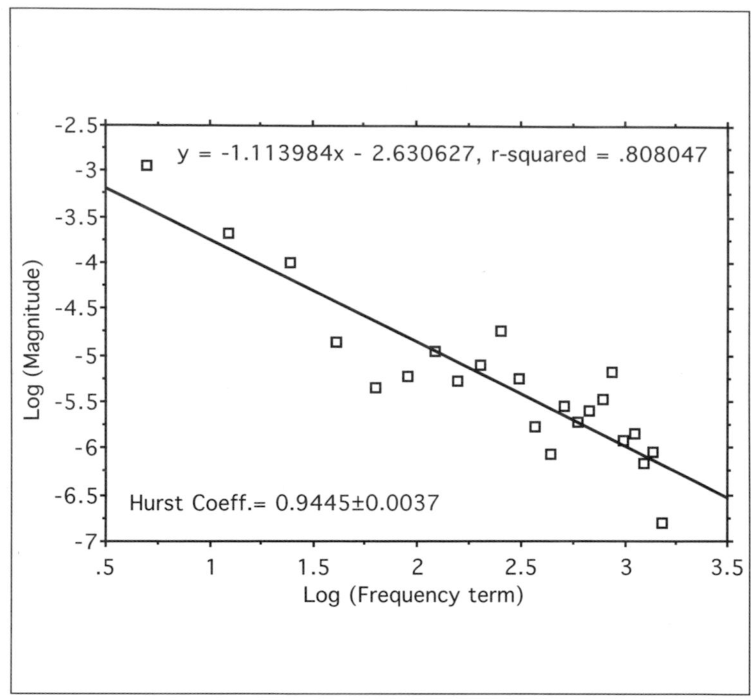

ponential decrease in magnitude of the terms in a Fourier expansion, as indeed had been predicted by Feder (1988). This correlation makes it practical to use the radial decrease of magnitude in a two-dimensional Fourier-transform image as a measure of roughness and the directional variation of that decrease as a measure of orientation (Mitchell & Bonnell, 1990; Russ, 1990b).

Correlating the slope is much more efficient than measuring and averaging Hurst coefficients along many individual brightness profiles in the original image. It also allows any periodic structures that may be present to be ignored, since these show up as discrete points in the frequency-transform image and can be skipped in determining the overall exponential decrease in the

Figure 36. Correlation between slope of the plot of log magnitude vs. log frequency curves for the frequency transform, and Hurst coefficient, for ten generated test lines.

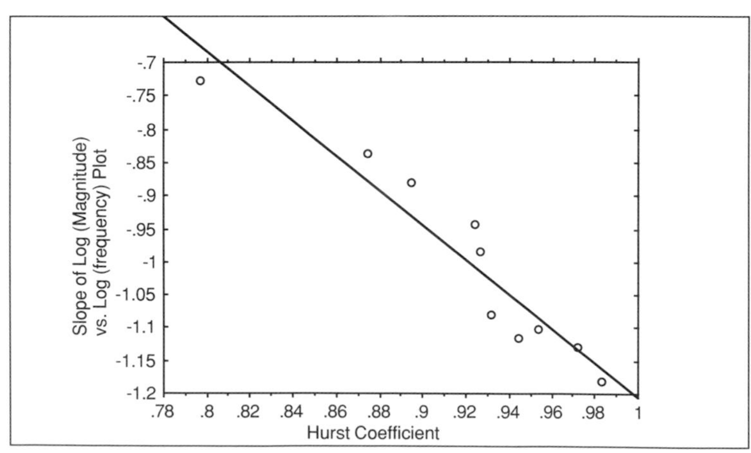

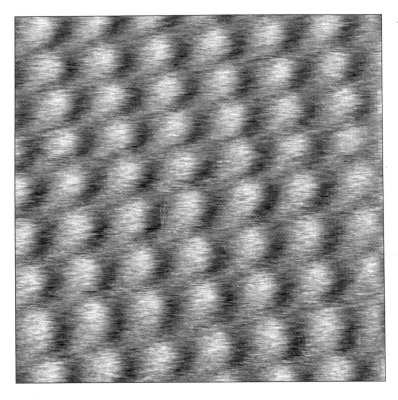

Figure 37. *STM image of pyrolytic graphite. (Image courtesy Richard Chapman, Microelectronics Center of North Carolina.)*

magnitude values. In other words, it is possible to look beyond the periodic structures or noise (e.g., arising from electronic components) in the images and still characterize the underlying chaotic nature of the surface, as shown in the image.

Figure 37 shows an image of surface elevation measured with a STM. The sample is an ion-implanted surface that has been altered by the interaction and motion of atoms under the ion beam. The periodic structure evident is the atomic lattice of the material, a hexagonal basal plane in pyrolytic graphite. Individual line profiles of the brightness (elevation) values in the image can be fit to determine a Hurst coefficient, as long as the bright points (atoms) are avoided. However, these are only samples of the surface; we would like to characterize the average roughness and its directional variation.

Figure 38 shows the two-dimensional Fourier transform of this image. The power spectrum image is shown with a logarithmic intensity scale, so we expect to find a linear decrease in brightness with the log of radius (frequency). **Figure 39** shows several plots in the horizontal direction on the transform, which do indeed follow this trend for log (magnitude) vs. log (frequency). Notice that the few high values corresponding to periodic peaks in the power spectrum can easily be skipped in performing the fit.

Figure 40 shows a plot of the same information in the vertical direction. These data do not fit the expected function, indicating

Figure 38. *Two-dimensional FFT of the image in Figure 37.*

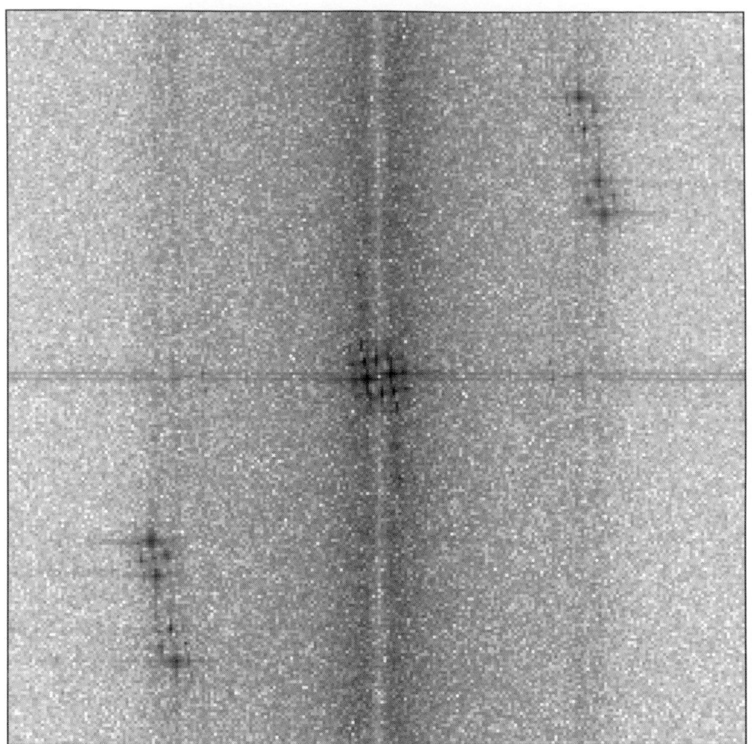

that the variation of measured brightness does not vary in a fractal pattern in this direction. The detailed interpretation of these results on a series of specimens has yet to be performed. It is likely, though, that the good fit to a Hurst relationship in the direction perpendicular to the raster lines in the scan reveals a source of time-correlated noise, arising from either electronic or mechanical sources in the microscope, which is not present along one scan line. Nevertheless, it is clear that a fractal analysis of two-dimensional surface roughness is possible and that the data can be obtained using frequency transforms of the original images.

Filtering images

Isolating periodic noise

Figure 41 shows two spatial-domain features having grey scales that together would add up to the same rectangular step function shown in Figure 13. The power spectrum displays of these two images are shown along with their sum **(Figure 42).** The sum is identical to that shown in **Figure 13** for the original rectangle. In other words, the frequency transform has a property of separability and additivity. Adding together the transforms of two original images or functions produces the same result as the transform of the sum of the originals.

This opens the way to using subtraction to remove unwanted parts of images. It is most commonly used to remove periodic noise, which can be introduced by the devices used to record or

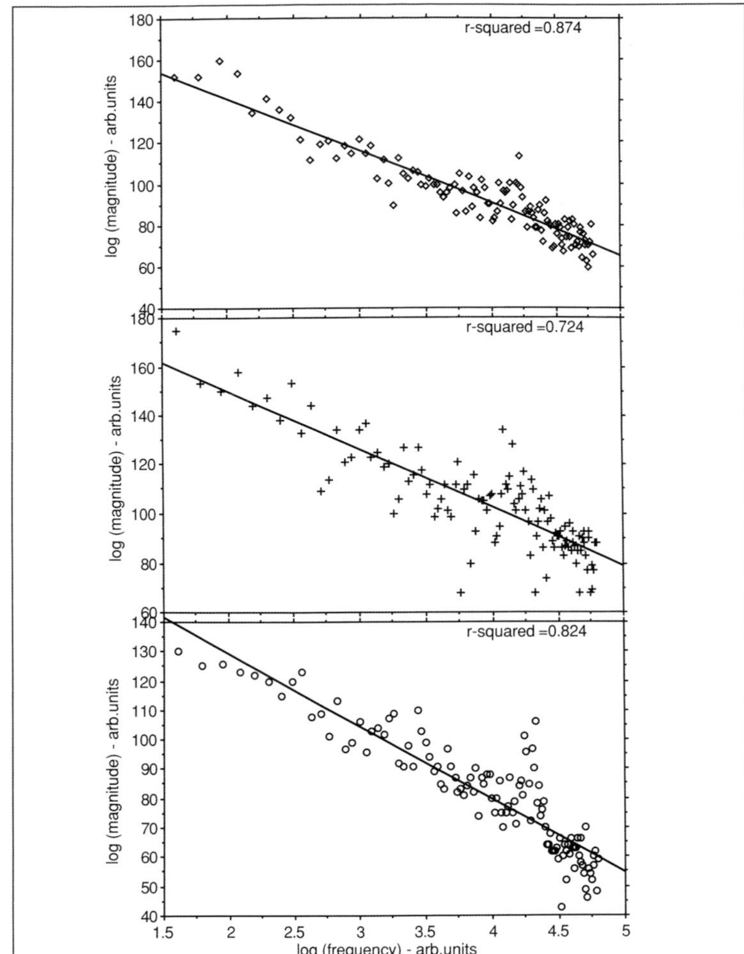

Figure 39. *Examples of log magnitude vs. log frequency plots for horizontal lines through frequency domain images in Figure 38, showing high correlation.*

transmit images. We will see some examples below. If the image of the noise or its Fourier transform can be determined, then subtracting the transform from that of the noisy image will leave only the desired part of the information. This can then be transformed back to the spatial domain (usually described as the inverse transform) to produce a noise-free image.

Figures 32 and **33** showed a resolution test pattern (as digitized by a video camera) and its two-dimensional Fourier-transform power spectrum. If a circle is used to limit the portion of the power spectrum to the center (low frequencies less than 9 pixels^{-1}), then the reconstruction shows the coarse spacings in the original, as shown in **Figure 43,** but it does not show the central portion of the original pattern, where the spacings are smaller and higher-frequency information is present. Conversely, reconstructing the portion of the power spectrum outside the same circle shows only the high-frequency portion of the original image **(Figure 43).** This consists of the central portion of the original pattern and the edges of the wider portions of the lines.

Figure 40. *Examples of log magnitude vs. log frequency plots for vertical lines through frequency domain images in Figure 38, showing lack of significant correlation.*

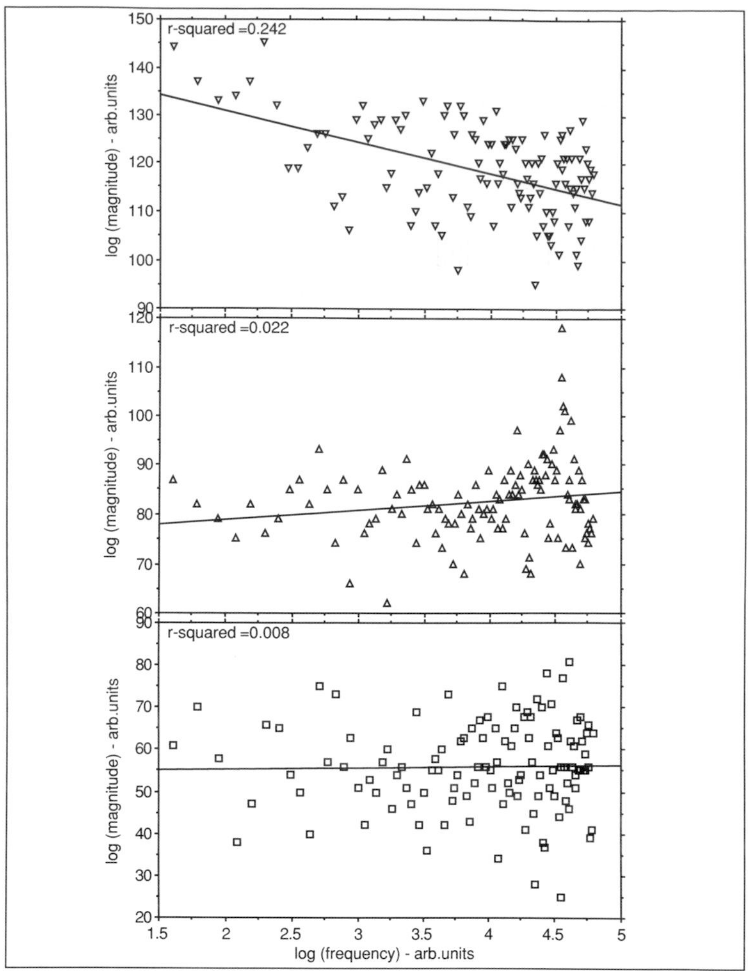

In this illustration of filtering, portions of the Fourier-transform image were selected based on frequency, which is why these filters are generally called low-pass and high-pass filters. Usually, selecting arbitrary regions of the frequency domain for reconstruction produces artefacts, unless some care is taken to shape the edges of the filter region to attenuate the data smoothly. This can be seen in the one-dimensional example of the step function in **Figure 1.** If only the first few terms are used (in addition to not modeling the steepness of the step), the reconstruction has oscillations near the edge, which are generally described as ringing.

It is necessary to shape the edge of the filter to prevent ringing at sharp discontinuities. This behavior is well-known in one-dimensional filtering (used in digital signal processing, for example). Several different shapes are commonly used. Over a specified width (usually given in pixels, but of course ultimately specified in terms of frequency or direction), the filter magnitude can be reduced from maximum to minimum using a weighting function. The simplest function is linear interpolation (also called

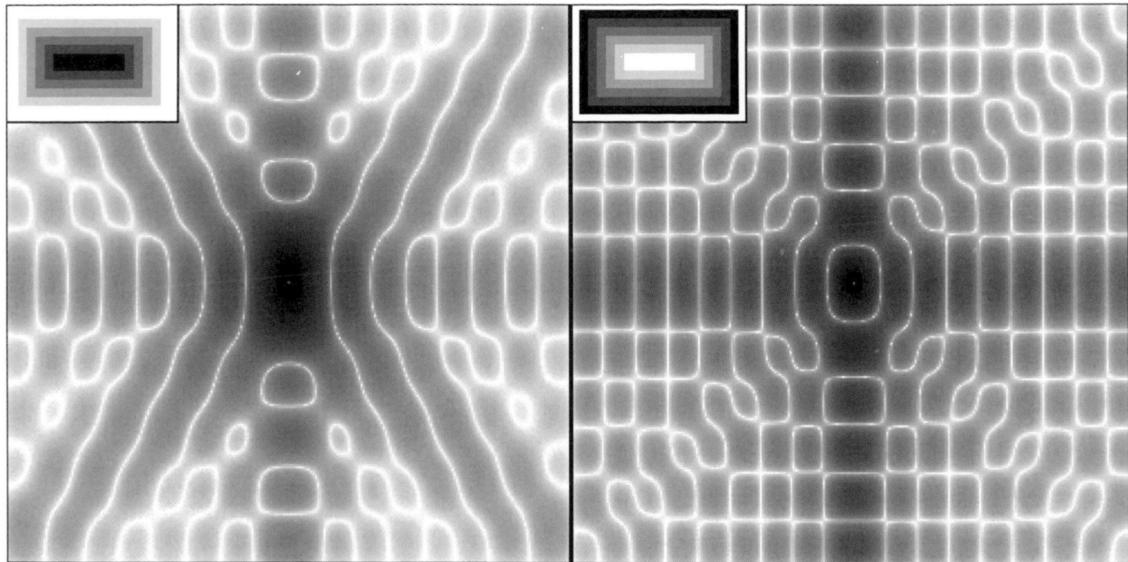

Figure 41. *Stepped (grey scale) rectangles (insets) and their frequency transforms.*

a Parzen window function). Better results can be obtained using a parabolic or cosine function (also called Welch and Hanning window functions, respectively, in this context). The most elaborate filter shapes do not drop to the zero or minimum value, but extend a very long tail beyond the cutoff point. One such

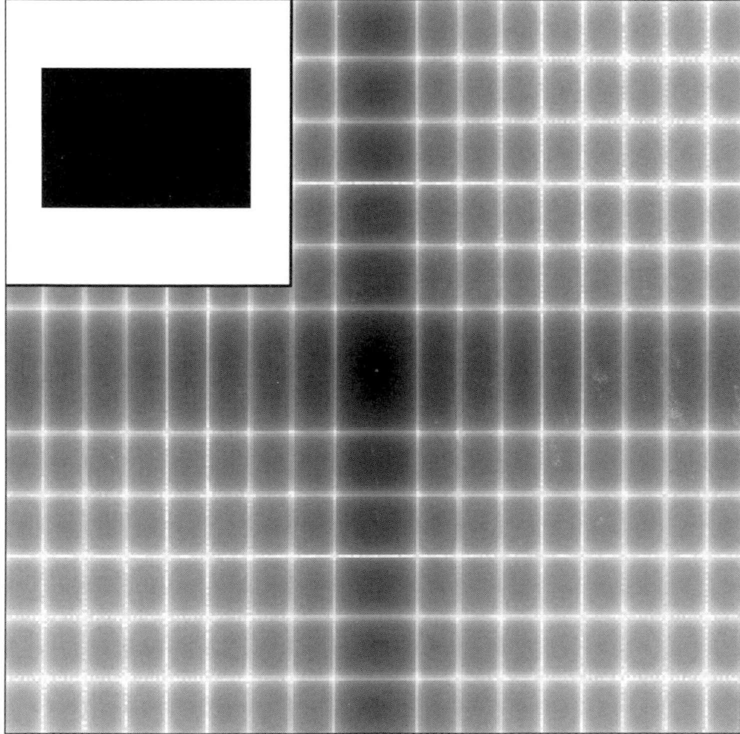

Figure 42. *The sum of the two rectangles in Figure 41 (a black and white rectangle, inset) and the sum of the individual frequency transforms.*

Figure 43. *Reconstructions of the image in Figure 32 through low-pass (left) and high-pass (right) filters.*

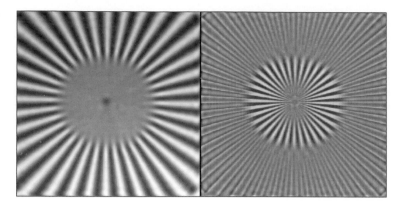

shape is a Gaussian. **Figure 44** shows several of these shapes. In **Figure 43,** a cosine cutoff 6 pixels wide was used.

Another filter shape often used in these applications is a Butterworth filter, whose magnitude can be written as

$$H = 1 / [1 + C \cdot (R/R_0)^{2n}]$$

where R is the distance from the center of the filter (usually the center of the frequency transform image, or zero-frequency point), and R_0 is the nominal filter cutoff value. The constant C is often set equal to 1.0 or to 0.414: the value defines the magnitude of the filter at the point where $R=R_0$ as either 50% or $1/\sqrt{2}$. The integer n is the order of the filter; its most common value is 1. **Figure 45** shows comparison profiles of several Butterworth low-pass filters (ones that attenuate high frequencies). The converse shape having negative values of n, which passes high frequencies and attenuates low ones, is also used.

To illustrate the effects of these filters on ringing at edges, **Figure 46** shows a simple test shape and its two-dimensional FFT power spectrum image. The orientation of principal terms perpendicu-

Figure 44. *Some common filter edge profiles.*

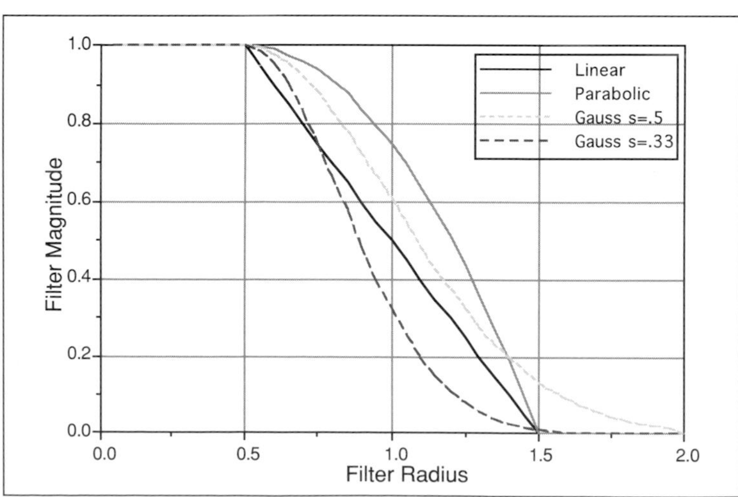

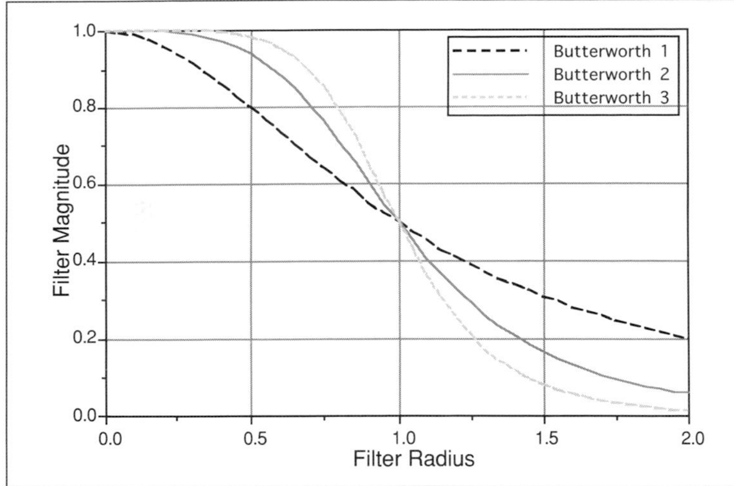

Figure 45. *Shapes for Butterworth filter profiles of order 1, 2, and 3.*

lar to the major edges in the spatial-domain image is evident. Performing a reconstruction using a simple aperture with a radius equal to 25 pixels (an ideal filter) produces the result shown in **Figure 47a.** The oscillations in brightness near the edges are quite visible.

Ringing can be reduced by shaping the edge of the filter, as discussed above. The magnitudes of frequency terms near the cutoff value are multiplied by factors less than one, whose values are based on a simple function. If a cosine function is used, which varies from 1 to 0 over a total width of 6 pixels, the result is improved **(Figure 47b).** In this example, the original 25-pixel radius used for the ideal filter (the sharp cutoff) is the point at which the magnitude of the weighting factor drops to 50%. The weights drop smoothly from 1.0 at a radius of 22 pixels to 0.0 at a radius of 28 pixels.

Increasing the distance over which the transition takes place further reduces the ringing, as shown in **Figure 47c.** Here, the 50% point is still at 25 pixels, but the range is from 15 to 35 pixels. Note that the improvement is achieved not simply by increasing the high-frequency limit–which would improve the sharpness of

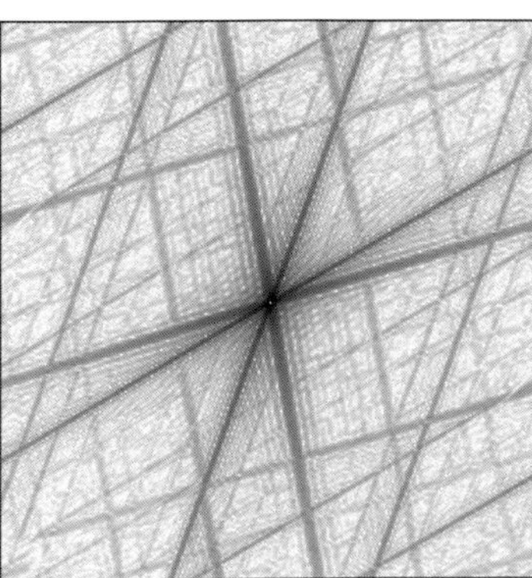

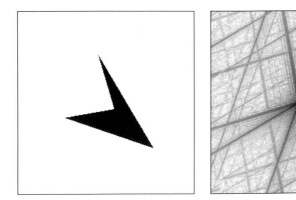

Figure 46. *Test shape with its frequency transform power spectrum.*

Figure 47. Reconstruction of shape from its frequency transform in Figure 46, using an aperture (mask or filter) diameter:

a) *ideal filter in which the cutoff at 25 pixels is exact and abrupt;*

b) *cosine-weighted edge shape in which the 50% radius is 25 pixels with a half-width of 3 pixels;*

c) *cosine-weighted edge shape in which the 50% radius is 25 pixels with a half-width of 10 pixels;*

d) *Butterworth second-degree shape with a 50% radius of 25 pixels.*

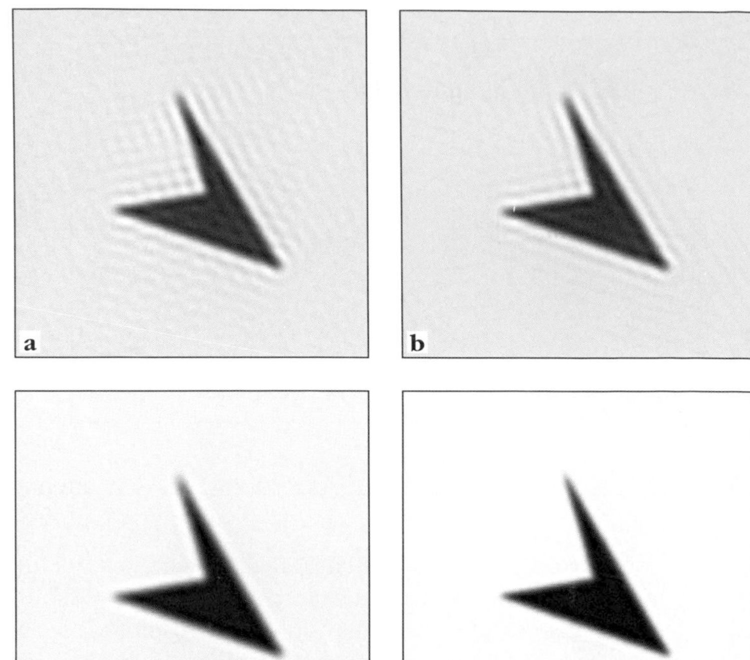

the feature edges but would not by itself reduce the ringing. **Figure 47d** shows the same reconstruction using a second-degree Butterworth filter shape whose 50% point is set at 25 pixels.

Figure 48 shows an image with both fine detail and some noise along with its frequency transform. Applying Butterworth low-pass filters with radii of 10 and 25 pixels in the frequency-domain image smooths the noise with some blurring of the high-frequency detail **(Figure 49),** while the application of Butterworth high-pass filters with the same radii emphasizes the edges and reduces the contrast in the large (low-frequency) regions **(Figure 50).** All of these filters were applied as multiplicative masks.

Figure 48. *Image and its transform used for filtering in Figures 49 and 50.*

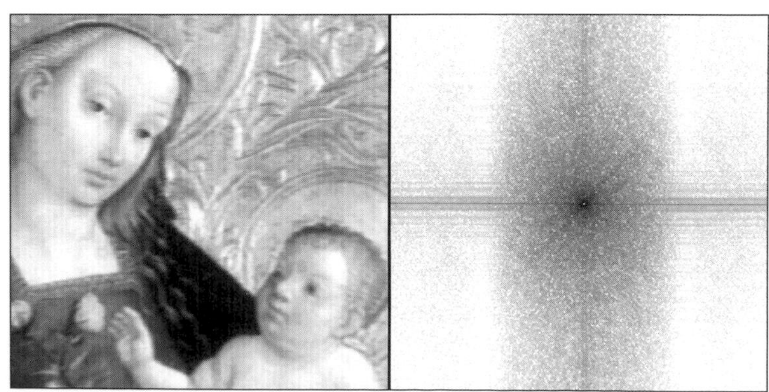

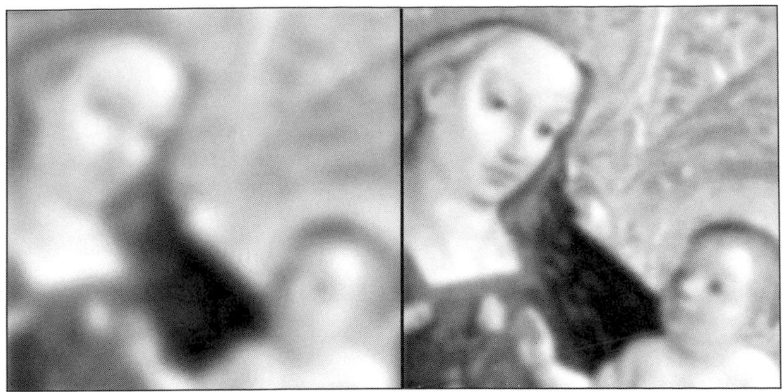

Figure 49. *Filtering of Figure 48 with low-pass Butterworth filters having 50% cutoff diameters of 10 (left) and 25 pixels (right).*

Of course, it is not necessary for the variation in magnitude to be from one to zero. Sometimes the lower limit is set to a fraction, so that the high (or low) frequencies are not completely attenuated. It is also possible to use values greater than one. A high-frequency emphasis filter with the low-frequency value set to a reduced value, such as 0.5, and a high-frequency value greater than 1, such as 2, is called a homomorphic filter. It is usually applied to an image whose brightness values have previously been converted to their logarithms (using a LUT). This filtering operation will simultaneously increase the high-frequency information, sharpening edges while reducing the overall brightness range to allow edge brightness values to show. The physical reasoning behind the homomorphic filter is a separation of illumination and reflectance components in the image. As with most of these filters, though, the real justification is that it improves the appearance of many images of practical interest.

It is also possible to select a region of the Fourier-transform image that is not symmetrical. **Figure 51** shows a selection of intermediate frequency values lying in a particular direction on the transform in **Figure 33,** along with the resulting reconstruction. This kind of filtering may be useful to select directional information from images. It also demonstrates the basic characteristic of Fourier-transform images: locations in the Fourier-transform im-

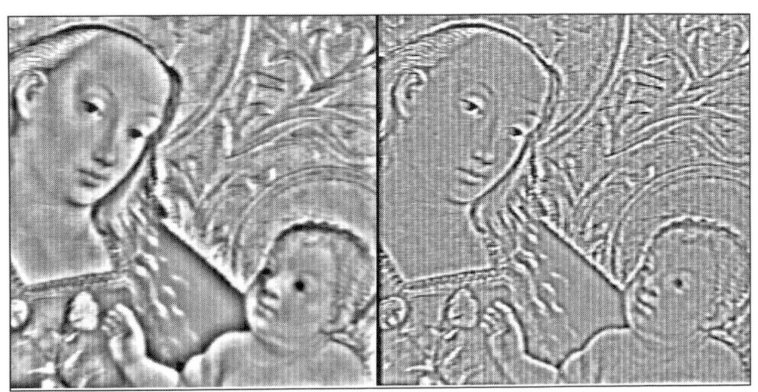

Figure 50. *Filtering of Figure 48 with high-pass Butterworth filters having 50% cutoff diameters of 10 (left) and 25 pixels (right).*

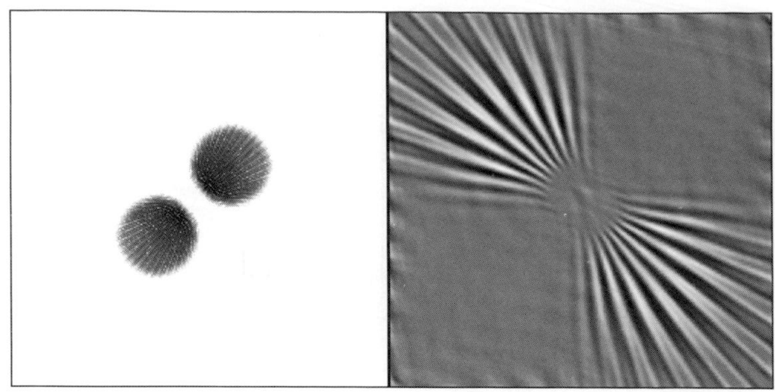

Figure 51. *Retransformation of Figure 32 (right) through a filter centered at a non-zero frequency and direction (left).*

age identify periodicity and orientation information from any or all parts of the spatial-domain image.

Masks and filters

Once the location of periodic noise in an original image is isolated into a single point in the Fourier-transform image, it becomes possible to remove it. A filter removes selected frequencies and orientations by reducing the magnitude values for those terms, either partially or to zero, while leaving the phase information alone (which is important in determining where in the image that information appears).

There are many different ways to specify and to apply this reduction. Sometimes it is practical to specify a range of frequencies and orientations numerically, but most often it will be convenient to do so directly, using the magnitude or power spectrum display of the Fourier-transform image. Drawing circular or pie-shaped regions on this display allows specific peaks in the power spectrum, corresponding to the periodic information, to be selected.

Properly, the regions should be shaped either as circles symmetrically centered on the origin (zero frequency point) or as pie-shaped regions of annuli bounded on the inside and outside by concentric circles whose radii specify frequencies and bounded on the other two sides by radial lines specifying directions. **Figure 52** illustrates several such wedges; note their symmetry about the origin. In practice, it is often more convenient to draw arbitrary shapes, such as circles or rectangles, to select the regions of the Fourier transform to be filtered. This usually requires eliminating a bit more of the original image information than the purely periodic noise. Except in those few cases in which the important information is very close in frequency and orientation to the noise, however, nothing of importance in the original image is lost.

More important is the use of a smoothing function, to ease the transition in magnitudes from outside the filtered region to inside. Instead of an abrupt cutoff, a variety of transition functions ranging from simple linear interpolation to cosine curves, Gauss-

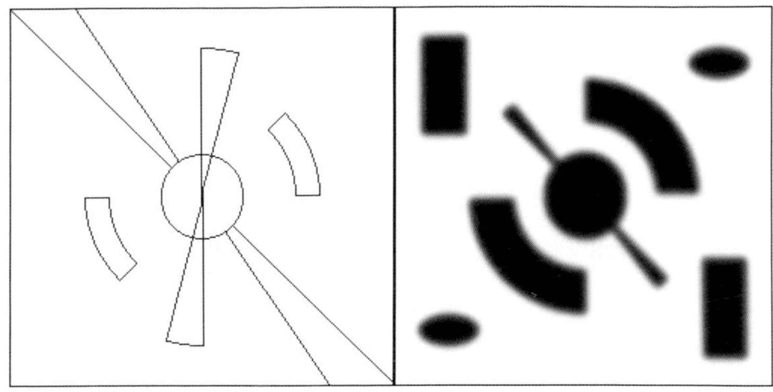

Figure 52. *Illustration of circular, annular, and wedge filter shapes (left) and edge shaping of similar regions (right).*

ian curves, etc. may be used, as mentioned before. When the transition takes place over a distance of only a few pixels, the differences between these transition curves are of little importance.

It can be difficult to calculate the reduction of magnitude in the transition edge zone of a filter region if the region is complex in shape, making it simpler to apply circular or rectangular filter regions. However, if the filter is considered as another image containing a mask of values to be multiplied by the original magnitude component of the Fourier transform (leaving the phase information untouched), then it becomes possible to modify the edges of the region using standard image processing tools, such as smoothing (Chapter 2), constructing a Euclidean distance map (Chapter 6), or manipulating the values with a nonlinear LUT (Chapter 3). **Figure 52** shows several regions of different shapes which have had their edge values reduced in this way. Multiplying this image (scaled to the range 0 to 1) by the original Fourier-transform magnitude and following with retransformation will remove any periodic information with the selected frequency and direction.

Usually, it is only by first examining the transform-image power spectrum that the presence and exact location of these points can be determined. **Figure 53** shows an image of a halftone print from a magazine. The pattern results from the halftone screen used in the printing process. In the frequency transform of the image, this regular pattern shows up as well-defined narrow peaks or spikes. Filtering removes the peaks by setting the magnitude at those locations to zero (but not altering any of the phase information). This allows the image to be retransformed without the noise. The filtered Fourier-transform image power spectrum shown in **Figure 54** shows the circular white spots where filtering was performed.

Figure 55 shows another example, this time a light microscope image that was also digitized from a printed brochure with halftone noise. The filtering and retransformation shown in **Figure 56** shows the use of notch filters, which remove large rectangular (or ideally, pie-shaped) regions of the power spec-

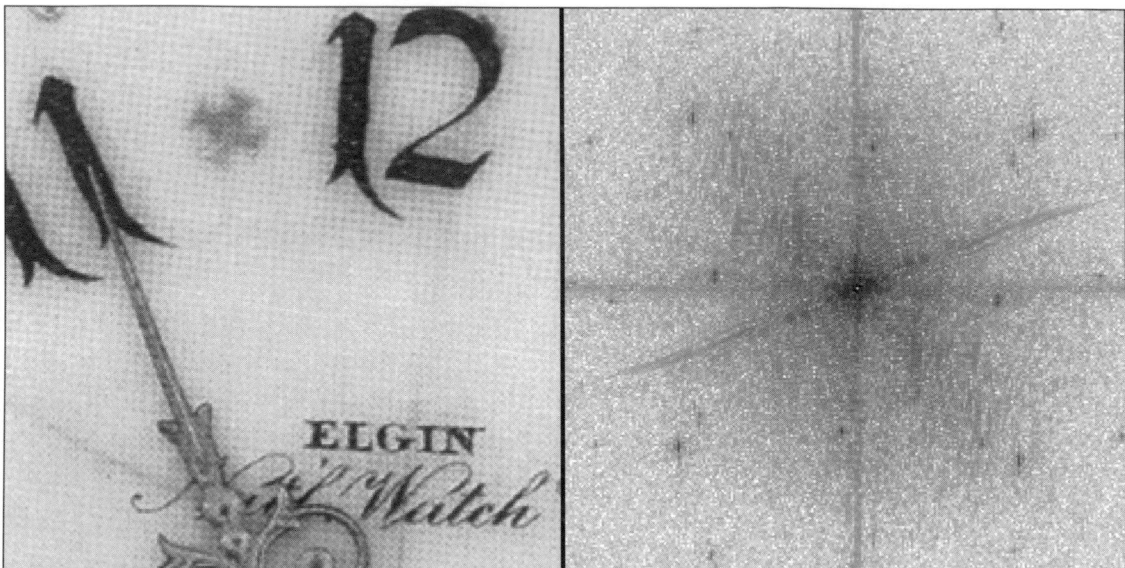

Figure 53. *A halftoned image (left) and its frequency transform (right).*

trum to clean up the noise. The notch filter is also applied in some cases to *keep* only a narrow range of frequencies or directions, rather than eliminate them. Discussed below, this simply requires the filter mask values to be inverted before multiplying. **Figure 57** illustrates the same removal of periodic noise from a reconnaissance photograph, in which the interference is due to electronic noise from transmission or recording. The principles are identical for macroscopic or microscopic images.

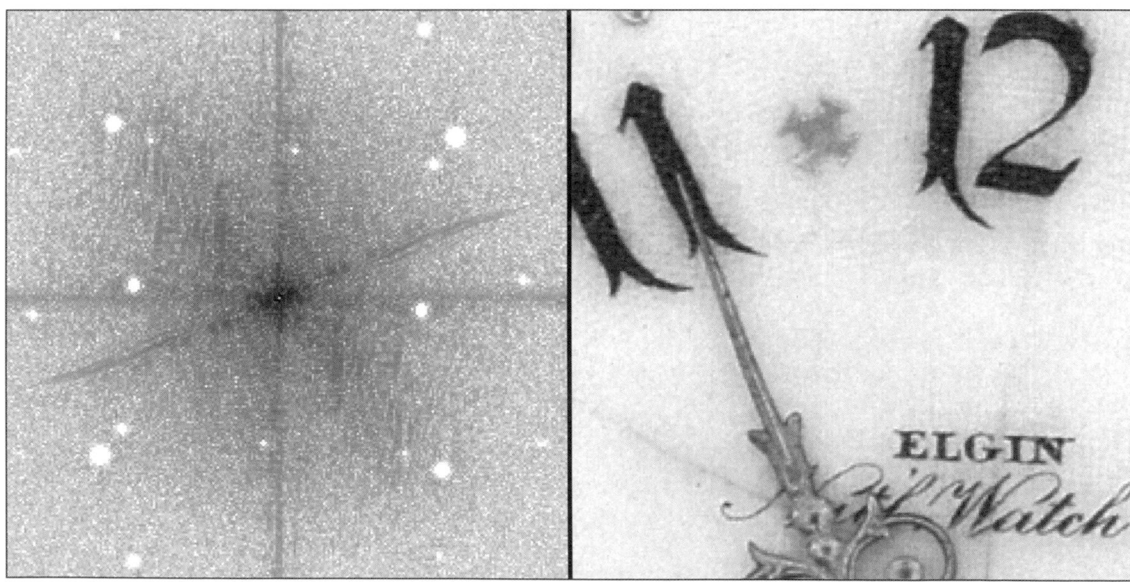

Figure 54. *Removal of periodic information from Figure 53 by reducing the magnitude (left) and retransforming (right).*

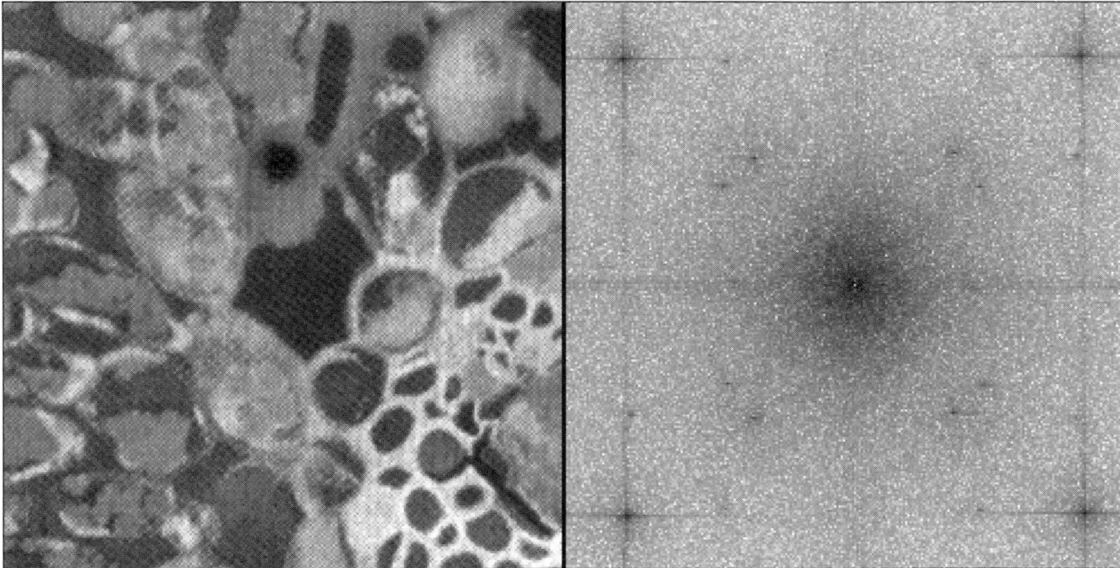

Figure 55. *A digitized microscope image (left) and its frequency transform (right).*

The preceding examples relied on human observation of the peaks in the Fourier-transform image, recognition that the peaks were responsible for the periodic noise, and outlining them to produce the filter. In some cases, it is possible to construct an appropriate image filter automatically from the Fourier-transform power spectrum. The guiding principle is to remove peaks in the power spectrum that are narrow and rise significantly above the local background. If the Fourier-transform magnitude image is treated like an ordinary spatial-domain grey scale image, this peak removal is easily accomplished using a rank filter.

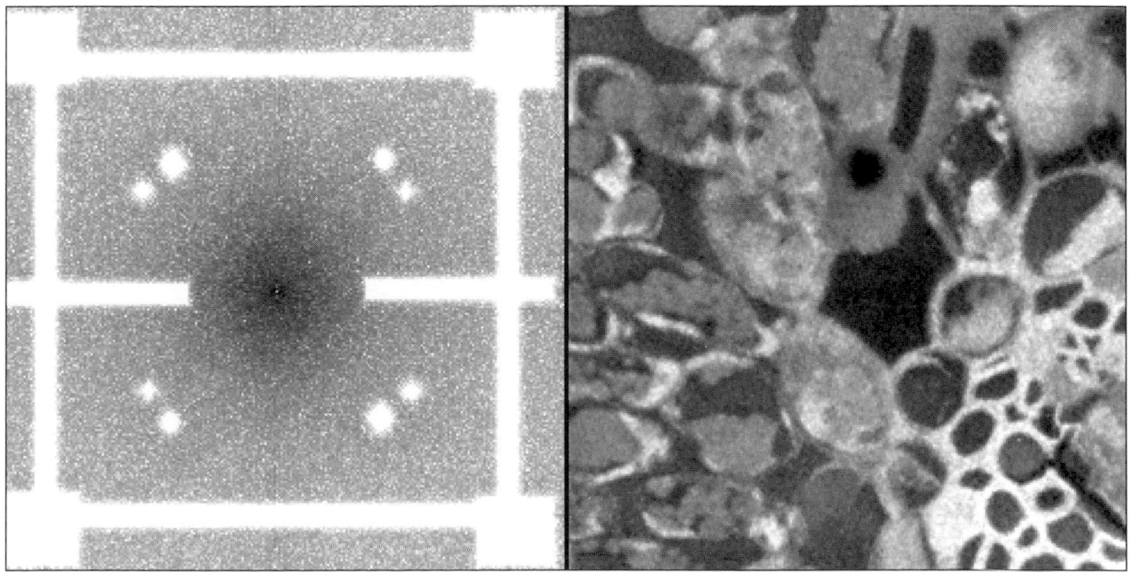

Figure 56. *Application of filters to Figure 55 (left) and retransformation (right).*

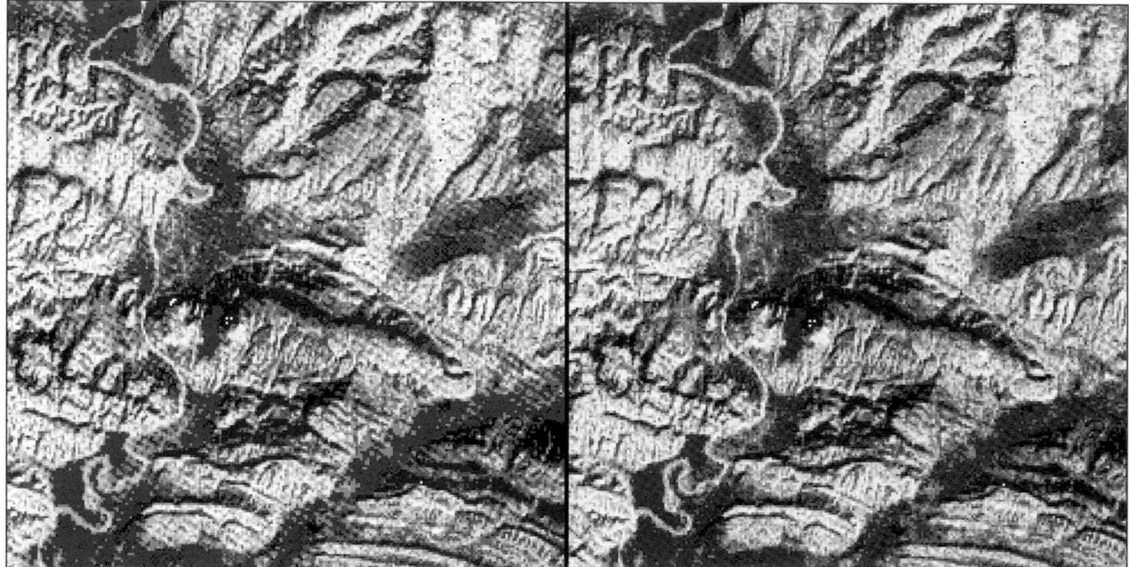

Figure 57. *Removal of periodic transmission noise from a reconnaissance photo (left: original; right: filtered).*

The rank filter replaces each pixel value with the minimum (or maximum) value found anywhere within some small defined region, such as a 5×5 or 7×7 square, or an octagon (approximating a circle). It will not change values in uniform or gradually varying regions, but will effectively erase any large variations that are smaller than the radius of the neighborhood. Since many Fourier-transform magnitude images are rather grainy, particularly at high frequencies, the direct application of a rank filter to the magnitude image may cause other artefacts to appear in the image. Consequently, it is more common to construct a mask by copying the magnitude image, performing some smoothing to reduce the graininess, and then using a rank filter. The difference between the original smoothed image and the rank-filtered one should contain just the peaks. The inverse of this difference image can be used as a multiplicative mask to completely remove peaks caused by periodic noise.

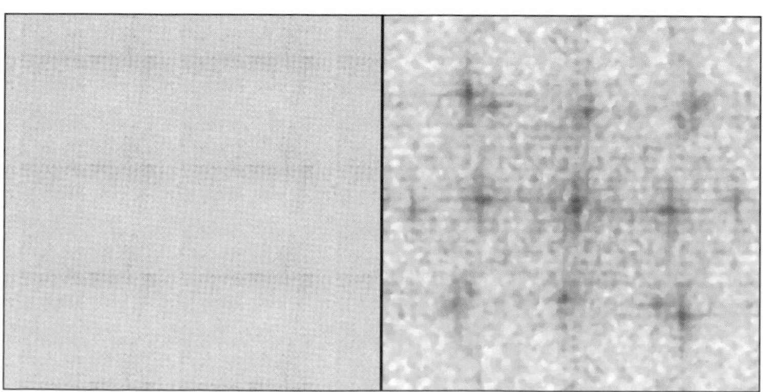

Figure 58. *Construction of a mask from the frequency transform of a tiled noise region. Left: repeated tiling of one section of noise in the original image; right: transform after rank filtering.*

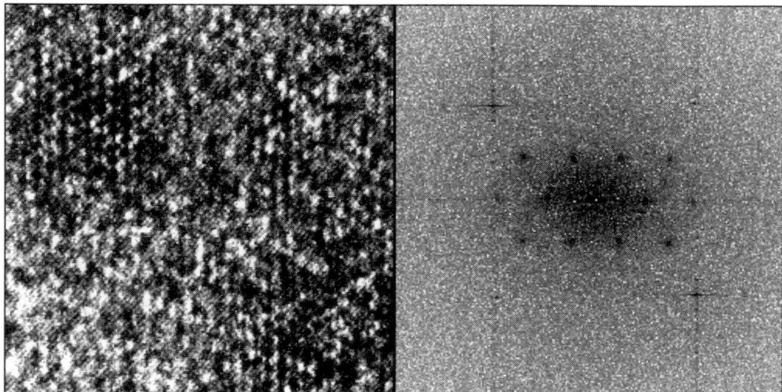

Figure 59. *High-resolution TEM lattice image (left) and its frequency transform (right).*

This sequence is demonstrated in **Figure 58** for the same image as in **Figures 53** and **54.** A region of halftone periodic noise is selected and tiled to fill the entire image area. The transform of this image is then processed using a maximum rank filter of size 9×9 (octagonal) to produce the mask shown in **Figure 58,** in which the peaks due to periodicity are clearly delineated. By tiling the image fragment (repeating it in all directions), the phase information from the position of the periodic structure is correctly preserved. The inverse of this mask is then multiplied by the frequency transform of the original image to produce the filtered result.

Selection of periodic information

In some types of images, it is the periodic information that is useful and the non-periodic noise that must be suppressed. The methods for locating the periodic peaks, constructing filters, smoothing the filter edges, etc. are unchanged. The only difference is that the filter sense is changed and in the case of a multiplicative mask, the values are inverted.

Figure 59 shows a high-resolution TEM lattice image from a crystalline ceramic (mullite). The periodicity of the lattice can be seen, but it is superimposed on a variable and noisy background that results from local variations in the thickness of the sample. This alters the local contrast, making it more difficult to observe the details in the rather complex unit cell of this material. The figure shows the Fourier-transform image, in which the peaks corresponding to the periodic structure can be seen. As noted before, this image is essentially the same as would be recorded photographically using the TEM to project the diffraction pattern of the specimen to the camera plane. Of course, it is not possible to retransform the spatial-domain image from the photographed diffraction pattern because the phase information has been lost. In addition, more control over the Fourier-transform display is possible because a log scale or other rule for converting magnitude to screen brightness can be selected.

A filter mask is constructed in **Figure 60** to select a circular region around each of the periodic spots. Multiplying this by the

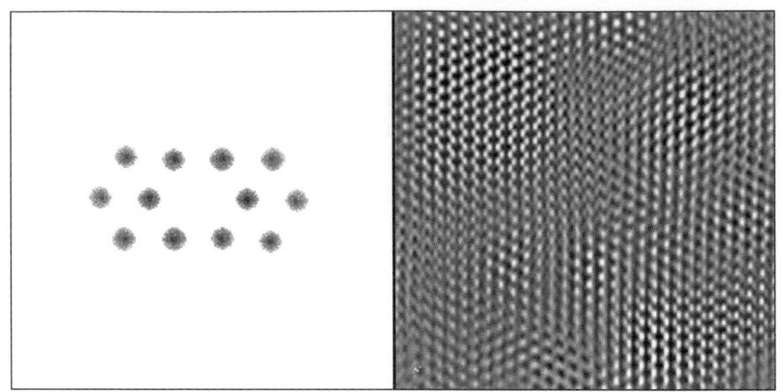

Figure 60. *Filtering of Figure 59 to keep the periodic signal (left) and retransformation (right).*

magnitude values reduces them to zero everywhere else. Retransforming this image produces the spatial-domain image shown. Filtering has removed all of the non-periodic noise, both the short-range (high-frequency) graininess and the gradual (low-frequency) variation in overall brightness. The resulting image clearly shows the lattice structure.

Figure 61 shows an even more dramatic example. In the original image (a cross section of muscle myofibrils) it is practically impossible to discern the periodic structure caused by the presence of noise. There are isolated locations where a few of the fibrils can be seen to have a regular spacing and arrangement, but human observers do not easily see through the noise and variability to find this regularity. The Fourier-transform image shows the peaks from the underlying regularity, however. Selecting only these peak points in the magnitude image (with their original phase information) and reducing all other magnitude values to zero produces the result shown in **Figure 62.** The retransformed image clearly shows the six-fold symmetry expected for the myofibril structure. The inset shows an enlargement of this structure in even finer detail, with both the thick and thin filaments shown. The latter, especially, cannot be seen clearly in the original image.

A caution is needed in using this type of filtering to extract periodic structures. It is possible to construct a mask that will eliminate real information from the image while keeping artefacts and

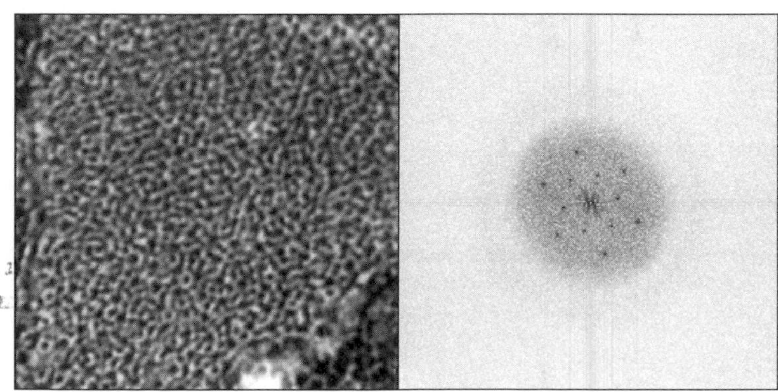

Figure 61. *Transmission electron microscope image of cross section of muscle myofibrils (left) and the frequency transform (right). (Image courtesy Arlo Reeves, Dartmouth Univ.)*

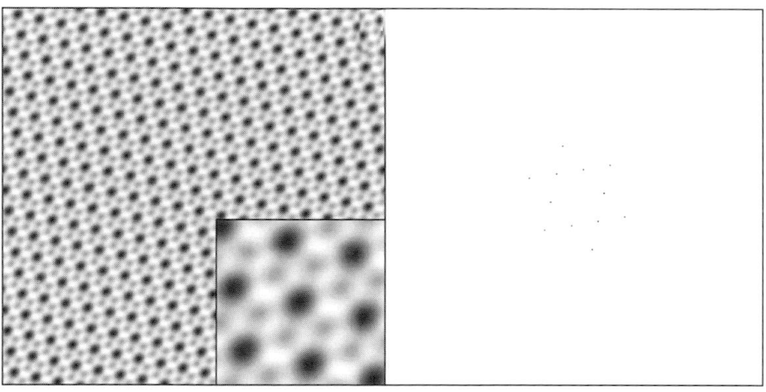

Figure 62. *Retransformation of Figure 61 (left) with only the six principal periodic peaks in the frequency transform (right).*

noise. Selecting the points in the power spectrum with six-fold symmetry insured that the filtered and retransformed spatial image would show periodic structure. This means that the critical step is the recognition and selection of the peaks in the Fourier-transform image. Fortunately, there are many suitable tools for finding and isolating such points, since they are narrow peaks that rise above a gradually varying local background. The top hat filter discussed in Chapter 3 is an example of this approach.

It is also possible to construct a filter to select a narrow range of spacings, such as the interatomic spacing in a high-resolution image. Called an annular filter, this makes it possible to selectively enhance a desired periodic structure. **Figure 63** shows a high-resolution TEM image of an atomic lattice. Applying an annular filter that blocks both the low and high frequencies produces the result shown, in which the atom positions are more clearly defined. However, if the filter also selects a particular orientation (a slit or pie-wedge filter), then the dislocation that is difficult to discern in the original image becomes clearly evident.

As for removing periodic noise, a filter that selects periodic information and reveals periodic structure can often be designed

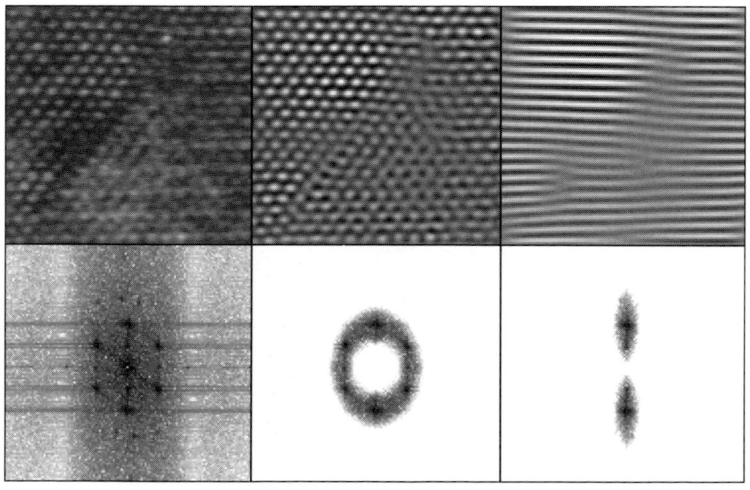

Figure 63. *Noisy high-resolution TEM image (left), and the results of applying an annular filter to select atomic spacings (center) and a slit filter to select vertical spacings only (right). Top images show the spatial domain, and bottom row shows frequency domain.*

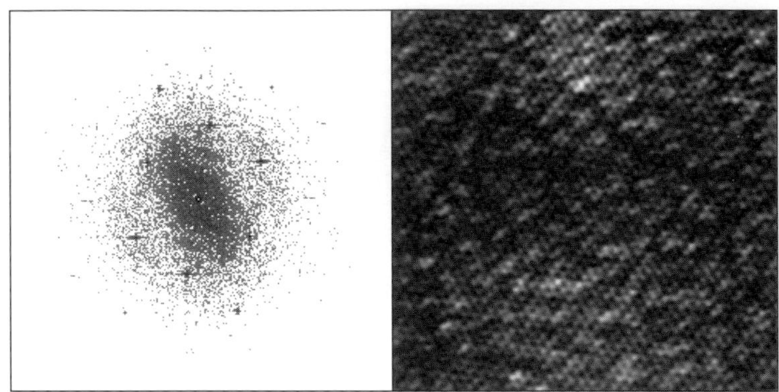

Figure 64. Thresholding of a frequency transform to select only points with a high magnitude (left) and retransformation (right).

by examining the Fourier-transform power spectrum image itself to locate peaks. The mask or filter can be constructed either manually or automatically. In some cases, there is *a priori* information available (such as lattice spacings of crystalline specimens).

Figures 64 and **65** compare two methods for masking the frequency transform. The original is a TEM image of a silicon lattice. Setting a threshold to choose only those points in the transform above a certain level tends to reject high-frequency points, producing some image smoothing, as shown in **Figure 64.** However, selection of the discrete periodic points with a mask produces a superior result, as shown in **Figure 65.**

Convolution and Correlation

Fundamentals of convolution

One of the most common operations on images that is performed in the spatial domain is convolution, in which a kernel of numbers is multiplied by each pixel and its neighbors in a small region, the results summed, and the result placed in the original pixel location. This is applied to all of the pixels in the image. In all cases, the original pixel values are used in the multiplication and addition and the new derived values are used to produce a new image. Sometimes this is performed a few lines at a time, so that the new image ultimately replaces the old one.

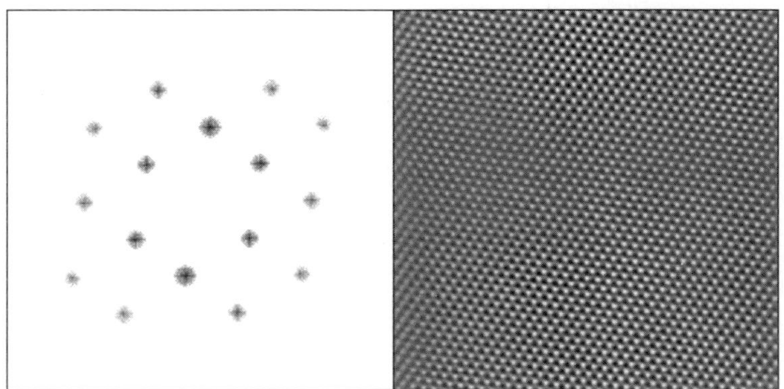

Figure 65. Masking of discrete periodic points (left) and retransformation (right); compare to Figure 64.

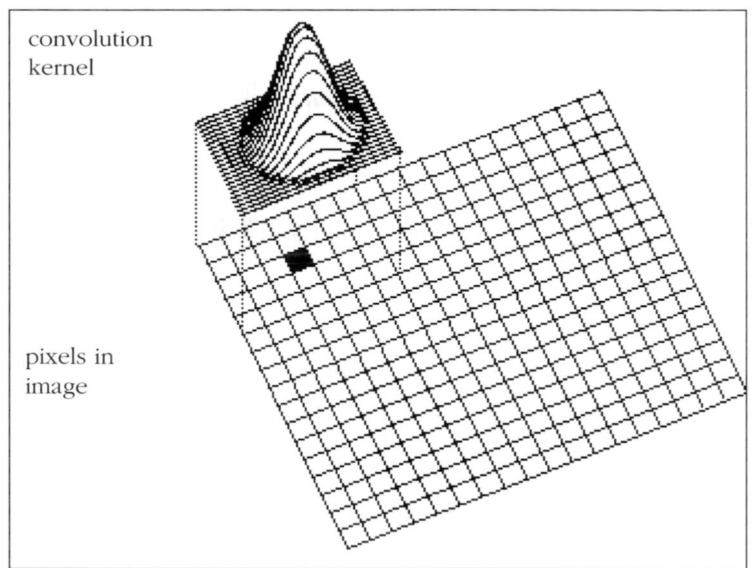

Figure 66. *Illustration of applying a convolution kernel to an image in the spatial domain.*

This type of convolution is particularly common for smoothing and derivative operations. For instance, a simple smoothing kernel might contain the following values:

1/16	2/16	1/16
2/16	4/16	2/16
1/16	2/16	1/16

In practice, the fastest implementation would be to multiply the pixel and its 8 immediate neighbors by the integers 1, 2, or 4, sum the products, then divide the total by 16. In this case, using integers that are powers of 2 allows the math to be extremely fast (involving only bit shifting) and the small size of the kernel (3×3) makes the application of the smoothing algorithm on the spatial-domain image very fast, as well.

There are many spatial-domain kernels, including ones that take first derivatives (for instance, to locate edges) and second derivatives (for instance, the Laplacian, which is a non-directional operator that acts as a high-pass filter to sharpen points and lines). They are usually presented as a set of integers, with it understood that there is a divisor (usually equal to the sum of all the positive values) that normalizes the result. Some of these operators may be significantly larger than the 3×3 example shown above, involving the adding together of the weighted sum of neighbors in a much larger region that is usually, but not necessarily, square.

Applying a large kernel takes time. **Figure 66** illustrates the process graphically for a single placement of the kernel. Even with very fast computers and with careful coding of the process to most efficiently carry out additions and multiplications in optimum order, performing the operation with a 25×25 kernel on a 512×512 image would require a significant amount of time

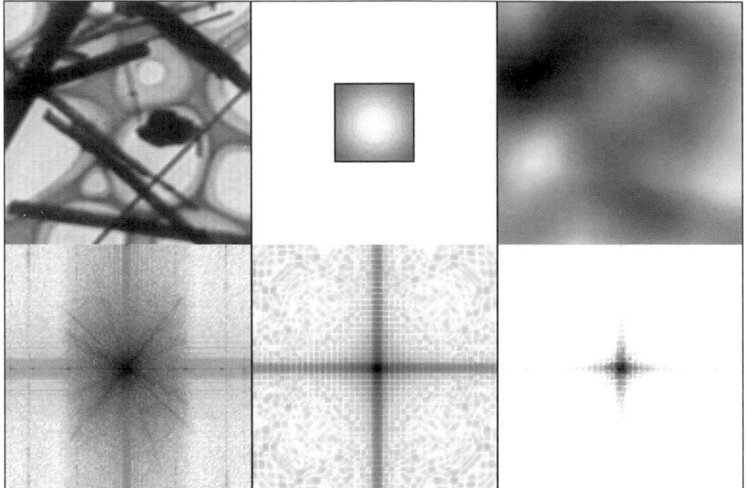

Figure 67. *Smoothing by applying a large kernel in the spatial domain, and convolution in the frequency domain. Top left: original image; bottom left: its frequency transform; top center: smoothing kernel; bottom center: its frequency transform; bottom right: convolution (product of the transforms); top right: smoothed image produced by spatial convolution with kernel or retransformation of product.*

(and even larger kernels and images are often encountered). Though it can be speeded up somewhat by the use of special hardware, such as a pipelined array processor, a special-purpose investment is required., Our interest here is in the algorithms, rather than in their implementation.

For any computer-based system, increasing the kernel size eventually reaches a point at which it is more efficient to perform the operation in the Fourier domain. The time needed to perform the FFT or FHT transformation from the spatial domain to the frequency domain and back is more than balanced by the speed with which the convolution can be carried out. If there are any other reasons to perform the transformation to the frequency-domain representation of the image, then even small kernels can be most efficiently applied there.

This is because the equivalent operation to spatial-domain convolution is a simple multiplication of each pixel in the magnitude image by the corresponding pixel in a transform of the kernel. Both the kernel and the transform can be obtained and stored beforehand. If the kernel is smaller than the image, it is padded with zeroes to the full image size. Without deriving a proof, it can be simply stated that convolution in the spatial domain is exactly equivalent to multiplication in the frequency domain. Using the notation presented before, in which the image is a function $f(x,y)$ and the kernel is $g(x,y)$, we would describe the convolution operation in which the kernel is positioned everywhere on the image and multiplied by it as

$$g(x,y) * f(x,y) = \int\int (f(\alpha,\beta) \cdot g(x-\alpha, y-\beta)\ d\alpha\ d\beta$$

where α and β are dummy variables for the integration, the range of which is across the entire image, and the symbol * indicates convolution. If the Fourier transforms of $f(x,y)$ and $g(x,y)$ are $F(u,v)$ and $G(u,v)$ respectively, then the convolution operation in the Fourier domain is simple point-by-point multiplication, or

$$g(x,y) * f(x,y) <=> G(u,v)\ F(u,v)$$

There are a few practical differences between the two operations. The usual application of a kernel in the spatial domain avoids the edge pixels (those nearer to the edge than the half-width of the kernel), since their neighbors do not exist. As a practical alternative, a different kernel, which is one-sided and has different weights, is applied near edges. In transforming the image to the frequency domain, the tacit assumption is made that the image wraps around at edges, so that the left edge is contiguous with the right and the top edge is contiguous with the bottom. Applying a convolution by multiplying in the frequency domain is equivalent to addressing pixels in this same wrap around manner when applying the kernel to the spatial image. It will usually produce some artefacts at the edges.

Figure 67 shows the equivalence of convolution in the spatial domain and multiplication in the frequency domain, for the case of a large smoothing kernel. The kernel is shown along with its transform. Applying the kernel to the image in the spatial domain produces the result shown in the example. Multiplying the kernel transform by the image transform produces the frequency-domain image, whose power spectrum is shown. Retransforming this image, in turn, produces the identical result to the spatial-domain operation. Large kernels such as this one are often used to smooth images, eliminating small features and obtaining a varying background that can be subtracted to isolate features.

Notice that the equivalence of frequency-domain multiplication to spatial-domain convolution is restricted to multiplicative or linear filters. Other neighborhood operations, such as rank filtering (saving the brightest, darkest, or median brightness value in a neighborhood), are nonlinear and have no frequency-domain equivalent.

Imaging system characteristics

Convolution can also be used as a tool to understand how imaging systems alter or degrade images. For example, the blurring introduced by imperfect lenses can be described by a function $H(u,v)$ which is multiplied by the frequency transform of the image **(Figure 68).** The operation of physical optics is readily modeled in the frequency domain. Sometimes it is possible to determine the separate characteristics of each component of the system; sometimes it is not. In a few cases, determining the point-spread function of the system (the degree to which a perfect point in the object plane is blurred in the image plane) may make it possible to sharpen the image by removing some of the blur. This is done by dividing by $H(u,v)$, the transform of the point-spread image.

Figure 68. *System characteristics introduce a point-spread function into the acquired image.*

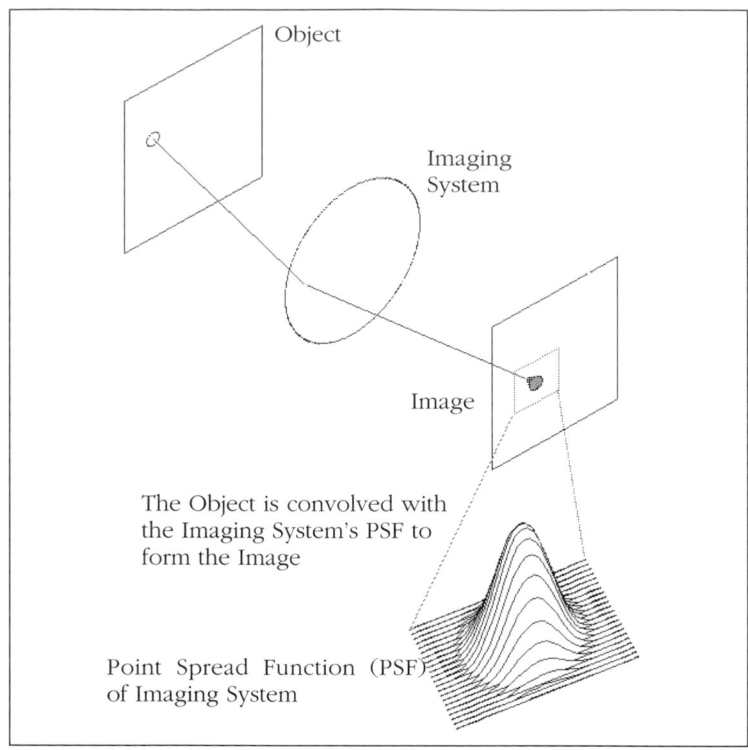

To illustrate this, we can use the simple resolution test pattern shown before. The radial lines become unresolved at the center of the pattern, even in the best-focus image shown in **Figure 32.** This is largely due to the limited resolution of the video camera used (a solid-state CCD array). The image was digitized as a 256×256 square. **Figure 33** showed the power spectrum (using a log scale) for the original in-focus image. The falloff in power at high frequencies is in agreement with the visual loss of resolution at the center of the pattern.

An intentionally out-of-focus image was obtained **(Figure 69)** by misadjusting the camera lens. In addition to blurring the lines, this also reduces the image contrast slightly. The point-spread function of the camera system was determined by placing a single black point in the center of the field of view, without dis-

Figure 69. *Blurred (out-of-focus) image of test pattern in Figure 32 (left) and its frequency transform (right).*

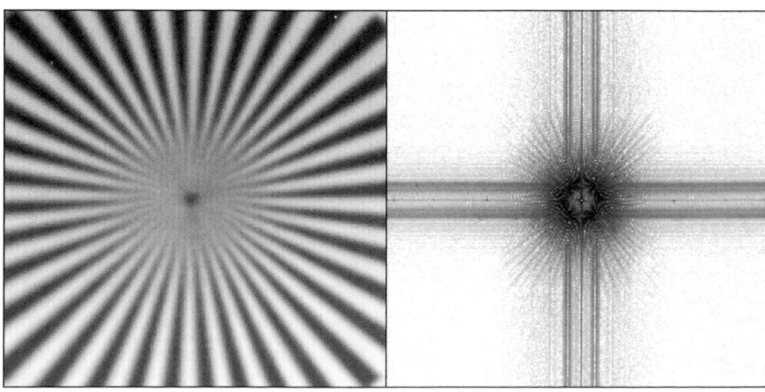

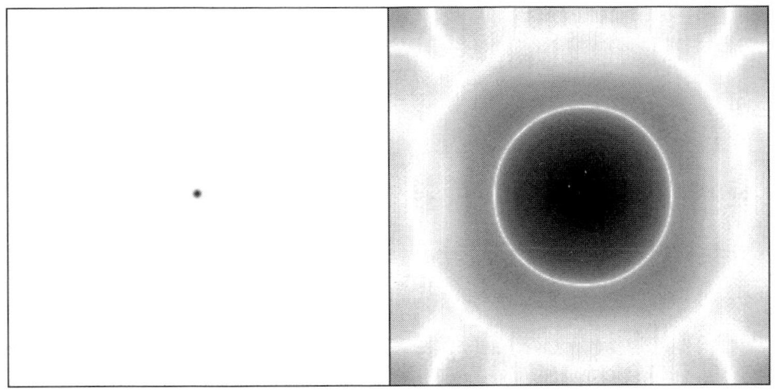

Figure 70. *Blurred (out-of-focus) image of a single point (left) and its frequency transform (right).*

turbing the lens focus, and acquiring the image shown in **Figure 70.**

Power spectra (using a logarithmic display scale) for the out-of-focus and point-spread images are shown in **Figures 69** and **70,** respectively. The magnitude of the point-spread function is sometimes called the imaging system's Modulation Transfer Function (MTF). The reduction in medium and high frequencies for the out-of-focus pattern is evident. For the symmetric point-spread function, the white ring at about one-third of the image width is a ring of zero values, which will become important in performing the deconvolution.

For deconvolution, we divide the complex frequency-domain image from the out-of-focus test pattern by that for the point-spread. Actually, this is done by dividing the magnitude values and subtracting the phase values, but it is usually handled directly by the software. The result of retransformation after performing the operation is shown in **Figure 71.** While some hint of the test pattern is evident, the retransformed image is dominated by a noise pattern. This results from the zeroes in the divisor, which cause numeric overflow problems for the program.

There are two approaches to dealing with this effect, both of which seek to restrict division to those pixels in the complex transform images that will not cause overflow. One is to place a physical restriction, such as a filter or mask, on the image (this is

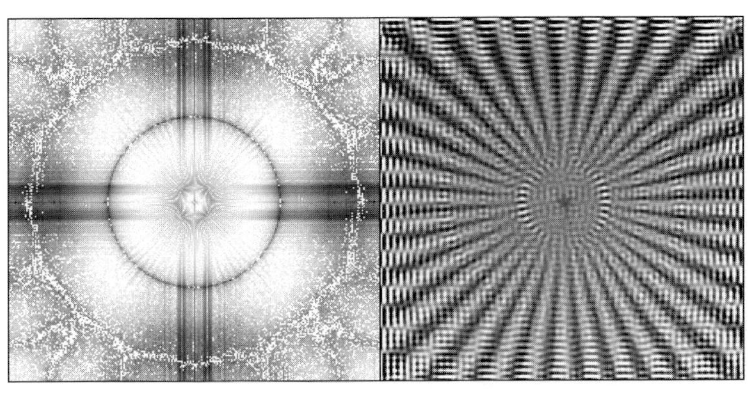

Figure 71. *Result of dividing the frequency transform in Figure 69 by that in Figure 70 (left) and retransforming (right).*

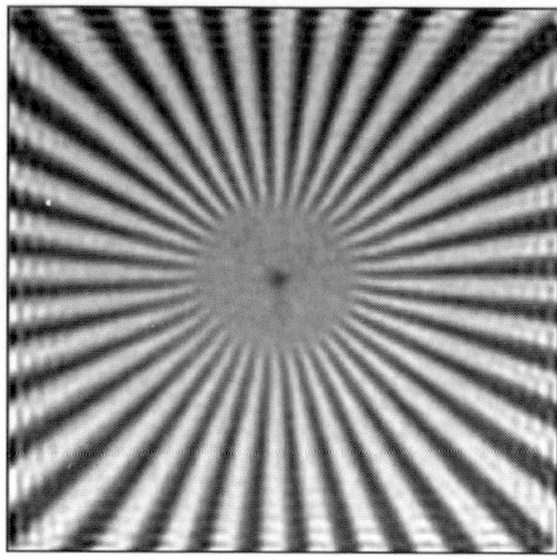

Figure 72. *Same procedure as in Figure 71 but restricting the range to avoid zeroes.*

often described as apodization). The other is to define a zero result for any division that causes numerical overflow. By defining a circular band along the line of zeroes, with cosine edge-weighting over a six-pixel-wide region, the zeroes were avoided. Retransformation produced the result shown in **Figure 72**. Most of the artefacts have been removed and the radial lines appear well-defined, although they are not as sharp as the original in-focus image of the test pattern.

There are potential pitfalls in this method. One problem is the finite representation of the complex numbers in the frequency-domain image. Division by small values can produce numerical overflow that can introduce serious artefacts into the image. Also, it is often very difficult to obtain a good point-spread function by recording a real image. If the noise contents of that image and the one to be sharpened are different, it can exacerbate the numerical precision and overflow problems. It is almost never possible to remove more than a small fraction of the blurring in a real image, but of course there are some situations where even a small improvement may be of considerable practical importance.

Division by the frequency transform of the blur is referred to as an inverse filter. Using the notation introduced previously, it can be written as

$$F(u,v) \approx \left[\frac{1}{H(u,v)}\right] \cdot G(u,v)$$

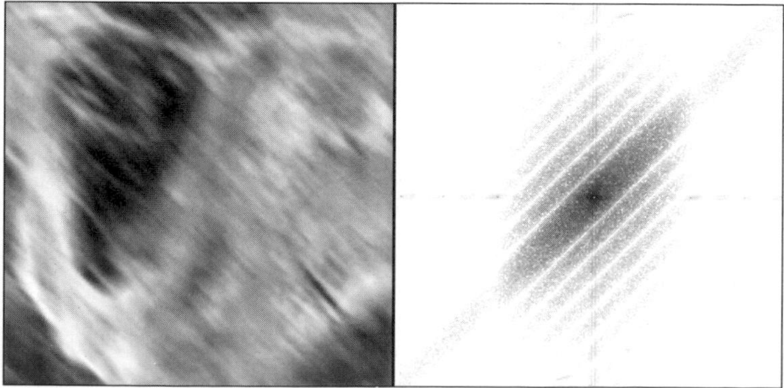

Figure 73. *Aerial photo blurred by motion (left) and its frequency transform (right).*

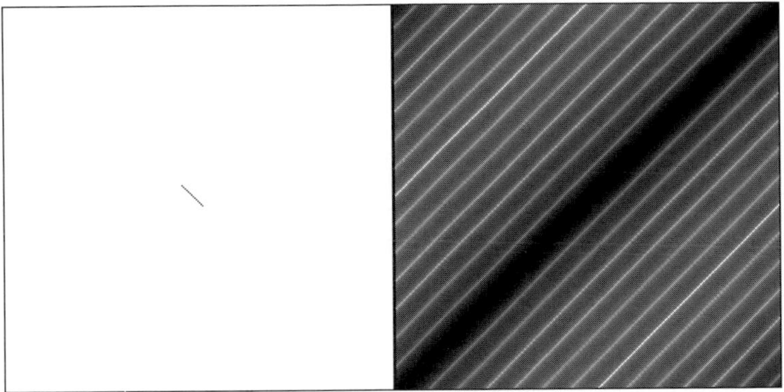

Figure 74. The blur vector for Figure 73 (left) and its frequency transform (right).

An approach to limiting the damage caused by very small values of H is to add a weighting factor, so that zeroes are avoided.

$$F(u,v) \approx \left[\frac{1}{H(u,v)}\right] \cdot \left[\frac{|H(u,v)|^2}{|H(u,v)|^2 + K}\right] \cdot G(u,v)$$

Ideally, K should be calculated from the statistical properties of the transforms (in which case it is known as a Wiener filter). However, when this is impractical, it is common to approximate K by trial and error to find a satisfactorily restored image in which the sharpness of edges from high-frequency terms is balanced against the noise from dividing by small numbers.

There are other ways to remove blur from images. One is the maximum-entropy method discussed in Chapter 2. This assumes some foreknowledge about the image, such as its noise properties. Information is expressed in a different way than the filter shape, but both methods represent practical compromises.

Removing motion blur and other defects

Additional defects besides out-of-focus optics can be corrected in the frequency domain as well. One of the most common is blur caused by motion. This is rarely a problem in microscopy applications, but can be very important in remote sensing, where light levels are low and exposure time must be long enough for significant camera motion to occur with respect to the scene. Fortunately, in most of these circumstances the amount and direction of motion is known. That makes it possible to draw a line in the spatial domain that defines the blur. The frequency transform of this line is then divided into the transform of the blurred image. Retransforming the resulting image restores the sharp result. **Figures 73** to **75** illustrate this method. **Figure 73** is the blurred image, **Figure 74** is the blur vector and its transform, and **Figure 75** is the reconstructed (deblurred) result.

It is important to note the similarity and the difference between this example and the removal of out-of-focus blur. Both involve dividing the transform of the blurred image by that of the defect. This follows directly from the equation presented for convolu-

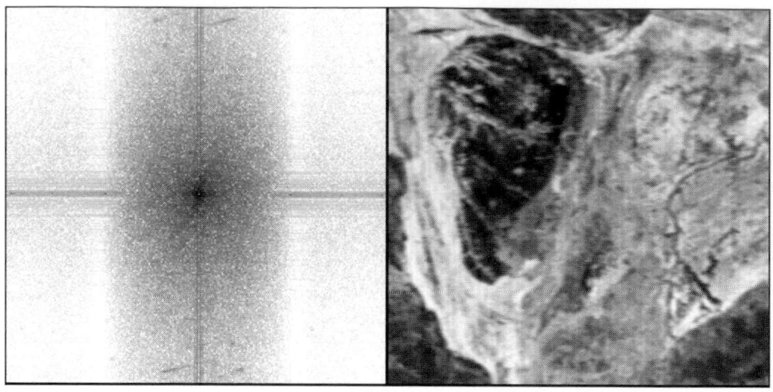

Figure 75. *The result of dividing Figure 73 by Figure 74 (left) and retransforming (right).*

tion, in which the transform of the convolved image is the product of those from the original image and the defect. The major difference is that in the motion blur case, we can calculate the exact blurring vector to be removed, while in the out-of-focus blur case, we must estimate the blur from an actual image. This introduces unavoidable noise in the image, which is greatly magnified by the division. Using a filter mask to limit the range of application of the division restricts the correction to lower frequencies and the amount of restoration is consequently limited. The greater the uncertainty in the defects introduced by the imaging system, the less the degree of restoration possible.

Additional limitations arise from the finite internal precision in computer implementation of the FFT or FHT and the storage of the complex frequency-transform image. Programs may use either floating-point or fixed-point notation, the latter requiring less storage space and offering somewhat greater speed. However, the minimum magnitude values that can be accurately recorded generally occur at higher frequencies, controlling how sharp edges appear in the spatial-domain image. Too small a precision also limits the ability to sharpen images by removing degrading blur due to the imaging system.

If the blur is not known *a priori*, it can often be estimated from the direction and spacing of the lines of zeroes in the frequency-domain power spectrum. To avoid the limitations shown above in attempting to remove out-of-focus blur using a measured point-spread function, it may be necessary to iteratively divide by several assumed blur directions and magnitudes to find an optimum result.

Template matching and correlation

Closely related to the spatial-domain application of a kernel for smoothing, etc. is the idea of template matching. In this case, a target pattern is shifted to every location in the image, the values are multiplied by the pixels that are overlaid, and the total is stored at that position to form an image showing where regions identical or similar to the target are located. **Figure 76** illustrates this process.

This method is used in many contexts to locate features within images. One is searching reconnaissance images for particular objects, such as vehicles. Tracking the motion of hurricanes in a series of weather satellite images or cells moving on a microscope slide can also use this approach. Modified to deal optimally with binary images, it can be used to find letters in text. When the target is a pattern of pixel brightness values from one image in a stereo pair and the searched image is the second image from the pair, the method has been used to perform fusion (locating matching points in the two images) to measure parallax and calculate range.

For continuous two-dimensional functions, the cross-correlation image is calculated as

$$c(i,j) = \int_{-\infty}^{+\infty}\int_{-\infty}^{+\infty} f(x,y)\, g(x-i, y-j)\, dx\, dy$$

Replacing the integrals by finite sums over the dimensions of the image gives the expression below. In order to normalize the result of this template matching or correlation without the absolute brightness value of the region biasing the results, the operation in the spatial domain is usually calculated as the sum of the products of the pixel brightnesses divided by their geometric mean.

$$\frac{\sum_i \sum_j f_{x+i,\, y+j} \cdot g_{i,j}}{\sqrt{\sum_i \sum_j f^2_{x+i,\, y+j} \cdot \sum_i \sum_k g^2_{i,j}}}$$

When the dimensions of the summation are large, this is a slow and inefficient process compared to the equivalent operation in frequency space. The frequency-space operation is simply

$$C(u,v) = F(u,v)\, G^*(u,v)$$

where * indicates the complex conjugate of the function values. The complex conjugate of the pixel values affects only the imaginary part (or, when magnitude and phase are used, the phase). The operation is thus seen to be very similar to convolution, and indeed it is often performed using many of the same program subroutines. Operations that involve two images (division for deconvolution, multiplication for convolution, and multiplication by the conjugate for correlation) are sometimes called dyadic operations, to distinguish them from filtering and masking operations (monadic operations) in which a single frequency transform image is operated on (the mask image is not a frequency-domain image).

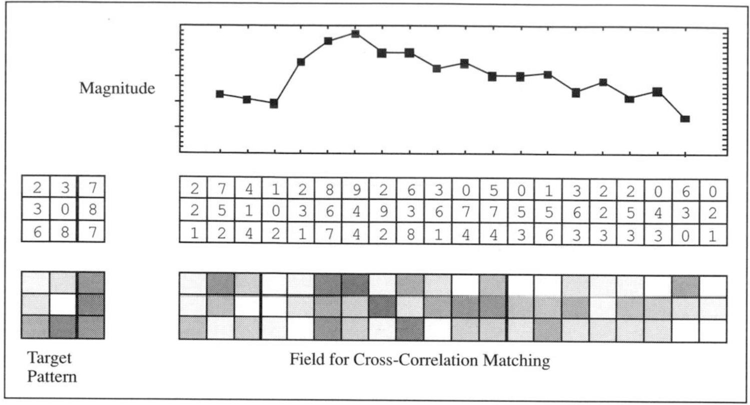

Figure 76. *Diagram of template matching. The target pattern is shifted across the image fragment and the cross-correlation value at each location is recorded as brightness.*

Usually, when correlation is performed, the wraparound assumption joining the left and right edges and the top and bottom of the image is not acceptable. In these cases, the image should be padded by surrounding it with zeroes to bring it to the next larger size for transformation (the next exact power of two, required for FFT and FHT calculations). Since the correlation operation also requires that the actual magnitude values of the transforms be used, slightly better mathematical precision can be achieved by padding with the average values of the original image brightnesses rather than with zeroes. It may also be useful to subtract the average brightness value from each pixel, which removes the zeroth (DC) term from the transformation. Since this value is usually the largest in the transform (it is the value at the central pixel), its elimination allows the transform data more dynamic range.

Correlation is primarily used for locating features in one image that appear in another. **Figures 77** to **79** show an example. The first image contains text, while the second contains the letter "e" by itself. The frequency transforms of the two images are shown in each figure. Since neither image has text crossing the image boundaries, no padding to a larger size was needed in this case. **Figure 79** shows the result of the cross-correlation after retransforming the image to the spatial domain and also shows the same image presented as an isometric display.

Note that the brightest points in the correlation image correspond to the occurrences of the letter "e." These have been found by the autocorrelation process. Note also that there are lower but still significant peaks corresponding to other letters with some similarity to the "e," particularly the "a" and the "o." Finally, note that the letter "e" in the upper sentence is not found by this method. This is because that text is set in a different font (sans serif Helvetica instead of serif Times Roman). Cross-correlation is sensitive to feature shape (and also size and orientation).

Autocorrelation

In the special case when the image functions f and g (and their transforms F and G) are the same, the correlation operation is

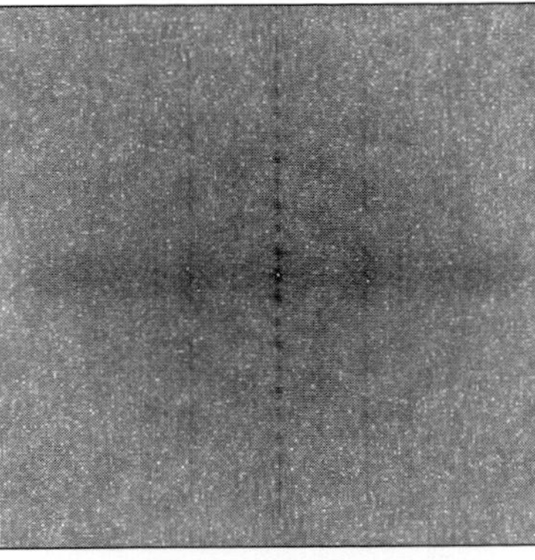

Figure 77. *Sample of text (left) and its frequency transform (right).*

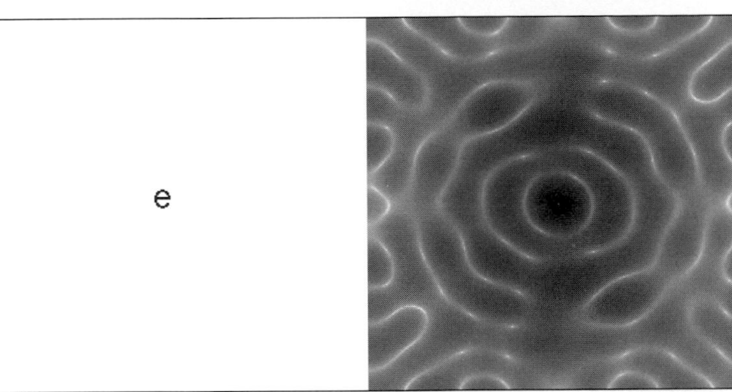

Figure 78. *The target letter "e" (left) and its frequency transform (right).*

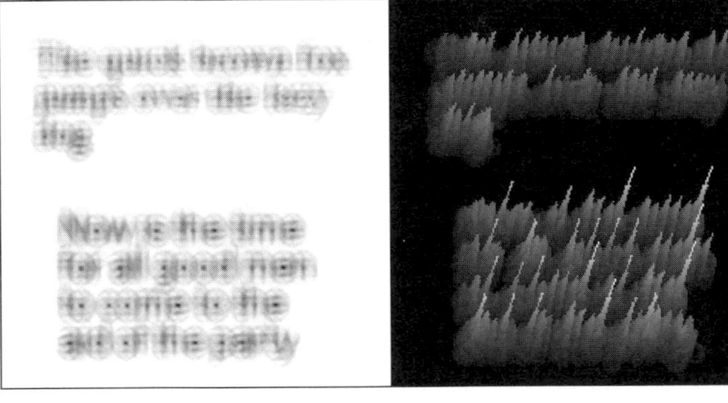

Figure 79. *The cross-correlation of Figures 77 and 78, shown as brightness (left) and as an isometric display (right).*

called autocorrelation. This is used to combine together all parts of the image, in order to find and average repetitive structures. **Figures 80** and **81** show one of the classic uses of this method: application to a TEM image of a lattice structure (mullite). Each individual repeating unit in the image contains some noise, but by averaging all repeats together, a better image of the fine structural details can be obtained.

The process is carried out as described above. The frequency transform of the image is multiplied by its own conjugate and the result retransformed, so that fine details down to atomic positions in this complex lattice can be seen. **Figure 82** shows another example, in which the repeating structure of muscle fibers in an insect flight muscle is averaged in the same way by auto-

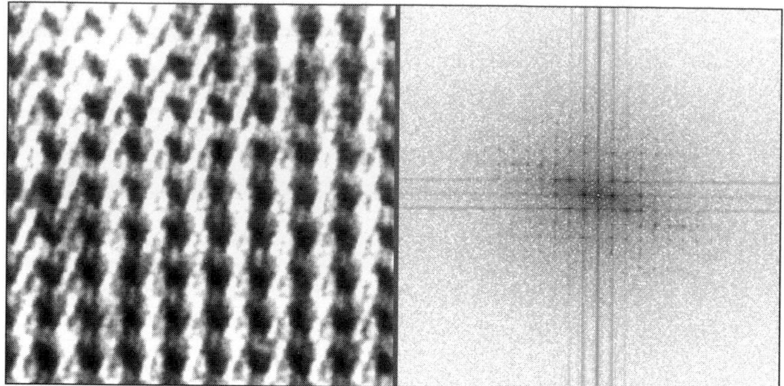

Figure 80. *High-resolution TEM image of mullite (left) and its frequency transform (right). (Image courtesy Sopa Cehvacharoenkul, Microelectronics Center of North Carolina.)*

correlation. In both these cases, padding was needed because the images do not wrap around at the edges.

To compare this method of removing noise with filtering, we can use the (quite noisy) STM image shown in **Figure 37** with its frequency transform. **Figure 83** compares the results of filtering by setting a mask to accept only the central (low-frequency) portion of the transform (12 pixels in diameter plus a 6-pixel-wide cosine edge shaping), with the result of autocorrelation. The filtered image is certainly smoother, since all high-frequency information (some of which has produced significant peaks in the transform image) is removed. The autocorrelation image shows more details of the shape of the response at the regularly spaced atoms by averaging all of the repetitions and keeping high-frequency information.

Figure 84 shows another use of the autocorrelation function, to measure preferred orientation. The image is a felted textile material. The fibers have neither a randomized nor uniform orientation due to the fabrication process. The frequency transform shown indicates a slightly asymmetric shape. Performing the cross-correlation and retransforming to the spatial domain gives the image shown in **Figure 85.** The brightness profiles of the central spot show the preferred orientation quantitatively. This is the same result achieved by cross-correlation in the spatial domain (sliding the image across itself and recording the area of

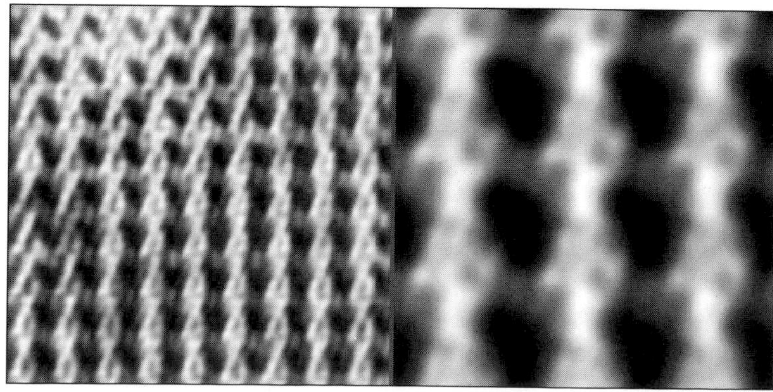

Figure 81. *Autocorrelation image from Figure 80 (left) and an enlarged view (right).*

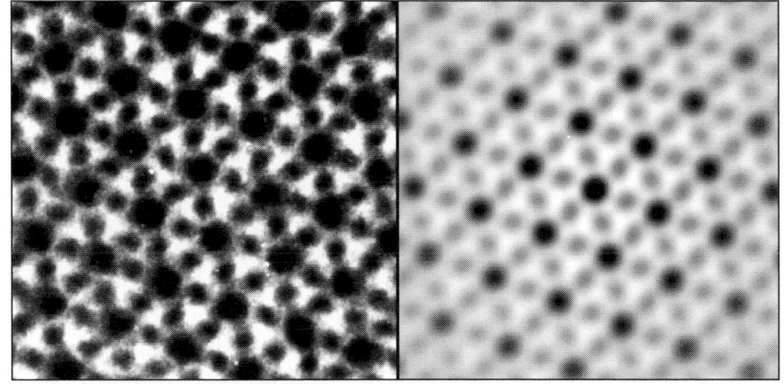

Figure 82. *TEM image of cross section of insect flight muscle (left) and the autocorrelation image (right). (Image courtesy of Mike Lamvik, Duke Univ.)*

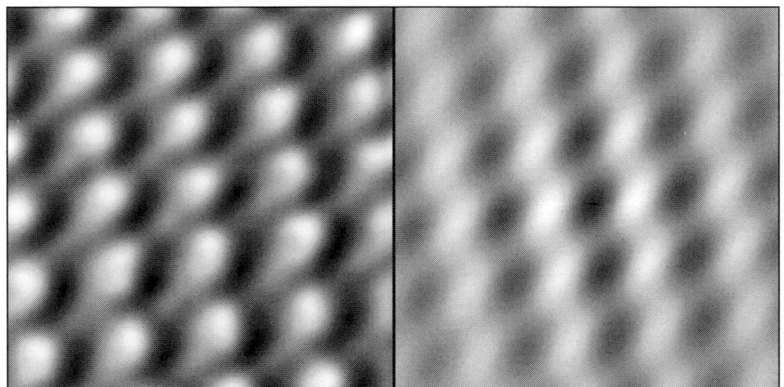

Figure 83. *Processing of Figure 37: comparison of smoothing with a low-pass filter (left) and autocorrelation (right).*

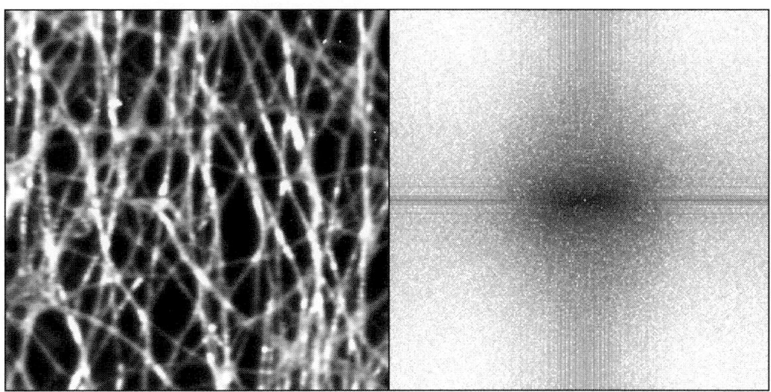

Figure 84. *Image of felted textile fibers (left) and the frequency transform (right).*

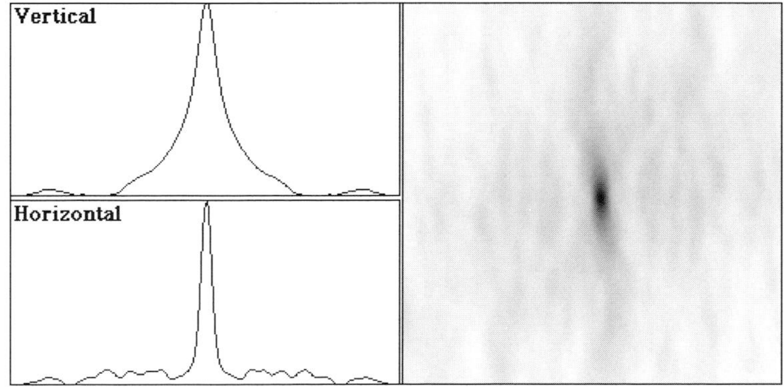

Figure 85. *Autocorrelation image from Figure 84 (right) and its horizontal and vertical brightness profiles (left).*

feature overlap as a function of relative offset) to determine preferred orientation.

Conclusion

Processing images in the frequency domain is useful for removing certain types of noise, applying large convolution kernels, enhancing periodic structures, and locating defined structures in images. It can also be used to measure images to determine periodicity or preferred orientation. All of these operations can be carried out in the spatial domain, but are often much more efficient in the frequency domain. The FFT (or FHT) operation is limited to images that are powers of two in size, but they can be efficiently computed in small (desktop) systems. This makes frequency-domain operations useful and important tools for image analysis.

5

Segmentation and Thresholding

One of the most widely used steps in the process of reducing images to information is segmentation: dividing the image up into regions that hopefully correspond to structural units in the scene or distinguish objects of interest. This is often described by analogy to visual processes as a foreground/background separation, implying that the selection procedure concentrates on a single kind of feature and discards the rest.

This is not quite true for computer systems, which can generally deal much better than humans with scenes containing more than one type of feature of interest. **Figure 1** shows a common optical illusion that can be seen as a vase or as two facing profiles, depending on whether we concentrate on the white or black areas as the foreground. It seems that humans are unable to see both interpretations at once, although we can flip rapidly back and forth between them once the two have been recognized.

This is true in many other illusions as well. **Figure 2** shows two others. The cube can be seen in either of two orientations, with the dark corner close to or far from the viewer; the sketch can be seen as either an old woman or a young girl. In both cases, we can switch between versions very quickly but we cannot perceive them both at the same time.

Thresholding

Selecting features within a scene or image is an important prerequisite for most kinds of measurement or scene understand-

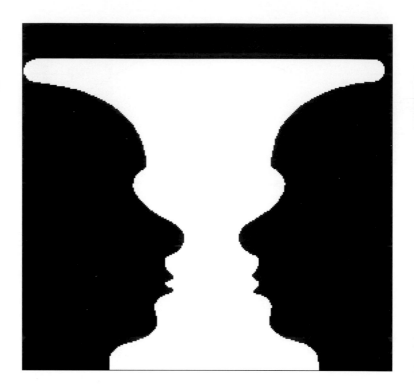

Figure 1. *The "vase" illusion. Viewers may see either a vase or two human profiles in this image, and can alternate between them, but cannot see both interpretations at the same time.*

ing. Traditionally, one simple way it has been accomplished is to define a range of brightness values in the original image, select the pixels within this range as belonging to the foreground, and reject all of the other pixels to the background. Such an image is then usually displayed as a binary or two-level image, using black and white or other colors to distinguish the regions. (There is no standard convention on whether the features of interest are white or black; the choice depends on the particular display hardware in use and the designer's preference.)

Such an operation is called thresholding. Thresholds may be set interactively by a user watching the image and using a colored overlay to show the result of turning a knob or otherwise adjusting the settings. The brightness histogram of the image (or a portion of it) is also useful for making adjustments. It is a plot of the number of pixels in the image having each brightness level. For a typical 8-bit monochrome image, this equals 2^8 or 256 grey scale values. The plot may be presented in a variety of formats, either vertical or horizontal, and some displays use color or grey scale coding to assist the viewer in distinguishing the white and black sides of the plot.

Examples of histograms have been given in earlier chapters. In the figures that follow, most are shown with a grey scale to identify the pixel brightness and lines whose length are proportional to the number of pixels with that brightness. Note that the histogram counts pixels in the entire image, losing all information about the original location of the pixels or the brightness values

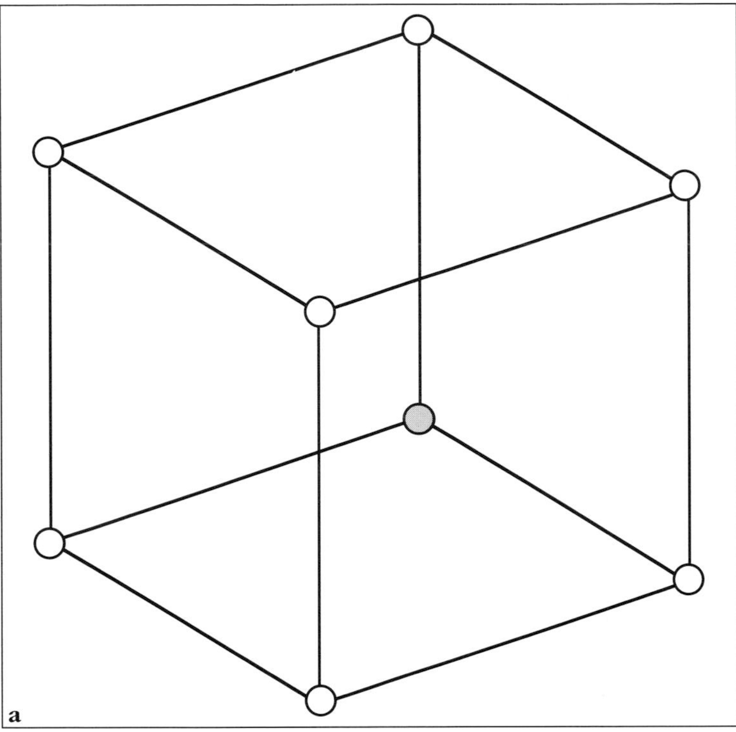

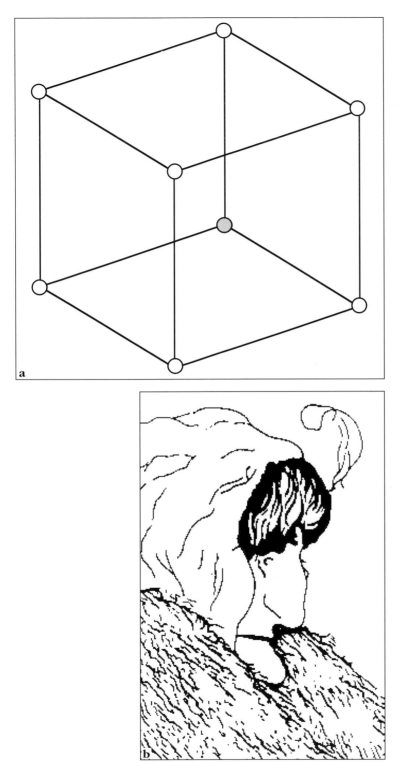

Figure 2. Examples of either/or interpretation:
a) *the Necker cube, in which the dark corner may appear close to or far from the viewer;*
b) *the "Old woman/Young girl" sketch.*

of their neighbors. Peaks in the histogram often identify the various homogeneous regions (often referred to as phases, although they correspond to a phase in the metallurgical sense only in a

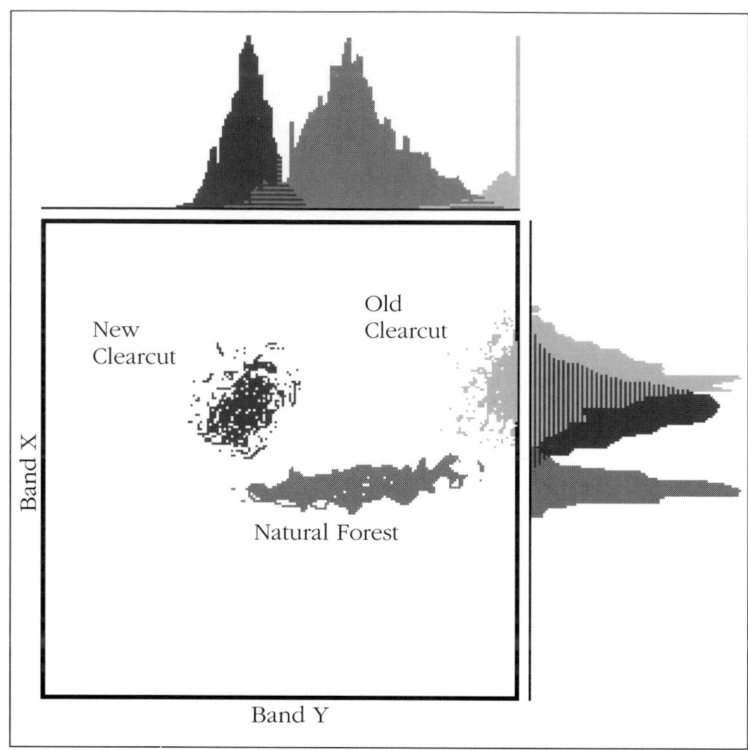

Figure 3. *Example of terrain classification from satellite imagery using multiple spectral bands.*

few applications) and thresholds can then be set between the peaks. There are also automatic methods to adjust threshold settings (Prewitt & Mendelsohn, 1966; Weszka, 1978; Russ & Russ, 1988a; Rigaut, 1988), using either the histogram or the image itself as a guide, as we will see below. Methods that compare to *a priori* knowledge the measurement parameters obtained from features in the image at many threshold levels (Wolf, 1991) are too complex and specialized for this discussion.

There are many images in which no clear-cut set of histogram peaks correspond to distinct phases or structures in the image. In some of these cases, direct thresholding of the image is still possible. In most, however, the brightness levels of individual pixels are not uniquely related to structure. In some of these instances, prior image processing can be used to transform the original brightness values in the image to a new image, in which pixel brightness represents some derived parameter such as the local brightness gradient or direction.

Multiband images

In some cases, segmentation can be performed using multiple original images of the same scene. The most familiar example is that of color imaging, which uses different wavelengths of light. For satellite imaging in particular, this may include several infrared bands containing important information for selecting regions according to vegetation, types of minerals, etc. (Haralick & Dinstein, 1975). **Figure 3** shows an example. It is more difficult to visualize, but a series of images obtained by performing different processing operations on the same original image can also be used in this way. Examples include combining one image containing brightness data, a second containing local texture information, etc.

In general, the more independent color bands or other images that are available, the easier and better the job of segmentation that can be performed. Points that are indistinguishable in one image may be fully distinct in another. However, with multi-spectral or multi-layer images, it can be difficult to specify the selection criteria. The logical extension of thresholding is simply to place brightness thresholds on each image, for instance to specify the range of red, green, and blue intensities. These multiple criteria are then usually combined with an AND operation (i.e., the pixel is defined as part of the foreground if its three R, G, B components all lie within the selected ranges). This is logically equivalent to segmenting each image plane individually, creating separate binary images, and then combining them with a Boolean AND operation afterward. Such operations to combine multiple binary images are discussed in Chapter 6.

The reason for wanting to combine the various selection criteria in a single process is to assist the user in defining the ranges for each. The optimum settings and their interaction are not particularly obvious when the individual color bands or other multiple image brightness values are set individually. Indeed, simply designing a user interface which makes it possible to select a specific range of colors for thresholding a typical visible light image (usually specified by the RGB components) is not easy. A variety of partial solutions are available for use.

This problem has several aspects. First, while red, green, and blue intensities represent the way the detector works and the way the data are stored internally, they do not correspond to the way that people recognize or react to color. As discussed in Chapter 1, a system based on hue, saturation, and intensity or lightness (HSI) is more familiar. A series of histograms for each of the RGB color planes may show peaks, but the user is not often able to judge which of the peaks correspond to individual features of interest.

Even if the RGB pixel values are converted to the equivalent HSI values and histograms are constructed in that space, the use of three separate histograms and sets of threshold levels still does nothing to help the user see which pixels have various combinations of values. For a single monochrome image, various interactive color-coding displays allow the user both to see which pixels are selected as the threshold levels are adjusted and also to select a pixel or cluster of pixels and see where they lie in the histogram. **Figure 4** shows an example, though because it con-

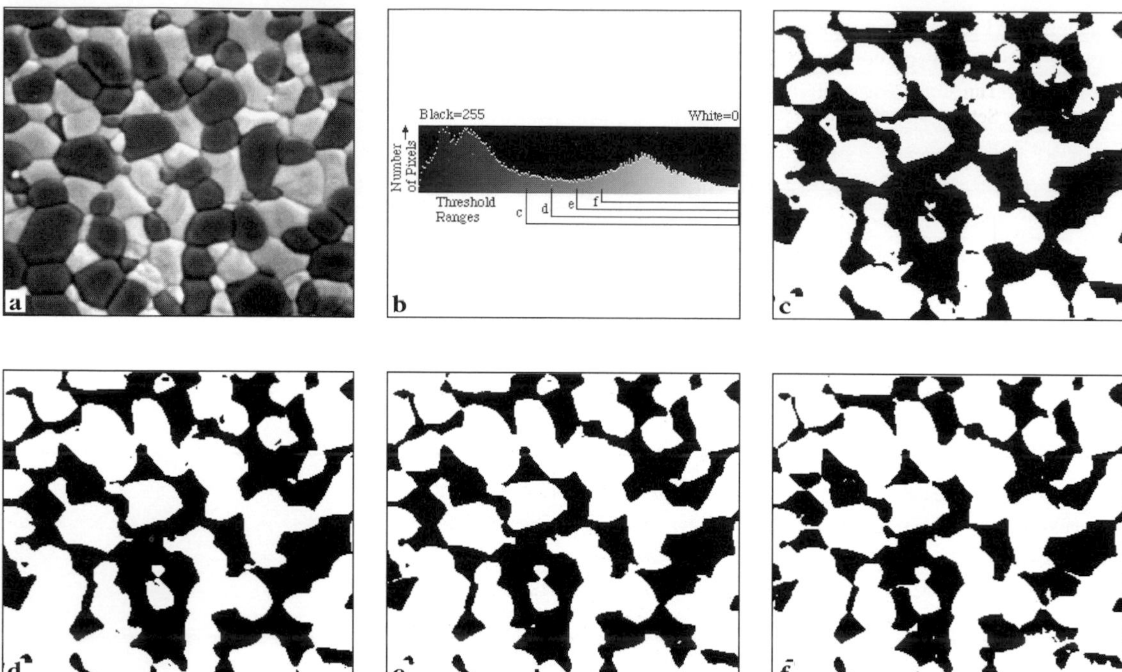

***Figure 4. A grey scale image:* (a)** *with its brightness histogram* **(b)** *and several binary images* **(c, d, e, f)** *produced by changing the settings of the threshold values used to select pixels, as shown on the histogram. The area fraction of the light phase varies with these setting from about 33 to 48%.*

sists of still images, it cannot show the live, real-time feedback possible in this situation.

For a three-dimensional color space, either RGB or HSI, this is not possible. There is no way with present display or control facilities to interactively enclose a region in three-dimensional space and see which pixels are selected, or to adjust that region and see the effect on the image. It is also difficult to mark a pixel or region in the image and see the color values (RGB or HSI) labeled directly in the color space. For more than three colors (e.g., the multiple bands sensed by satellite imagery), the situation is even worse.

Using three one-dimensional histograms and sets of threshold levels, for instance in the RGB case, and combining the three criteria with a logical AND selects pixels that lie within a portion of the color space that is a simple prism, as shown in **Figure 5.** If the actual distribution of color values has some other shape in the color space, for instance if it is elongated in a direction not parallel to one axis, then this simple rectangular prism is quite inadequate to enclose some shapes and exclude others.

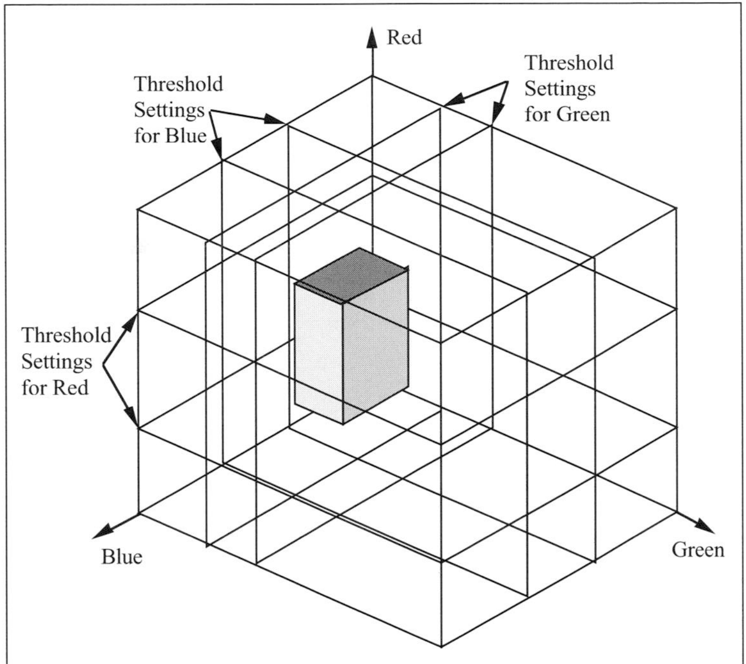

Figure 5. *Illustration of the combination of separate thresholds on individual color planes. The shaded region is the AND of the three threshold settings for red, green, and blue. The only shape that can be formed in the three-dimensional space is a rectangular prism.*

Two-dimensional thresholds

A somewhat better bound can be set by using a two-dimensional threshold. This can be done in any color coordinates (RGB, HSI, etc.), but in RGB space it is difficult to interpret the meaning of the settings. This is one of the arguments against the use of RGB for color images. However, the method is well-suited for color images encoded by hue and saturation. The HS plane is usually represented as a circle, in which direction (angle) is proportional to hue and radius is proportional to saturation **(Figure 6).** The intensity, or lightness, of the image is perpendicular to this plane and requires another dimension to show or to control.

Similar histogram displays and threshold settings can be accomplished using other planes and coordinates. For color images, the HS plane is sometimes shown as a hexagon (with red, yellow, green, cyan, blue, and magenta corners). The CIE color diagram shown in Chapter 1 is also a candidate for this purpose. For some satellite images, the near and far infrared intensities form a plane in which combinations of thermal and reflected IR can be displayed and selected.

As a practical matter, the HS plane is sometimes plotted as a square face on a cube that represents the HSI space. This is simpler for the computer graphics display and is used in several of the examples which follow. However, the HSI cube with square faces is topologically different from the cone or bi-cone used to represent HSI space in Chapter 1, and the square HS plane is topologically different from the circle in **Figure 6.** In the square, the minimum and maximum hue edges (400 nm = red and 700

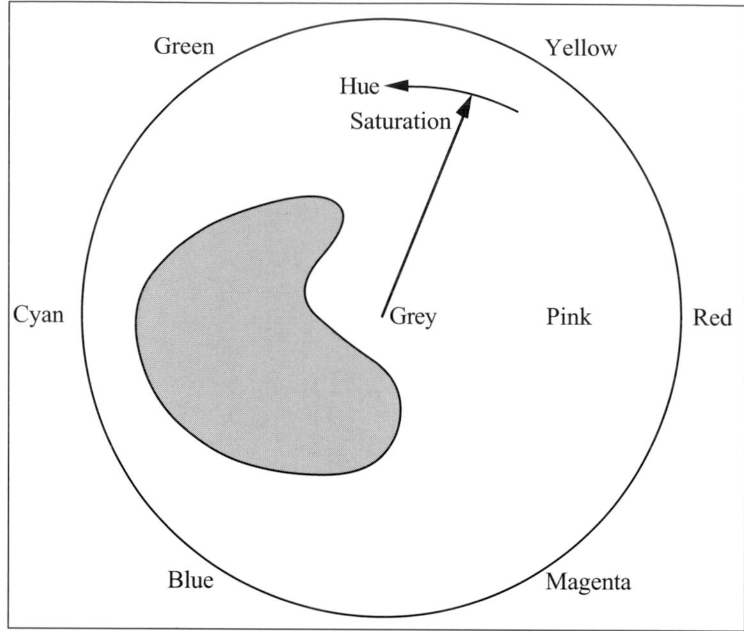

Figure 6. *Illustration of selecting an arbitrary region in a two-dimensional parameter space (here the hue/saturation plane) to define a combination of color in two image planes to be selected for thresholding.*

nm = violet) are far apart, whereas in the circle, hue is a continuous function that wraps around. This makes using the square for thresholding somewhat less intuitive, but it is still superior in most cases to the use of RGB color space.

An analog to a one-dimensional histogram of brightness in a monochrome image is a two-dimensional display in the HS plane. The number of pixels with each pair of values of hue and saturation can be plotted on this plane using brightness or color. Thresholds can be set by drawing an outline that is not necessarily simple or even convex, and so can be adapted to the distribution of the actual data. **Figure 6** illustrates this schematically. Automatic methods are available for drawing or adjusting the boundary based on the data. Indeed, they are very similar to methods for locating clusters for feature recognition, which is discussed below.

It is also possible to mark locations in this plane of individual pixels or regions of pixels in the image, as a guide to the user in the process of defining the boundary. This is often done by having the user point to or encircle pixels in the image and then highlight the location of the color values on the various display planes.

For the two-dimensional square plot, the axes may have unusual meanings, but the ability to display a histogram of points based on the combination of values and to select threshold boundaries based on the histogram is a significant advantage over multiple one-dimensional histograms and thresholds, even if it does not generalize easily to the n-dimensional case.

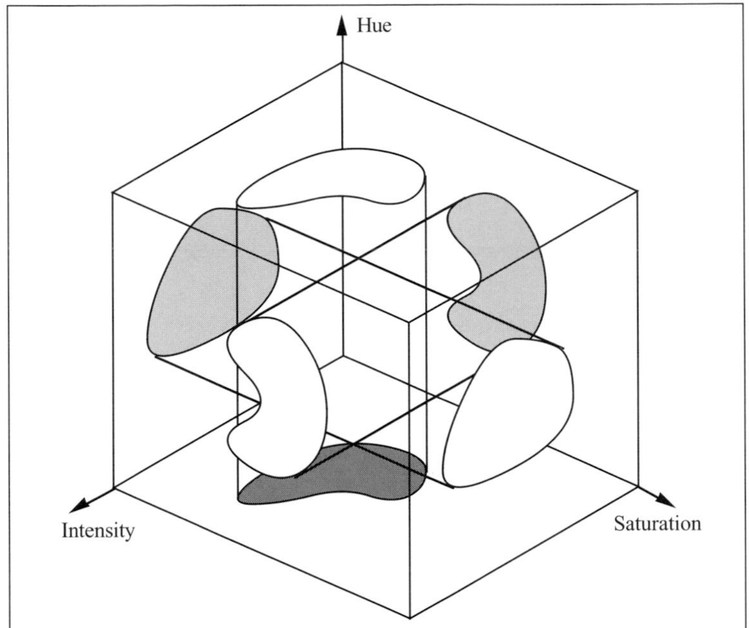

Figure 7. *Illustration of the combination of two-parameter threshold settings. Outlining of regions in each plane defines a shape in the three-dimensional space which is more adjustable than the Boolean combination of simple one-dimensional thresholds in Figure 5, but still cannot conform to arbitrary three-dimensional cluster shapes.*

The dimensions of the histogram array are usually somewhat reduced from the actual resolution (typically one part in 256) of the various RGB or HSI values for the stored image. This is not only because the array size would become very large (256^2 = 65,536 for the square, 256^3 = 16,777,216 for the cube). Another reason is that for a typical real image, there are simply not that many distinct pairs or triples of values present, and a useful display showing the locations of peaks and clusters can be presented using fewer bins. The examples shown below use 32×32 bins for each of the square faces of the RGB or HSI cubes, each of which thus requires 32^2 = 1,024 words of storage.

It is possible to imagine a system in which each of the two-dimensional planes defined by pairs of signals is used to draw a contour threshold, then project all of these contours back through the multi-dimensional space to define the thresholding, as shown in **Figure 7.** However, as the dimensionality increases, so does the complexity for the user and the AND region defined by the multiple projections still cannot fit irregular or skewed regions very satisfactorily.

Multiband thresholding

Plate 6 in Chapter 1 showed a color image from a light microscope. The microtomed thin specimen of intestine has been stained with two different colors, so that there are variations in shade, tint, and tone. **Figure 8** shows the individual red, green, and blue values. The next series of figures illustrates how this image can be segmented by thresholding to isolate a particular structure using this information.

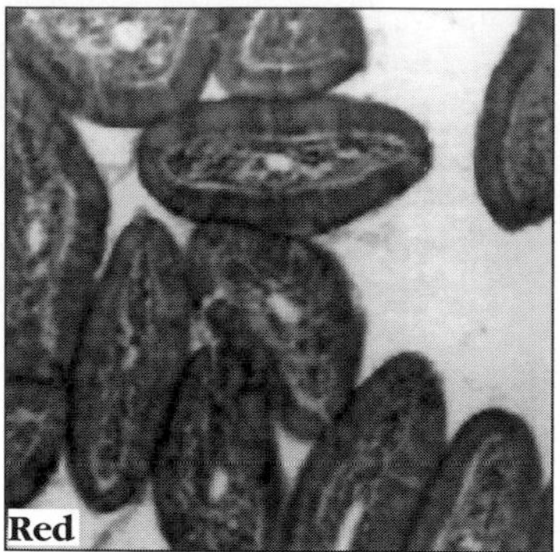

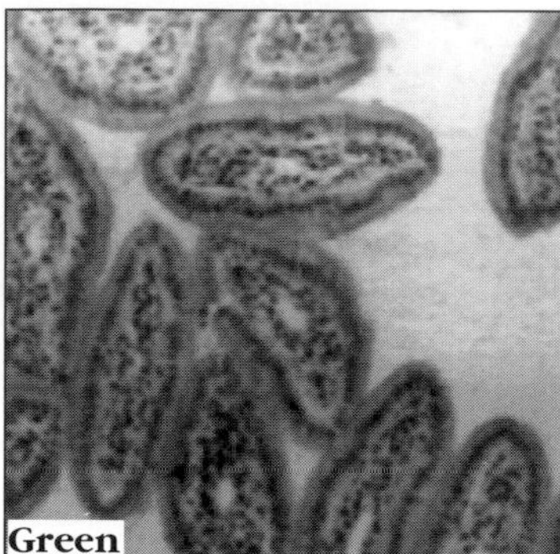

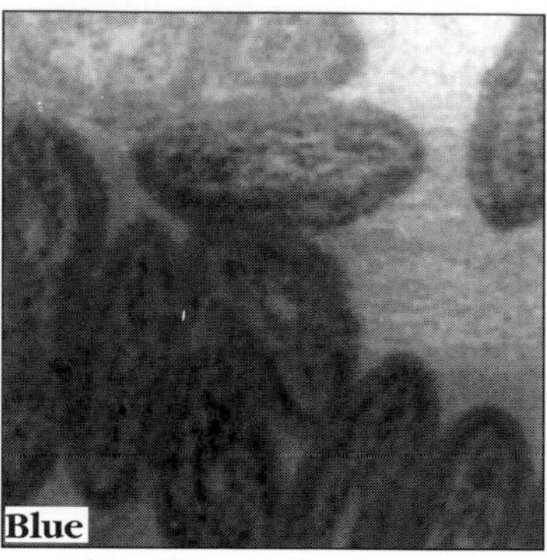

Figure 8. *Red, green, and blue color planes from the image in Plate 6 discussed in Chapter 1.*

Figure 9. *Brightness histograms for the color plane images in Figure 8.*

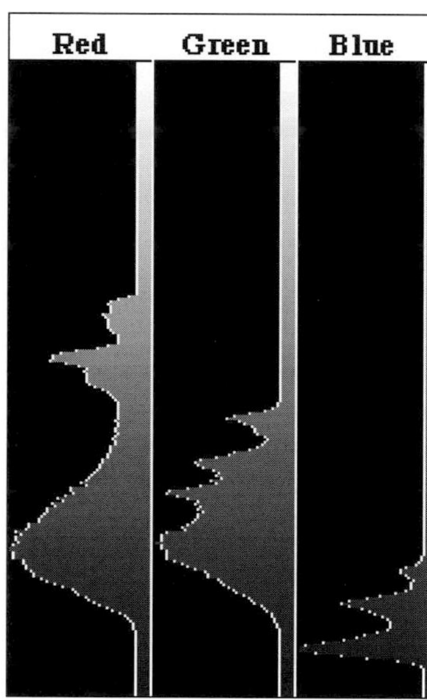

Figure 10. *Pairs of values for the pixels in the images of Figure 8, projected onto RG, BG, and RB planes.*

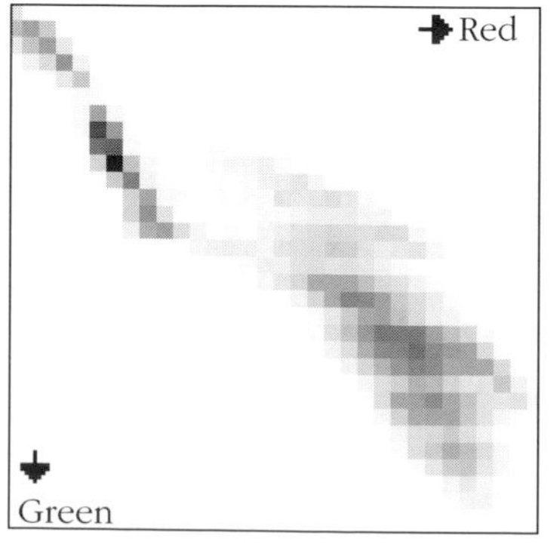

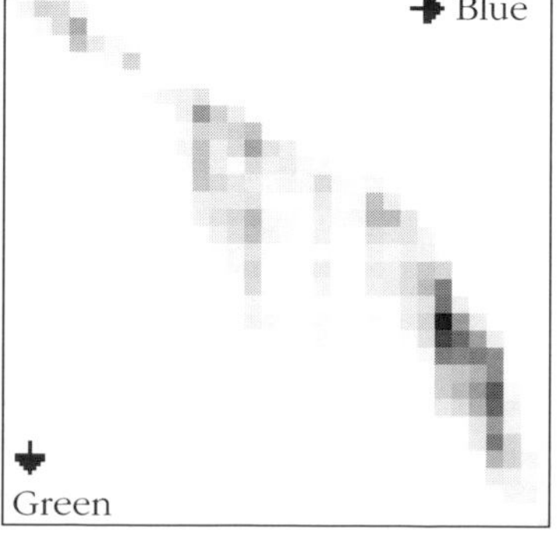

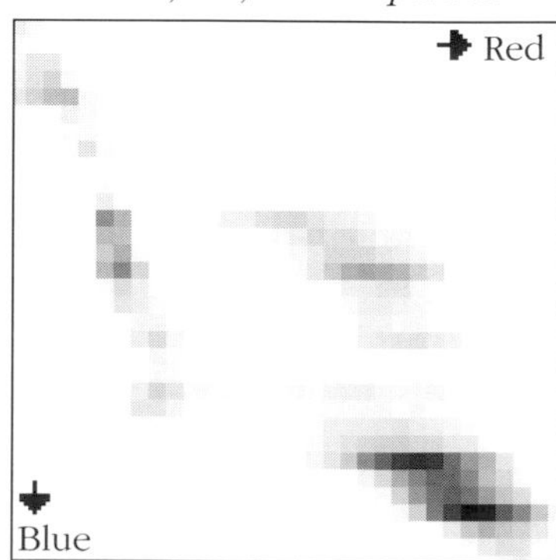

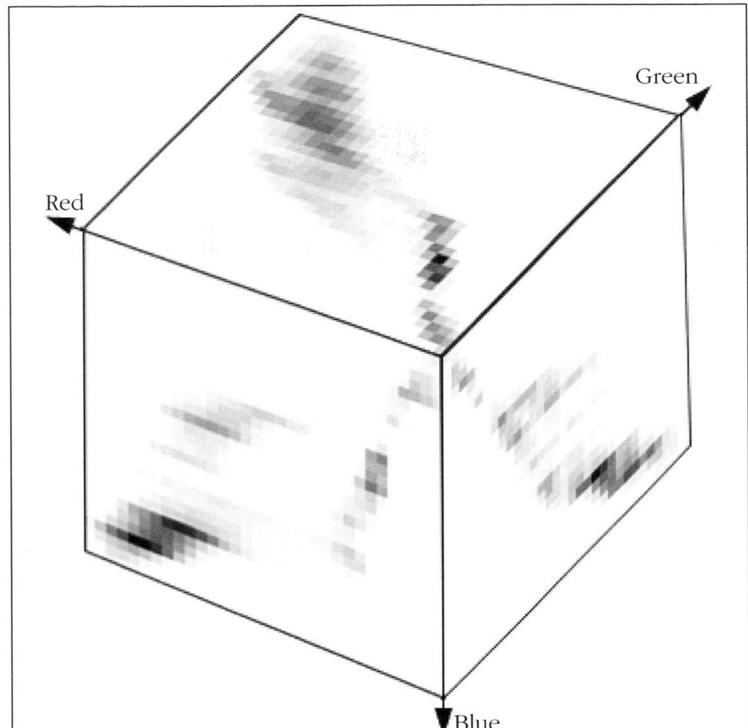

Figure 11. *The data from Figure 10 projected onto the faces of a cube.*

Figure 9 shows the individual brightness histograms of the red, green, and blue color planes in **Figure 8. Figure 10** shows the histograms of pixel values in the image, projected onto the red/green, green/blue, and blue/red faces of the RGB color cube. **Figure 11** presents this data as a perspective view on the cube. Notice that there is a trend on all faces for the majority of pixels in the image to cluster along the central diagonal in the cube. In other words, for most pixels, the trend toward more of any one color is part of a general increase in brightness by increasing the values of all colors. This means that RGB space poorly disperses the various color values and does not facilitate setting thresholds to discriminate the different regions present.

Figure 12 shows the conversion of the color information from **Figure 8** into hue, saturation, and intensity images, and **Figure 13** shows the individual brightness histograms for these planes. **Figure 14** shows the values projected onto individual two-dimensional hue/saturation, saturation/intensity, and intensity/hue square plots. **Figure 15** combines these values into the total cube. Notice how the much greater dispersion of peaks in the various histograms uses more of the color space and separates several different clusters of values.

Figure 16 compares two different thresholded binary images. The pixels selected from their hue values alone include both the general background of the slide and the structures in the villi. However, a two-dimensional threshold set using the saturation

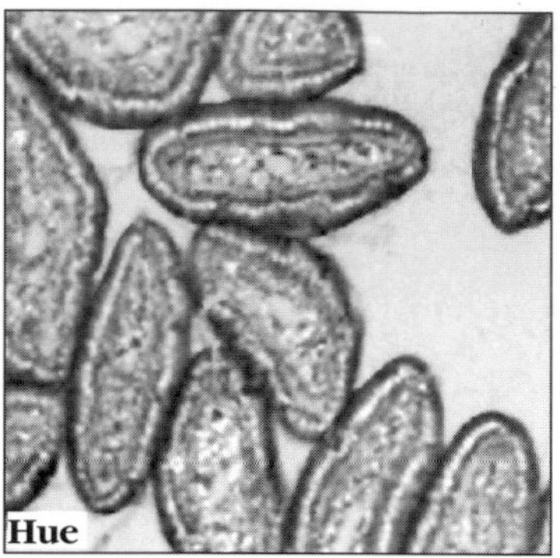

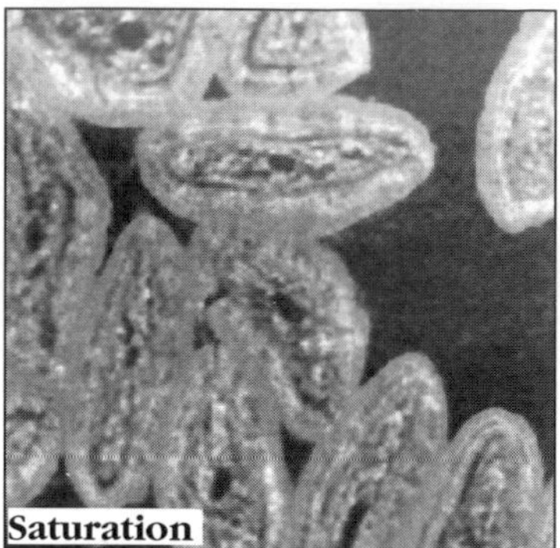

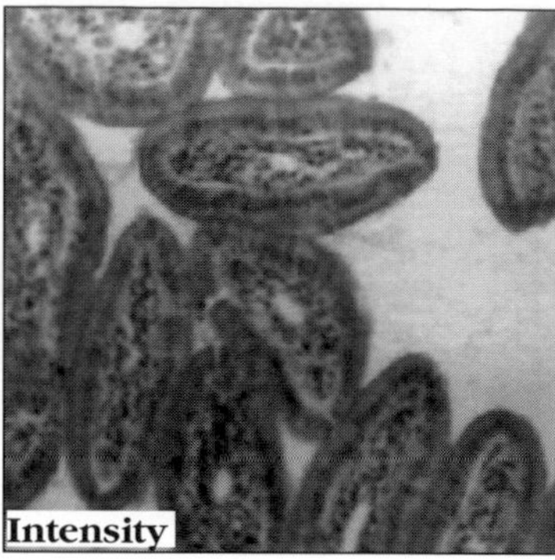

Figure 12. *The same color information as in Figure 8, converted to hue, saturation, and intensity components.*

Figure 13. *Brightness histograms for the color plane images in Figure 12.*

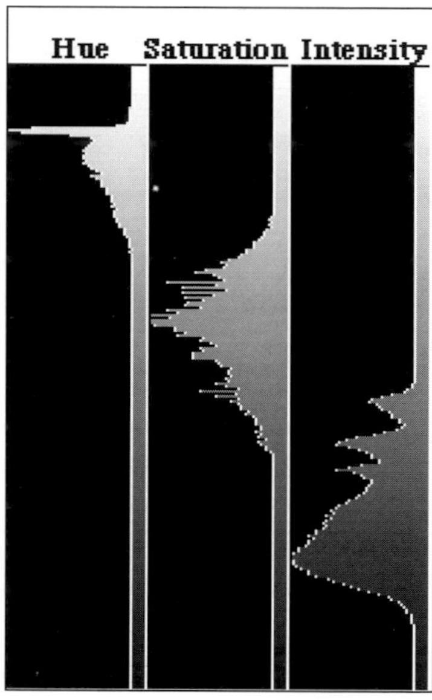

Figure 14. *Hue, saturation, and intensity values for the pixels in Figure 12, projected onto HI, HS, and SI planes. Note that the hue-saturation plane is topologically different from the usual HS circle.*

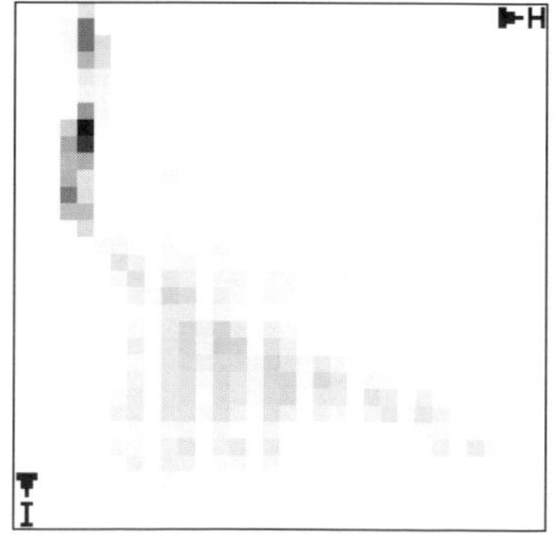

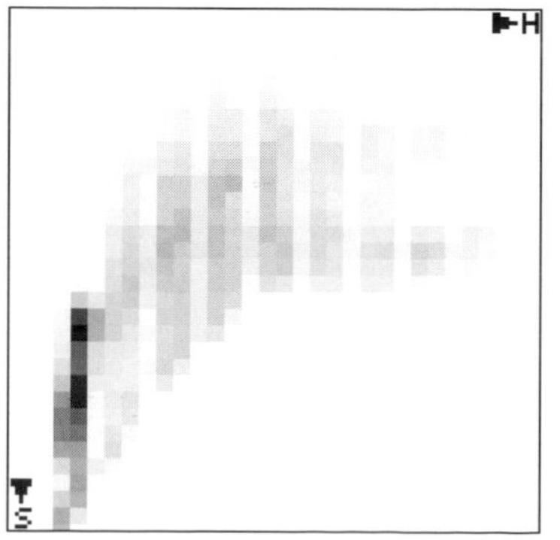

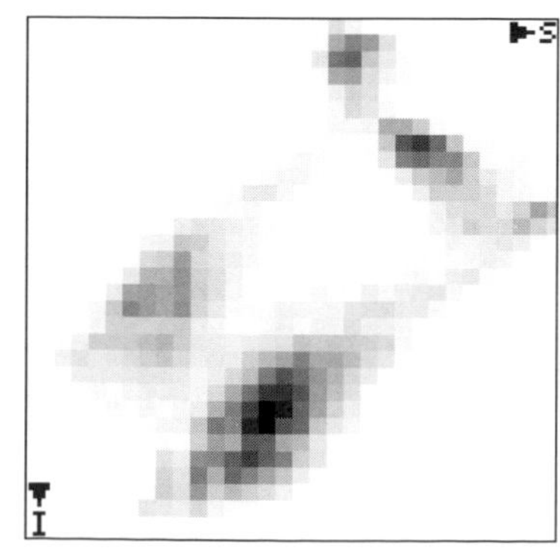

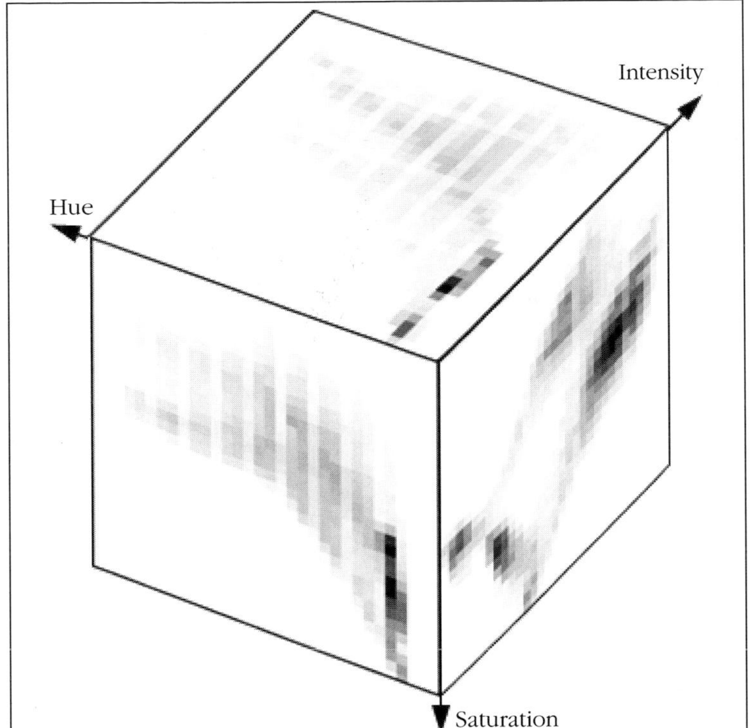

Figure 15. The data from Figure 14 projected onto the faces of a cube. Note that this cube is topologically different from the usual HSI biconical space (see text).

and intensity values allows only the villi to be selected, eliminating the general background. This is a more specific image and hence is more useful for further measurement.

Multiband images are not always simply different colors. A very common example is the use of multiple elemental X-ray maps from the SEM, which can be combined to select phases of interest based on composition. In many cases, this combination can be accomplished simply by separately thresholding each individual image and then applying Boolean logic to combine the images. Of course, the rather noisy original X-ray maps may first require image processing, such as smoothing, to reduce the statistical variations from pixel to pixel (as discussed in Chapters 2 and 3), and binary image processing (as illustrated in Chapter 6).

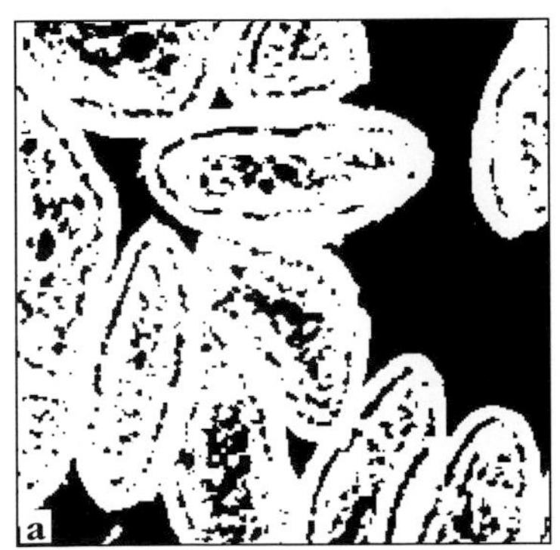

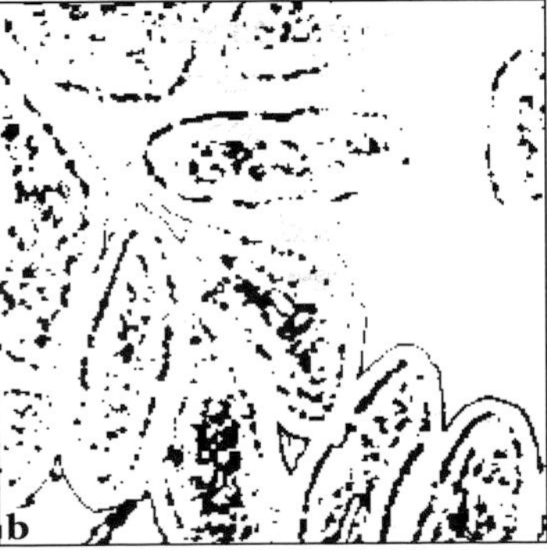

Figure 16. Thresholded binary images from the color figure represented in Figures 8 and 12:
a) *thresholded on hue, which includes both the structures within the villi and the background in the slide;*
b) *thresholded by a region in the two-dimensional saturation/intensity histogram, which selects just the villi.*

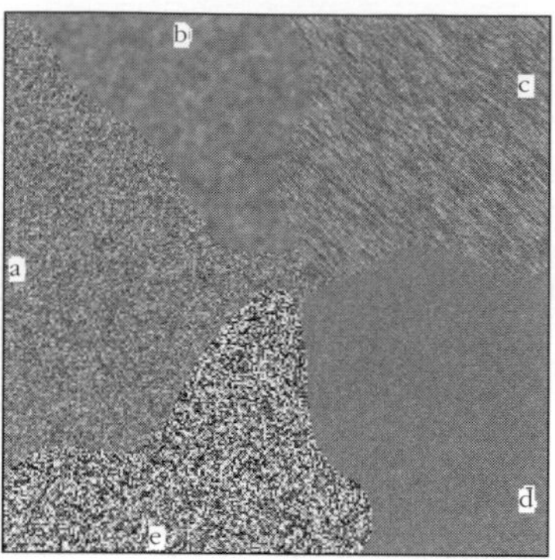

Figure 17. *Test image containing five different regions to be distinguished by differences in the textures. The average brightness of each region is the same.*

Using X-rays or other element-specific signals, such as secondary ions or Auger electrons, essentially the entire periodic table can be detected. It becomes possible to specify very complicated combinations of elements that must be present or absent, or the approximate intensity levels needed (since intensities are generally roughly proportional to elemental concentration) to specify the region of interest. Thresholding these combinations of elemental images produces results that are sometimes described as chemical maps. Of course, the fact that several elements may be present in the same area of a specimen, such as a metal, mineral, or block of biological tissue, does not directly imply that they are chemically combined, however.

In principle, it is possible to store an entire analytical spectrum for each pixel in an image and then use appropriate computation to derive actual compositional information at each point, which is eventually used in a thresholding operation to select regions of interest. At present, this approach is limited in application by the large amount of storage and lengthy calculations required. However, as faster and larger computers and storage devices become common, such methods will become more widely used.

Visualization programs used to analyze complex data may also employ Boolean logic to combine multiple parameters. A simple example would be a geographical information system, in which such diverse data as population density, mean income level, and other census data were recorded for each city block (which would be treated as a single pixel). Combining these different values to select regions for test marketing commercial products is a standard technique. Another example is the rendering of calculated tensor properties in metal beams subject to loading, as modeled in a computer program. Supercomputer simulations of complex dynamical systems, such as evolving thunderstorms, produce rich data sets that may benefit from such analysis.

There are other uses of image processing that derive additional information from a single original grey scale image to aid in performing selective thresholding of a region of interest. The processing produces additional images, which can be treated as multiband images useful for segmentation.

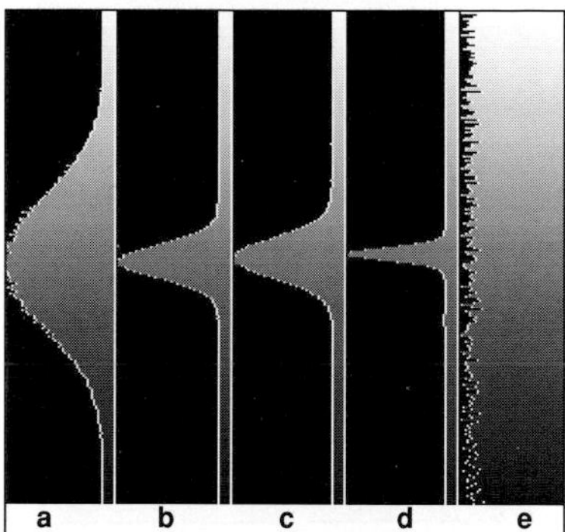

Figure 18. Brightness histograms of each area in Figure 17.

Thresholding from texture

Few real images of practical interest can be satisfactorily thresholded using simply the original brightness values in a monochrome image. The texture information present in images is one of the most powerful additional tools available. Several kinds of texture may be encountered, including different ranges of brightness, different spatial frequencies, and different orientations (Haralick et al., 1973). The next few figures show example images that illustrate these variables and the tools available to utilize them.

Figure 17 shows a test image containing five irregular regions that can be visually distinguished by texture. The average brightness of each of the regions is identical, as shown by the brightness histograms in **Figure 18.** Region (e) contains pixels with uniformly random brightness values covering the entire 0 to 255 range. Regions (a) through (d) have Gaussian brightness variations, which for regions (a) and (d) are also randomly assigned to pixel locations. For region (b) the values have been spatially averaged with a Gaussian smooth, which also reduces the amount of variation. For region (c) the pixels have been averaged together in one direction to create a directional texture.

One tool that is often recommended for textural characterization is the two-dimensional frequency transform. **Figure 19** shows these power spectra for each of the patterns in **Figure 21.** The smoothing in region (b) acts as a low-pass filter, so the high frequencies are attenuated. In region (c) the directionality is visible in the frequency transform image. For the other regions, the random pixel assignments do not create any distinctive patterns in the frequency transforms. They cannot be used to select the different regions in this case.

Several spatial-domain, texture-sensitive operators are applied to the image in **Figure 20.** The Laplacian shown in (a) is a 3×3 neighborhood operator; it responds to very local texture values and does not enhance the distinctions between the textures present here. All of the other operators act on a 5×5 pixel octagonal neighborhood and transform the textures to grey scale values

Figure 19. *Two-dimensional FFT power spectra of the pattern in each area of Figure 18. While some minor differences are seen (e.g., the loss of high frequencies in region b and the directionality in region c), these cannot be used with a filter for segmentation.*

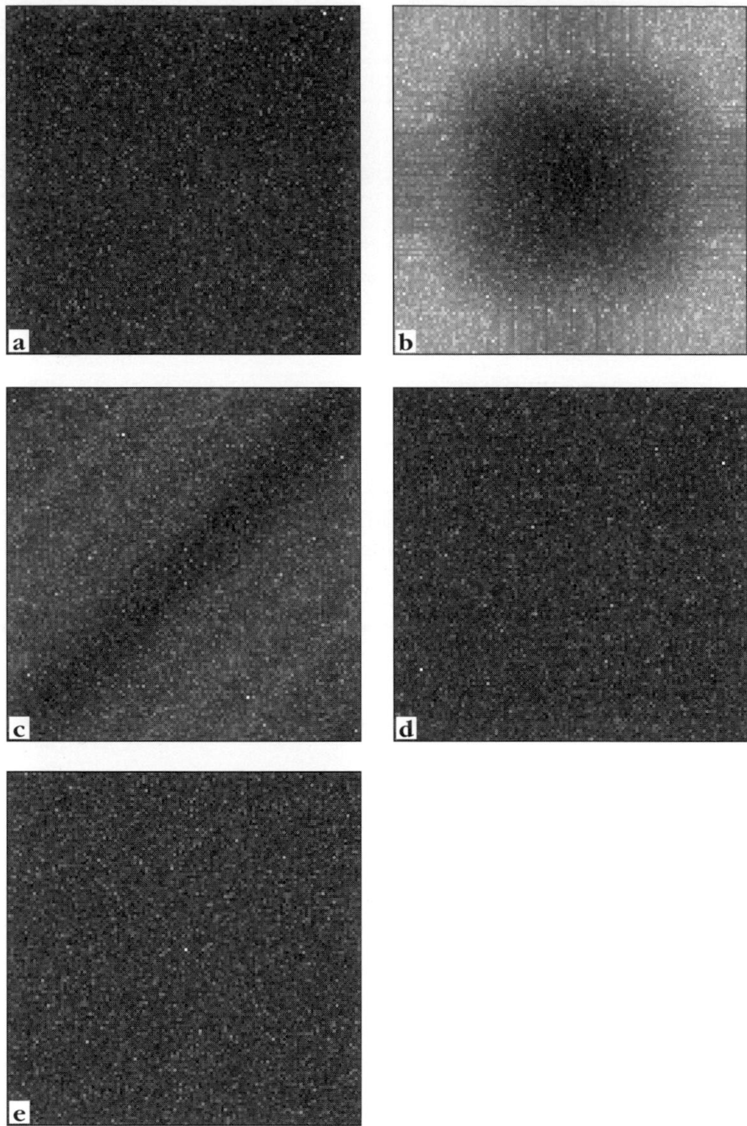

with somewhat different levels of success. Range (d) and variance (f) give the best distinction between the different regions.

There is still some variation in the grey values assigned to the different regions by the texture operators, because they work in relatively small neighborhoods where only a small number of pixel values control the result. Smoothing the variance image **(Figure 21a)** produces an improved image that has unique grey scale values for each region. **Figure 22** shows the brightness histogram of the original variance image and the result after smoothing. The spatial smoothing narrows the peak for each region by reducing the variation within it. The five peaks are separated and allow direct thresholding. **Figure 23** shows a composite image with each region selected by thresholding the smoothed variance image.

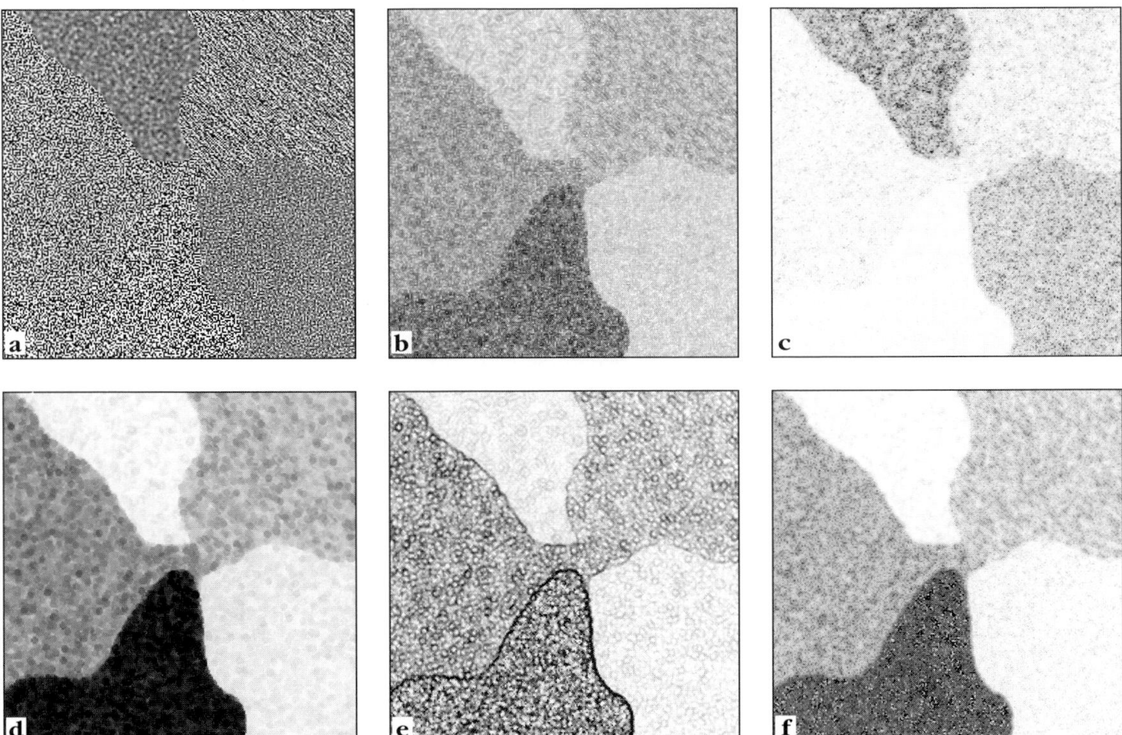

Figure 20. Application of various texture-sensitive operators to the image in Figure 17: ***a)*** *Laplacian;* ***b)*** *Frei and Chen;* ***c)*** *Haralick;* ***d)*** *range;* ***e)*** *Hurst;* ***f)*** *variance.*

Figure 21b shows the application of a Sobel edge (gradient) operator to the smoothed gradient image. Thresholding and skeletonizing (as discussed in Chapter 6) produces a set of boundary lines, which are shown superimposed on the original image in **Figure 24.** Notice that because the spatial scale of the texture is several pixels wide, the location of the boundaries of regions is necessarily uncertain by several pixels. It is also difficult to visually estimate the proper location, for the same reason.

Figure 25 shows a typical image obtained in microscopy. The preparation technique has used a chemical etch to reveal the microstructure of a metal sample. The lamellae indicate islands of

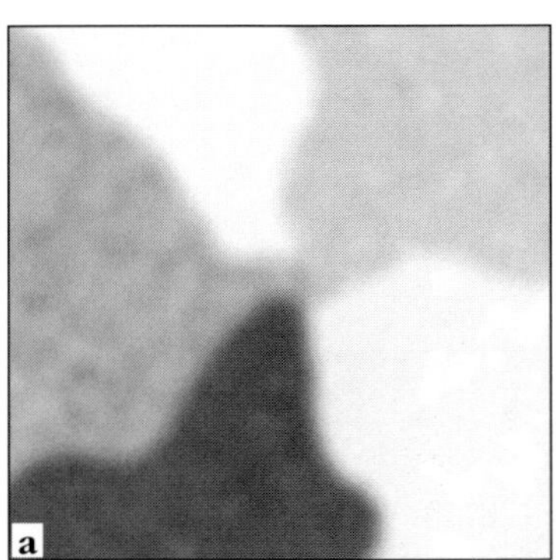

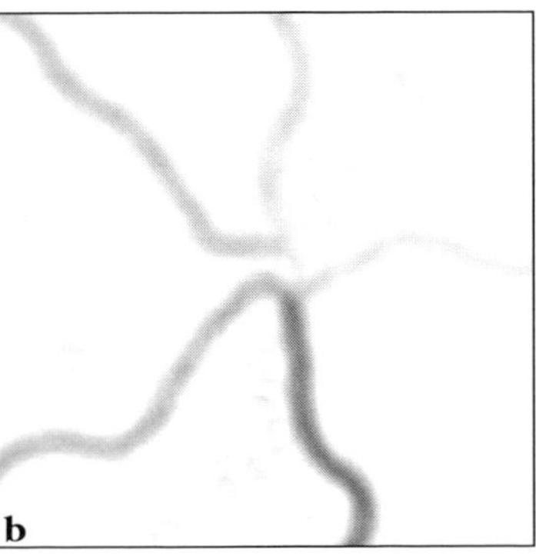

Figure 21. *Result of smoothing the variance image (Figure 20f) with a Gaussian kernel with standard deviation equal to 1.6 pixels (a), and the Sobel edge detector applied to the smoothed image (b).*

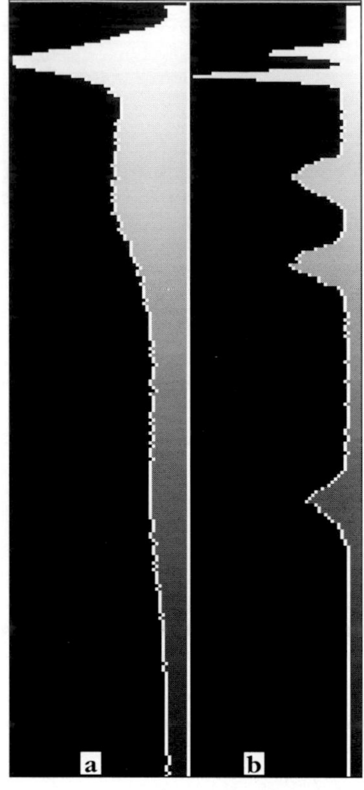

Figure 22. *Histograms of the variance image (Figure 20f) before (a) and after (b) smoothing the image with a Gaussian kernel with 1.6 pixel standard deviation. The five regions are now different in brightness and can be thresholded.*

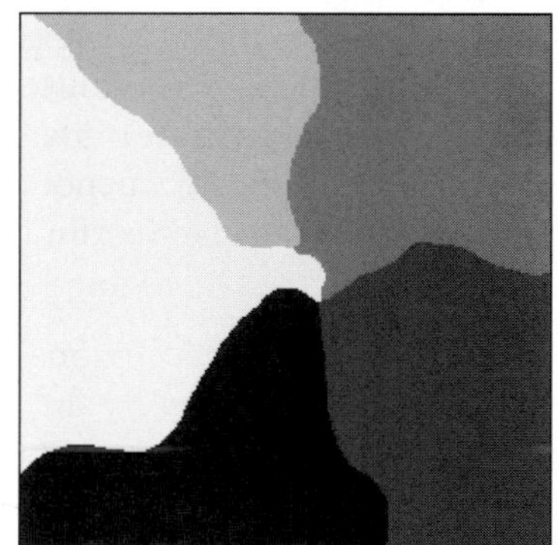

Figure 23. *Thresholding the smoothed variance image for each of the peaks in the histogram delineates the different texture regions.*

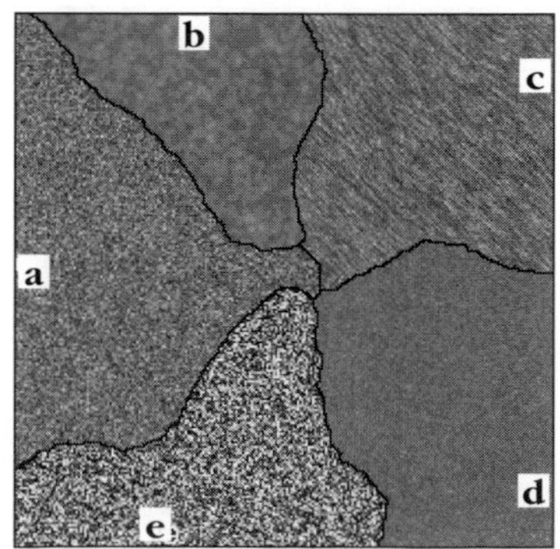

Figure 24. *Results of segmentation by skeletonizing the edge from the Sobel operator in Figure 21b.*

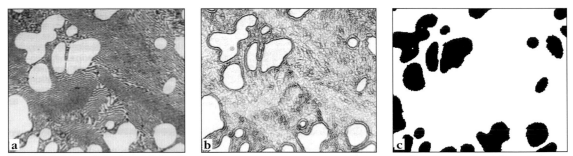

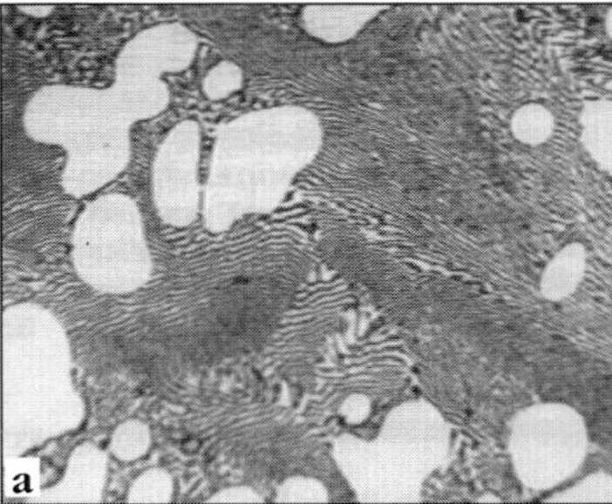

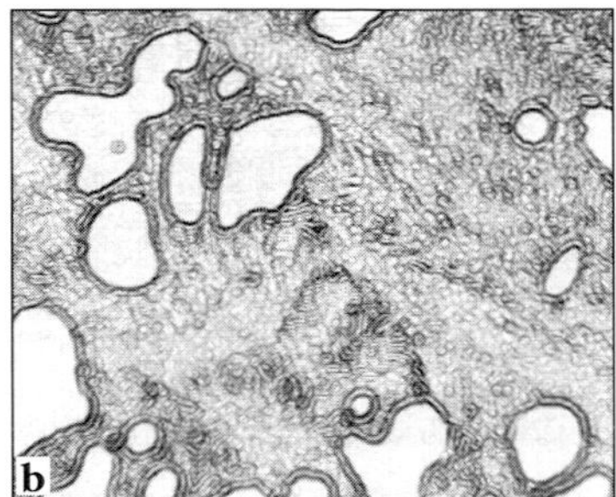

Figure 25. Application of the Hurst texture operator to a microscope image of a metal containing a eutectic:
a) *original image, with light single-phase regions and lamellae corresponding to the eutectic;*
b) *application of a Hurst operator (discussed in Chapter 3) to show the local texture in image a;*
c) *binary image formed by thresholding image b to select the low-texture (single-phase) regions.*

eutectic structure, which are to be separated from the uniform light regions to determine the volume fraction of each. The brightness values in regions of the original image are not distinct, but a texture operator is able to convert the image to one that can be thresholded.

Multiple thresholding criteria

Figure 26 shows a somewhat more complex test image, in which some of the regions are distinguished by a different spatial texture and some by a different mean brightness. No single parameter can be used to discriminate all four regions. The texture values are produced by assigning Gaussian random values to the pixels. As before, a variance operator applied to a 5×5 octagonal neighborhood produces a useful grey scale distinction. **Figure 27** shows the result of smoothing the brightness values and the variance image.

It is necessary to use both images to select individual regions. This can be done by thresholding each region separately and then using Boolean logic (discussed in Chapter 6) to combine the two binary images in various ways. Another approach is to use the same kind of two-dimensional histogram as described

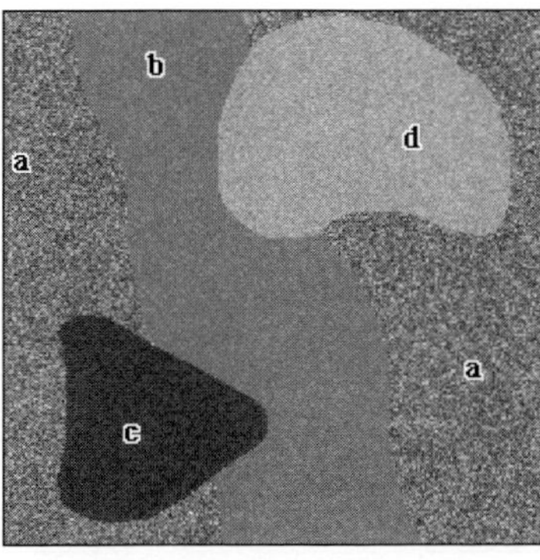

Figure 26. *Another segmentation test image, in which some regions have different textures and some different mean brightness.*

Figure 27. The brightness (a) and variance (b) images from Figure 26, and the results of smoothing with a Gaussian filter, standard deviation = 1.6 pixels.

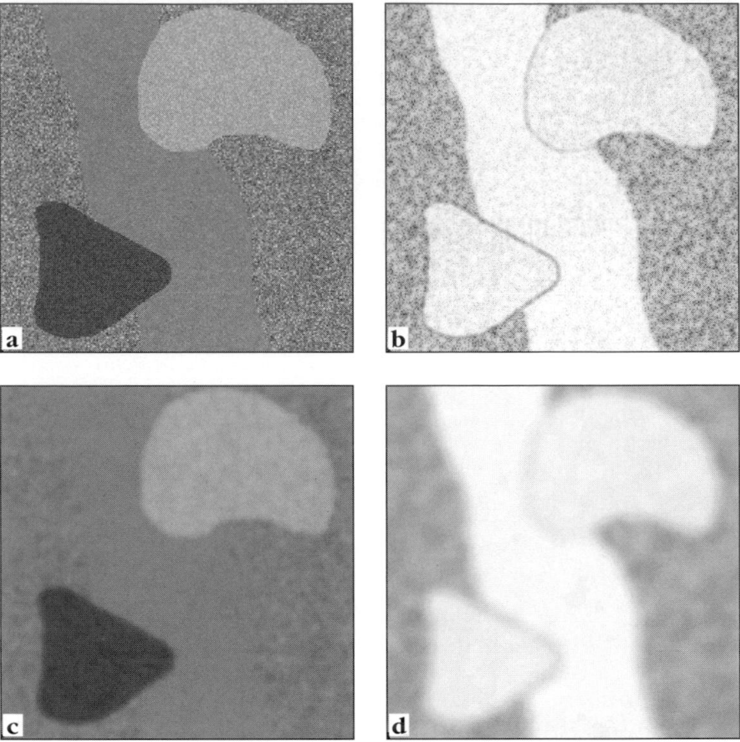

above for color images (Panda & Rosenfeld, 1978). **Figure 28** shows the individual image-brightness histograms and the two-dimensional histogram. In each of the individual histograms, only three peaks are present because the regions are not all distinct in either brightness or variance. In the two-dimensional histogram, individual peaks are visible for each of the four regions.

Figure 28. Histograms of the individual images in Figure 27c (brightness) and d (variance as a measure of texture) and the two-way histogram of the pixels showing the separation of the four regions.

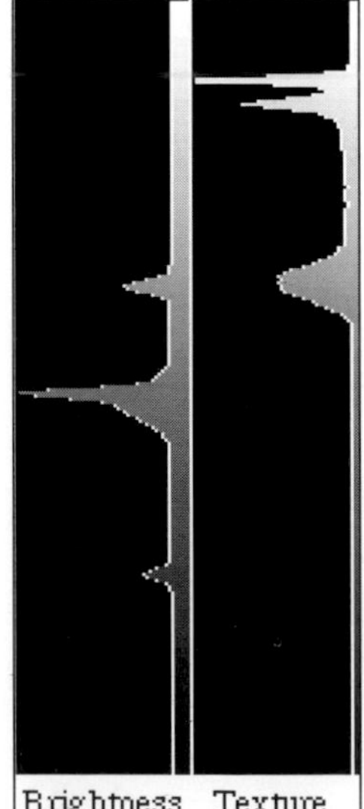

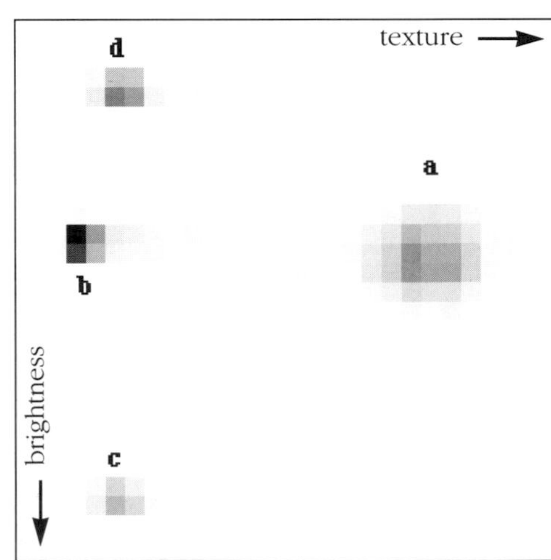

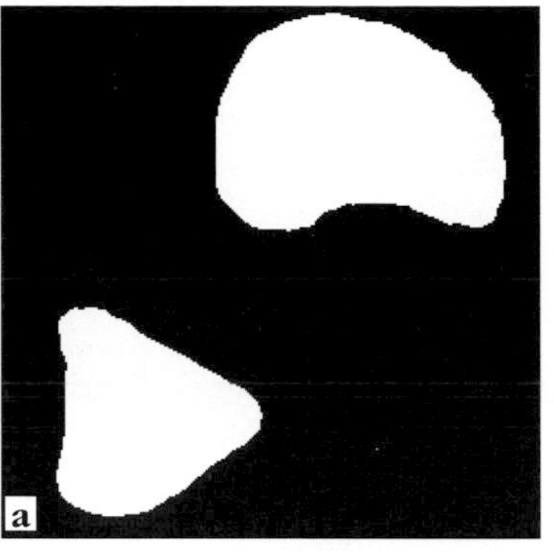

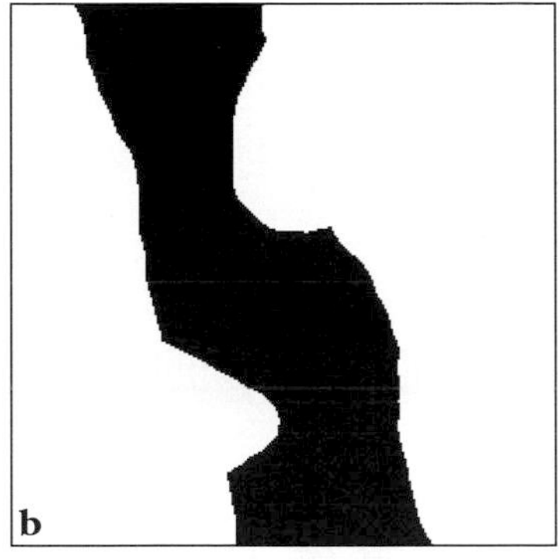

Figure 29. Thresholding of images in Figure 27:
a) *selecting intermediate brightness values (regions a and b);*
b) *selecting only region b by its brightness and texture.*

Figure 29a shows the result of thresholding the intermediate peak in the histogram of the brightness image, which selects two of the regions of medium brightness. **Figure 29b** shows the result of selecting a peak in the two-dimensional histogram to select only a single region. The outlines around each of the regions selected in this way are shown superimposed on the original image in **Figure 30.**

The different derived images used to successfully segment an image such as this one are sometimes displayed using different color planes. This is purely a visual effect, of course, since the data represented have nothing to do with color. However, it does take advantage of the fact that human vision uses color information for segmentation. **Plate 11** shows the information from the image in **Figure 26,** with the original image in the intensity plane, the smoothed brightness values in the hue plane, and the texture information from the variance operator in the saturation plane of a color image.

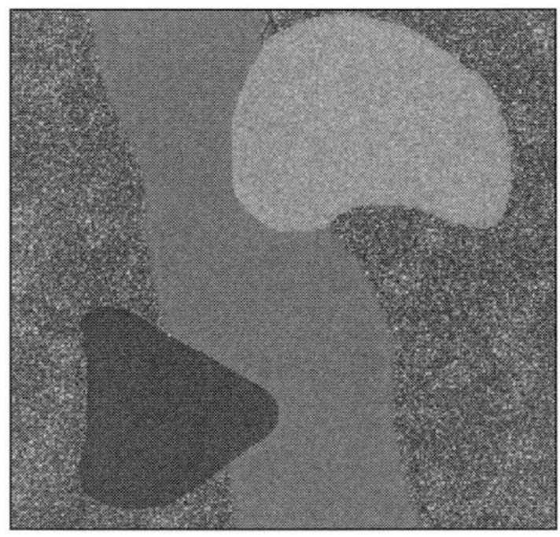

Plate 11. *See color plate, page VI. Color plates appear following page 246.*

Textural orientation

Figure 31 shows another test image containing regions having different textural orientations but identical mean brightness, brightness distribution, and spatial scale of the local variation. This rather subtle texture is evident in a two-dimensional fre-

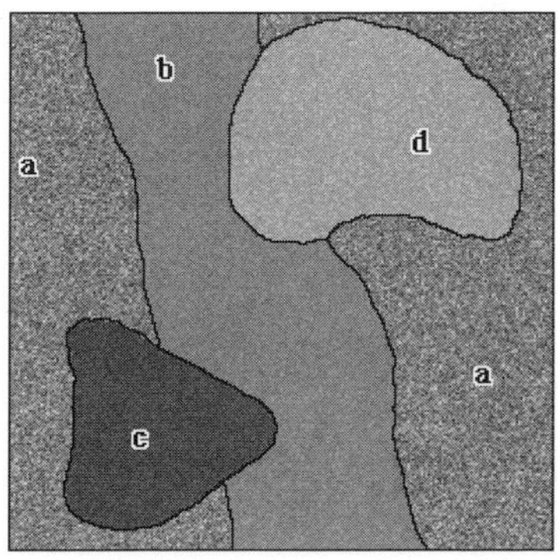

Figure 30. *Result of segmenting Figure 26 by thresholding on two-dimensional histogram or by ANDing binary images thresholded individually.*

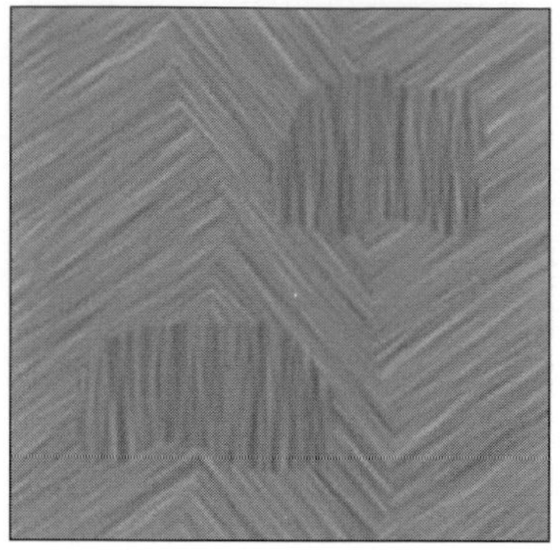

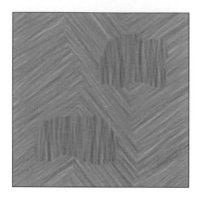

Figure 31. *An image containing regions which have different textural orientations, but the same average brightness, standard deviation, and spatial scale.*

quency transform, as shown in **Figure 31a.** The three ranges of spatial-domain orientation are revealed in the three spokes in the transform.

Using a selective wedge-shaped mask with smoothed edges to select each of the spokes and re-transform the image produces the three spatial-domain images shown in **Figure 32.** Each texture orientation in the original image is isolated, having a uniform grey background in other locations. These images cannot be directly thresholded because the brightness values in the textured regions cover a range that includes the surroundings. Applying a range operator to a 5×5-pixel octagonal neighborhood, as shown in **Figure 33,** suppresses the uniform background regions and highlights the individual texture regions.

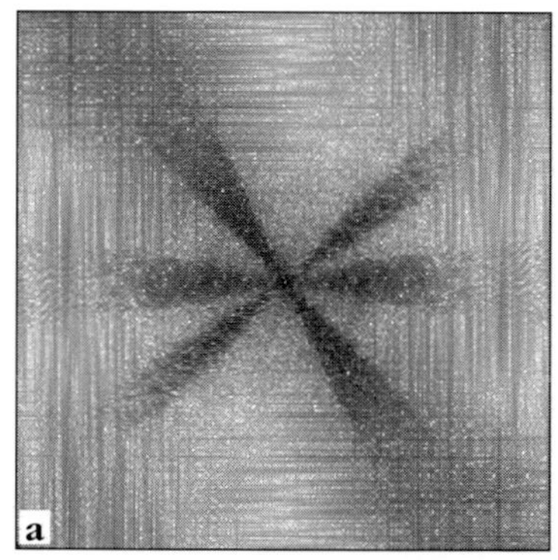

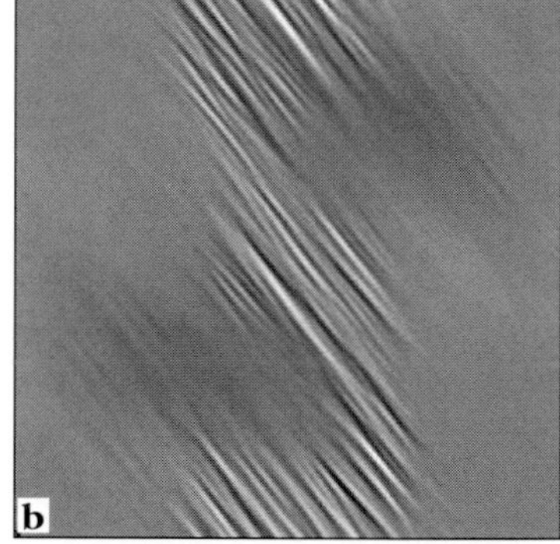

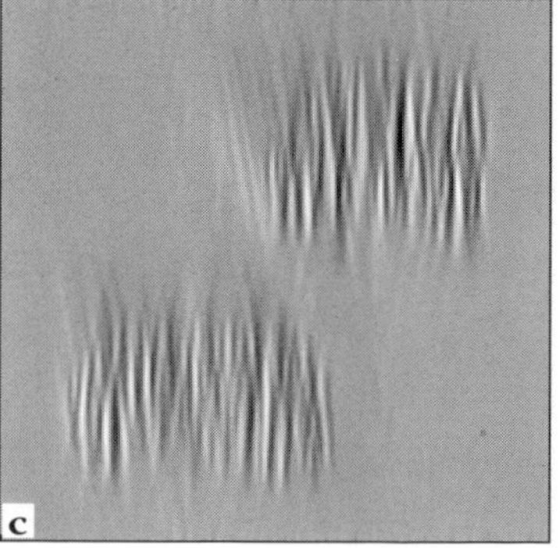

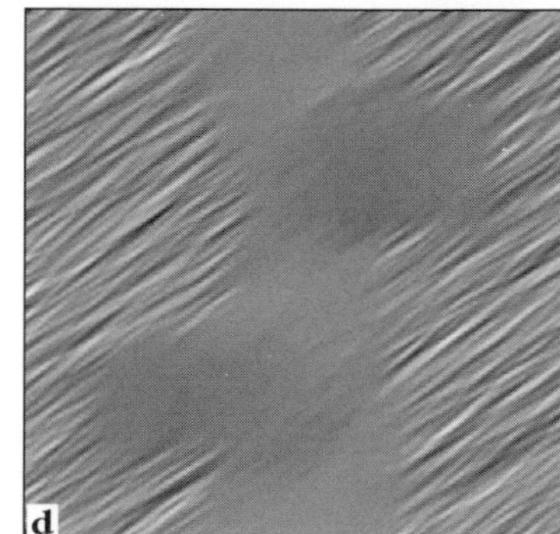

Figure 32. Isolating the directional texture in frequency space:
a) *two-dimensional frequency transform of the image in Figure 31, showing the radial spokes corresponding to each textural alignment;*
b, c, & d) *retransformation using masks to select each of the orientations.*

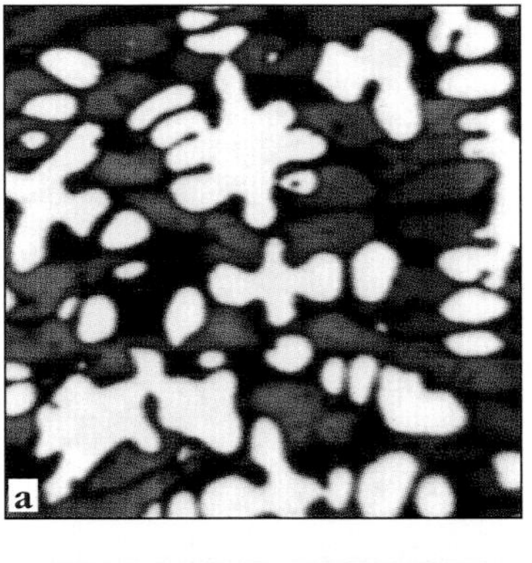

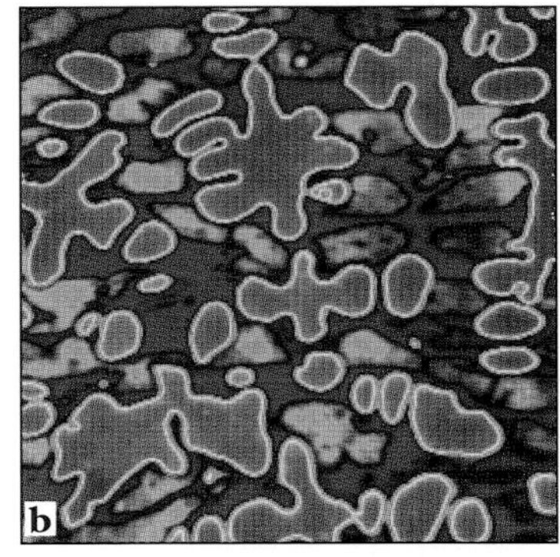

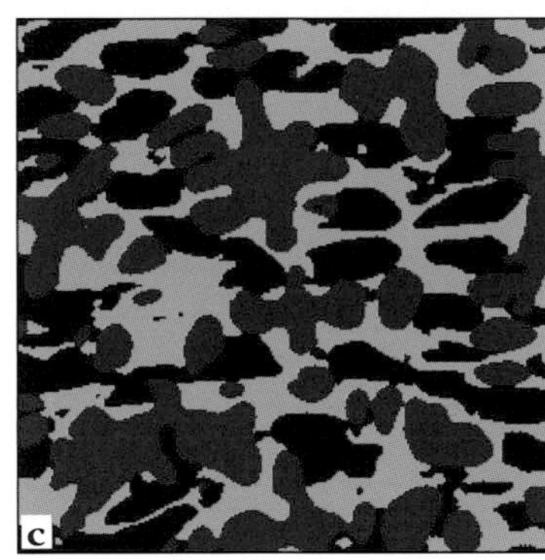

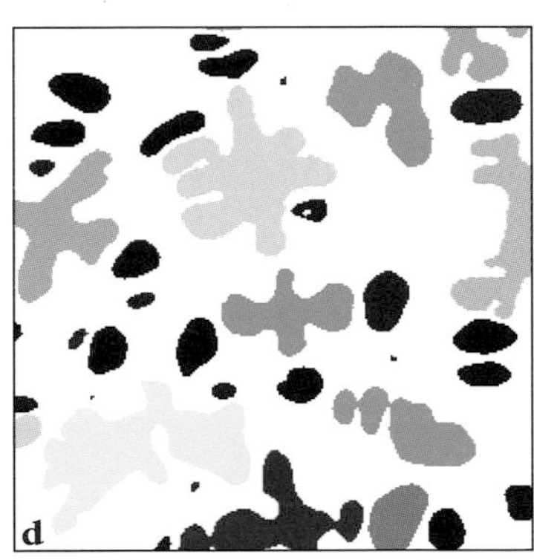

Plate 1. Uses for pseudo-color displays:

a) *Portion of a grey scale microscope image of a polished metallographic specimen with three phases having different average brightnesses.*

b) *Image a with pseudo-color palette or LUT which replaces grey values with colors. Note the misleading colors along boundaries between light and dark phases.*

c) *Image a with colors assigned to phases. This requires segmentation of the image by thresholding and other logic to assign each pixel to a phase based on grey scale brightness and neighboring pixel classification.*

d) *Lightest features from image a with colors assigned based on feature size. This requires the steps to create feature c, plus collection of all touching pixels into a feature and the measurement of that feature.*

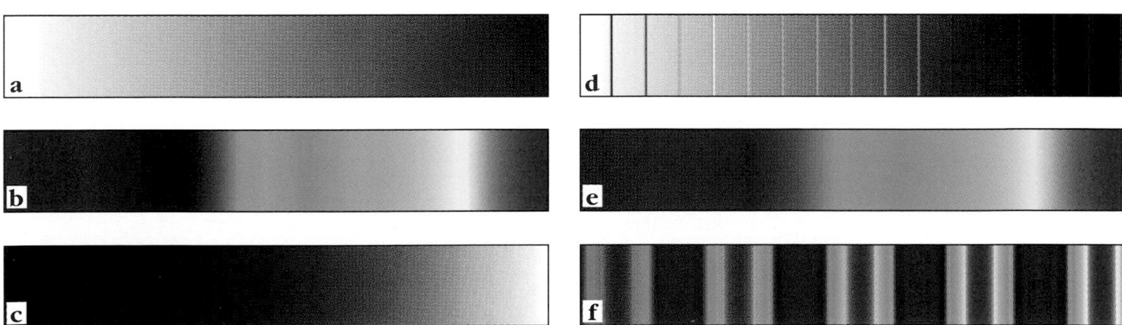

Plate 2. Six examples of display look-up tables (LUTs):

a) *monochrome (grey scale);*

b) *spectrum or rainbow (linear variation of hue, maximum saturation, and intensity);*

c) *heat scale;*

d) *monochrome with contour lines (rainbow colors substituted every 16th value);*

e) *linear variation of hue, saturation, and intensity;*

f) *sinusoidal variation of hue with linear variation of saturation and intensity.*

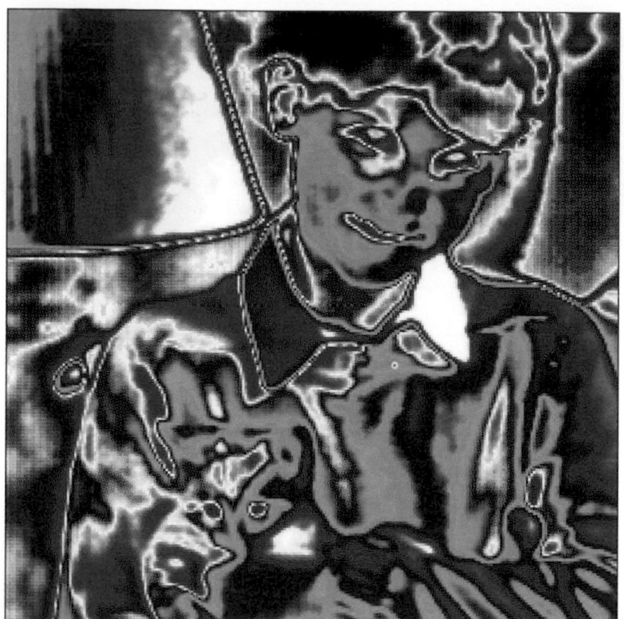

Plate 3. *The same image used in Figures 25 and 26 of Chapter 1, with a pseudo-color display LUT. The Gestalt contents of the image are obscured.*

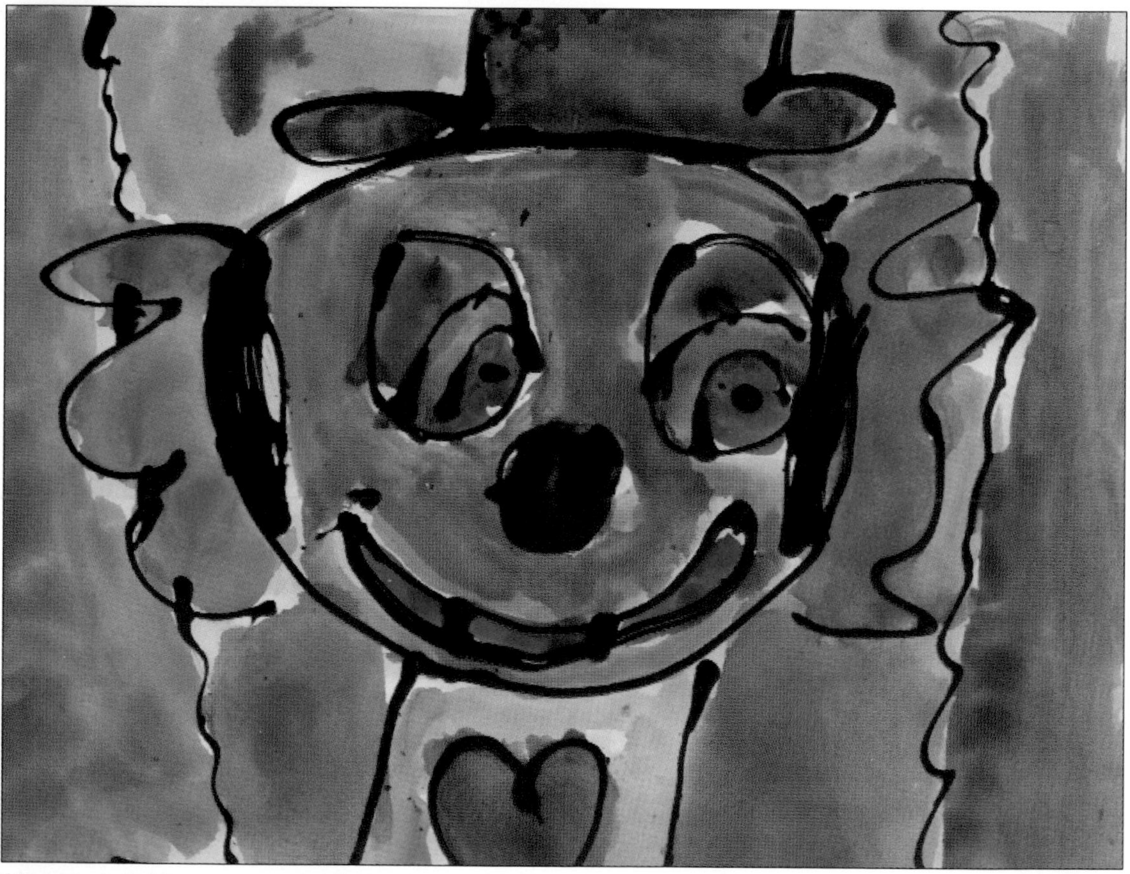

Plate 4. *A child's painting of a clown. Notice that the colors are unrealistic, but their relative intensities are correct, and that the painted areas are not exactly bounded by the lines. The dark lines nevertheless give the dimensions and shape to the features, and we are not confused by the colors which extend beyond their regions.*

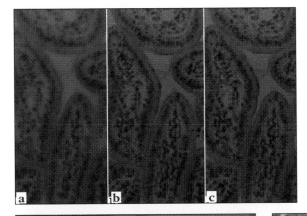

Plate 5. Portion of the color image described in Plate 6, expanded to show individual pixels:

***a)** original image;*

***b)** filtered to sharpen the image using the red, green, and blue planes; note the appearance of false colors near boundaries;*

***c)** filtered to sharpen the image by processing the hue, saturation, and intensity components.*

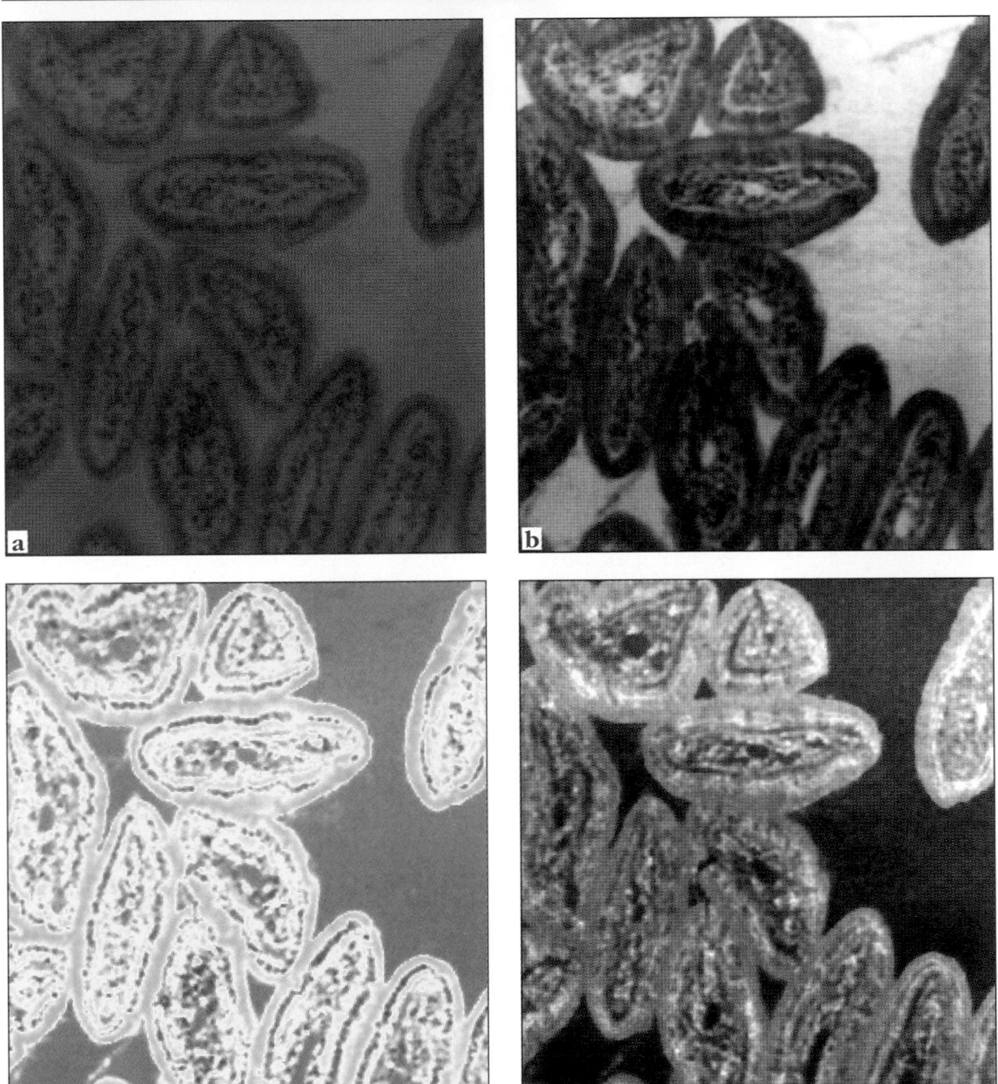

Plate 6. Microtomed tissue section of paraffin-embedded mouse intestine, Feulgen stained and counterstained with fast green, Bouin's fixative (specimen courtesy of Dr. Barbara Grimes, Div. of Interdisciplinary Studies, North Carolina State Univ., Raleigh, NC):

***a)** original color image; **b)** intensity component of image a;*

***c)** hue component of image a; **d)** saturation component of image a.*

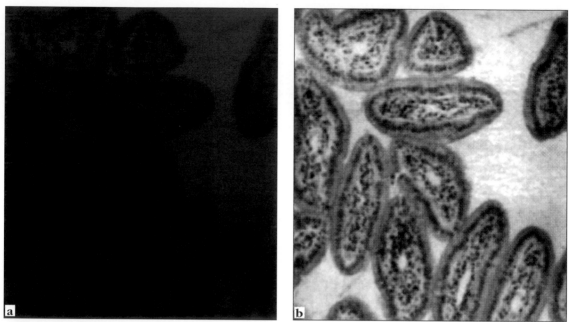

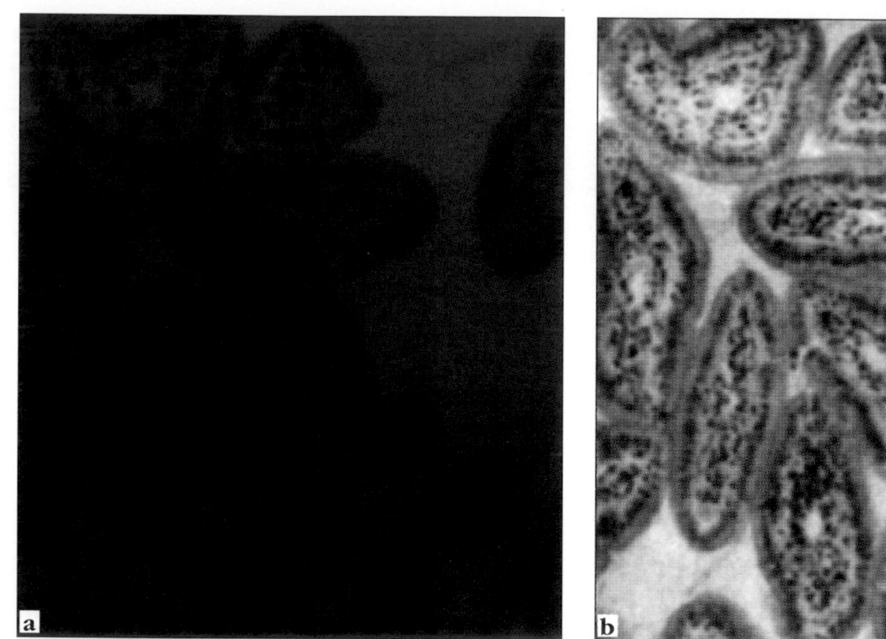

Plate 7. Filtering of the image in Plate 6:
a) *application of a 480-nm filter to the original color image;* ***b)*** *monochrome intensity from image c.*

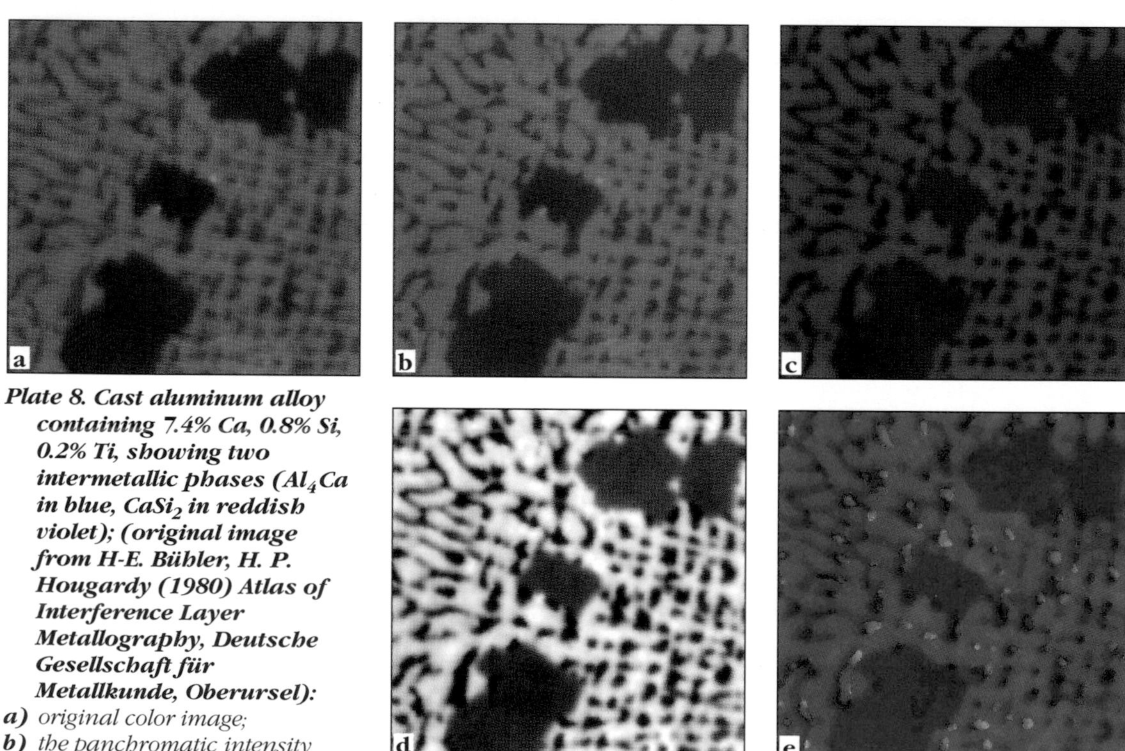

Plate 8. Cast aluminum alloy containing 7.4% Ca, 0.8% Si, 0.2% Ti, showing two intermetallic phases (Al_4Ca in blue, $CaSi_2$ in reddish violet); (original image from H-E. Bühler, H. P. Hougardy (1980) Atlas of Interference Layer Metallography, Deutsche Gesellschaft für Metallkunde, Oberursel):

- ***a)*** *original color image;*
- ***b)*** *the panchromatic intensity component of image a showing inability to distinguish two of the phases;*
- ***c)*** *application of a 590-nm filter;*
- ***d)*** *monochrome intensity from image c;*
- ***e)*** *the hue component of image a.*

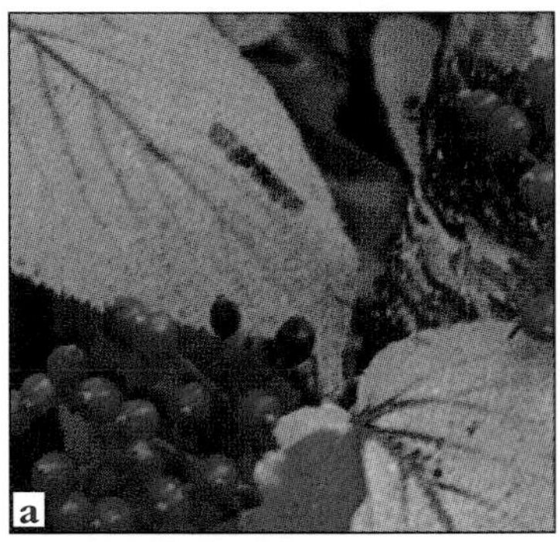

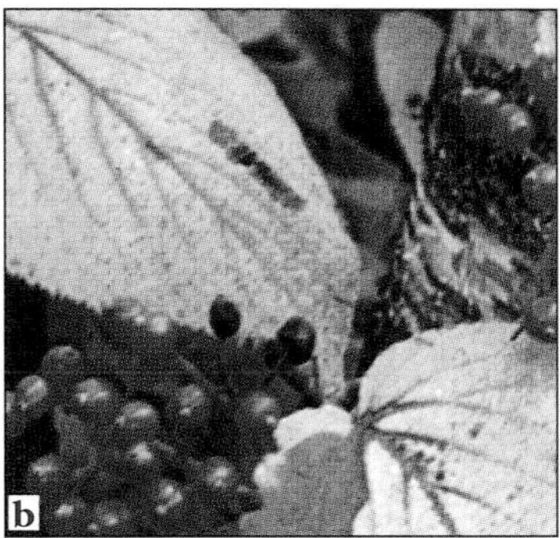

Plate 9. *Compression of a color image. The original image (a) shows fine details, sharp boundaries for colored regions, and gradual variation in color (hue and saturation) which are degraded by compression (b). However, the disk file for the compressed image is smaller by a factor of 16:1, occupying 14 kilobytes instead of 224 kilobytes.*

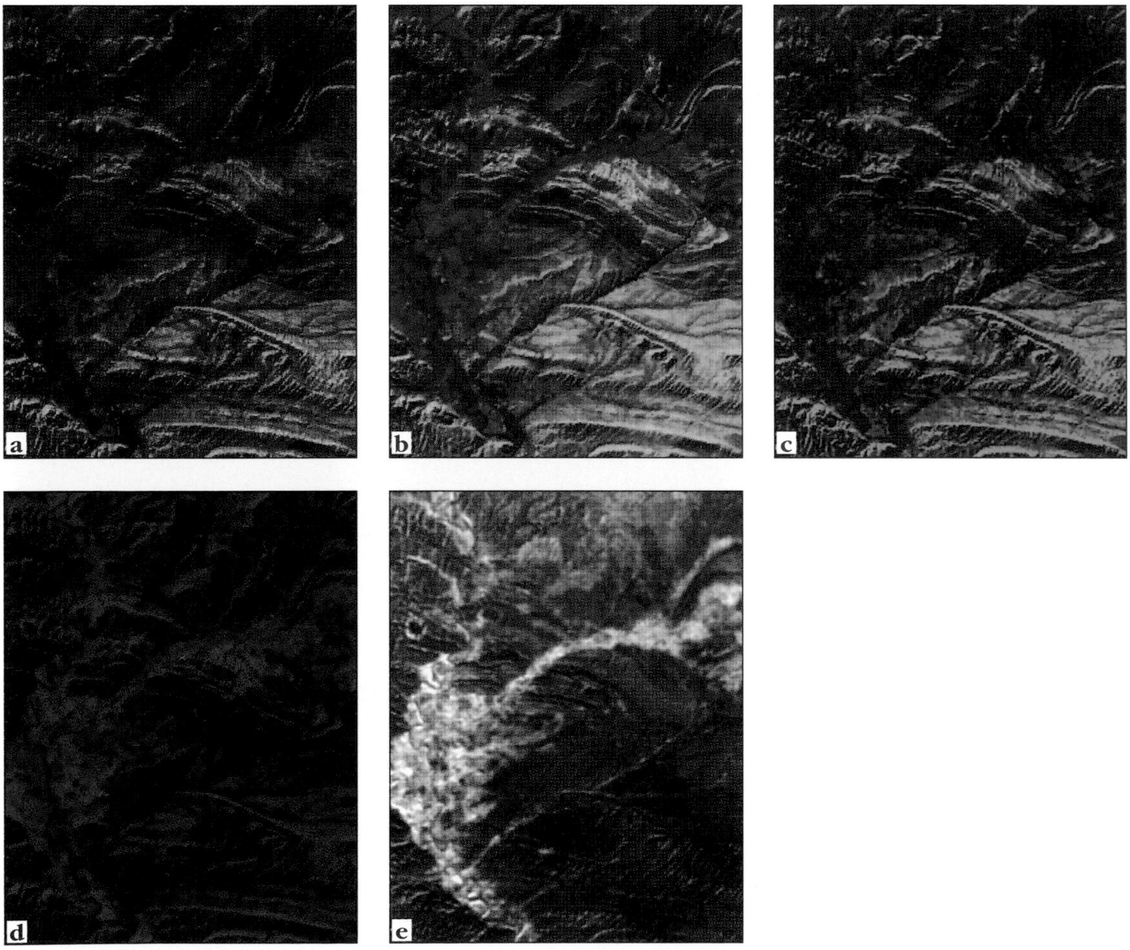

Plate 10. *Landsat Thematic Mapper images in visual and infrared color (20-km region at Thermopolis, Wyoming); (original image from F. F. Sabins (1987) Remote Sensing: Principles and Interpretation, W. H. Freeman, New York):*
a) *visible light;* ***b)*** *infrared light;* ***c)*** *result of filtering the visible image at 520 nm;*
d) *filtering the infrared image at 1100 nm;* ***e)*** *the ratio of the green (visible) to red (IR) filtered intensities.*

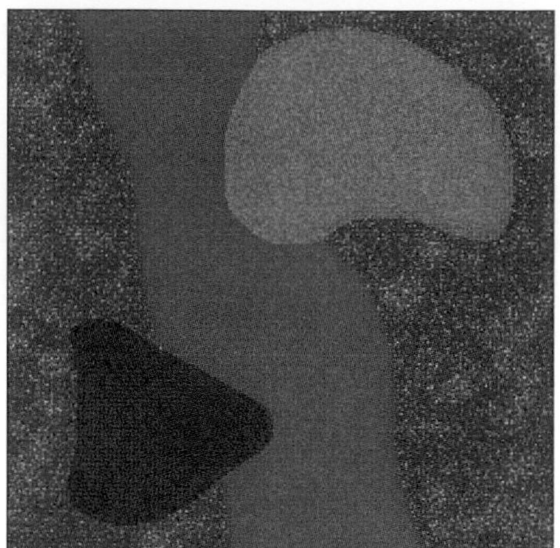

Plate 11. *Multiband coding of data from the image in Figure 24 in Chapter 5. The intensity plane shows the original image, the hue plane contains smoothed brightness values, and the saturation plane contains the texture information from a variance operator.*

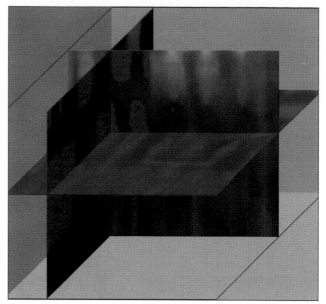

Plate 12. *Color coding of elemental intensity from SIMS images. The multiband three-dimensional data set is sectioned on x, y, and z planes, and the 256-level (8-bit) brightness scale for the elements aluminum, boron, and oxygen is assigned to red, green, and blue, respectively.*

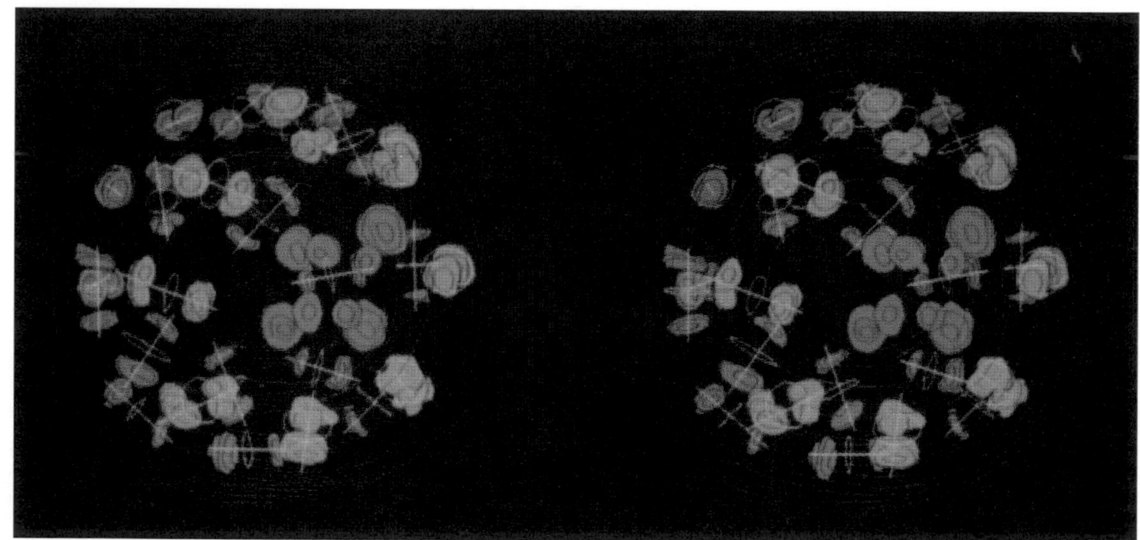

Plate 13. *Stereo view of the data set from Chapter 8, Figure 27, but surface rendered and color coded. The surface image shows contours within each section which render the surfaces of the chromosomal masses but obscure any internal detail or structures to the rear. Contour lines for the embryo are also shown. (Image courtesy of R. G. Summers, Dept. of Anatomical Sciences, State University of New York at Buffalo.)*

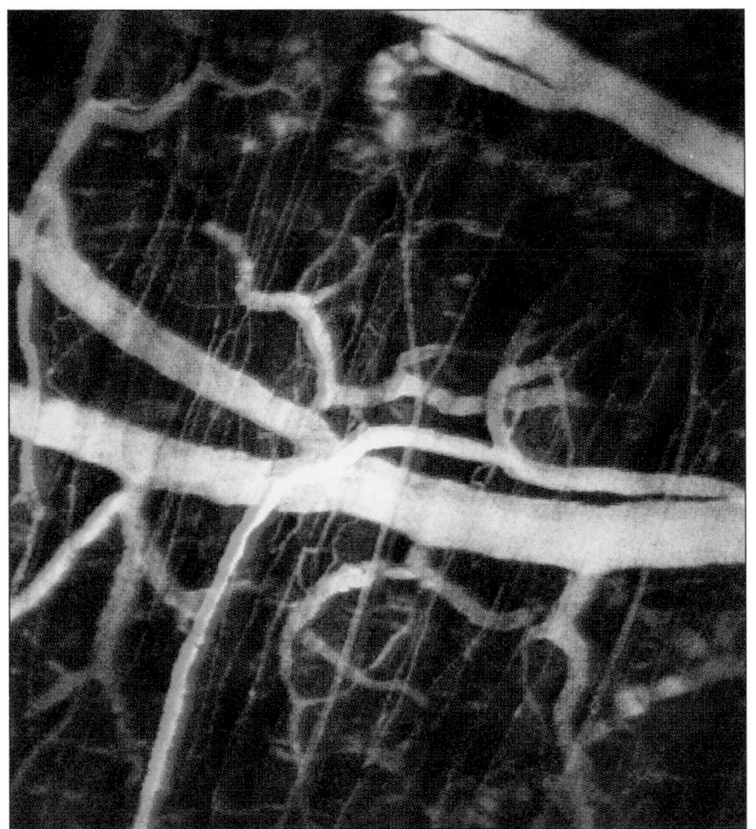

Plate 14. *Stereo pair of the same image pair shown in Chapter 8, Figure 21, using red and green for the different eye views. This allows viewing the image with normal eye vergence, using glasses (red lens on left eye, green on right).*

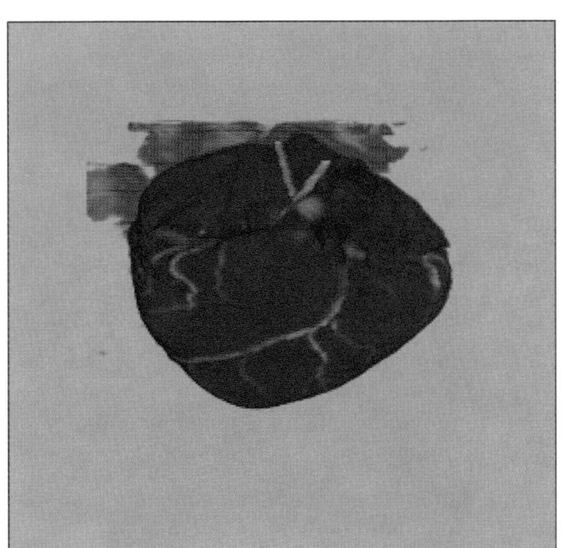

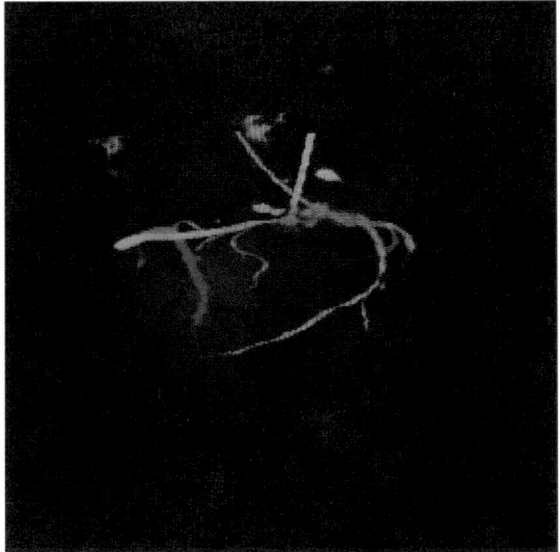

Plate 15. *Volumetric rendering of MRI data. Specimen is a hog heart (data courtesy B. Knosp, R. Frank, M. Marcus, R. Weiss, Univ. of Iowa Image Analysis Facility and Dept. of Internal Medicine). Changing the arbitrary relationship between voxel value and display opacity for the voxels allows selectively showing the heart muscle or blood vessels.*

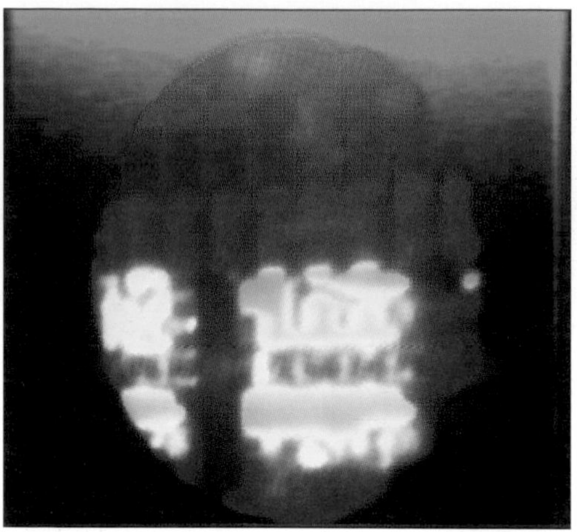

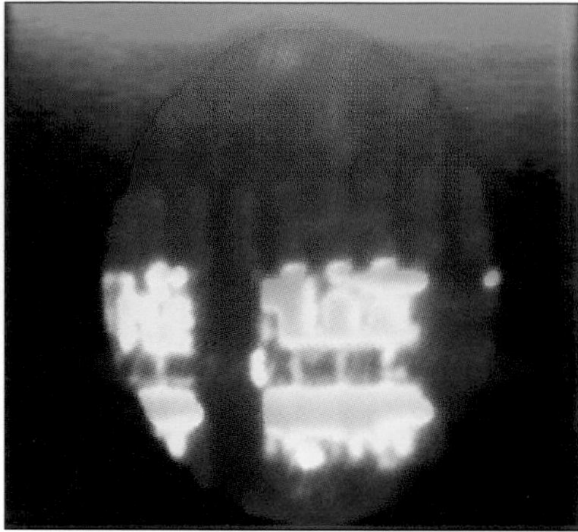

Plate 16. *Stereo pair of volumetric images from the SIMS data set. Colors assigned to the different elements are red = aluminum, green = boron, and blue = oxygen, with 256 brightness levels of each. The use of color for elemental information precludes color coding of views as in Plate 13. The density of information in this display is so great that fusing the images to see the depth is quite difficult.*

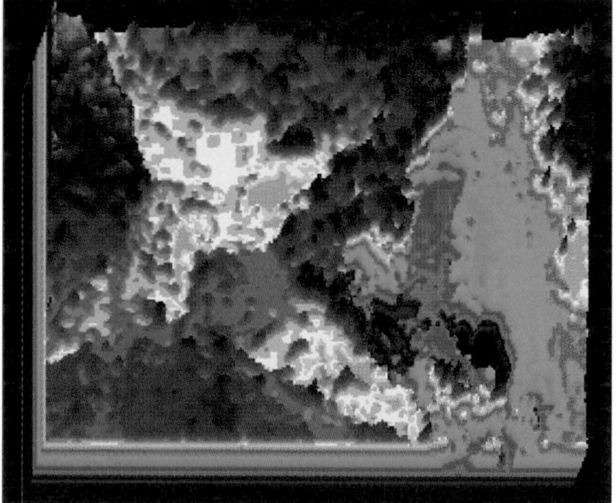

Plate 17. *Isometric view of elevation data for the alumina fracture surface shown in Chapter 2, Figures 57 and 58 and Chapter 8, Figure 24. A color palette is used to facilitate comparison.*

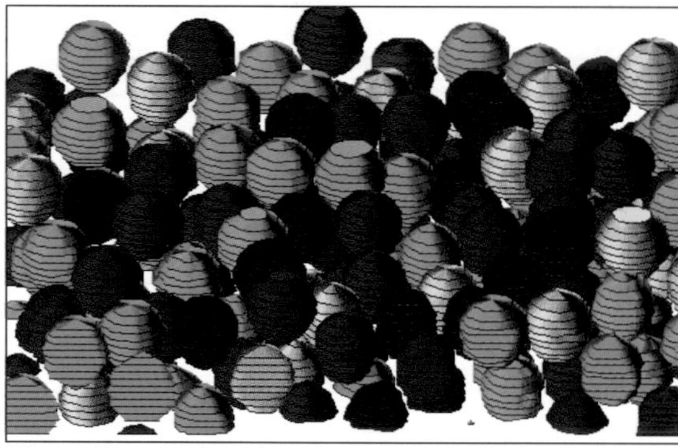

Plate 18. *Rendered surface image of spherical particles from tomographic reconstruction (Chapter 7, Figures 40 to 42) created by interpolating surface tiles between the slices shown in Chapter 8, Figure 19 and assigning arbitrary colors to each feature.*

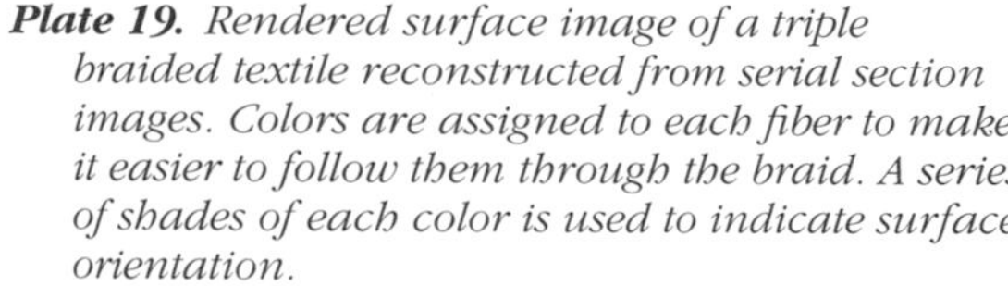

Plate 19. *Rendered surface image of a triple braided textile reconstructed from serial section images. Colors are assigned to each fiber to make it easier to follow them through the braid. A series of shades of each color is used to indicate surface orientation.*

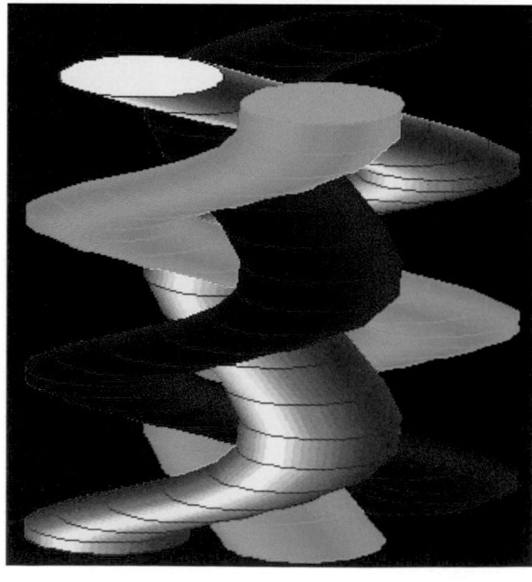

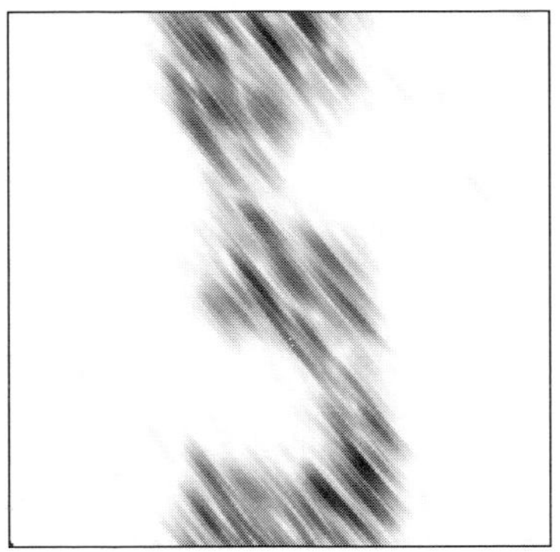
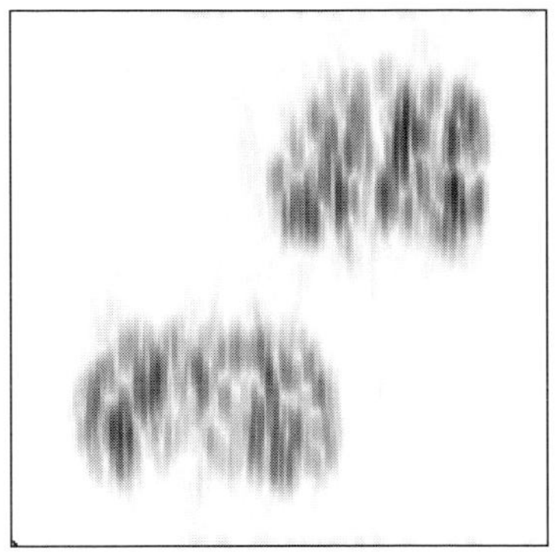
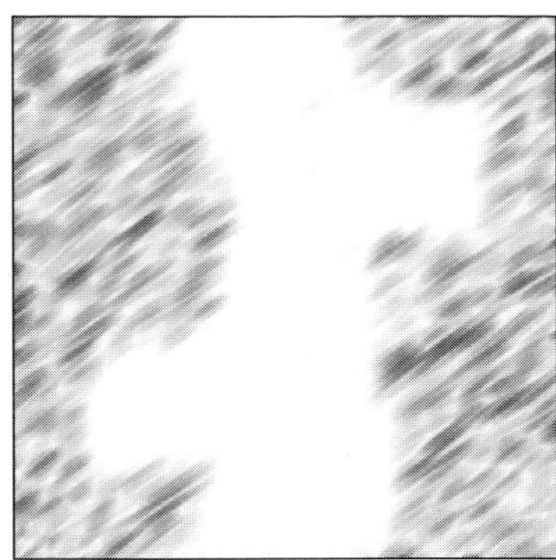

Figure 33. *Application of a range operator to the images in Figure 32b, c, and d.*

Thresholding these images and applying a closing operation (a dilation followed by an erosion, as discussed in Chapter 6) to fill in internal gaps and smooth boundaries produces images of each region. **Figure 34** shows the composite result. Notice that the edges of the image are poorly delineated, which is a consequence of the inability of the frequency transform method to preserve edge details, as discussed in Chapter 4. Also, the boundaries of the regions are rather irregular and only approximately rendered in this result.

In many cases, spatial-domain processing is preferred for texture orientation. **Figure 35** shows the result from applying a Sobel operator to the image, as discussed in Chapter 3. Two directional first derivatives in the x and y directions are obtained using a 3×3 neighborhood operator. These are then combined using the arc tangent function to obtain an angle that is the direction of maximum brightness gradient. The resulting angle is scaled to fit the 0 to 255 brightness range of the image.

The brightness histogram shown in **Figure 35** shows six peaks. These occur in pairs 180 degrees apart, since in each texture region the direction of maximum gradient may lie in either of two opposite directions. This image can be reduced to three directions in several ways. One is to use a grey scale LUT, as discussed in Chapter 3, which assigns the same grey scale values to

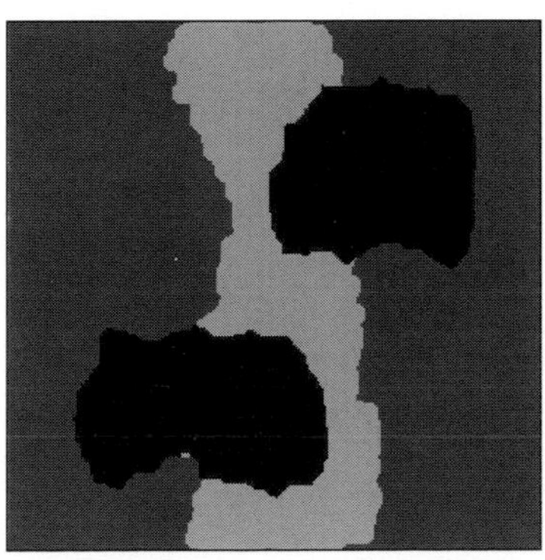

Figure 34. *Regions from Figure 31 selected by thresholding the images in Figure 33.*

Figure 35. Application of the Sobel operator to the image in Figure 31, calculating the orientation of the gradient at each pixel by assigning a grey level to the arc tangent of $(\partial B/\partial y)/(\partial B/\partial x)$. The brightness histogram shows six peaks, in pairs for each principal textural orientation, since the directions are complementary.

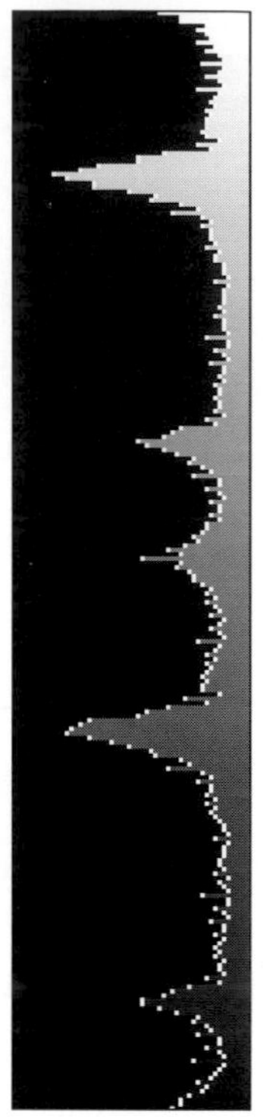

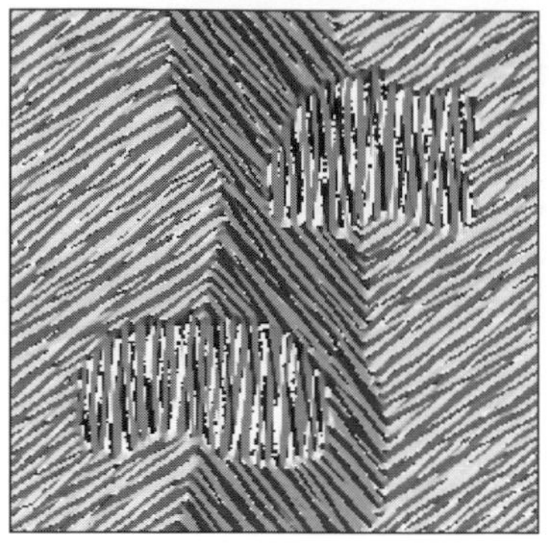

the highest and lowest halves of the original brightness (or angle) range, followed by thresholding the single peak for each direction. A second method is to set two different threshold ranges on the paired peaks and then combine the two resulting binary images using a Boolean OR operation (see Chapter 6). A third approach is to set a multiple-threshold range on the two complementary peaks. All of these are functionally equivalent.

Figure 36 shows the results of three thresholding operations to select each of the three textural orientations. There is some noise in these images, consisting of white pixels within the dark re-

Figure 36. Thresholded binary images from Figure 35, selecting the grey values corresponding to each pair of complementary directions (or performing two separate thresholds and ORing the results).

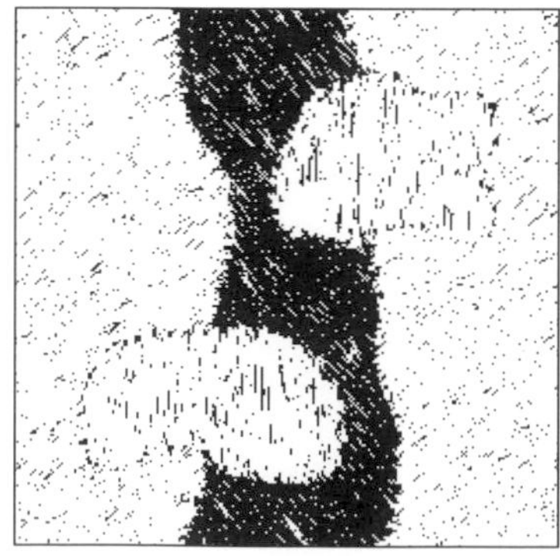

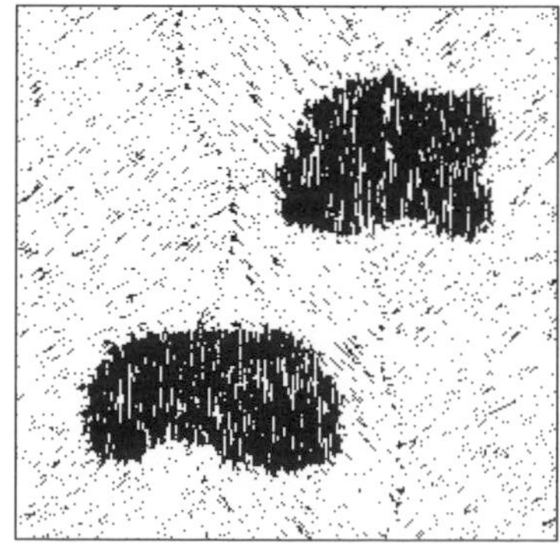

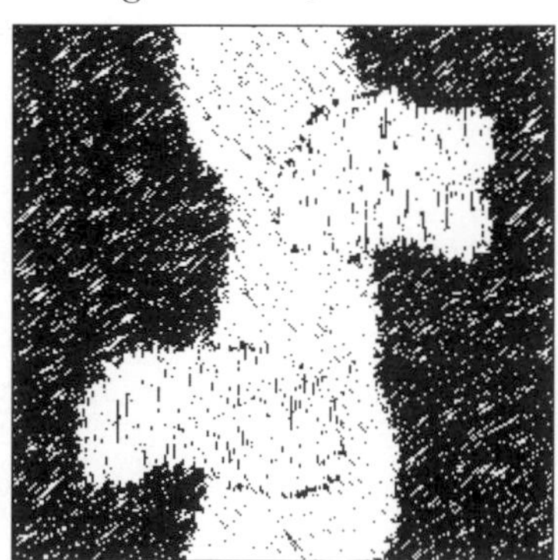

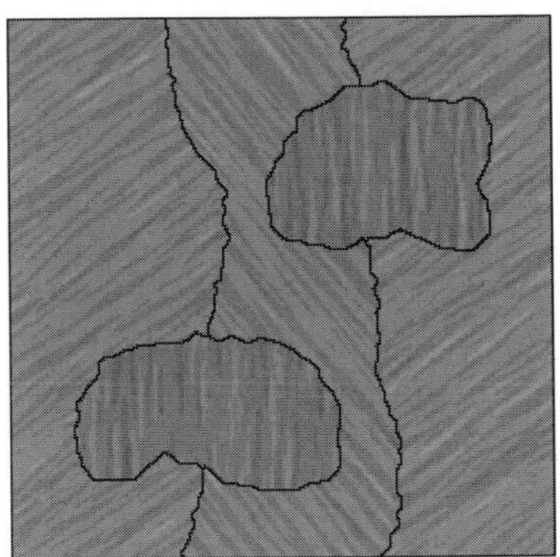

Figure 37. Outlines showing the regions defined by applying a closing (dilation and erosion) operation to each of the images in Figure 36.

gions and vice versa, but these are much fewer and smaller than in the case of thresholding the results from the frequency-transform method shown above. After applying a closing operation (a dilation followed by an erosion, as discussed in Chapter 6), the regions are well delineated, as shown by the superimposition of the outlines on the original image **(Figure 37).** This result is superior to the frequency transform and has smoother boundaries, better agreement with the visual judgement of location, and no problems at the image edges.

A more concrete example of the use of texture is shown in **Figure 38.** This is an image of bone marrow from the light microscope with a second image of the same area produced by applying a variance operator, as discussed in Chapter 3. This responds to the local texture in the image, rather than absolute brightness. **Figure 39** shows the individual histograms of the two images and the two-dimensional histogram of pixel values in both images.

Simple thresholding on the bright pixels in the original image does not select the large white areas, because the small spaces between the dark cells are equally bright **(Figure 40).** However, these regions are also low in texture (relatively smooth in appearance, with little local change in brightness).

Thresholding on the texture image and combining that result with the binary image from **Figure 40** produces a better repre-

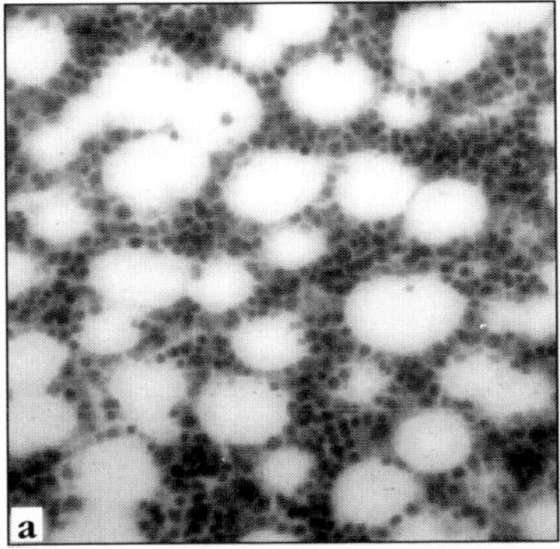

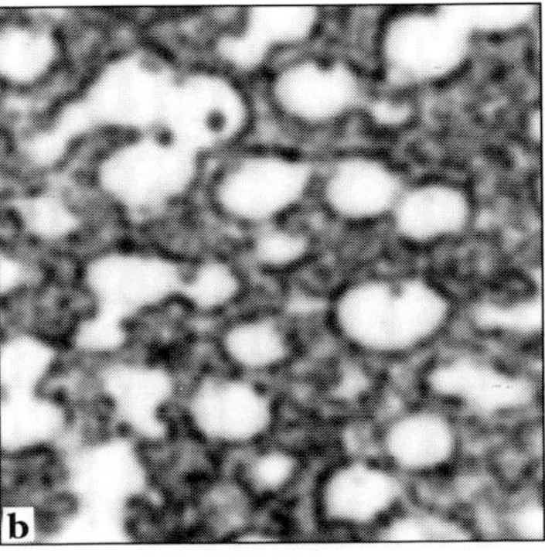

Figure 38. Light microscope image of bone marrow (a) and the result of applying a variance operator to characterize the texture in the image (b).

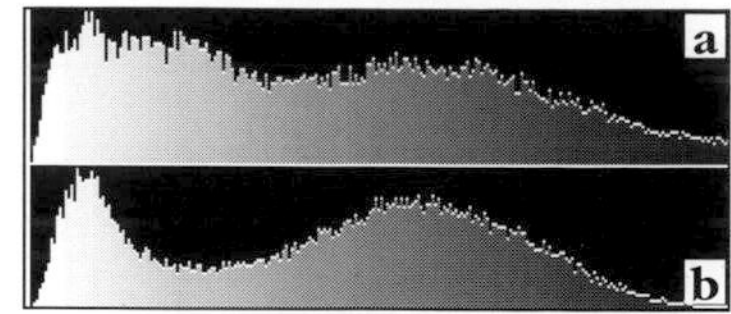

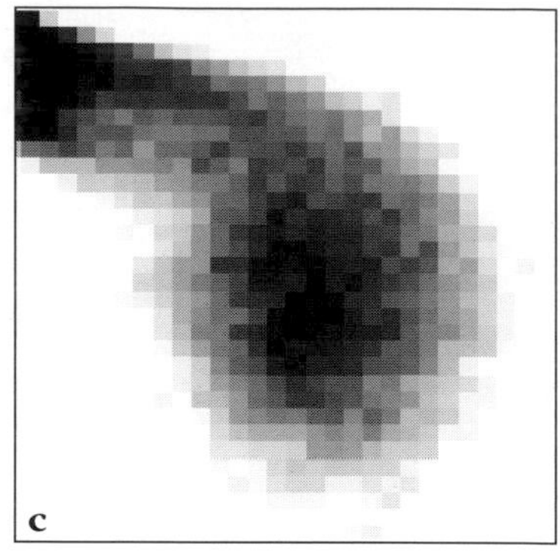

Figure 39. *Brightness histograms (a and b) for the images in Figure 38, and the two-dimensional histogram showing the frequency of pairs of values of brightness (vertical) and texture (horizontal) for pixels at the same location in both images (c).*

sentation, as shown in **Figure 41a.** This is equivalent to selecting pixels whose brightness and texture values fall within a rectangle in the texture/brightness histogram. Selecting a non-rectangular region in that plane produces an improved result, as shown in **Figure 41b.** Additional examples of thresholding a derived texture image to produce a binary image are shown in Chapter 3.

Accuracy and reproducibility

In one or more dimensions, the selection of threshold values discussed so far has been manual. An operator interactively sets the cutoff values so that the resulting image is visually satisfying and the correspondence between what the user sees in the image and the pixels the thresholds select is as close as possible. This is not always consistent from one operator to another, or even for the same person over a period of time. The difficulty and variability of thresholding represents a serious source of error for further image analysis.

There are two slightly different requirements for setting threshold values. Both have to do with the typical use of binary images for feature measurement. One is to achieve reproducibility, so that variations due to the operator, lighting, etc. do not affect the results. The second goal of setting threshold values is to achieve accurate boundary delineation. For quality-control work, as one

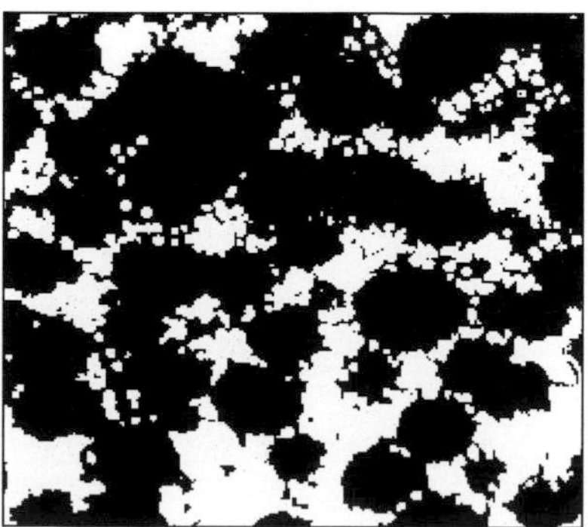

Figure 40. *Binary image produced by thresholding Figure 38a to select white areas.*

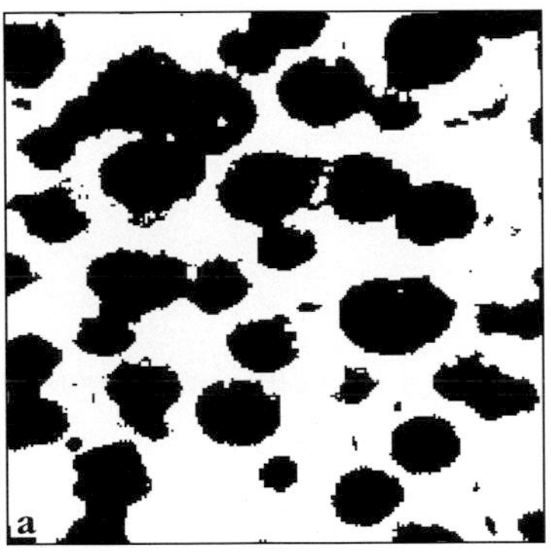

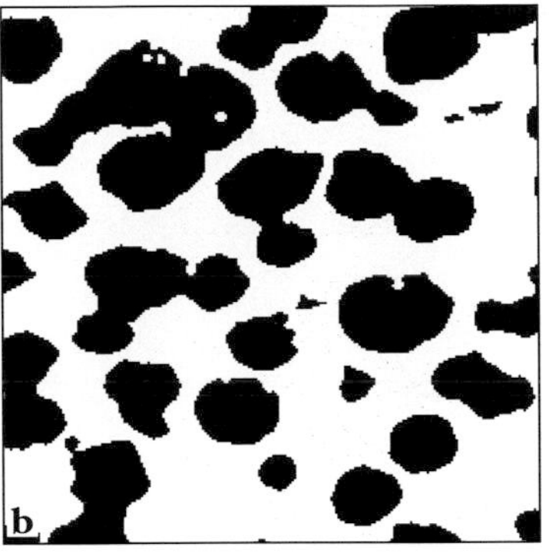

Figure 41. Two-dimensional thresholding to select regions in Figure 38:
a) *ANDing together binary images selected by thresholding the two images individually;*
b) *using a non-rectangular threshold region directly on the two-dimensional histogram.*

example, this latter requirement of accuracy is somewhat less important than precision.

Since pixel-based images represent at best an approximation to the continuous real scene being represented, and since thresholding classifies each pixel as either part of the foreground or the background, there is only a certain level of accuracy that can be achieved. An alternate representation of features based on the boundary line can be more accurate. This is a polygon with many sides and corner points defined as x,y coordinates of arbitrary accuracy, as compared to the comparatively coarse pixel spacing.

The boundary-line representation is superior for accurate measurement because the line itself has no width. However, determining the line is far from easy. The location of individual points can be determined by interpolation between pixels, perhaps fitting mathematical functions to pixels on either side of the boundary to improve the results. This type of approach is commonly used in metrology applications, such as measuring dimensions of microelectronic circuit elements on silicon wafers. This type of application goes beyond the typical image processing operations dealt with in this text.

Thresholding produces a pixel-based representation of the image, which assigns each pixel to either the feature(s) or the surroundings. The finite size of the pixels allows the representation only a finite accuracy, but we would prefer to have no bias in the result. This means that performing the same operation on many repeated images of the same scene should produce an average result that approaches the true value for size or other feature measurements. This is not necessary for quality-control applications in which reproducibility is of greater concern than accuracy, and some bias (as long as it is consistent) can be tolerated.

Many things can contribute to bias in setting thresholds. Human operators are not very good at setting threshold levels without bias. In most cases, they are more tolerant of settings that include additional pixels from the background region along with the features than they are of settings that exclude some pixels

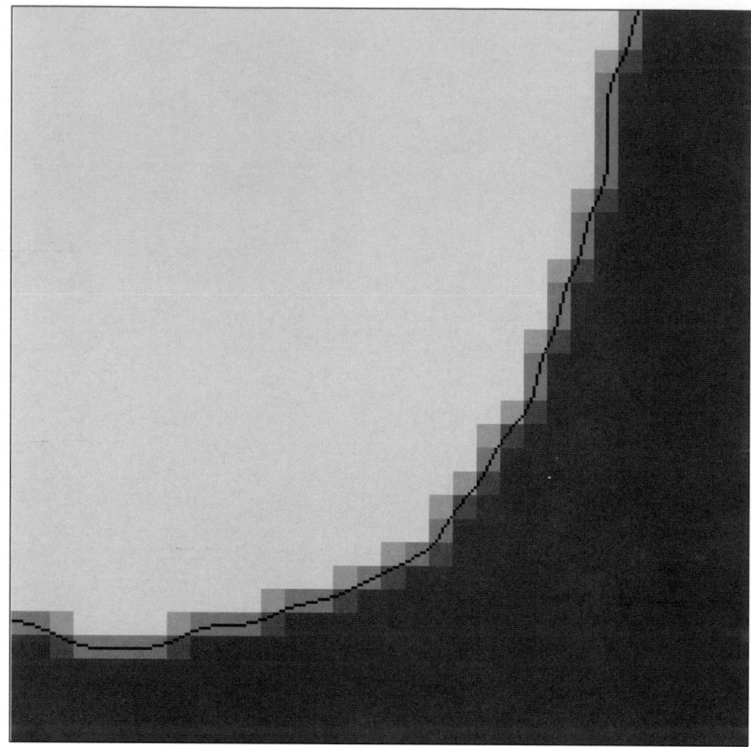

Figure 42. *Example of finite pixels straddling a boundary line, with brightness values that average those of the two sampled regions.*

from the features. They are also not particularly consistent at choosing a brightness value for the threshold that is midway between two levels characteristic of feature and background. This is particularly true if the brightness scale is not logarithmic, either because of the detector or camera response, or prior image processing.

As indicated at the beginning of this chapter, the brightness histogram from the image is an important tool for setting threshold levels. In many cases, it will show distinct and separated peaks from the various phases or structures present in the field of view, or it can be made to do so by prior image processing steps. In this case, it seems that setting the threshold level midway between the peaks should produce consistent, and perhaps even accurate, results.

Unfortunately, this idea is easier to state than to accomplish. In many real images, the peaks corresponding to particular structures are not perfectly symmetrical or ideally sharp, particularly when there may be shading either of the entire image or within the features (e.g., a brightness gradient from center to edge). Changing the field of view or even the illumination may cause the peak to shift and/or to change shape. Nonlinear camera response or automatic gain circuits can further distort the brightness histogram. If the area fraction of the image that is the bright (or dark) phase changes from one field of view to another, some

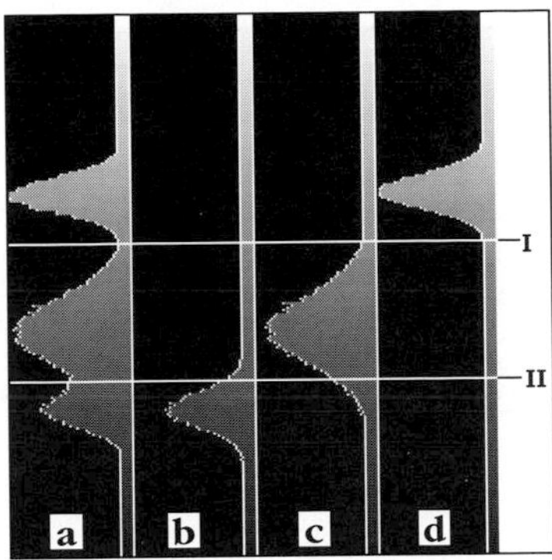

Figure 43. *An example histogram from a specimen with three distinct regions. The minimum at level I cleanly separates the two peaks, while the one at level II does not because the brightness values in the two regions have variations that overlap.*

method is needed to maintain a threshold setting that adapts to these changes and preserves precision and accuracy.

If the peaks are consistent and well-defined, then choosing an arbitrary location at some fixed fraction of the distance between them is a rapid method often satisfactory for quality-control work. In many cases, it is necessary to consider the pixels whose brightness values lie between the peaks in the brightness histogram. In most instances, these are pixels that straddle the boundary and have averaged together the two principal brightness levels in proportion to the area subtended within the pixel, as indicated in **Figure 42.**

Asymmetric boundaries (for example, a metallographic specimen in which etching has attacked the softer of two phases so that the boundary is skewed) can introduce bias in these brightness values. So can prior processing steps, such as those responding to texture in the image. Many of these operations work on a finite and perhaps rather large neighborhood, so the boundary position becomes somewhat uncertain. If the processing operation responds nonlinearly to differences, as the variance operator does, the apparent boundary location will shift toward the most different pixel in the neighborhood.

Including position information

The histogram display shows only the frequency of occurrence of different values and does not preserve any information about position, the brightness of neighboring pixels, etc. Yet it is this spatial information that is important for determining boundary location. It is possible, in principle, to build a co-occurrence matrix for the image, in which all possible combinations of pixel brightness are counted in terms of the distance between them. This information is used to select the pixels that are part of the feature instead of simply the pixel brightness values, but this is equivalent to a processing operation that uses the same co-occurrence matrix to construct a texture image for which simple thresholding can be used.

Another possible algorithm for threshold settings is to pick the minimum point in the histogram **(Figure 43).** This should cor-

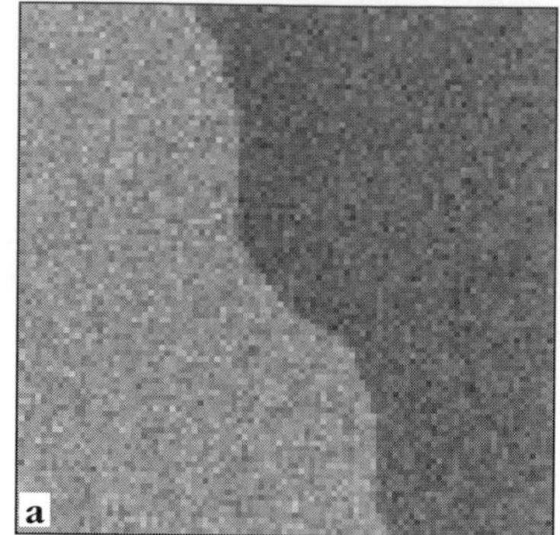

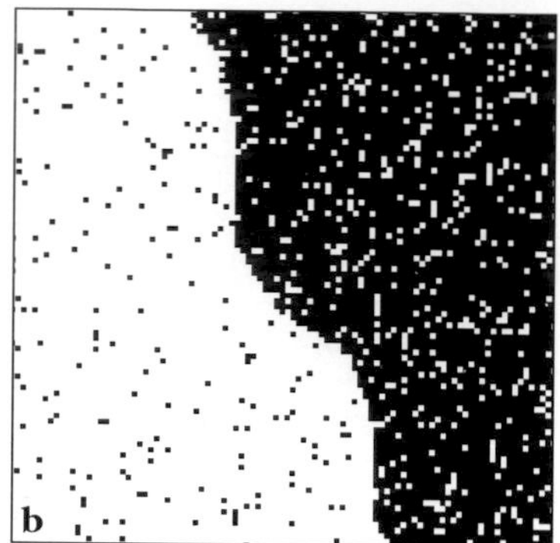

Figure 44. A test image containing two regions whose mean brightness levels are different, but which have variations in individual pixels that overlap:

a) *original image (enlarged to show pixels);*

b) *result of setting a simple threshold at the minimum point.*

respond to the value that affects the fewest pixels and thus gives the lowest expected error in pixel classification when the image is segmented into features and background. The difficulty is that because this region of the histogram is (hopefully) very low, with few pixels having these values, the counting statistics are poor and the shape of the curve in the histogram is poorly defined. Consequently, the minimum value is hard to locate and may move about considerably with only tiny changes in overall illumination, a change in the field of view to include objects with a different shape, or more or fewer pixels along the boundary.

Figure 44 shows an image having two visibly obvious regions. Each contains a Gaussian noise pattern with the same standard deviation but a different mean, though the brightness values in

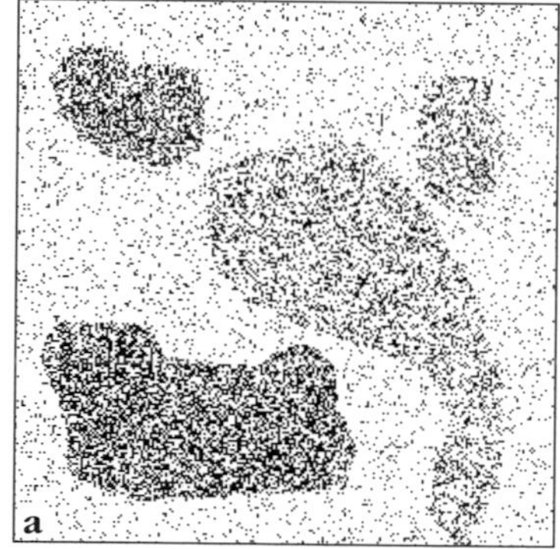

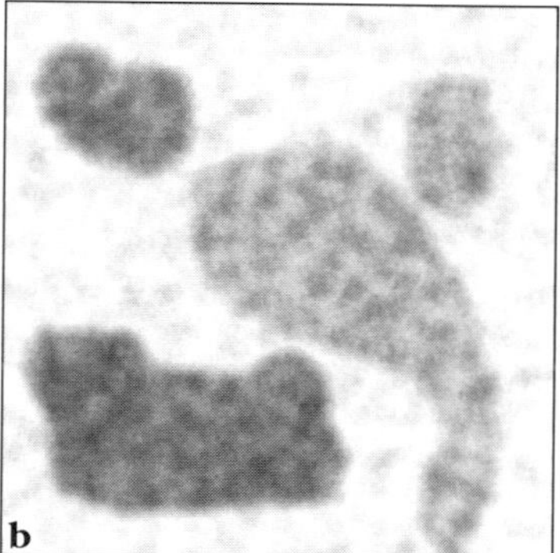

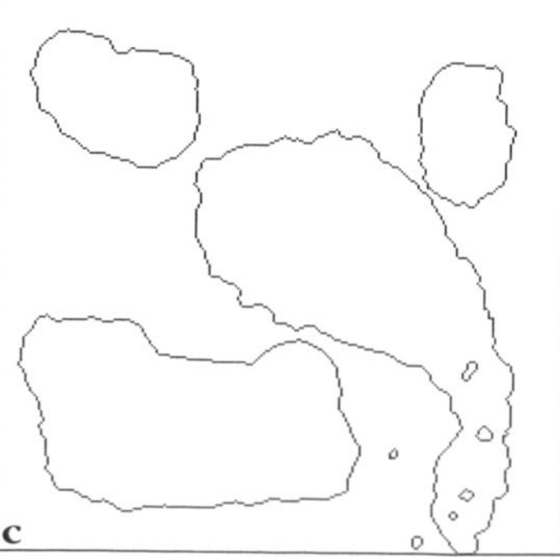

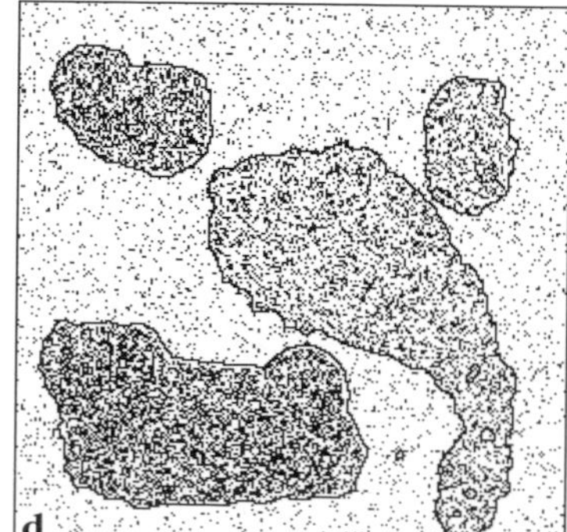

Figure 45. Thresholding sparse or noisy images may require processing first:

a) *a sparse X-ray dot map;*

b) *a grey scale image formed by counting the dots within a 15-pixel-diameter circle around each pixel;*

c) *boundary determined by thresholding image (b);*

d) *superposition of the boundary from (c) on the original.*

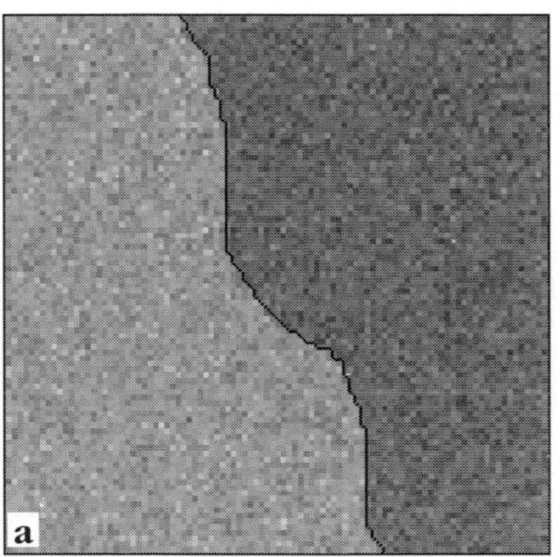

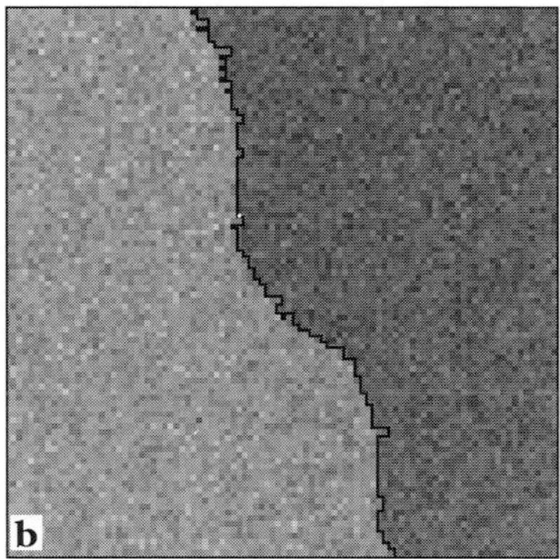

Figure 46. The boundary in the image of Figure 44:
a) *thresholding at the minimum point in the histogram followed by closing (dilation and erosion);*
b) *iteratively setting the minimum entropy point.*

the two regions overlap. This means that setting a threshold value at the minimum between the two peaks causes some pixels in each region to be misclassified, as shown in the figure.

This type of image often results from situations in which the total number of photons or other signals is low and counting statistics cause a variation in the brightness of pixels in uniform areas. Counting statistics produces a Poisson distribution, but when moderately large numbers are involved, this is very close to the more convenient Gaussian function used in these images. For extremely noisy images, such as X-ray dot maps from the SEM, some additional processing in the spatial domain may be required before attempting thresholding (O'Callaghan, 1974).

Figure 45 shows a typical sparse dot map. Most of the pixels contain 0 counts, and a few contain 1 count. The boundaries in the image are visually evident, but their exact location is at best approximate, requiring the human visual computer to group the dots together. Imaging processing can do this by counting the number of dots in a circular neighborhood around each pixel. Convolution with a kernel consisting of 1's in a 15-pixel-diameter circle accomplishes this, producing the result shown. This grey scale image can be thresholded to locate the boundaries shown, but there is inadequate data to decide whether the small regions, voids, and irregularities in the boundaries are real or simply due to the limited counting statistics.

Several possible approaches may be used to improve the segmentation of noisy regions, using **Figure 44** as a test case. Chapter 6 discusses binary image editing operations, including morphological processing. The sequence of a dilation followed by an erosion, known as a closing, fills holes, erases isolated pixels, and smooths the boundary line to produce the result shown in **Figure 46a.** By contrast, a much more complicated operation reassigns pixels from one region to the other to achieve minimum entropy in each of the two regions. Entropy methods are generally a very computer-intensive approach to image restoration when a blur function is known. They function to improve degraded grey scale images, as discussed in Chapter 2.

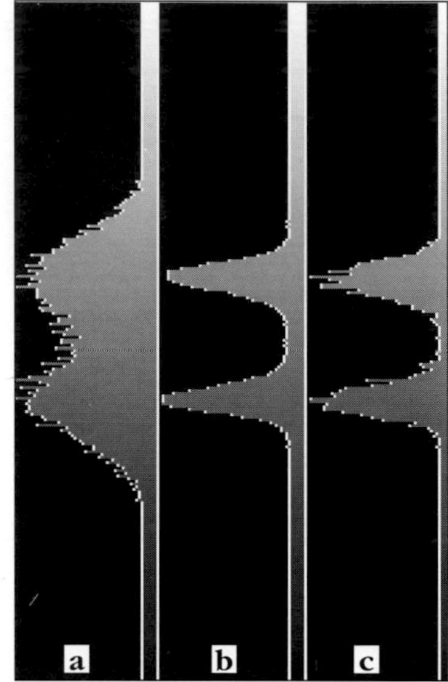

Figure 47. Histogram of the image in Figure 44:
a) *original, with overlapped peaks;*
b) *after smoothing;*
c) *after median filtering.*

In this case, the collection of pixels into two regions can be described as an entropy problem as follows (Kanpur et al., 1985): The total entropy in each region is calculated as $-\Sigma p_i \log_e p_i$, where p_i is the number of pixels having brightness i. Solving for the boundary, which classifies each pixel into one of two groups to minimize this function for the two regions (subject to the constraint that the pixels in each region must touch each other), produces the boundary line shown in **Figure 46b.** Additional constraints, such as minimizing the number of touching pixels in different classes, would smooth the boundary. The problem is that such constraints are ad hoc, make the solution of the problem very difficult, and can usually be applied more efficiently in other ways (for instance by smoothing the binary image).

Setting a threshold value at the minimum in the histogram is sometimes described as selecting for minimum area sensitivity in the value (Weszka, 1978; Wall et al., 1974). This means that changing the threshold value causes the least change in the feature (or background) area, although as noted above this says nothing about the spatial arrangement of the pixels that are thereby added to or removed from the features. Indeed, the definition of the histogram makes any minimum in the plot a point of minimum area sensitivity.

For the image shown in **Figure 44,** the histogram can be changed to produce a minimum that is deeper, broader, and has a more stable minimum value by processing the image. **Figure 47** shows the results of smoothing the image (using a Gaussian kernel with a standard deviation of 1 pixel) or applying a median filter (both methods are discussed in Chapters 2 and 3). The peaks are narrower and the valley is broader and deeper. The consequences for the image and the boundary, which is selected

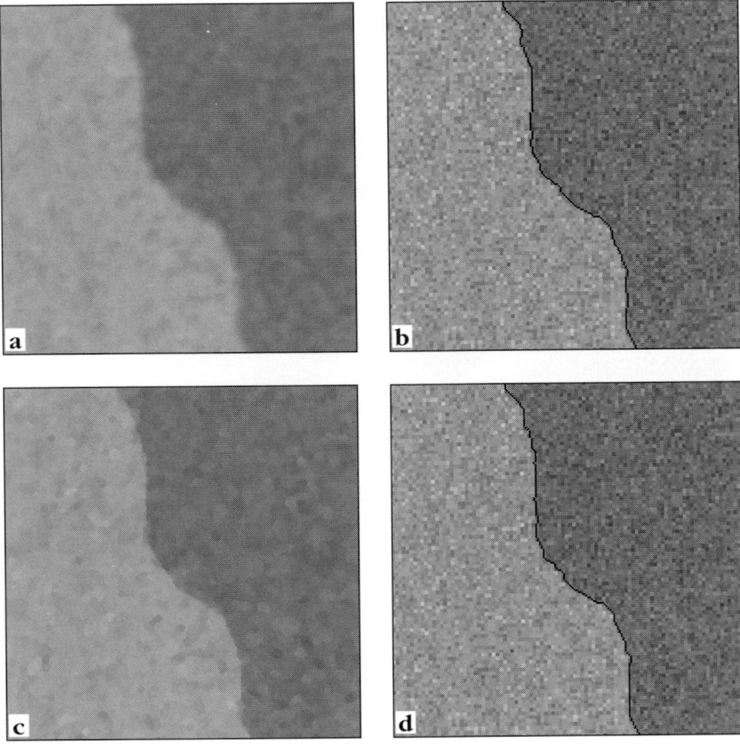

Figure 48. Processing the image in Figure 44 to modify the histogram:
a) *smoothing with a Guassian kernel, standard deviation = 1 pixel;*
b) *the boundary produced by thresholding image a, superimposed on the original;*
c) *median processing (iteratively applied until no further changes occurred);*
d) *the boundary produced by thresholding image c, superimposed on the original.*

by setting the threshold level between the peaks, are shown in **Figure 48.**

This seems not to be the criterion used by human operators, who can watch an image and interactively adjust a threshold value. Instead of the total area of features changing least with adjustment, which is difficult for humans to judge, we can instead use the total change in perimeter length around the features (Russ & Russ, 1988a). This may in fact be the criterion actually used by skilled operators. The variation in total perimeter length with respect to threshold value provides an objective criterion that can be efficiently calculated. The minimum in this response curve provides a way to set the thresholds that is reproducible, adapts to varying illumination, etc., and mimics to some extent the way humans set the values. For the case in which both upper and lower threshold levels are to be adjusted, this produces a response surface in two dimensions (the upper and lower values), which can be solved to find the minimum point as indicated in **Figure 49.**

Figure 49 shows an image whose brightness threshold has been automatically refined to minimize the variation in total boundary length. The brightness histogram shown in the figure has a very long valley between the two phase peaks, neither of which has a symmetric or Gaussian shape. The lowest point in the histogram does not necessarily correspond to the best threshold setting.

Figure 49. A two-way plot of the change in perimeter length vs. the settings of upper and lower level brightness thresholds. The minimum indicates the optimal settings.

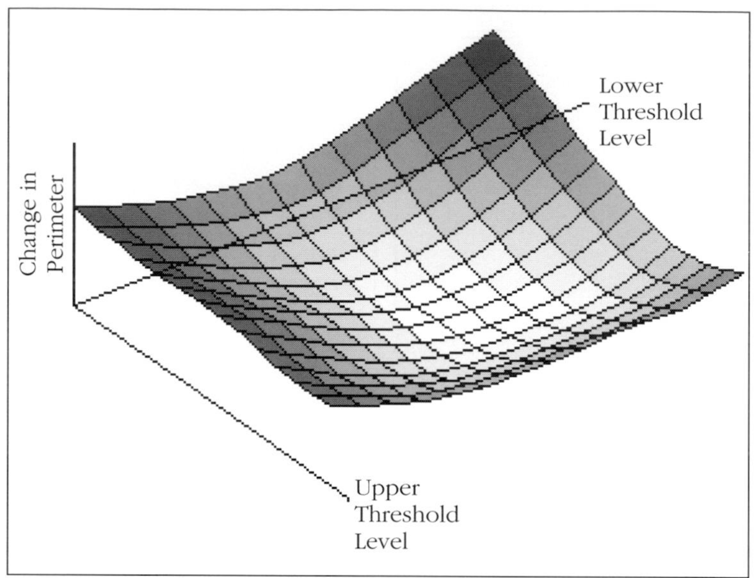

Figure 51 shows several plots derived from the histogram and image of **Figure 50.** Graphs plotting the area of the dark phase vs. the threshold setting and the total boundary perimeter vs. the threshold setting are not helpful in finding an optimum or stable setting, but the derivatives of these curves are. The minimum point in the plot of change of area vs. setting occurs at a bright-

Figure 50. A test image for automatic threshold adjustment, and its brightness histogram. The range from brightness values 100 through 165 is used in the plots of Figure 51.

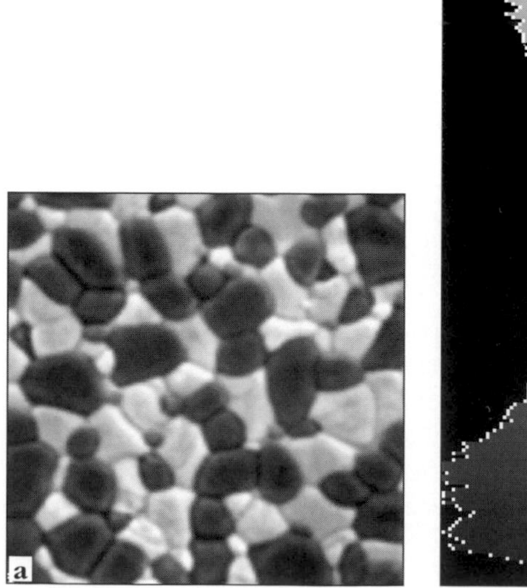

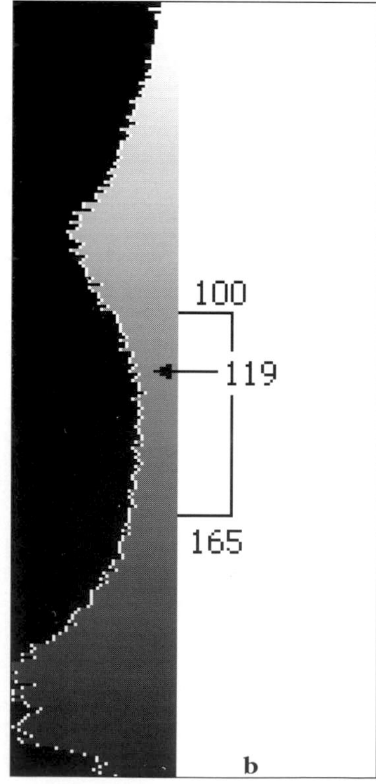

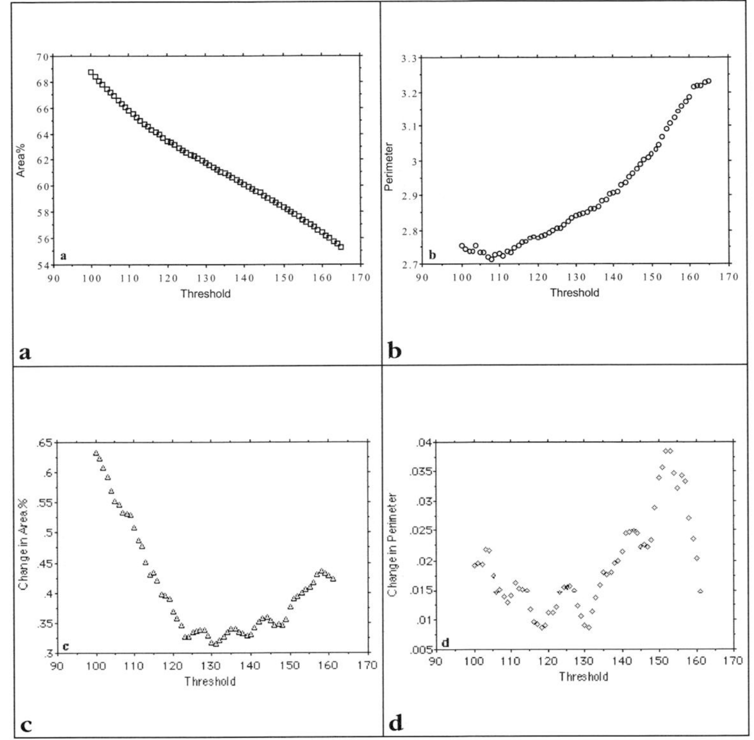

Figure 51. Plots of
a) *total area of the dark phase;*
b) *total boundary perimeter;*
c) *change in area; and*
d) *change in perimeter, for threshold settings from 100 to 165 on the image of Figure 50.*

ness value of 131. The two minima in the plot of change of perimeter vs. setting occur at 119 and 131. The two binary images produced by thresholding at these levels are shown in **Figure 52.** The 119 value appears to produce good representation of the phase boundaries, as shown in **Figure 53.**

Repeated measurements using this algorithm on many images of the same objects show that the reproducibility in the presence of finite image noise and changing illumination is rather good. Length variations for irregular objects varied less than 0.5%, or 1 pixel in 200 across the major diameter of the object.

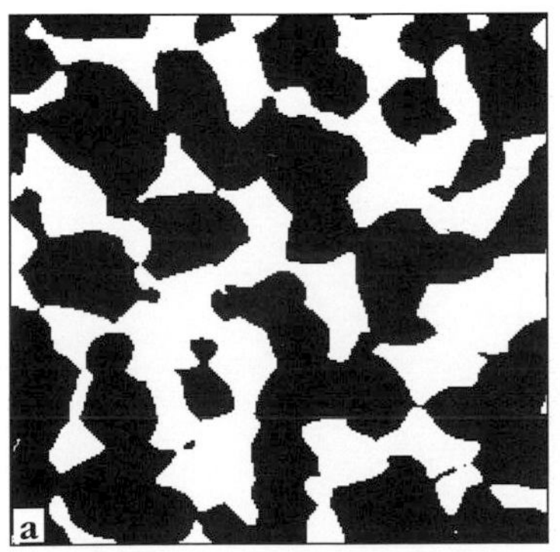

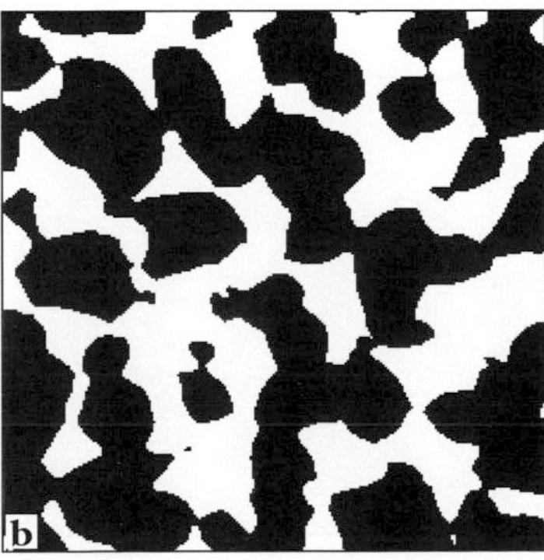

Figure 52. Binary images produced from Figure 50 by the application of thresholds at brightness levels of
a) *119 and*
b) *131, which are the minima in the plot of Figure 51d.*

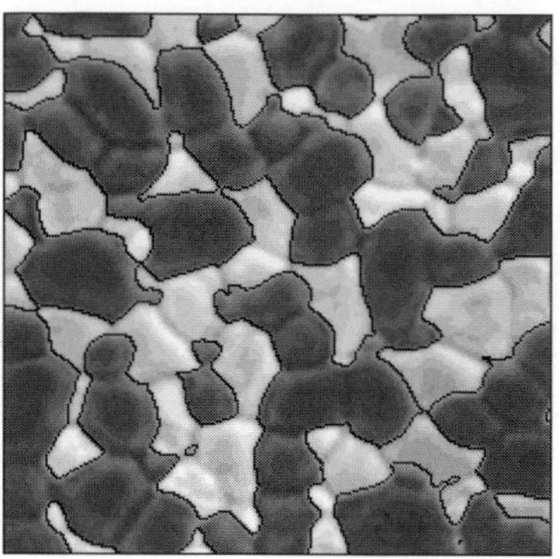

Figure 53. *Superposition of the boundary selected with a threshold setting of 119 (minimum perimeter sensitivity) on the original image from Figure 50.*

Selective histograms

Most of the difficulties with selecting the optimum threshold brightness value between two peaks in a typical histogram arise from the intermediate brightness values of the histogram. These pixels lie along the boundaries of the two regions, so methods that eliminate them from the histogram will contain only peaks from the uniform regions and can be used to select the proper threshold value (Weszka & Rosenfeld, 1979; Milgram & Herman, 1979).

One way to perform this selection is to use another derived image, such as the Sobel gradient or any of the other edge-finding operators discussed in Chapter 3. Pixels having a high gradient value can be eliminated from the histogram of the original image to reduce the background level in the range between the two phase peaks. **Figure 54** shows an example. The original image contains three phases with visually distinct grey levels.

Several methods can be used to eliminate edge pixels. A two-dimensional histogram of the original and gradient images is not a good choice here, because the coarser bins may distort the peak shape and reduce resolution in the histogram. Instead, it is more straightforward to threshold the gradient image, selecting pixels with a high value. This produces a binary image that can be used as a mask, as discussed in Chapter 6. This mask either restricts which pixels in the original image are to be used or replaces

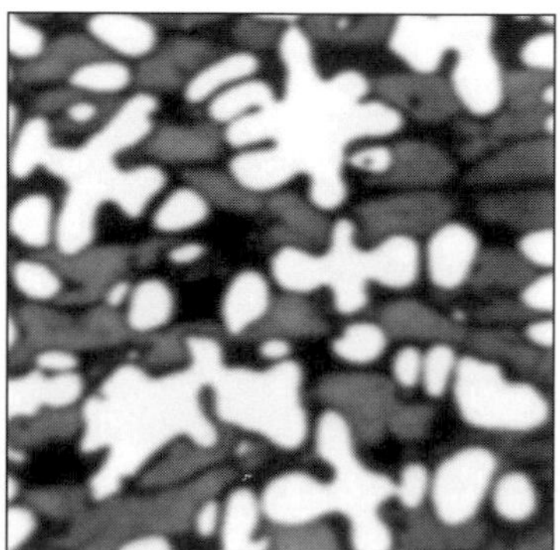

Figure 54. *A test image containing three visually distinct phase regions with different mean grey levels.*

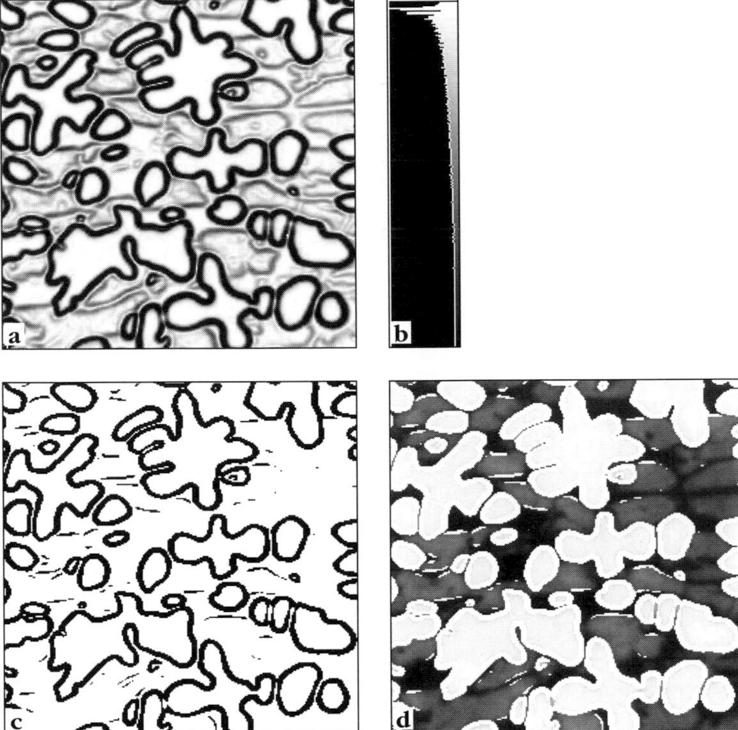

Figure 55. *Application of a gradient operator (Sobel) to the image of Figure 54 (a). The histogram (b) of the gradient does not show any useful structure. Thresholding image a to select the 20% of the pixels with the largest gradient (c) produces a mask which can be used to eliminate many of the edge-straddling pixels in the original image (d).*

their brightness values with black or white so that they are effectively removed from the portion of the histogram to be analyzed.

As an example, using the image from **Figure 54,** the 20% of the pixels with the largest magnitude in the Sobel gradient image are selected by thresholding to produce a mask, which is used to remove those pixels from the original image **(Figure 55).** The result, shown in **Figure 56,** is the reduction of those portions of the histogram between peaks, with the peaks themselves little affected. This makes it easier to characterize the shapes of the peaks from the phases and select a consistent point between them.

Of course, this requires setting a threshold on the gradient image to select the pixels to be bypassed. As shown in the example of **Figure 55,** this histogram rarely contains a peak, since the gradient magnitudes in the image vary widely. The most often used technique is simply to choose some fixed percentage of the pixels with the highest gradient value and eliminate them from the histogram of the original image.

In this case, however, the gradient operator responds more strongly to the larger difference between the white and grey regions than to the smaller difference between the grey and dark regions. Hence the edge-straddling pixels (and their background in the histogram) are reduced much more between the white and grey peaks than between the grey and black peaks. **Figure 57**

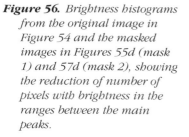

Figure 56. *Brightness histograms from the original image in Figure 54 and the masked images in Figures 55d (mask 1) and 57d (mask 2), showing the reduction of number of pixels with brightness in the ranges between the main peaks.*

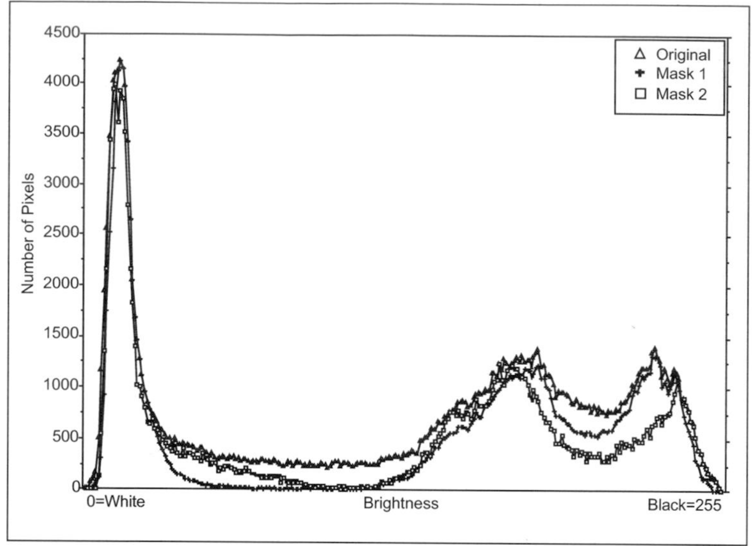

shows another method which alleviates the problem in this image. Beginning with a range image (the difference between the darkest and brightest pixels in a 5-pixel-wide octagonal neighborhood), non-maximum suppression (also known as grey scale skeletonization, or ridge-finding) is used to narrow the boundaries and eliminate pixels that are not actually on the boundary. Then thresholding is used to select the darkest 20% of the remaining pixels to form a mask, which is applied to the original image.

The plot of the resulting histogram, also in **Figure 56,** shows a much greater suppression of the valley between the grey and black peaks. Since the same total fraction of pixels has been removed, this also affects the background near the white peak. All of these methods are somewhat ad hoc; the particular combination of different region brightnesses present in an image will dictate what edge-finding operation will work best and what fraction of the pixels should be removed.

Boundary lines

One of the shortcomings of thresholding is that the pixels are selected mainly by brightness, and only secondarily by location. This means that there is no requirement for regions to be continuous. Instead of defining a region as a collection of pixels whose brightness values are similar in one or more images, an alternate definition can be based on a boundary.

Manually outlining regions for measurement is one way to use this approach. Various interactive pointing devices, such as graphics tablets, touch screens, mice, light pens, etc., may be used and the drawing may take place while the viewer looks at the computer screen, at a photographic print on a tablet, or

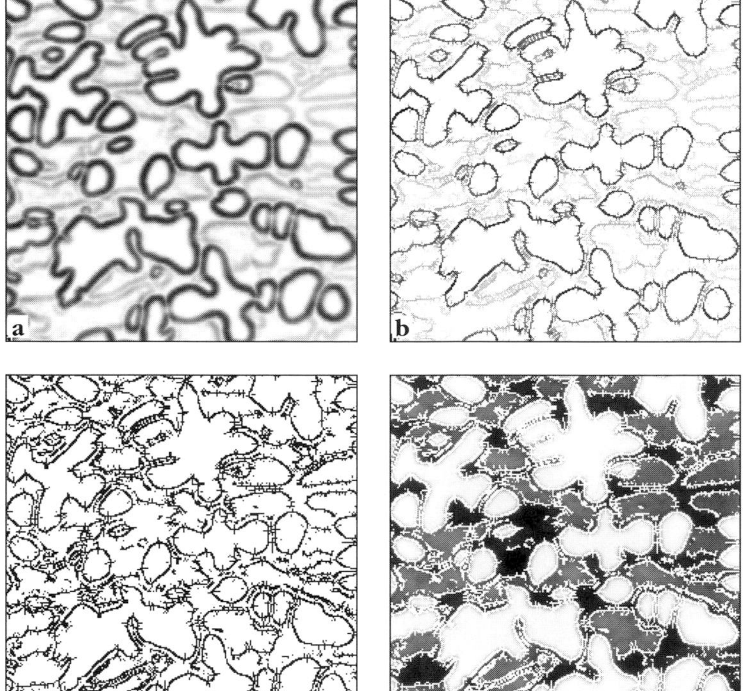

Figure 57. Another gradient mask for the image in Figure 54:
a) *application of a 5-pixel-wide octagonal range operator;*
b) *non-maximum suppression (grey scale skeletonization or ridge finding) applied to image (a);*
c) *thresholding of image (b) to keep the darkest 20% of the pixels;*
d) *masking of original image with image (c).*

through the microscope, while the pointer device is optically superimposed. None of these methods is without problems. Video displays have rather limited resolution. Drawing on the image in a microscope does not provide a record of where you have been. Mice are clumsy pointing devices, light pens lose precision in dark areas of the display, touch screens have poor resolution (and your finger gets in the way), and so on.

It is beyond our purpose here to describe the operation or compare the utility of these different approaches. Regardless of what physical device is used for manual outlining, the method relies on the human visual image processor to locate boundaries and produces a result that consists of a polygonal approximation to the region outline. Most people tend to draw just outside the actual boundary, making dimensions larger than they should be, and the amount of error is a function of the contrast at the edge. (There are exceptions to this, of course. Some people draw inside the boundary. But bias is commonly present in manually drawn outlines.)

Attempts to emulate the human outlining operation with a computer algorithm require a starting point, usually provided by the human. Then the program examines each adjoining pixel to find which has the characteristics of a boundary, usually defined as a step in brightness. Whichever pixel has the highest value of local gradient is selected and added to the growing polygon, and then the procedure is repeated. Sometimes, a constraint is added

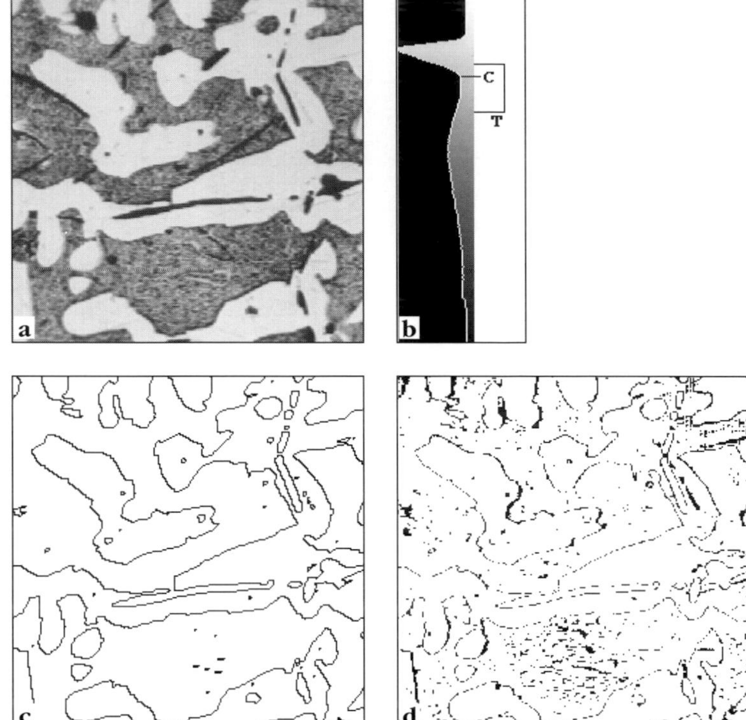

Figure 58. Cast iron (light micrograph) with ferrite (white) and graphite (black):
a) *original image;*
b) *brightness histogram showing levels used for contour (C) and threshold (T);*
c) *contour lines drawn using the value shown in (b);*
d) *pixels selected by the threshold setting shown in (b).*

to minimize sharp turns, such as weighting the pixel values according to direction.

Automatic edge following suffers from several problems. First, the edge definition is essentially local. People have a rather adaptable capability to look ahead various distances to find pieces of edge to be connected together. Gestalt psychologists describe this as grouping. Such a response is difficult for an algorithm that looks only within a small neighborhood. Even in rather simple images, there may be places along boundaries where the local gradient or other measure of edgeness drops.

In addition, edges may touch where regions abut. The algorithm is equally likely to follow either edge, which of course gives a nonsensical result. There may also be a problem of when to end the process. If the edge is a single, simple line, then it ends when it reaches the starting point. If the line reaches another feature that already has a defined boundary (from a previous application of the routine) or if it reaches the edge of the field of view, then there is no way to complete the outline.

The major problems with edge following, though, are: a) it cannot by itself complete the segmentation of the image because it has to be given each new starting point and cannot determine whether there are more outlines to be followed and b) the same edge-defining criteria used for following edges can be applied more easily by processing the entire image and then thresholding. This produces a line of pixels that may be broken and incomplete (if the edge following would have been unable to continue) or may branch (if several boundaries touch). However, there are methods discussed in Chapter 6 that apply erosion/dilation logic to deal with some of these deficiencies. The global application of the processing operation finds all of the boundaries.

Contours

One type of line that may provide boundary information and is guaranteed to be continuous is a contour line. This is analogous to the iso-elevation contour lines drawn on topographic maps. The line marks a constant elevation, or in our case a constant brightness in the image. These lines cannot end, although they may branch or loop back upon themselves. In a continuous image or an actual topographic surface, there is always a point through which the line can pass. For a discrete image, the brightness value of the line may not happen to correspond to any specific pixel value. Nevertheless, if there is a pair of pixels with one value brighter than and one value darker than the contour level, then the line must pass somewhere between them.

The contour line can, in principle, be fit as a polygon through the points interpolated between pixel centers for all such pairs of pixels that bracket the contour value. This actually permits measuring the locations of these lines, and the boundaries that they may represent, to less than the dimensions of one pixel, called sub-pixel sampling or measurement. This is rarely done for an entire image because of the amount of work involved and the difficulty in representing the boundary by such a series of points, which must be assembled into a polygon.

Instead, the most common use of contour lines is to mark the pixels that lie closest to, or closest to and above, the line. These pixels approximate the contour line to the resolution of the pixels in the original image, form a continuous band of touching pixels (touching in an 8-neighbor sense, as discussed below), and can be used to delineate features in many instances. Creating the line from the image is simply a matter of scanning the pixels once, comparing each pixel and its neighbors above and to the left to the contour value, and marking the pixel if its values are above or below the test value.

Figure 58 shows a grey scale image with several contour lines, superimposed at arbitrarily chosen brightness values, marked on the histogram. Notice that setting a threshold range at this same brightness level, even with a fairly large range, does not produce a continuous line, because the brightness gradient in some regions is quite steep and no pixels fall within the range. The brightness gradient is very gradual in other regions, so a gradient image **(Figure 59)** obtained from the same original by applying a Sobel operator does not show all of the same boundaries.

Figure 59. Gradient image obtained by applying a Sobel operator to Figure 58 (a), and the pixels selected by thresholding the 20% darkest (highest gradient) values.

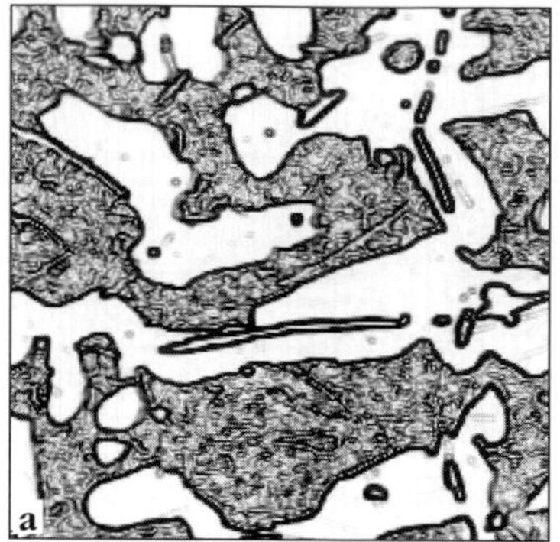

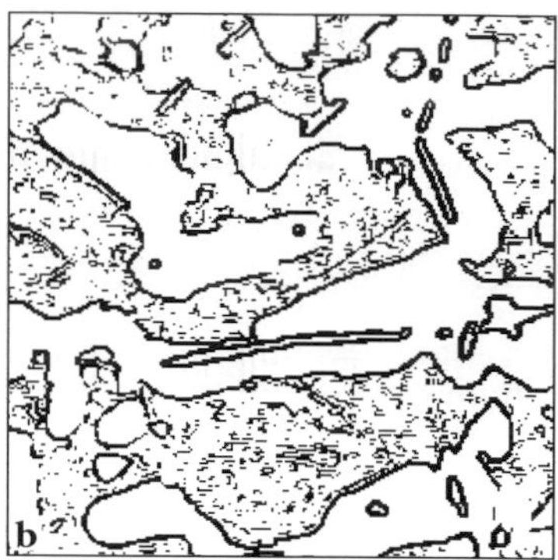

Drawing a series of contour lines on an image can be an effective way to show minor variations in brightness, as shown in **Figure 60.** Converting an image to a series of contour lines **(Figure 61)** is equivalent to creating a topographic map. Indeed, such a set of lines is a topographic map for a range image, in which the brightness values of pixels are their elevations. Such images may result from radar imaging, the CSLM, interferometry, the STM or atomic force microscope, and other devices.

They may also be produced by surface elevation measurements, as shown in **Figure 62.** This image has elevation contours calculated from stereo pair views of a specimen in the TEM, where the "mountains" are deposited contamination spots. The information from the contour lines can be used to generate a rendered surface, as shown in the figure and discussed in Chapter 8, to illustrate the surface topography.

Figure 63 shows an image containing features to be measured. The contours drawn by selecting a brightness value (marked on the histogram) provide the same outline information as the edge pixels in regions determined by thresholding with the same value. The contour lines can be filled in to provide a pixel representation of the feature, using the logic discussed in Chapter 6. Conversely, the solid regions can be converted to an outline by a different set of binary image processes.

If the contour line is defined by pixel values, the information is

Figure 60. Ion microprobe image of boron implanted in a silicon wafer:
***a)** original image, in which brightness is proportional to concentration;*
***b)** two iso-brightness or iso-concentration contour values which make it easier to compare values in different parts of the image.*

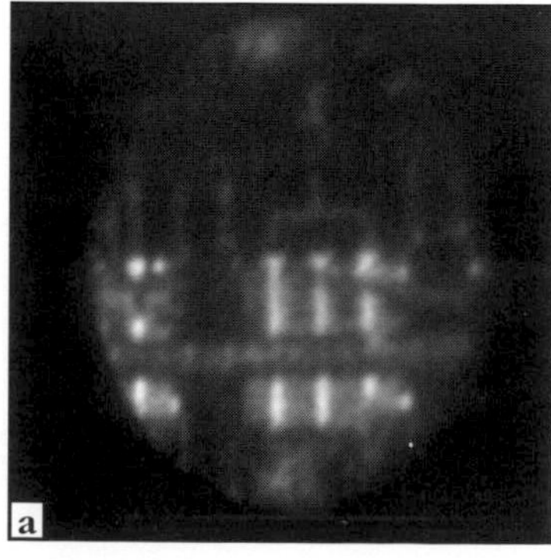

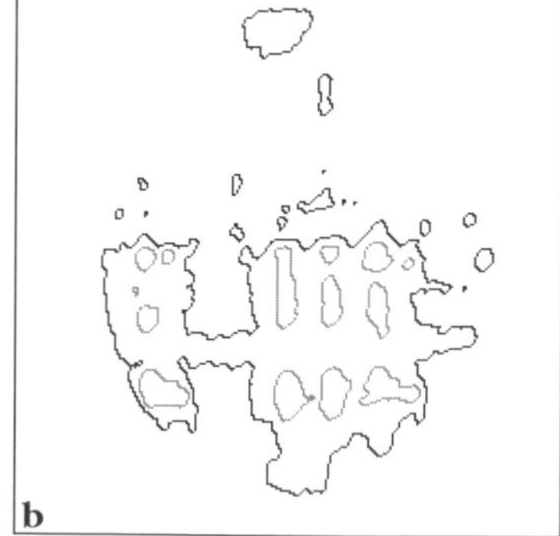

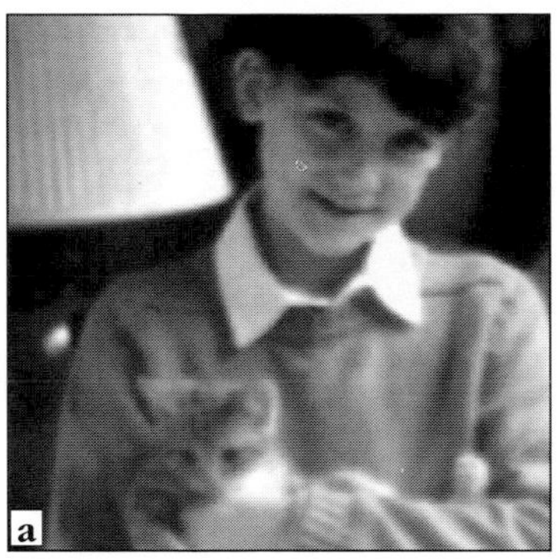
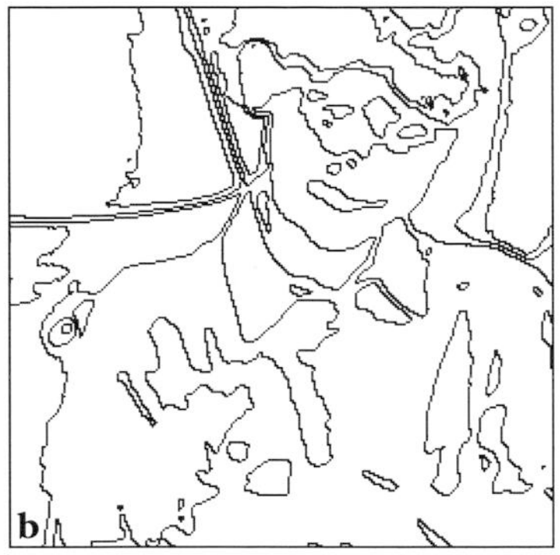

Figure 61. Real-world image (a) and four contour lines drawn at selected brightness values (b). However irregular they become, the lines are always continuous and distinct.

identical to the thresholded regions. If sub-pixel interpolation has been used, then the resolution of the features may be better. The two formats for image representation are entirely complementary, although they have different advantages for storage, measurement, etc.

Image representation

Different representations of the binary image are possible; some are more useful than others for specific purposes. Most measurements, such as feature area and position, can be directly calculated from a pixel-based representation by simple counting procedures. This can be stored in less space than the original array of pixels by using run-length encoding (also called chord encoding). This treats the image as a series of scan lines. For each sequential line across each region or feature, it stores the line number, start position, and length of the line. **Figure 64** illustrates this schematically.

For typical images, the pixels are not randomly scattered, but collected together into regions or features so that the run-length encoded stable is much smaller than the original image. This is the method used, for instance, to transmit fax messages over telephone lines. The run-length table can be used directly for area and position measurements, with even less arithmetic than the pixel array. Since the chords are in the order in which the raster

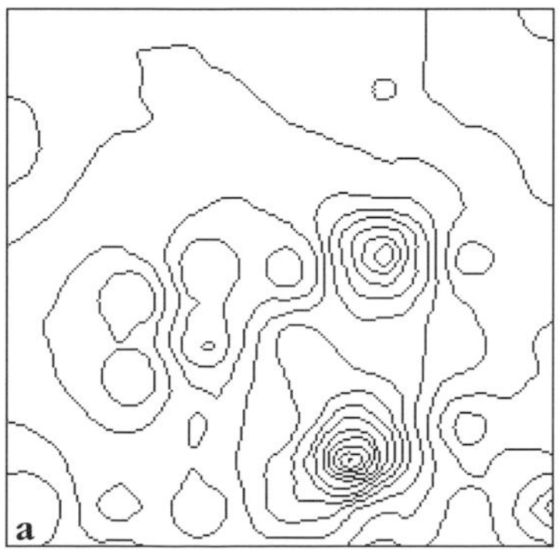
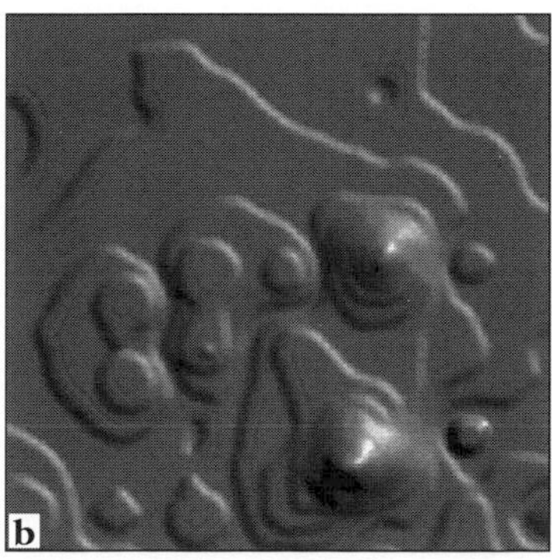

Figure 62. Elevation contour map from a range image (a) in which pixel brightness represents surface elevation and a reconstructed and rendered view of the surface (b) as discussed in Chapter 8.

Figure 63. ***Selection of features in an image:***
a) *light micrograph of a cross section of a coating on a metal;*
b) *outlines of particles and voids obtained by setting a contour level;*
c) *features or regions obtained by thresholding with the same brightness value as in (b);*
d) *regions obtained by automatically filling the boundaries from (b);*
e) *outlines obtained by taking the custer of (c).*

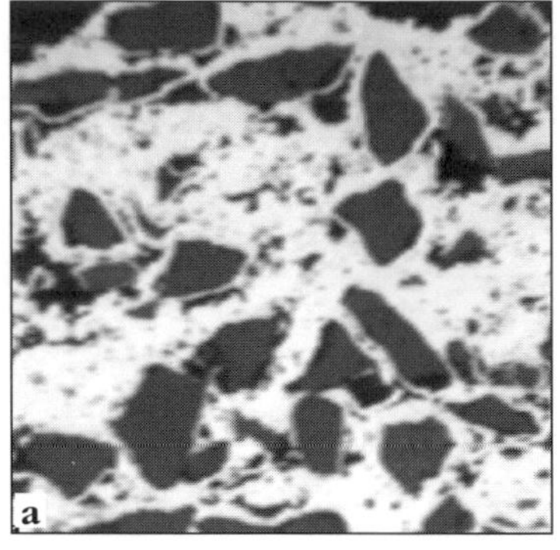

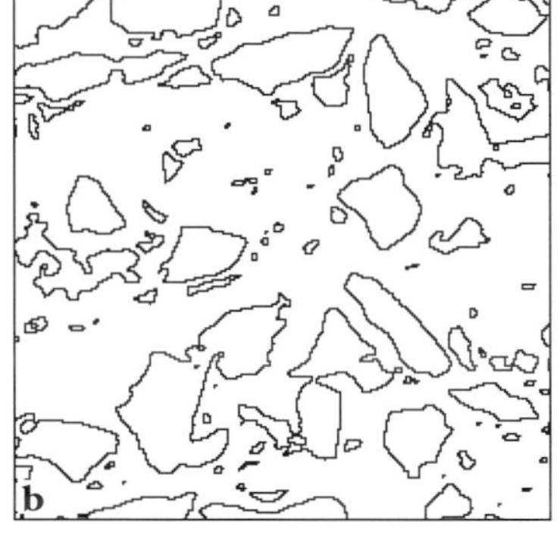

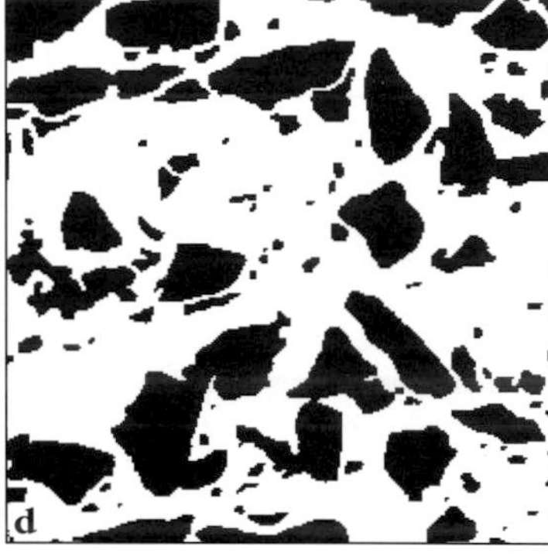

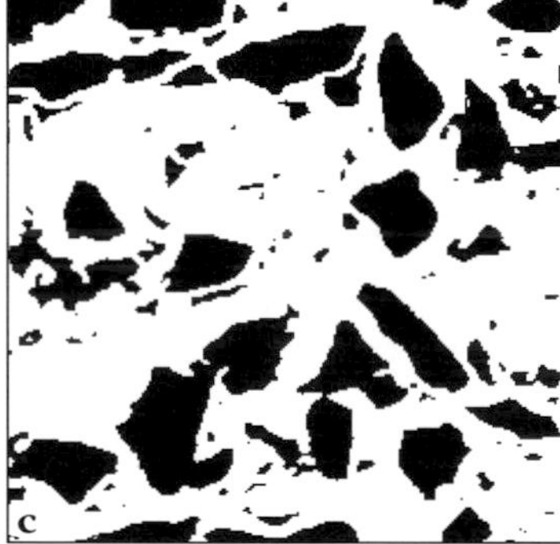

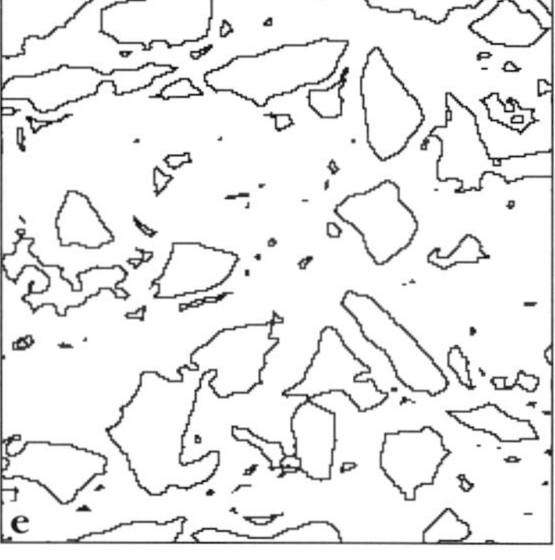

crosses the features, some logic is required to identify the chords with the features, but this is often done as the table is built.

The chord table is poorly suited for measuring feature perimeters or shape. Boundary representation, consisting of the coordinates of the polygon comprising the boundary, is superior for this task. However, it is awkward for dealing with regions containing internal holes, since there is nothing to relate the interior boundary to the exterior. Again, logic must be used to identify the internal boundaries, keep track of which ones are exterior and which are interior, and assess a hierarchy of features within features, if needed.

A simple polygonal approximation to the boundary can be produced from the run-length table by using the end points of the

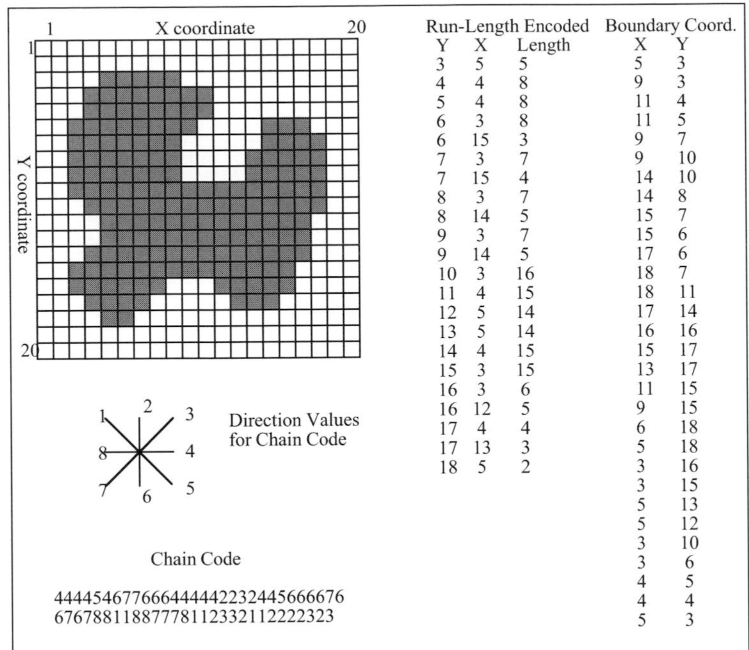

1
X coordinate
20
1
Y coordinate
20
1
2
3
8
4
7
6
5
Direction Values
for Chain Code
Chain Code
444454677666444442232445666676
67678811887778112332112222323
Run-Length Encoded
Y X Length
3 5 5
4 4 8
5 4 8
6 3 8
6 15 3
7 3 7
7 15 4
8 3 7
8 14 5
9 3 7
9 14 5
10 3 16
11 4 15
12 5 14
13 5 14
14 4 15
15 3 15
16 3 6
16 12 5
17 4 4
17 13 3
18 5 2
Boundary Coord.
X Y
5 3
9 3
11 4
11 5
9 7
9 10
14 10
14 8
15 7
15 6
17 6
18 7
18 11
17 14
16 16
15 17
13 17
11 15
9 15
6 18
5 18
3 16
3 15
5 13
5 12
3 10
3 6
4 5
4 4
5 3

Figure 64. *Encoding the same region in a binary image by run-length encoding, boundary polygonal representaton, or chain code.*

series of chords, as shown in **Figure 64.** A special form of this polygon can be formed from all of the boundary points, consisting of a series of short vectors from one boundary point to the next. On a square pixel array, each of these lines is either 1 or $\sqrt{2}$ pixels long and can only have 1 of 8 directions. Assigning a digit from 0 to 7 (or 1 to 8) to each direction and writing all of the numbers for the closed boundary in order produces chain code, also shown in **Figure 64.**

This form is particularly well-suited for calculating perimeter or describing shape (Freeman, 1961, 1974; Cederberg, 1979). The perimeter is determined by counting the number of even and odd digits, multiplying the number of odd ones by $\sqrt{2}$ to correct for diagonal directions, and adding. The chain code also contains shape information, which can be used to locate corners, simplify the shape of the outline, match features independent of orientation, or calculate various shape descriptors. These measurement techniques are beyond the scope of this text.

Most current-generation imaging systems use an array of square pixels, because it is well suited both to raster-scan acquisition devices and to processing images and performing measurements. If rectangular pixels are acquired by using a different pixel spacing along the scan lines than between the lines, processing with either neighborhood spatial domain or frequency transforms becomes much more difficult, because the different pixel distances as a function of orientation must be taken into account. This also impedes measurements.

Figure 65. ***Ambiguous images:***
a) *if the pixels are assumed to touch at their corners, then this shows a line which separates the background pixels on either side, but those pixels also touch at their corners. If eight-connectedness or four-connectedness is selected for feature pixels, then the opposite convention applies to background pixels;*
b) *this shows either four separate features or one containing an internal hole, depending on the touching convention.*

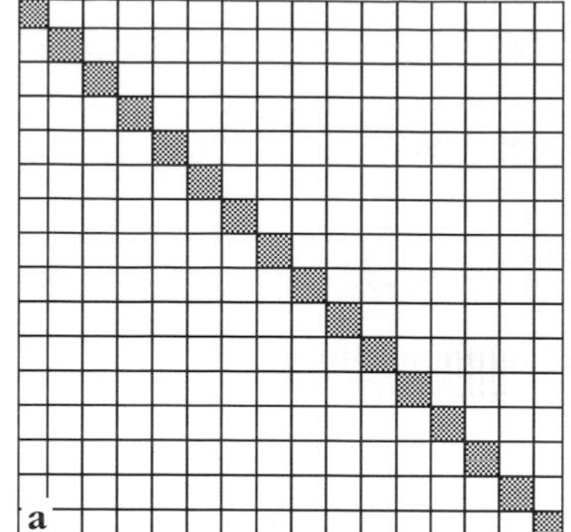

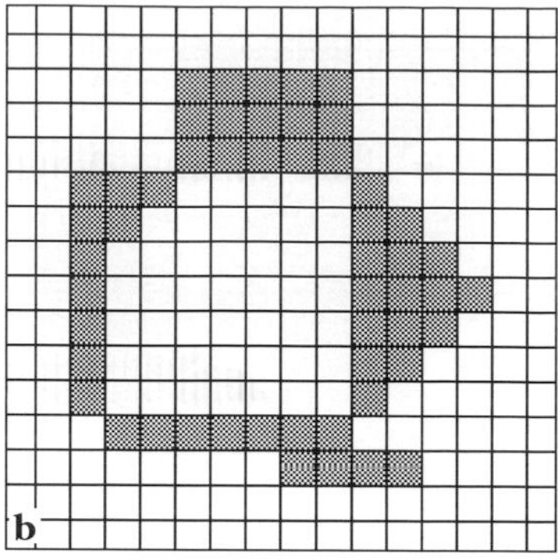

With a square pixel array, there is a minor problem that we have already seen in the previous chapters on image processing: the four pixels diagonally adjacent to a central pixel are actually farther away than the four sharing an edge. An alternative arrangement that has been used in a few systems is to place the pixels in a hexagonal array. This has the advantage of equal spacing between all neighboring pixels, which simplifies processing and calculations. Its great disadvantage, however, is that standard cameras and other acquisition devices do not operate that way.

For a traditional square pixel array, it is necessary to decide whether pixels adjacent at a corner are actually touching. This will be important for the binary processing operations in Chapter 6. It is necessary in order to link pixels together into features or follow points around a boundary, as discussed above. While it is not evident whether one choice is superior to the other, whichever one is made, the background (the pixels which surround the features) must have the opposite relationship.

Figure 65 shows this dual situation. If pixels within a feature are assumed to touch any of their eight adjacent neighbors (called eight-connectedness), then the line of pixels in **Figure 65a** separates the background on either side and the background pixels that are diagonally adjacent do not touch. They are therefore four-connected. Conversely, if the background pixels touch diagonally, the pixels are isolated and only touch along their faces. For the second image fragment shown, choosing an eight-connected rule for features (dark pixels) produces a single feature with an internal hole. If a four-connected rule is used, there are four features and the background, now eight-connected, is continuous.

This means that simply inverting an image (interchanging white and black) does not reverse the meaning of the features and background. **Figure 66** shows a situation in which the holes within a feature (separated from the background) become part of a single region in the reversed image. This can cause confusion in measurements and binary image processing. When feature dimensions as small as one pixel are important, there is some basic uncertainty, and perhaps also sensitivity, to how the feature

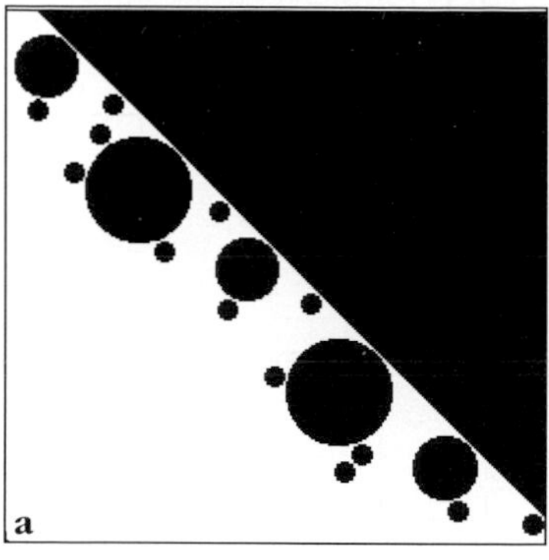

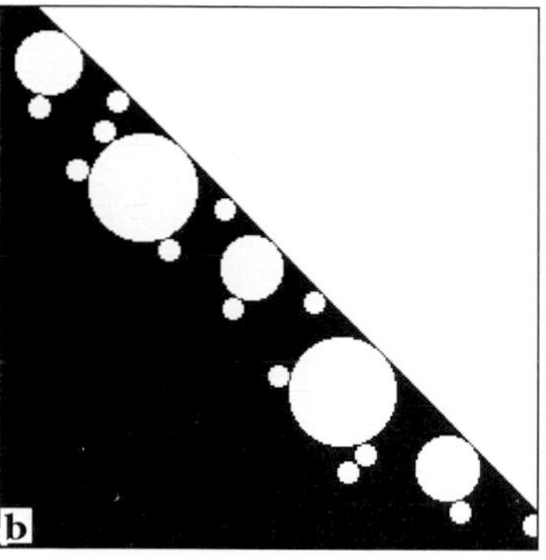

Figure 66. *Reversing an image (interchanging features and background) without changing the connectedness rules alters meaning. In image a the black pixels all touch at corners (eight-connectedness) and so this is one feature with an irregular boundary. In image b the white pixels do not touch (four-connectedness) and so these are separate holes within the feature.*

happens to lie along the raster orientation. This is unavoidable and argues for using large arrays of small pixels to accurately define small dimensions.

Other segmentation methods

There are other methods used for image segmentation besides the ones based on thresholding discussed above. These are generally associated with fairly powerful computer systems and with attempts to understand images in the sense of machine vision and robotics (Ballard & Brown, 1982; Wilson & Spann, 1988). Two of the most widely described are split-and-merge and region growing, which seem to lie at opposite extremes in method.

Split-and-merge is a top-down method that begins with the entire image. Some image property is selected as a criterion to decide whether everything is uniform. This is often based on the statistics from the brightness histogram. If the histogram is multimodal, or has a high standard deviation, etc., then the region is assumed to be nonuniform and is divided into four quadrants. Each quadrant is examined in the same way and subdivided again if necessary. The procedure continues until the individual pixel level is reached. The relationship between the parent region and the four quadrants, or children, is typically encoded in a quadtree structure, another name sometimes applied to this approach.

It should be noted that this is not the only way to subdivide the parent image and encode the resulting data structure. Thresholding can be used to divide each region into arbitrary subregions, which can be subdivided iteratively. This can produce final results having less blocky boundaries, but the data structure is much more complex, since all of the regions must be defined, and the time required for the process is much greater.

If subdividing regions were the only operation, it would not create useful image segmentation. After each iteration of subdividing, each region is compared to adjacent ones but lying in a different square at a higher level in the hierarchy. If they are similar, they are merged together. The definition of similar may use the same tests applied to the splitting operation, or comparisons may

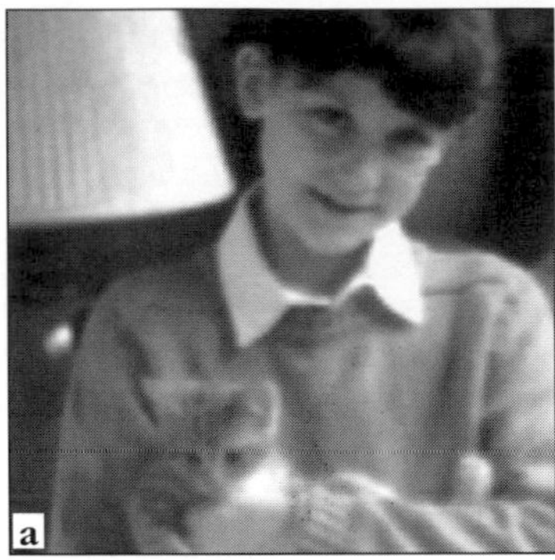

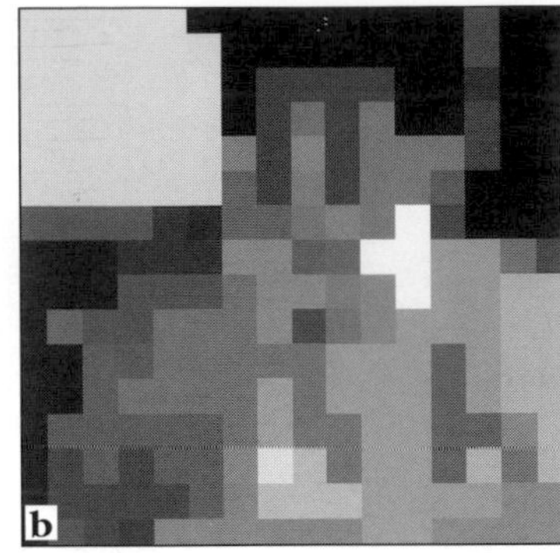

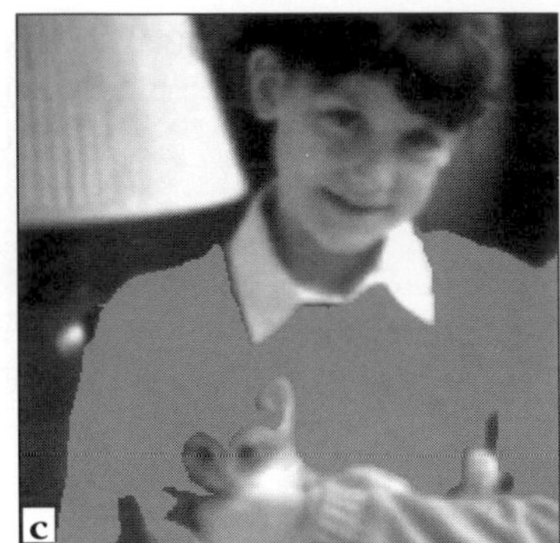

Figure 67. Other segmentation methods:
a) *original grey scale image;*
b) *split-and-merge after four iterations;*
c) *region growing from a point in the girl's sweater.*

be made only for pixels along the common edge. The latter has the advantage of tolerating gradual changes across the image.

Figure 67 shows an example, in which only four iterations have been performed. A few large areas have already merged and their edges will be refined as the iterations proceed. Other parts of the image contain individual squares that require additional subdivision before regions become visible.

An advantage to this approach is that a complete segmentation is achieved after a finite number of iterations (for instance, a 512-pixel-square image takes 9 iterations to reach individual pixels, since $2^9 = 512$). Also, the quadtree list of regions and subregions can be used for some measurements, and the segmentation identifies all of the different types of regions at one time. By comparison, thresholding methods typically isolate one type of region or feature at a time. They must be applied several times to deal with images containing more than one class of objects.

On the other hand, the split-and-merge approach depends on the quality of the test used to detect inhomogeneity in each region. Small subregions within large uniform areas can easily be missed with this method. Standard statistical tests that assume, for example, a normal distribution of pixel brightness within regions are rarely appropriate for real images, so more complicated procedures must be used (Yakimovsky, 1976). Tests used for subdividing and merging regions can also be expressed as image processing operations. A processed image can reveal the same edges and texture used for the split-and-merge tests in a way that allows direct thresholding. This is potentially less efficient, since time-consuming calculations may be applied to parts of the image that are uniform, but the results are the same. Thresholding also has the advantage of identifying similar objects in different parts of the field of view as the same, which may not occur with split-and-merge.

Region growing starts from the bottom, or individual pixel level, and works upwards. Starting at some seed location (usually provided by the operator), neighboring pixels are examined one at a time and added to the growing region if they are sufficiently similar. Again, the comparison may be made to the entire region or just to the local pixels, with the latter method allowing gradual variations in brightness. The procedure continues until no more pixels can be added. **Figure 67c** shows an example in which one region has been identified; notice that it includes part of the cat as well as the girl's sweater. Then a new region is begun at another location.

If the same comparison tests are implemented to decide whether a pixel belongs to a region, the result is the same as top-down split-and-merge. The difficulty with this approach is that the starting point for each region must be provided. Depending on the comparison tests employed, different starting points may not grow into identical regions. Also, there is no ideal structure to encode the data from this procedure, beyond keeping the entire pixel array until classification is complete, and the complete classification is slow, since each pixel must be examined individually.

Region growing also suffers from the conflicting needs to keep the test local, to see if an individual pixel should be added to the growing region, and to make it larger in scale, if not truly global, to ensure that the region has some unifying and distinct identity. If too small a test region is used, a common result is that regions leak out into adjoining areas or merge with different regions. This can occur if even a single pixel on the boundary can form a bridge.

Finally, there is no easy way to decide when the procedure is complete and all of the meaningful regions in the image have been found. Region growing may be a useful method for selecting a few regions in an image, as compared to manual tracing or edge following, for example, but it is rarely the method of choice for complex images containing many regions (Zucker, 1976).

The general classification problem

The various methods described so far have relied on human judgement to recognize the presence of regions and to define them by delineating the boundary or selecting a range of brightness values. Methods have been discussed that can start with an incomplete definition and refine the segmentation to achieve greater accuracy or consistency.

There are also fully automatic techniques that determine how many classes of objects are present and fully subdivide the image to isolate them. However, they are little used in small computer-based systems and are often much less efficient than using some human input. The task of general image segmentation can be

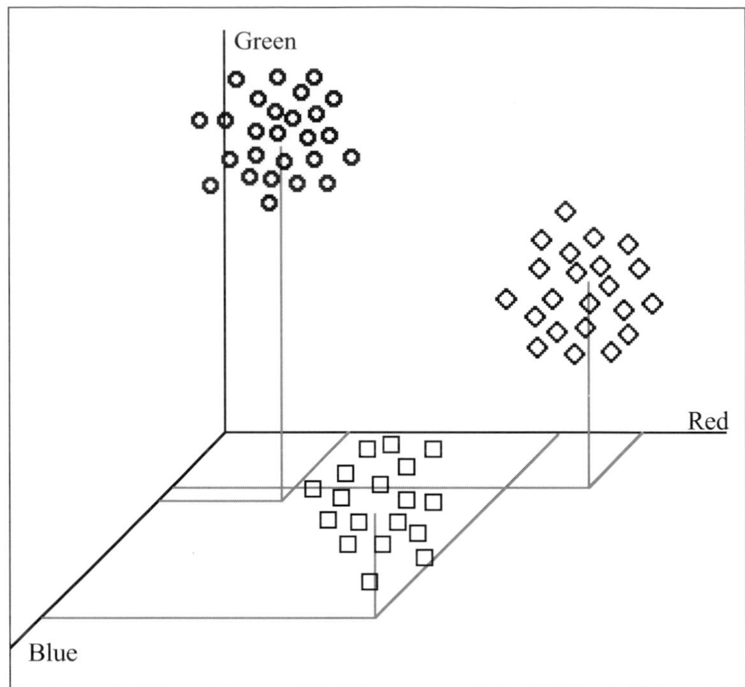

Figure 68. Schematic illustration of pixel classification in color space. Each pixel is plotted according to its color values, and clusters identify the various regions present.

treated as an example of a classification problem. Like most techniques involving elements or artificial intelligence, it may not use the same inputs or decision methods that a human employs, but it seeks to (and often succeeds in) duplicating the results.

One successful approach to general classification has been used with satellite imagery, in which many wavelength bands of data are available (Reeves, 1975). If each pixel in the image is plotted in a high-dimensionality space, where each axis is the measured brightness in one of the wavelength bands, it is expected that points corresponding to different classes of land use, crop type, soil or rock type, etc. will cluster together and the clusters will be well separated from each other, as indicated in **Figure 68.** The problem then reduces to finding the clusters and fitting boundaries between them that can be used for classification.

Reduced to a single dimension (a simple grey scale image), this produces the brightness histogram. The cluster analysis looks for peaks and tries to draw thresholds between them. This is successful in a tiny handful of specialized tasks, such as counting cells of one type on a microscope slide. As the number of dimensions increases, for instance using the RGB or HSI data from color imagery or adding values from a derived texture or gradient image, the separation of the clusters usually becomes more distinct. Satellite imagery with several discrete visible and infrared wavelength bands is especially well suited to this approach.

Clusters are easier to recognize when they contain many similar points, but minor regions or uncommon objects may be overlooked. Also, the number of background points surrounding the clusters (or more often lying along lines between them) confuse the automatic algorithms. These points arise from the finite size of pixels that straddle the boundaries between regions. Finding a few major clusters may be straightforward. Being sure that all have been found is not.

Even after the clusters have been identified (and here some *a priori* knowledge or input from a human can be of great assistance), there are different strategies to using this information to classify new points. One is to surround each cluster with a boundary, typically either a polyhedron formed by planes lying perpendicular to the lines between the cluster centers, or n-dimensional ellipsoids. Points falling inside any of these regions are immediately classified.

Particularly for the ellipsoid case, it is also possible to have a series of concentric boundaries that enclose different percentages of the points in the cluster, which can be used to give a probability of classification to new points. This is sometimes described as a "fuzzy" classification method.

A third approach is to find the nearest classified point to each new point and assign that identity to the new one. This has several drawbacks, particularly when there are some densely populated clusters and others with very few members or when the clusters are close or overlapping. It requires considerable time to search through a large universe of existing points to locate the closest one, as well. An extension of this technique is also used, in which a small number of nearest neighbors are identified and vote for the identity of the new point.

Segmentation of grey scale images into regions for measurement or recognition is probably the most important single problem area for image analysis. Many novel techniques have been used, many of which are rather ad hoc and narrow in their range of applicability. Review articles by Fu and Mui (1981) and Haralick and Shapiro (1988) present good guides to the literature. Most standard image analysis textbooks, such as Rosenfeld and Kak (1982), Castleman (1979), Gonzalez and Wintz (1987), Russ (1990b), and Pratt (1991) also contain sections on segmentation.

All of these various methods and modifications are used extensively in other artificial intelligence situations (see for example Fukunaga, 1990). They may be implemented in hardware, software, or some combination of the two. Only limited application of any of these techniques has been made to the segmentation problem. However, it is likely that this will increase in the future as more color or multiband imaging is done and readily accessible computer power continues to increase.

6

Processing Binary Images

Binary images, as discussed in the preceding chapter, consist of groups of pixels selected on the basis of some property. The selection may be performed by thresholding brightness values, perhaps using several grey scale images containing different color bands, or processed to extract texture or other information. The goal of binarization is to separate features from background, so that counting, measurement, or matching operations can be performed.

However, as shown by the examples in Chapter 5, the result of the segmentation operation is rarely perfect. For images of realistic complexity, even the most elaborate segmentation routines misclassify some pixels as foreground or background. These may either be pixels along the boundaries of regions or patches of noise within regions. The major tools for working with binary images fit broadly into two groups: Boolean operations, for combining images, and morphological operations which modify individual pixels within images.

Boolean operations

In the section on thresholding color images, in Chapter 5, a Boolean operation was introduced to combine the data from individual color plane images. Setting thresholds on brightness values in each of the RGB planes allows pixels to be selected that fall into those ranges. This produces three binary images, which can then be combined with a logical AND operation. The pro-

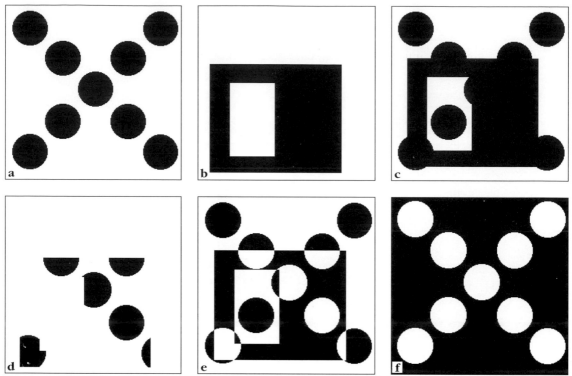

Figure 1. Simple Boolean operations: ***a, b)*** *two binary images;* ***c)*** *A OR B;* ***d)*** *A AND B;* ***e)*** *A Ex-OR B;* ***f)*** *NOT A.*

cedure examines the three images pixel by pixel, keeping pixels for the selected regions if they are turned ON in all three images.

An aside: The terminology used here will be that of ON (pixels that are part of the selected foreground features) and OFF (the remaining pixels, which are part of the background). There is no universal standard defining whether the selected pixels are displayed as white, black, or some other color. In many cases, systems that portray the selected regions as white on a black background on the display screen may reverse this and print hardcopy of the same image with black features on a white background. This apparently arises from the fact that in each case, the selection of foreground pixels is associated with some positive action in the display (turning on the electron beam) or printout (depositing ink on the paper). It seems to cause most users little difficulty, provided that something is known about the image. Since many of the images used here are not common objects and some are made-up examples, we must try to be consistent in defining the foreground pixels (those of interest) in each case.

Returning to our desire to combine the information from several image planes, the AND operation requires that a pixel at location *i,j* be ON in each individual plane to show up in the result. Pixels having the correct amount of blue but not of red will be omit-

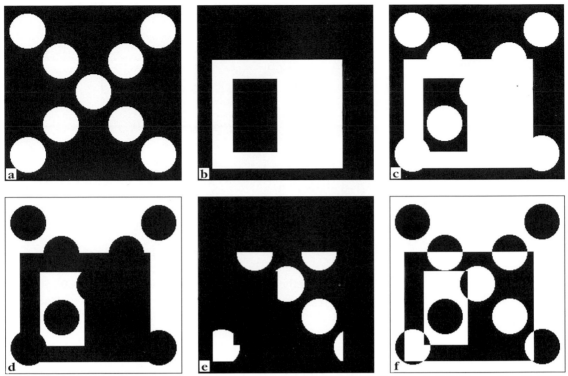

Figure 2. Combined Boolean operations: a) *NOT A;* ***b)*** *NOT B;* ***c)*** *(Image a) AND (Image b);* ***d)*** *NOT (Image c);* ***e)*** *NOT (A AND B);* ***f)*** *(Image d) AND (Image e), or (NOT (A AND B)) AND (NOT (NOT A) AND (NOT B)))—compare this to A Ex-OR B in Figure 1e.*

ted, and vice versa. As was noted before, this marks out a rectangle in two dimensions, or a rectangular prism in higher dimensions, for the pixel values to be included. More complicated combinations of color values can be described by delineating an irregular region in n dimensions for pixel selection. The advantage of simply ANDing discrete ranges is that it can be performed very efficiently and quickly using binary images.

Other Boolean logical rules can be employed to combine binary images. The four possibilities are AND, OR, Ex-OR (Exclusive OR), and NOT. **Figure 1** illustrates each of these basic operations, and **Figure 2** shows a few of the possible combinations. All are performed pixel-by-pixel. The illustrations are based on combining two images at a time, since any logical rule involving more than two images can be broken down to a series of steps using just two at once. The illustrations in the figures are identical to the Venn diagrams used in logic.

As described above, AND requires that pixels be ON in both of the original images in order to be ON in the result. Pixels that are ON in only one or the other original image are OFF in the result. The OR operator turns a pixel ON in the result if it is ON in either of the original images. Ex-OR turns a pixel ON in the result

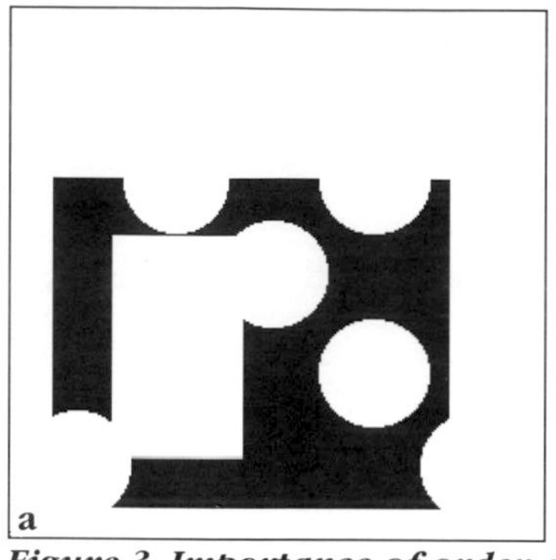

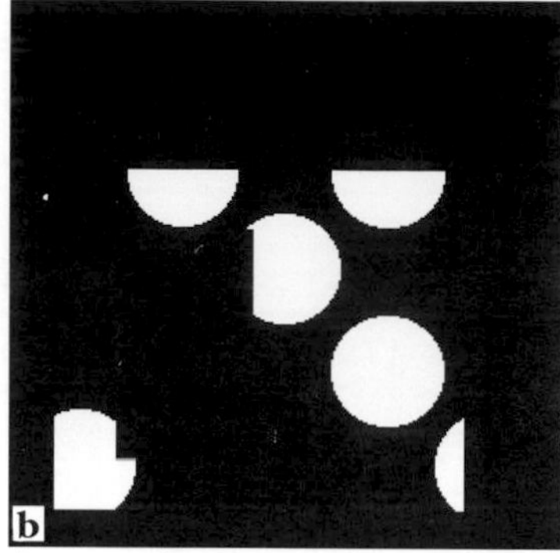

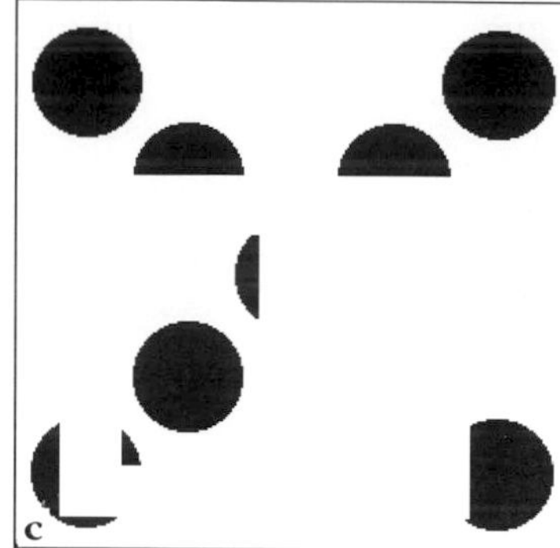

Figure 3. Importance of order and parentheses: a) *(NOT A) AND B;* ***b)*** *NOT (A AND B);* ***c)*** *A AND (NOT B).*

if it is ON in either of the original images, but not if it is ON in both. That means that combining (with an OR) the results of ANDing together two images with those from Ex-ORing them produces the same result as an OR in the first place. There are, in fact, many ways to join different combinations of the four Boolean operators to produce identical results (e.g., compare **Figure 2f** to **Figure 1e**).

AND, OR and Ex-OR require two original images and produce a single image as a result. NOT requires only a single image. It simply reverses each pixel, turning pixels that were ON to OFF and vice versa. Some systems implement NOT by swapping black and white values for each pixel. As long as we are dealing with pixel-level detail, it works correctly. Later, when feature-level combinations are described, the difference between an eight-connected feature and its four-connected background (discussed in Chapter 5) will have to be taken into account.

Given two binary images A and B, the combination (NOT A) AND B will produce an image containing pixels that lie within B but outside A. This is quite different from NOT (A AND B), which selects pixels that are not ON in both A and B and also from A AND NOT B (**Figure 3**). The order of operators is important and the use of parentheses to clarify the order and scope of operations is crucial.

Combining Boolean operations

Actually, the four operations discussed above are redundant. Three would be enough to produce all of the same results. **Figure 2f** and **Figure 4** show ways that the results of an Ex-OR operation can also be produced by a sequence of AND, OR, and NOT operators. Consequently, some systems may omit one of them (usually Ex-OR). For simplicity, however, all four will be used in the examples that follow.

When multiple criteria are available for selecting the pixels to be

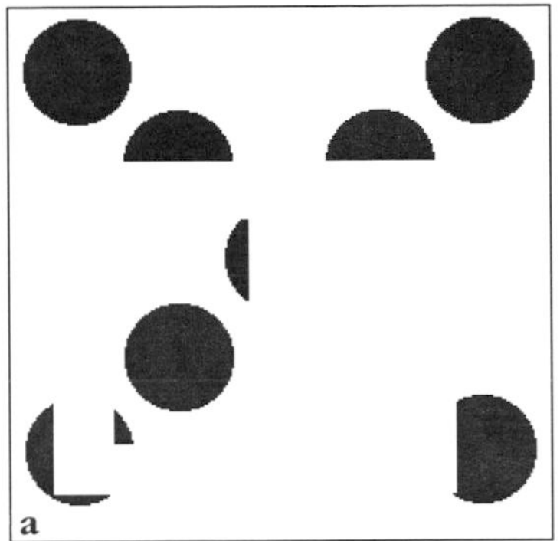

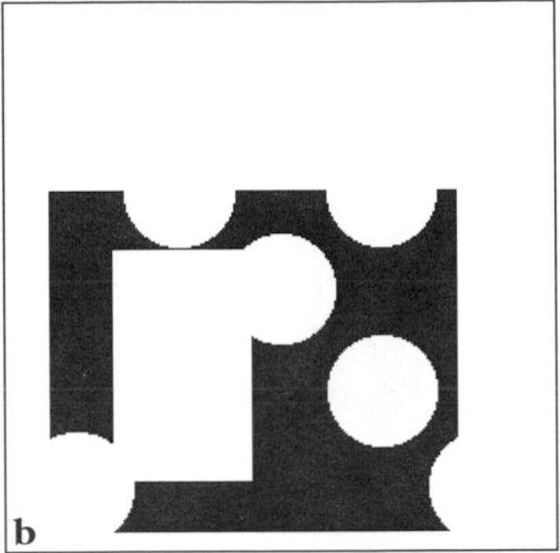

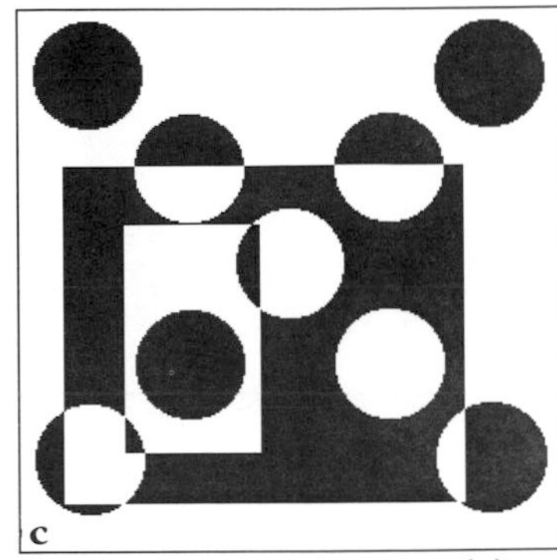

Figure 4. Equivalence of Boolean combinations: a) *A AND NOT B;* ***b)*** *B AND NOT A;* ***c)*** *Image (a) AND Image (b), or ((A AND NOT B) OR (NOT A AND B)). Compare this to A Ex-OR B in Image 1e.*

kept as foreground, they may be combined using any of these Boolean combinations. The most common situations are multi-band images, such as produced by a satellite or an SEM. In the case of the SEM, an X-ray detector is often used to create an image (called an X-ray dot map) showing the spatial distribution of a selected element. These images may be quite noisy (Chapter 2) and difficult to threshold (Chapter 5). However, by suitable long-term integration or spatial smoothing, they can lead to useful binary images that indicate locations where the concentration of the element is above some user-selected level.

This selection is usually performed by comparing measured X-ray intensity to some arbitrary threshold, since there is a finite level of background signal resulting from the process of slowing down the electrons in the sample. The physical background of this phenomenon is not important here. The very poor statistical characteristics of the dot map (hence the name) make it difficult to directly specify a concentration level as a threshold. The X-ray intensity in one part of the image may vary from another region, either because of a change in that element's concentration or the presence of another element that selectively absorbs or fluoresces the first element's radiation, or because of a change in specimen density or surface orientation. Comparison of one specimen to another is further hampered by the difficulty in exactly reproducing instrument conditions. These effects all complicate the relationship between elemental concentration and recorded intensity.

Furthermore, the very poor statistics of the images (due to the extremely low efficiency for producing X-rays with an electron beam and the low beam intensity required for good spatial resolution in SEM images) mean that these images often require processing, either as grey scale images (e.g., smoothing) or after binarization (using the morphological tools discussed below). For our present purpose, we will assume that binary images showing the spatial distribution of some meaningful concentration level of several elements can be obtained.

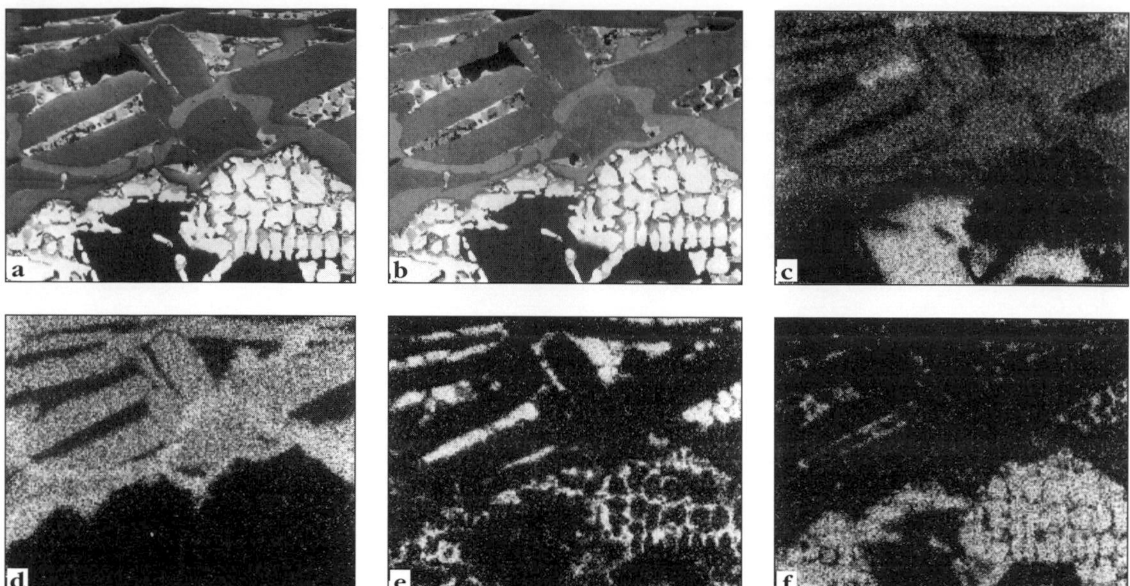

Figure 5. SEM results from a mineral: ***a)*** *backscattered electrons;* ***b)*** *secondary electrons;* ***c)*** *silicon (Si) X-ray map;* ***d)*** *iron (Fe) X-ray map;* ***e)*** *copper (Cu) X-ray map.*

As shown in **Figure 5,** the SEM also produces more conventional images using secondary or backscattered electrons. These have superior spatial resolution and better feature shape definition, but with less elemental specificity. The binary images from these sources will also be combined with the X-ray or elemental information.

Figure 6 shows one example. The X-ray maps for iron (Fe) and silicon (Si) were obtained by smoothing and thresholding the grey scale image. Notice that in the grey scale images, there is a just-discernible difference in the intensity level of the Fe X-rays in two different areas. This is too small a difference for reliable thresholding. Even the larger differences in Si intensity are difficult to separate. However, Boolean logic easily combines the images to produce an image of the region containing Fe but not Si.

Figure 7 shows another example from the same data. The re-

Figure 6:
a) *iron;*
b) *iron AND NOT silicon.*

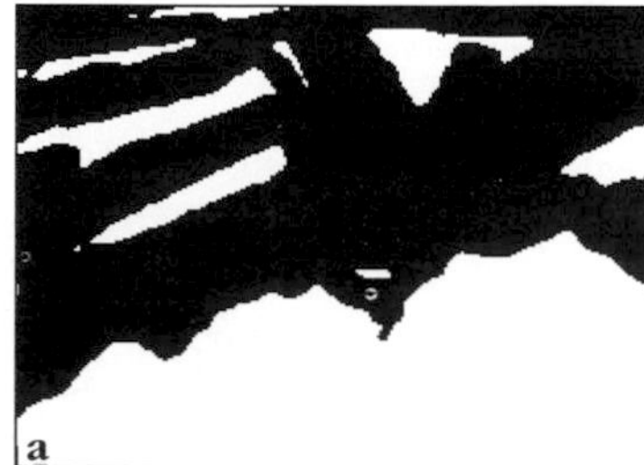

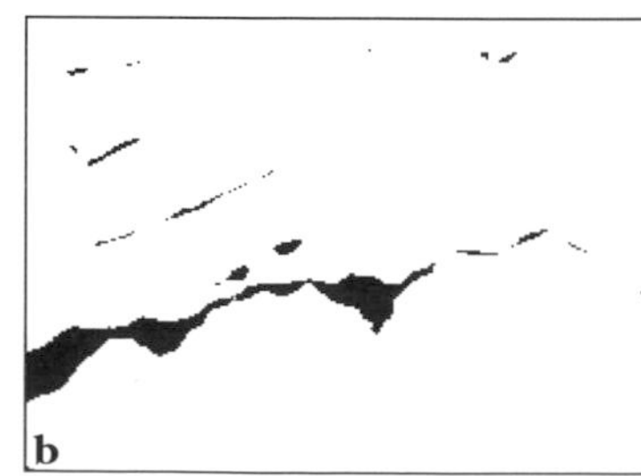

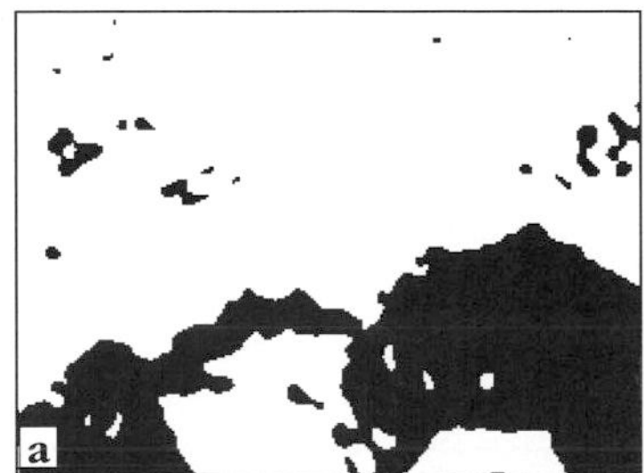

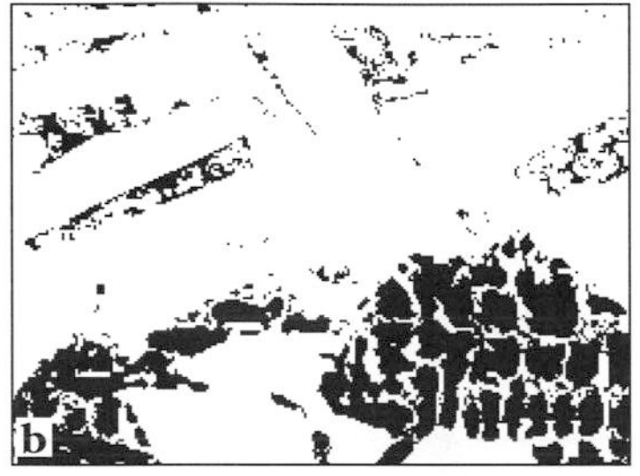

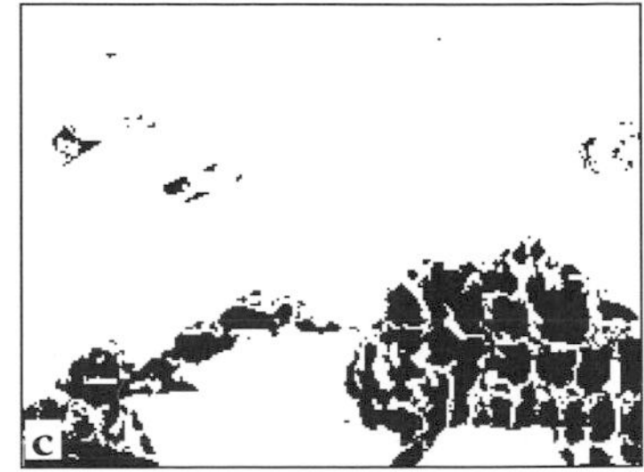

Figure 7: ***a)*** *silver;* ***b)*** *bright levels from backscattered electron image;* ***c)*** *image a AND image b.*

gions containing silver (Ag) are generally bright in the backscattered electron image, but some other areas are also bright. On the other hand, the Ag X-ray map does not have precise region boundaries because of the poor statistics. Combining the two binary images with an AND produces the desired regions. More complicated sequences of Boolean logical operations can easily be imagined (**Figure 8**).

It is straightforward to imagine a complex specimen containing many elements. Paint pigment particles with a diverse range of compositions provide one example. In order to count or measure a particular class of particles (pigments, as opposed to brighteners or extenders), it might be necessary to specify those containing iron or chromium or aluminum, but not titanium or sulfur. This would be written as

(Fe OR Cr OR Al) AND (NOT (Ti OR S))

The resulting image might then be ANDed with a higher-resolution binary produced by thresholding a secondary or backscattered electron image to delineate particle boundaries.

Masks

The above description of using Boolean logic to combine images makes the assumption that both images are binary; that is, black and white. It is also possible to use a binary image as a mask to modify a grey scale image. This is most often done to blank out (to either white or black) some portion of the grey scale image, either to create a display in which only the regions of interest are visible or to select regions whose brightness, density, etc. are to be measured.

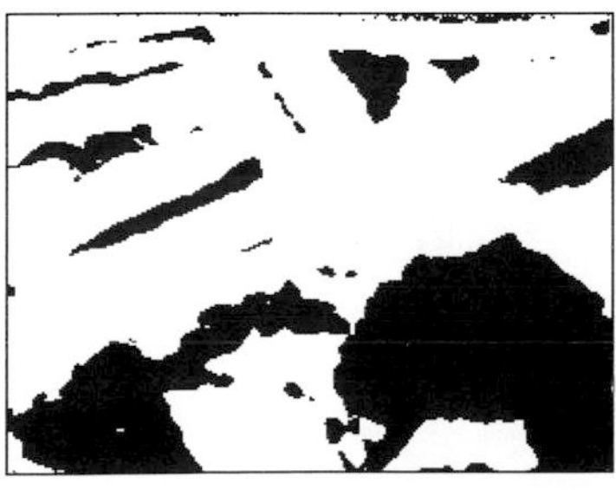

Figure 8. *Further combination to delineate structure: (Cu OR Ag) AND NOT (Fe).*

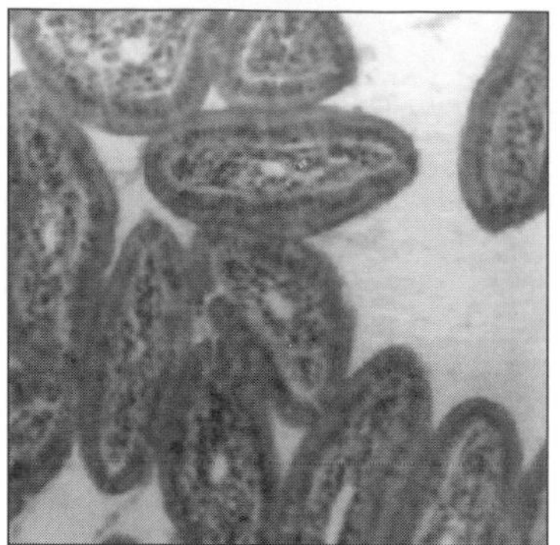
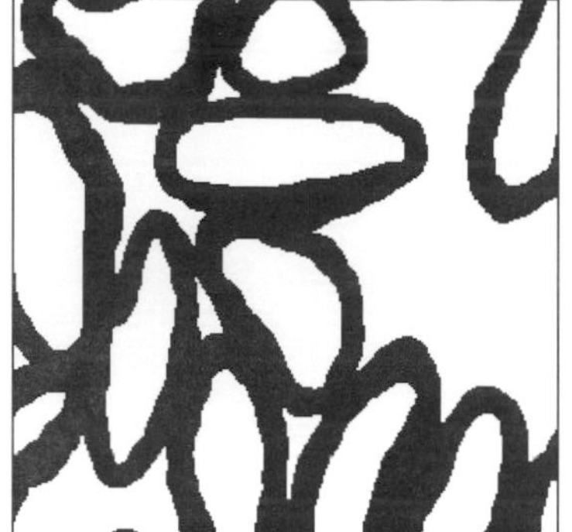
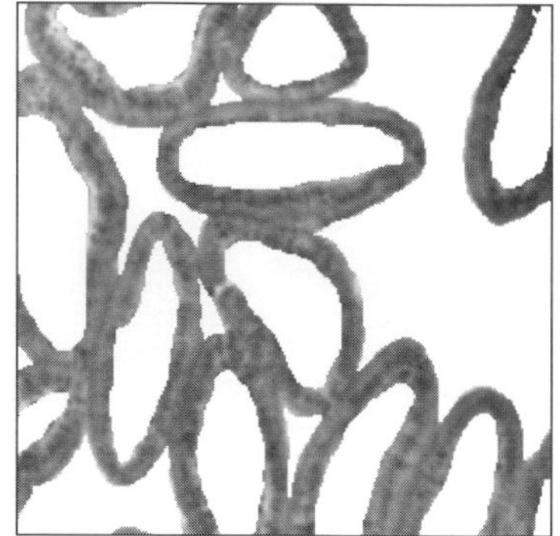

Figure 9. *Masking to show a portion of a grey scale image. The displayed villi are selected with a mask obtained by thresholding a combination of the hue and saturation images (see Plate 6).*

There are several physical ways that this operation can be performed. The binary mask can be used in an overlay, or alpha channel, memory in the display hardware to prevent pixels from being displayed if the hardware supports that capability. It is also possible, and somewhat more common, to use the mask to modify the stored image. This can done using Boolean logic to set pixels in the grey scale image to the value of the binary image if it is non-zero. It is possible to produce the same result by multiplying the grey scale image by the binary image, with the convention that the binary image values are 0 (OFF) or 1 (ON) at each pixel.

This capability has been used extensively in earlier chapters to display the results of various processing and thresholding operations. It is easier to judge the performance of thresholding by viewing selected pixels with the original grey scale information, rather than just looking at the binary image. This format can be seen in the examples of texture operators in **Figure 43** of Chapter 3, for instance.

It is also possible to use a mask obtained by thresholding one version of an image to view another version. For instance, **Figure 9** shows the region along the villi of a mouse intestine. The displayed pixels have the grey scale intensity values, but the thresholding to create the mask used to select these pixels is based on a combination of hue and saturation data.

Figure 10. *Masking one image with another. The direction of a Sobel gradient applied to the light microscope image of an aluminum alloy is shown only in the regions where the magnitude of the gradient is large.*

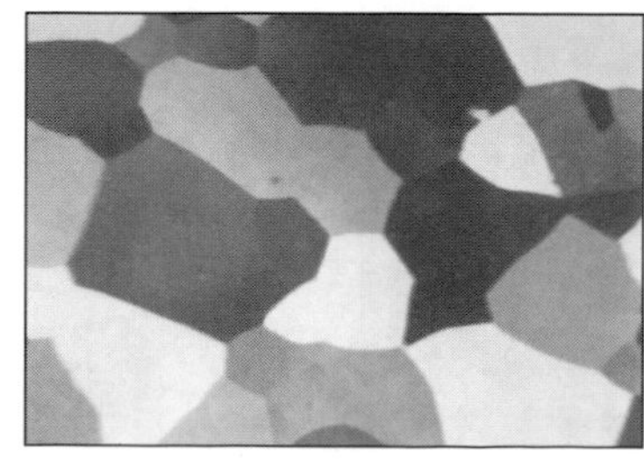
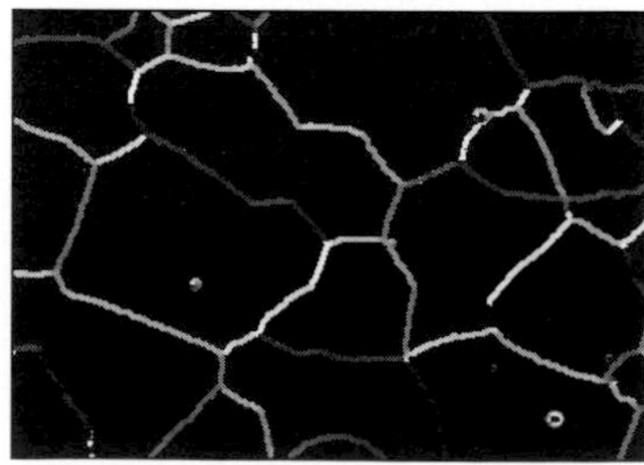

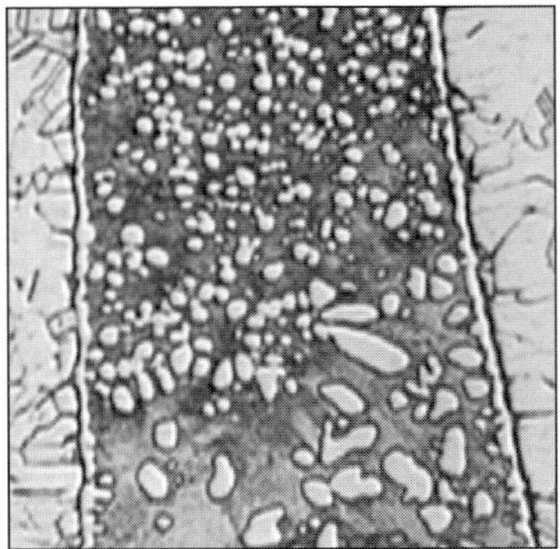

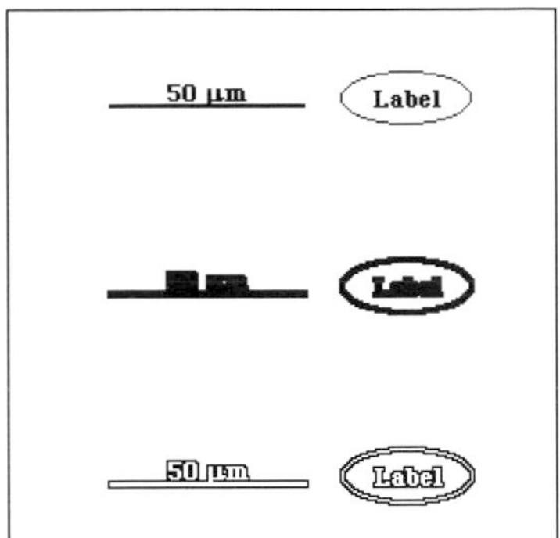

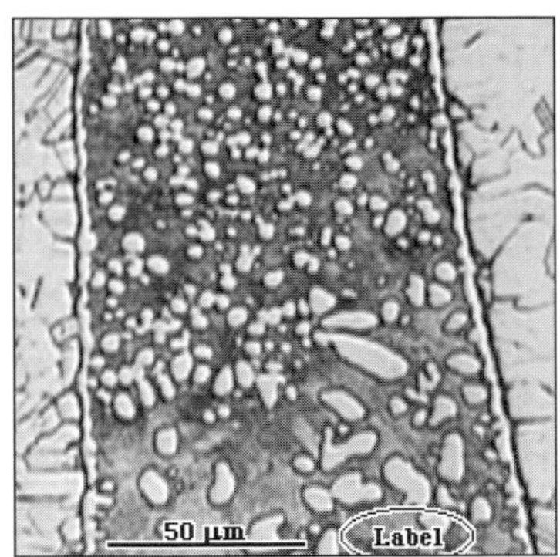

Figure 11. *Using a mask to apply a label to an image. The original image contains both white and black areas, so that simple superimposition of text will not be visible. A mask is created by dilating the label and Ex-ORing that with the original. The composite is then superimposed on the grey scale image.*

Masking one derived image with another produces results such as those shown in **Figure 10**. Grey scale values represent the orientation angle (from the Sobel derivative) of grain boundaries in the aluminum alloy, masked by thresholding the magnitude of the gradient to isolate only the boundaries. A similar example was shown in **Figure 24** of Chapter 3.

Another use of masking and Boolean image combination is shown in **Figure 11.** An essentially cosmetic application, it is still useful and widely employed. A label superimposed on an image using either black or white may be difficult to read if the image contains a full range of brightness values. In this example, the label is used to create a mask that is one pixel larger in all directions, using dilation (discussed below). This mask is then used to erase the pixels in the grey scale image to white before writing in the label in black (or vice versa). The result maintains legibility for the label while obscuring a minimum amount of the image.

Finally, a binary image mask can be used to combine portions of two (or more) grey scale images. This is shown in **Figure 12**. The composite image represents, in a very simple way, the kind

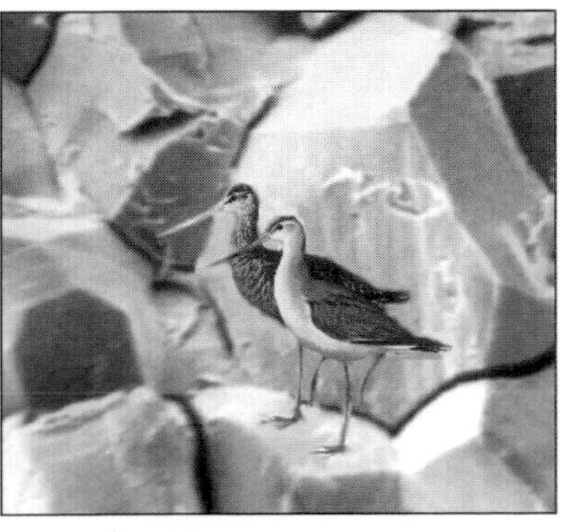

Figure 12. *Hudsonian Godwits searching for a nesting site on an SEM image of an alumina fracture surface.*

of image overlays and combinations common in printing, advertising, and commercial graphic arts. While rarely suitable for scientific applications, this example will perhaps serve to remind us that modifying images to create things that are not real is very easy with modern computer technology. This justifies a certain skepticism in examining images, which were once considered iron-clad evidence of the truth.

From pixels to features

The Boolean operations described above deal with individual pixels in the image. For some purposes it is necessary to identify the pixels forming part of a connected whole. As discussed in Chapter 5, it is possible to adopt a convention for touching that is either eight-connected or four-connected for the pixels in a single feature (sometimes referred to as a blob, to indicate that no interpretation of the connected group of pixels has been inferred as representing anything specific in the image). Whichever convention is adopted, grouping pixels into features is an important step.

It is possible to imagine starting with one pixel (any ON pixel, selected at random) and checking its 4 or 8 neighbor positions, labeling each pixel that is ON as part of the same feature, and then iteratively repeating the operation until no neighbors remain. Then a new unlabeled pixel would be chosen and the operation repeated, continuing until every ON pixel in the image was labeled as part of some feature. The usual way of proceeding with this deeply recursive operation is to create a stack to place pixel locations as they are found to be neighbors of already labeled pixels. Pixels are removed from the stack as their neighbors are examined. The process ends when the stack is empty.

It is more efficient to deal with pixels in groups. If the image has already been run-length or chord encoded, as discussed in Chapter 5, then all of the pixels within the chord are known to touch, touching any of them is equivalent to touching all, and the only candidates for touching are those on adjacent lines. This makes possible a very straightforward labeling algorithm that passes one time through the image. Each chord's end points are compared to those of chords in the preceding line; if they touch or overlap (based on a simple comparison of values), the label from the preceding line is attached to this chord. If not, then a new label is used.

If a chord touches two chords in the previous line that had different labels, then the two labels are identified with each other (this handles the bottom of a letter U, for example). All of the occurrences of one label can be changed to the other, either immediately or later. When the pass through the image or the list of chords is complete, all of the chords, and therefore all of the pix-

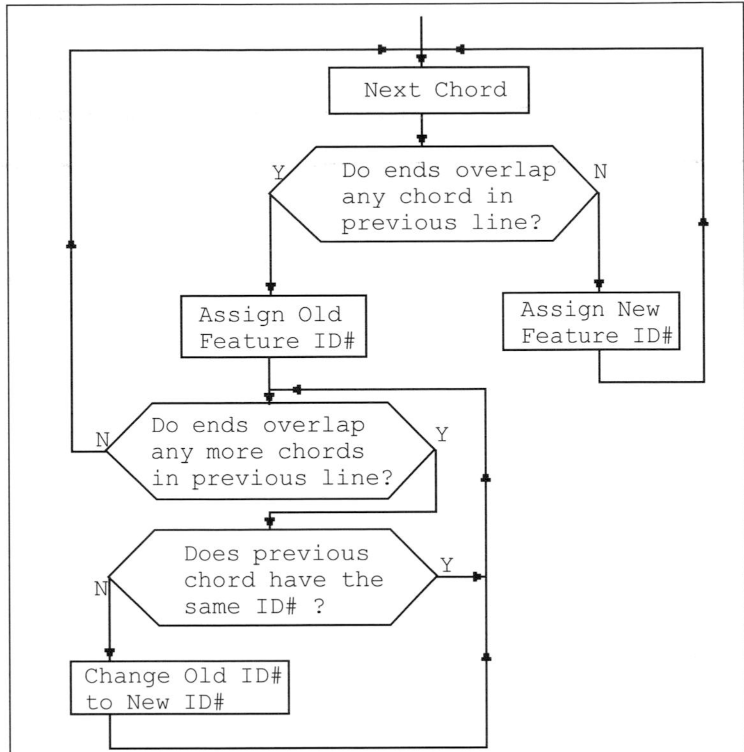

Figure 13. *Flow chart for grouping touching pixels in a run-length or chord-encoded array into features and assigning ID numbers.*

els, are identified and the total number of labels (and therefore features) is known. **Figure 13** shows this logic in the form of a flow chart.

For boundary representation (including the special case of chain code), the analysis is partially completed, since the boundary already represents a closed path around a feature. If features contained no holes and no feature could ever be surrounded by another, it would provide complete information. Unfortunately, this is not always the case. It is usually necessary to reconstruct the pixel array to identify pixels with feature labels.

In any case, once the individual features have been labeled, several additional Boolean operations are possible. One is to find and fill holes within features. Any pixel that is part of a hole is defined as OFF (i.e., part of the background) and is surrounded by ON pixels. For boundary representation, that means the pixel is within a boundary. For pixel representation, it means it is not connected to other pixels eventually forming a path to the edge of the field of view.

Recalling that the convention for touching (eight- or four-connectedness) must be different for the background than for the foreground, we can separate the two most easily by inverting the image (replacing white with black and vice versa) and labeling the resulting pixels as though they were features. Features in this inverted image that do not touch any side of the field of view are

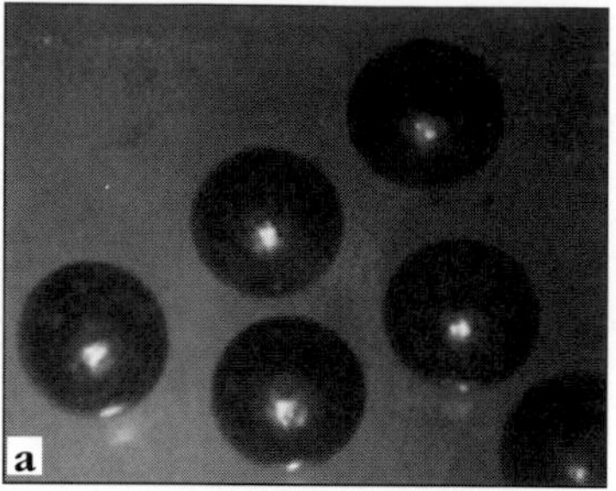

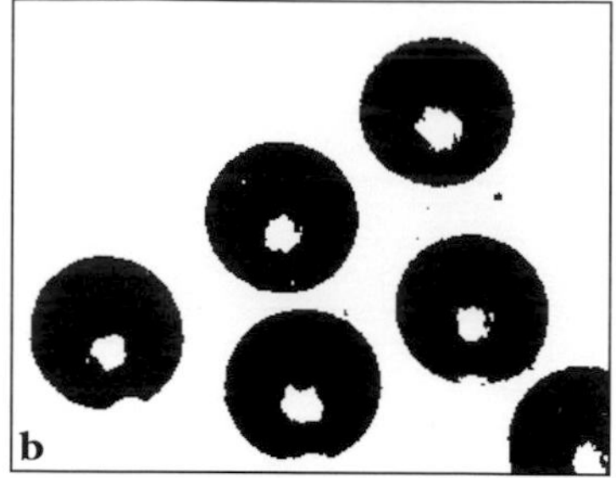

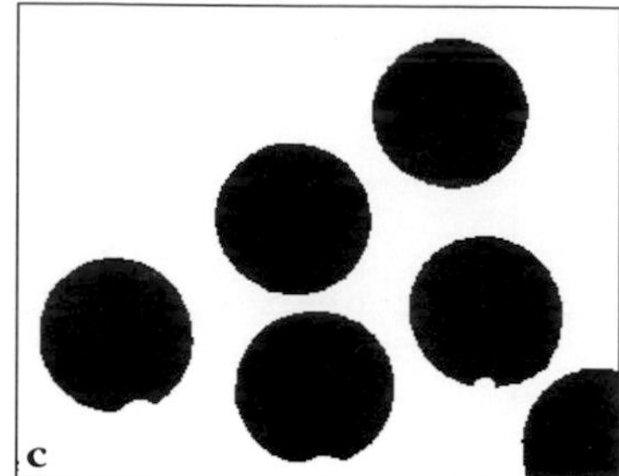

Figure 14. Image of buckshot with near-vertical incident illumination:
a) *original grey scale image;*
b) *brightness thresholded after leveling illumination;*
c) *internal holes filled and small regions (noise) in background removed by erosion.*

the original holes. If the pixels are added back to the original image (using a Boolean OR), the result is to fill any internal holes in the original features.

One very simple example of the application of this technique is shown in **Figure 14.** In this image of spherical particles, the center of each feature has a brightness very close to that of the substrate due to the lighting. Thresholding the brightness values gives a good delineation of the outer boundary of the particles, but the centers have holes. Filling them as described produces a corrected representation of the particles, which can be measured. This type of processing is commonly required for SEM images, whose brightness varies as a function of local surface slope so that particles frequently appear with bright edges and dark centers (see for instance **Figure 48** in Chapter 1).

This problem is not restricted to convex surfaces. **Figure 15** shows a light microscope image of spherical pores in an enamel coating. The light spots in the center of many of the pores vary in brightness, depending on the depth of the pore. They must be corrected by filling the features in a thresholded binary image.

Figure 16 shows a more complicated situation requiring several operations. The SEM image shows the boundaries of the spores clearly to a human viewer, but they cannot be directly revealed by thresholding because the shades of grey are also present in the substrate. Applying an edge-finding algorithm (in this example, a Frei and Chen operator) delineates the boundaries, and it

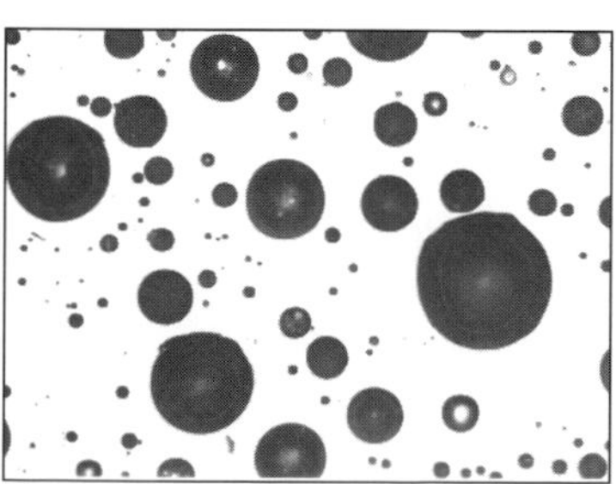

Figure 15. *Light microscope image of a polished section through an enamel coating on steel (courtesy V. Benes, Research Inst. for Metals, Panenské Brezany, Czechoslovakia) shows bright spots of reflected light within many pores (depending on their depth).*

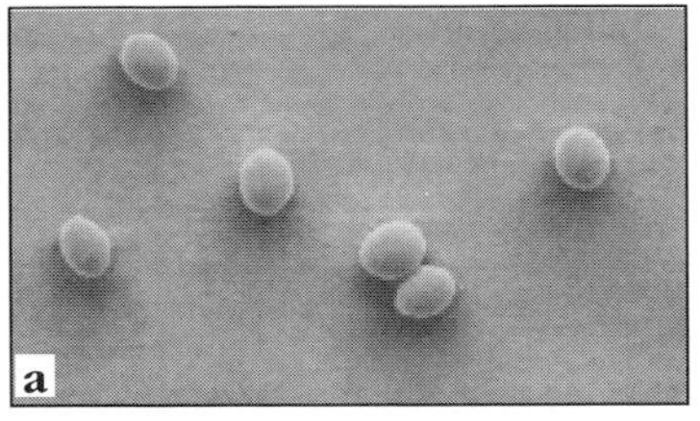

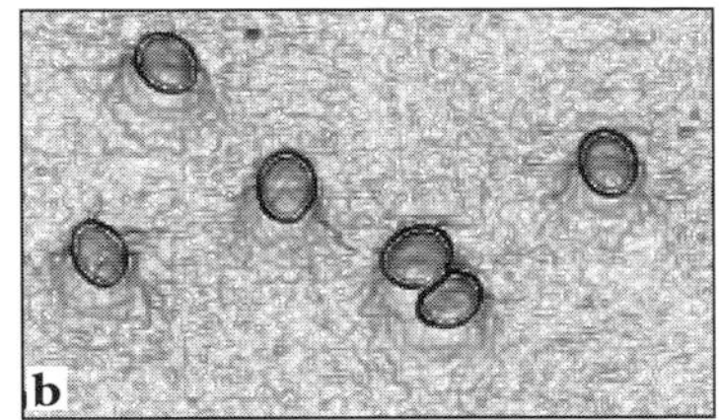

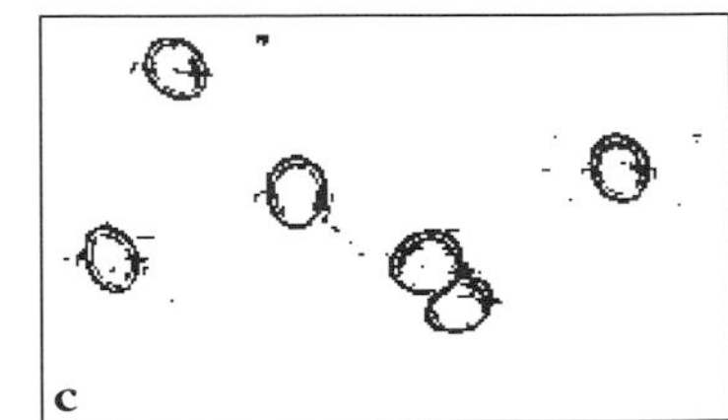

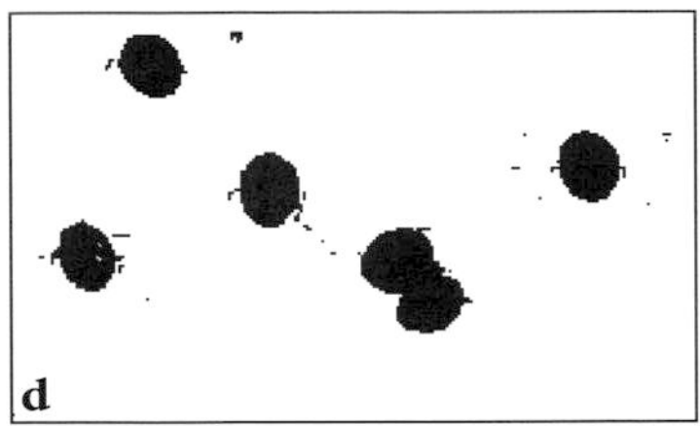

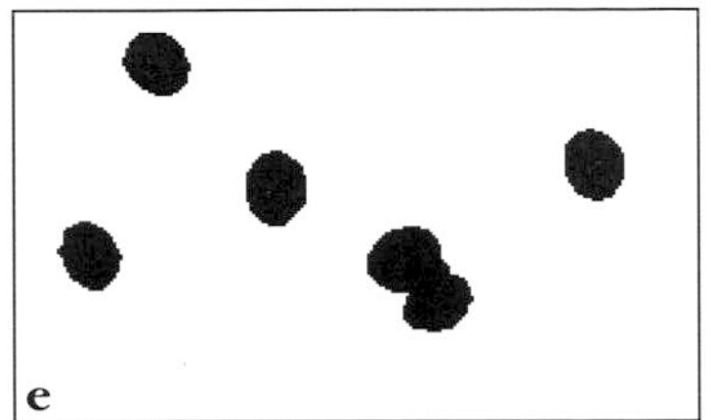

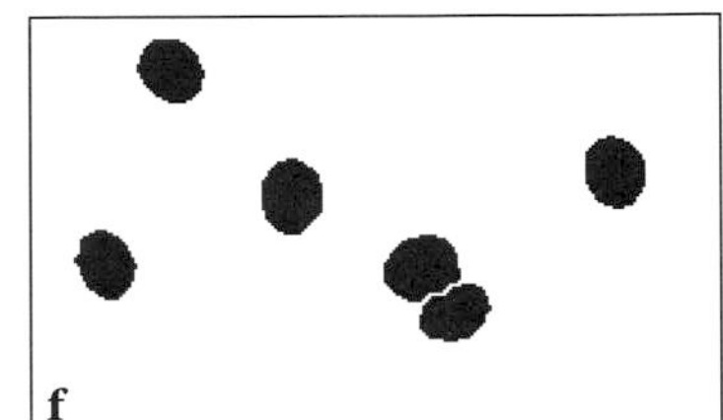

Figure 16. Segmentation of an image using multiple steps:
a) *original SEM image of spores on a glass slide;*
b) *application of a Frei and Chen edge operator to (a);*
c) *thresholding of image (b);*
d) *filling of holes in the binary image of the edges;*
e) *erosion to remove the extraneous pixels in (d);*
f) *watershed segmentation to separate touching features in (e).*

is then possible to threshold them to obtain feature outlines, as shown. These must be filled using the method described above. Further operations are then needed before measurement: erosion, to remove the other thresholded pixels in the image, and watershed segmentation, to separate the touching objects, are both described later in this chapter.

The Boolean AND operation is also widely used to apply measurement templates to images. For instance, consider the measurement of coating thickness on a wire or plate viewed in cross section. We will presume for the moment that the coating can be readily thresholded, but it is not uniform in thickness. In order to obtain a series of discrete thickness values for statistical interpretation, it is easy to AND the binary image of the coating with a template or grid, consisting of lines normal to the coating. **Figure 17** shows a schematic example, both for the case of a flat surface, in which the lines are vertical, and a wire, in which the lines are radial. The AND results in a series of line segments that sample the coating and are easily measured.

Figure 18 illustrates this for an actual case, consisting of coated particles embedded in a metallographic mount and sectioned. In this case, the distribution of the intercept lengths must be interpreted stereologically to measure the actual boundary thickness, since the plane of polish does not go through the center of the particle. Therefore, the coating appears thicker than it actually is. This is handled by a set of random lines in the template. The distribution of line intercept lengths is directly related to that of the coating thickness in the normal direction and the average coating thickness is just 2/3 of the average intercept length.

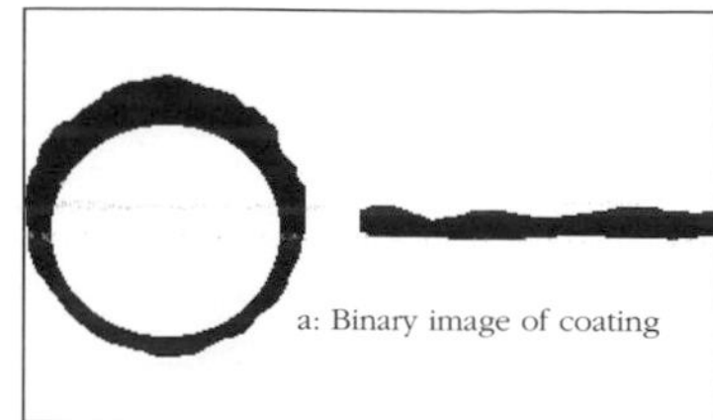

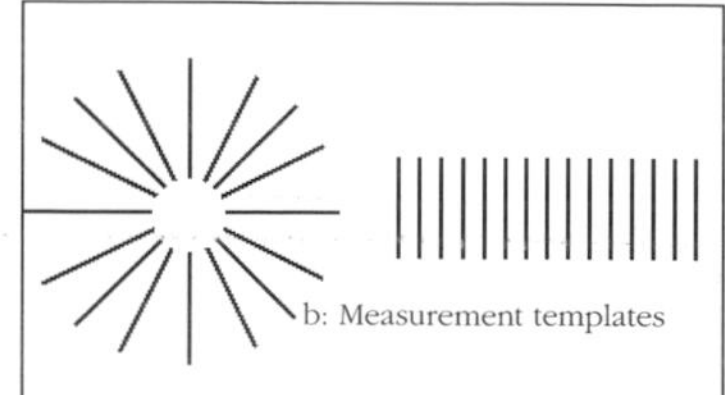

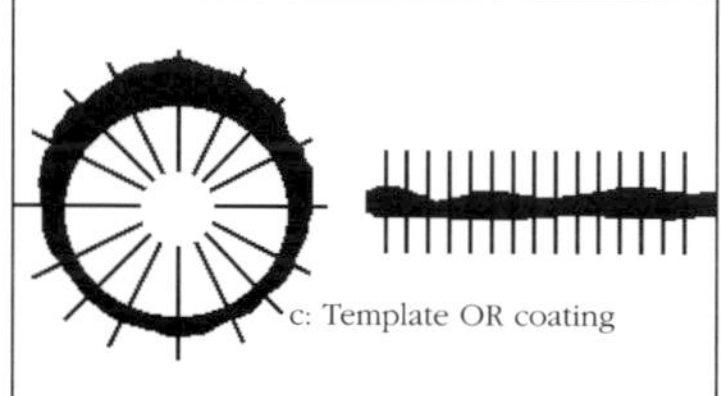

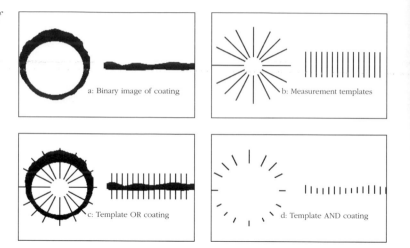

Figure 17. *Schematic diagram of ANDing a measurement template with a binary image of coating on flat or round substrate to obtain a series of line segments which measure the coating thickness.*

Boolean logic with features

Having identified or labeled the pixel groupings as features, it is possible to carry out Boolean logic at the feature level, rather than at the pixel level. **Figure 19** shows the principle of a feature-based AND. Instead of simply keeping the pixels that are common to the two images, entire features are kept if any part of them touches. This preserves the entire feature, so that it can be correctly counted or measured if it is selected by the second image.

This capability can be useful when using X-ray images to select particles in SEM images, for instance if the X-ray signal comes only from the portion of the particle visible to the X-ray detector. The entire particle image can be preserved if any part of it generates an identifying X-ray signal (which may require processing itself, as discussed above in the context of combining images and below in the context of merging isolated spots with dilation).

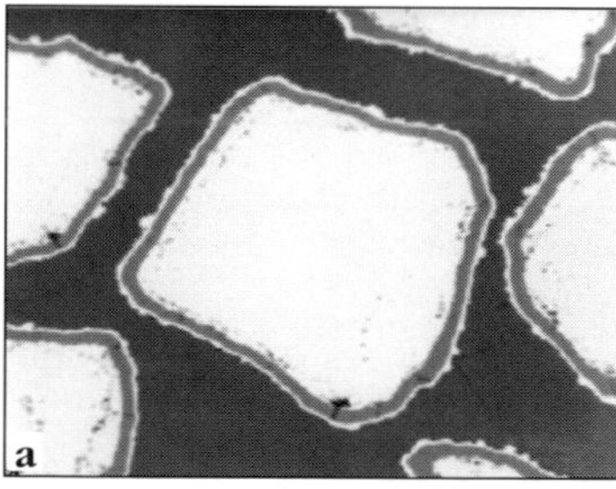

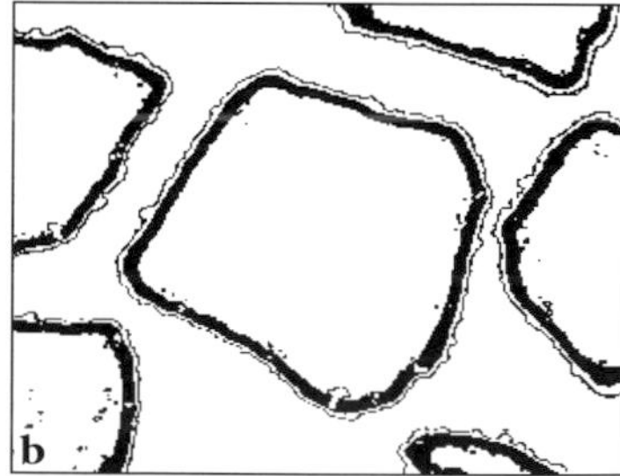

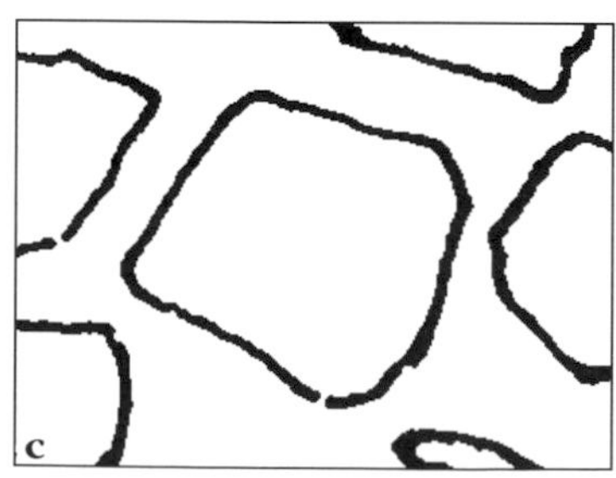

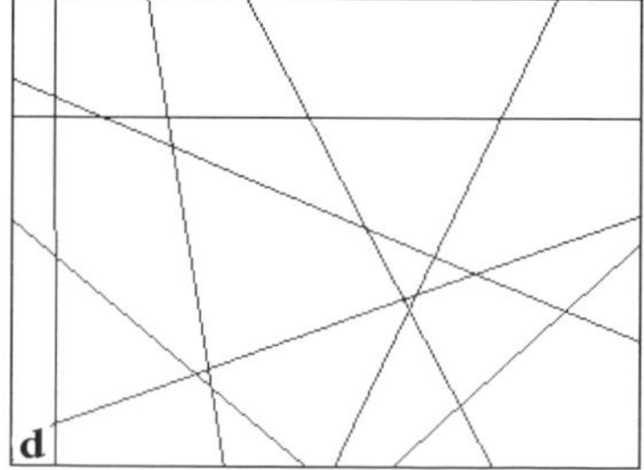

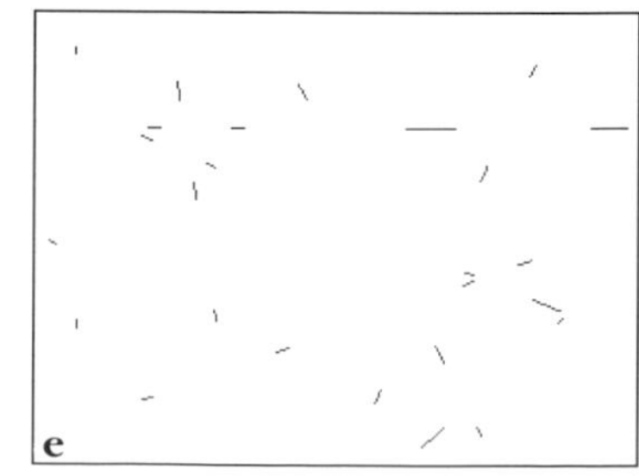

Figure 18. Measuring coating thickness on particles:
a) *original grey scale image of a random section through embedded, coated particles;*
b) *thresholded binary image of the coating of interest (note the additional lines of pixels which straddle the white and dark phase boundary);*
c) *removal of the straddle pixels by application of an opening (coefficient = 4, depth = 4) as discussed later in this chapter;*
d) *template consisting of random lines;*
e) *AND of image (c) and (d) showing line segments whose length distribution gives the actual coating thickness in a normal direction.*

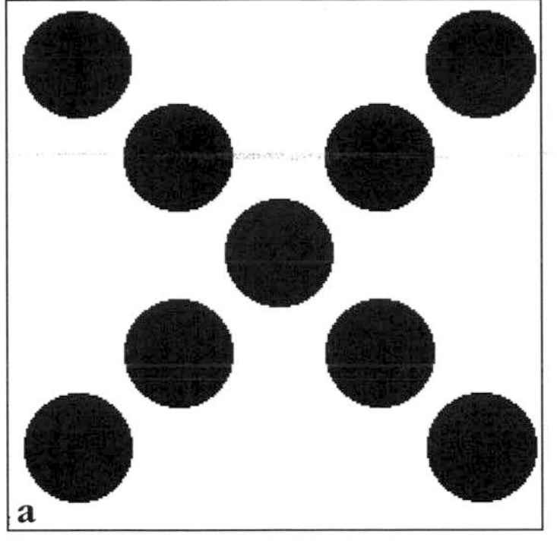

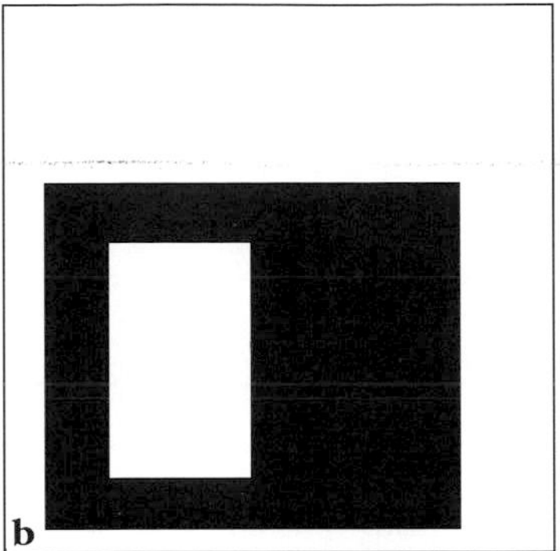

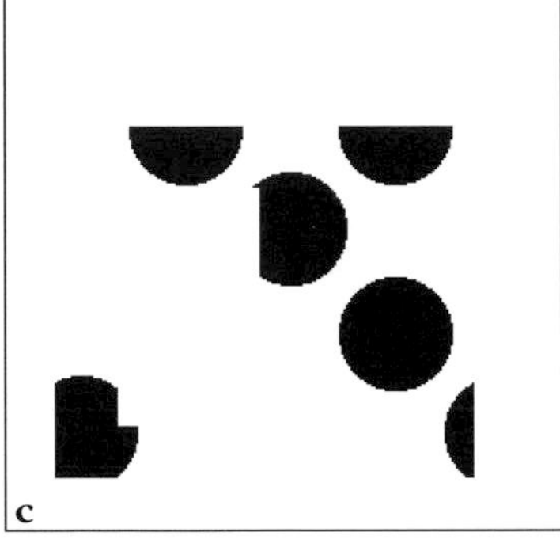

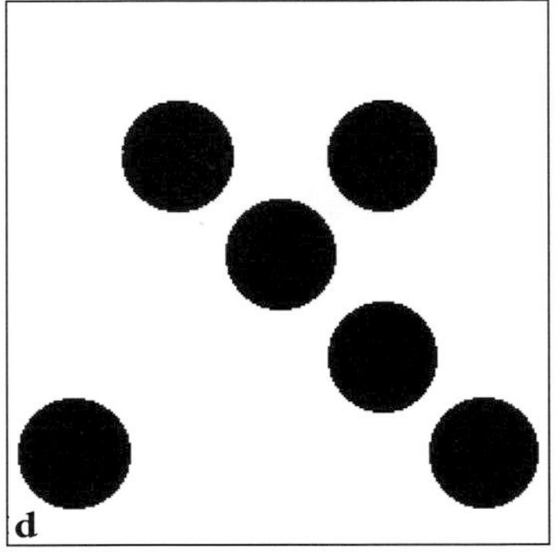

Figure 19. Schematic diagram of feature-based AND:
a, b) *test images;*
c) *pixel-based Boolean AND of images a and b;*
d) *feature-based AND of image a with image b.*

Feature AND is also useful when used in conjunction with images that map regions according to distance. We will see below that dilating a line, such as a grain boundary or cell wall, can produce a broad line of selected thickness. Using this line to select features that touch it selects those features which, regardless of size or shape, come within that distance of the original boundary. Counting these for different thickness lines provides a way to classify or count features as a function of distance from irregular boundaries. **Figure 20** shows a diagram and **Figure 21** shows an actual image measuring grain-boundary depletion.

Figure 22 shows a similar situation, a metallurgical specimen of a plasma-sprayed coating applied to a turbine blade. There is always a certain amount of oxide present in such coatings, which in general causes no difficulties. But if the oxide, which is a readily identifiable shade of grey, is preferentially situated at the coating-substrate interface, it can produce a plane of weakness that may fracture and cause spalling of the coating. Thresholding the image to select the oxide, then ANDing this with the line representing the interface (itself obtained by thresholding the substrate phase, dilating, and Ex-ORing to get the custer, discussed below) gives a direct measurement of the fraction of the contaminated interface.

An aperture or mask image can be used to restrict the analysis of a second image to only those areas within the aperture. Consider

Figure 20. ***Comparison of pixel- and feature-AND:***
a) *diagram of an image containing features and a boundary;*
b) *the boundary line, made thicker by dilation;*
c) *pixel-based AND of image b and a (incomplete features and one divided into two parts);*
d) *feature-AND of image b and a (all features within a specified distance of the boundary).*

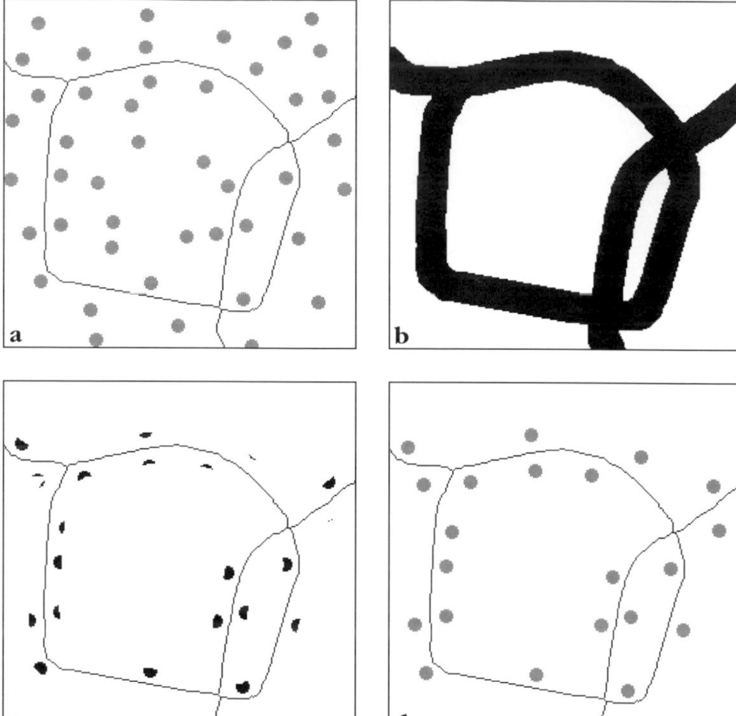

counting spots on a leaf: either spots due to an aerial spraying operation to assess uniformity of coverage, or perhaps spots of fungus or mold to assess the extent of disease. The acquired image is normally rectangular, but the leaf is not. There may well be regions outside the leaf that are similar in brightness to the spots. Creating a binary image of the leaf, then Feature ANDing it with the total image selects those spots lying on the leaf itself. If the spots are small enough, this could be done as a pixel-based AND. However, if the spots can touch the edge of the leaf, the feature-based operation is safer. Counting can then provide the desired information, normally expressed as number-per-unit area, where the area of the leaf forms the denominator.

Figure 23 shows another situation, in which two different

Figure 21. *Light-microscope image of polished section through a steel used at high temperature in boiler tubes. Notice the depletion of carbides (black dots) in the region near grain boundaries. This effect can be measured as discussed in the text.*

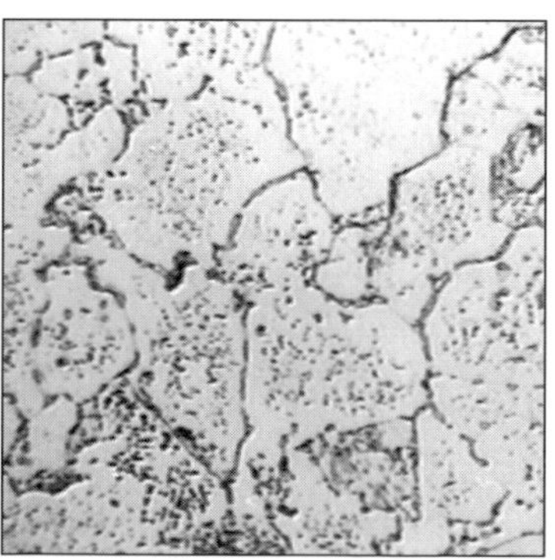

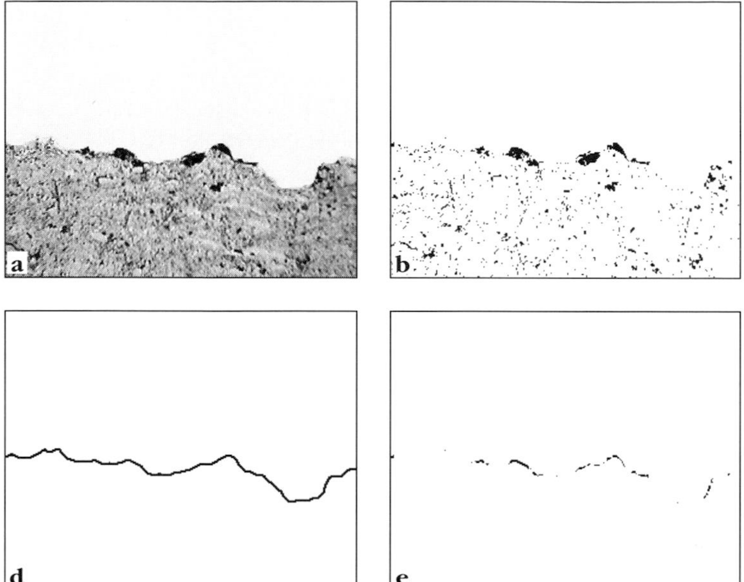

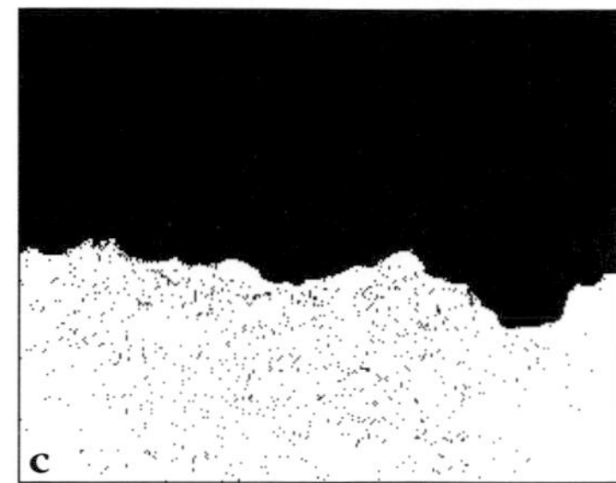

Figure 22. Isolating the oxide in a coating/substrate boundary:
a) *original grey scale microscope image of a cross section of the plasma-sprayed coating (bottom) on steel;*
b) *thresholding of the dark oxide in the coating, including that lying in the interface;*
c) *thresholding of the substrate;*
d) *boundary line obtained by applying an opening (coefficient 3, depth 2) to remove noise pixels, then dilating the binary image (coefficient 0, depth 2) and Ex-ORing the result with the original;*
e) *AND of image d with image b, showing just the fraction of the interface which is occupied by oxide.*

thresholding operations and a logical combination are used to select features of interest. The specimen is a polished cross section of an enamel coating on steel. The two distinct layers are different colored enamels containing different size distributions of spherical pores. Thresholding the darker layer includes several of the pores in the lighter layer, which have the same range of brightness values, but the layer can be selected by discarding features that are small or do not touch both edges of the field. This image then forms a mask, which can be used to select only the pores in the layer of interest. Similar logic can be employed to select the pores in the light layer. Pores along the interface will generally be included in both sets, unless additional feature-based logic is employed.

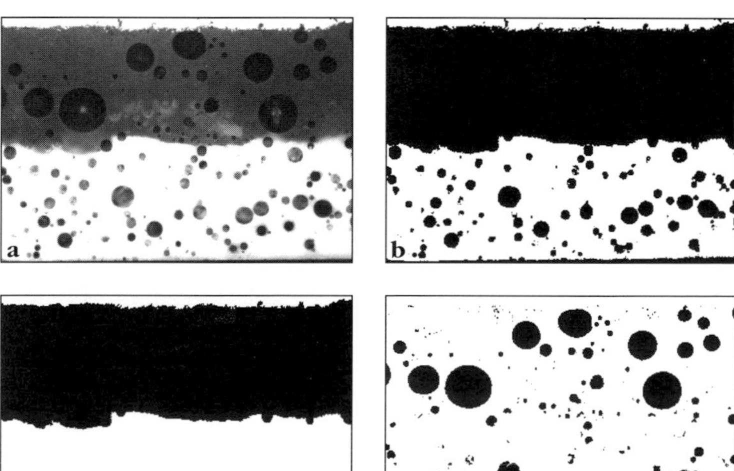

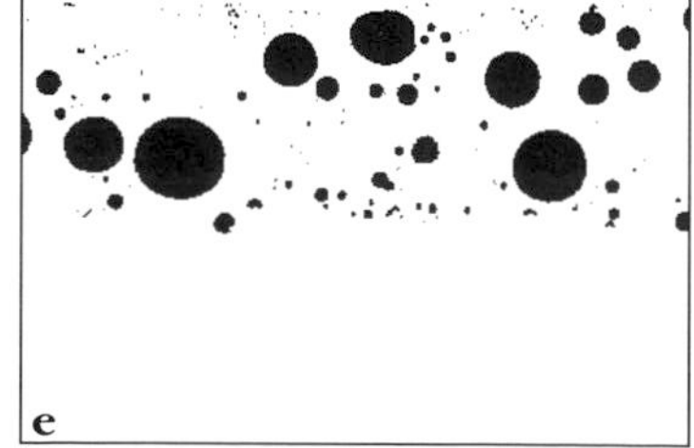

Figure 23. Selecting pores in one layer of enamel on steel:
a) *original light-microscope image (courtesy V. Benes, Research Inst. for Metals, Panenské Brezany, Czechoslovakia);*
b) *image a thresholded to select dark pixels;*
c) *discarding all features from image b which do not extend from one side to the other leaves just the layer of interest;*
d) *thresholding the original image to select only dark pores produces a binary image containing more pores than those in the layer;*
e) *combining images b and d with a Boolean AND leaves only the pores within the dark layer.*

The same Boolean operations (AND, OR, Ex-OR, NOT) used with pixel-based logic can also be used for feature-based combinations. The implementation of these operations is usually performed at the pixel level. Then, the feature label for each pixel is used to restore any pixels within the feature which have been removed. Applications include identifying grains in ores which are contained within other minerals. For instance, they can determine the fraction locked within a harder matrix which cannot easily be recovered by mechanical or chemical treatment, as opposed to those that are not so enclosed and are easily liberated from the matrix. This is often done by creating an image of the matrix phase, filling any holes, and then Ex-ORing that image with one of the desired grains.

Erosion and dilation

The most extensive class of binary image processing operations is sometimes collectively described as morphological operations (Serra, 1982; Coster & Chermant, 1985). These include erosion and dilation, and modifications and combinations of these operations. All are fundamentally neighbor operations, as were discussed in Chapters 2 and 3 to process grey scale images in the spatial domain. Because the values of pixels in the binary images are restricted to 0 or 1, the operations are simpler and usually involve counting rather than weighted multiplication and addition. However, the basic ideas are the same and it is possible to perform these procedures using the same specialized array-processor hardware sometimes employed for grey scale kernel operations.

There is a rich literature, much of it French, in the field of mathematical morphology. It has developed a specific notation for the operations and is generally discussed in terms of set theory. A much simpler and more empirical approach is taken here. Operations can be described simply in terms of adding or removing pixels from the binary image according to certain rules, which depend on the pattern of neighboring pixels. Each operation is performed on each pixel in the original image, using the original pattern of pixels. In practice, this may not need to create an entirely new image, but can replace the existing image in memory by copying out a few lines at a time, though none of the new pixel values are used in evaluating the neighbor pattern.

Erosion removes pixels from an image or, equivalently, turns pixels that were originally ON to OFF. The purpose is to remove pixels that should not be there. The simplest example is pixels that have been selected by thresholding because they fell into the brightness range of interest, but do not lie within the regions of that brightness. Instead, they may have that brightness value either accidentally, because of finite noise in the image, or because they happen to straddle a boundary between a lighter and darker region and thus have an averaged brightness that happens to lie in the range selected by thresholding.

Such pixels cannot be distinguished by simple thresholding because their brightness value is the same as that of the desired regions. It may be possible to ignore them by using two-dimensional thresholding, for instance using the grey level as one axis and the gradient as a second one, and requiring that the pixels to be kept have the desired grey level and a low gradient. However, for our purposes here we will assume that the binary image has already been formed and that extraneous pixels are present.

The simplest kind of erosion, sometimes referred to as classical erosion, is to remove (set to OFF) any pixel touching another pixel that is part of the background (is already OFF). This removes a layer of pixels from around the periphery of all features and regions, which will cause some shrinking of dimensions and may create other problems if it causes a feature to break up into parts. We will deal with these difficulties below. Erosion will also remove extraneous pixels altogether because these defects are normally only a single pixel wide.

Instead of removing pixels from features, a complementary operation known as dilation (or sometimes dilatation) can be used to add pixels. The classical dilation rule, analogous to that for erosion, is to add (set to ON) any background pixel that touches another pixel already part of a region. This will add a layer of pixels around the periphery of all features and regions, which will cause some increase in dimensions and may cause features to merge. It also fills in small holes within features.

Because erosion and dilation cause a reduction or increase in the size of regions, respectively, they are sometimes known as etching and plating or shrinking and growing. There are a variety of rules for deciding which pixels to add or remove and for forming combinations of erosion and dilation.

In the rather simple example described above and illustrated in **Figure 24,** erosion to remove the extraneous lines of pixels between light and dark phases also caused a shrinking of the features. Following the erosion with a dilation will more or less restore the pixels around the feature periphery, so that the dimensions are (approximately) restored. However, isolated pixels that have been completely removed do not cause any new pixels to be added. They have been permanently erased from the image.

Opening and closing

The combination of an erosion followed by a dilation is called an opening, referring to the ability of this combination to open up spaces between just-touching features, as shown in **Figure 25.** It is one of the most commonly used sequences for removing pixel noise from binary images. There are several parameters that can be used to adjust erosion and dilation operations, particularly the

__Figure 24:__ ***Removal of lines of pixels which straddle a boundary:***
a) *original grey scale microscope image of a three-phase metal;*
b) *binary image obtained by thresholding on the intermediate grey phase;*
c) *erosion of image (b) using two steps (coefficient = 0 and coefficient = 1);*
d) *dilation of image (c) using the same coefficients.*

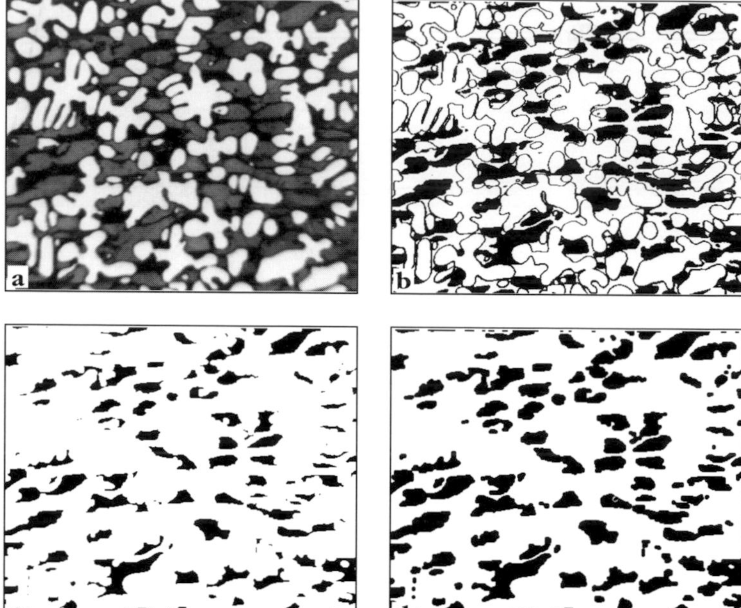

neighbor pattern and the number of iterations, as discussed below. In most opening operations, these are kept the same for both the erosion and the dilation.

In the example shown in **Figure 25,** the features are all similar in size. This makes it possible to continue the erosion until all features have separated but none have been completely erased. After the separation is complete, dilation grows the features back toward their original size. They would merge again unless logic is used to prevent it. A rule that prevents turning a pixel ON if its neighbors belong to different features maintains the separation shown in the figure. This requires performing feature identification for the pixels, so the logic discussed above is required at each step of the dilation.

Notice also that the features do not revert to their original shape during dilation, but instead take on the shape imposed by the neighbor tests (in this case, an octagon). Continuing the dilation beyond the number of erosion cycles to make the features larger than their original size, followed by ANDing with the original to restore the feature outlines, produces an image with the original features separated. If the features had different original sizes, the separation lines would not lie correctly at the junctions. The watershed segmentation technique discussed later in this chapter performs better in such cases.

If the sequence is performed in the other order, that is, a dilation followed by an erosion, the result is not the same. Instead of removing isolated pixels that are ON, the result is to fill in places where isolated pixels are OFF, missing pixels within features or narrow gaps between portions of a feature. **Figure 26** shows an

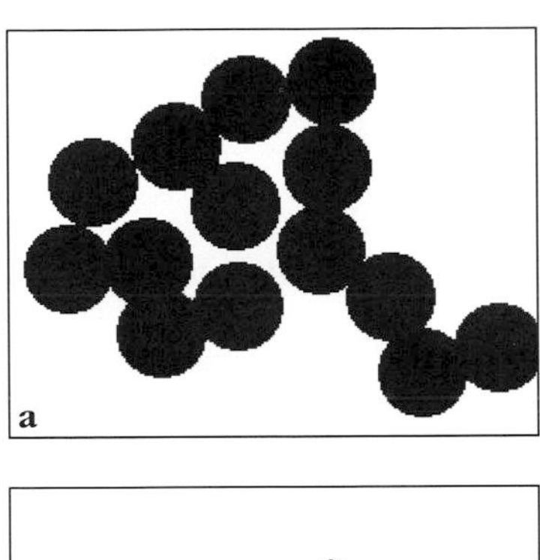
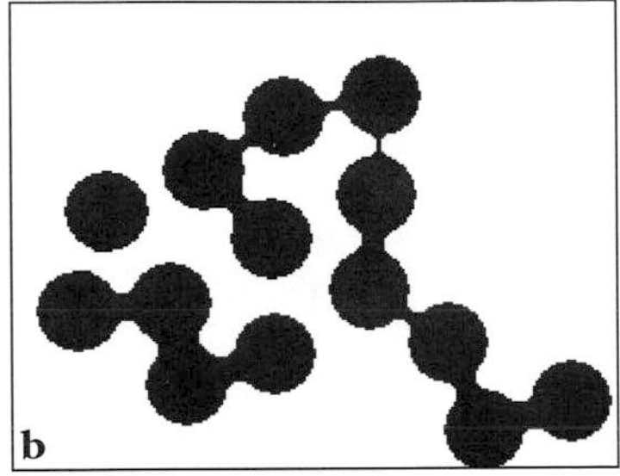
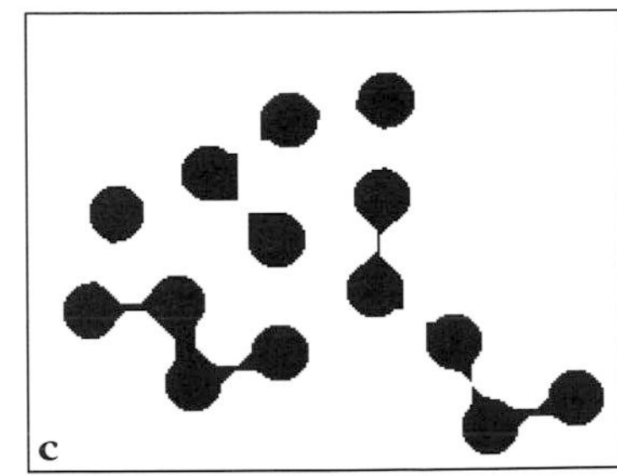
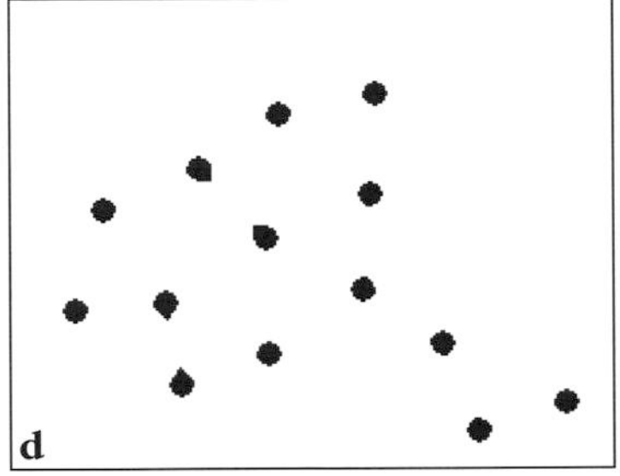
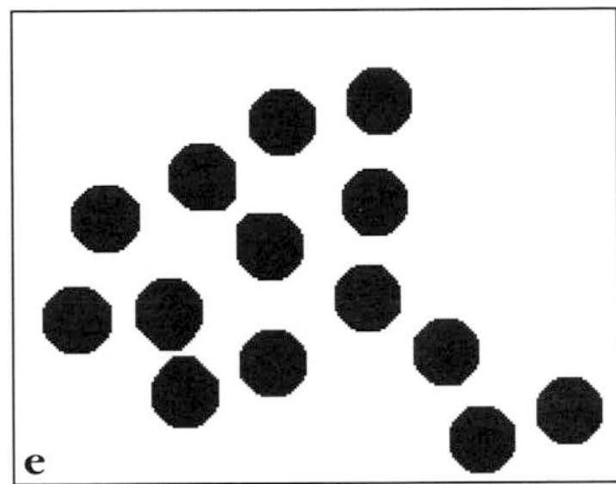
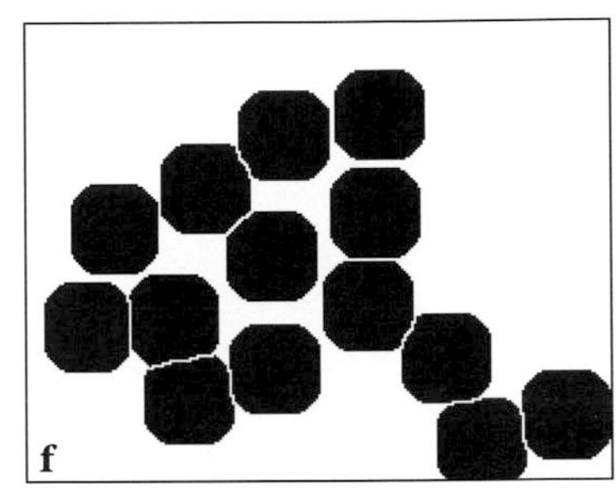
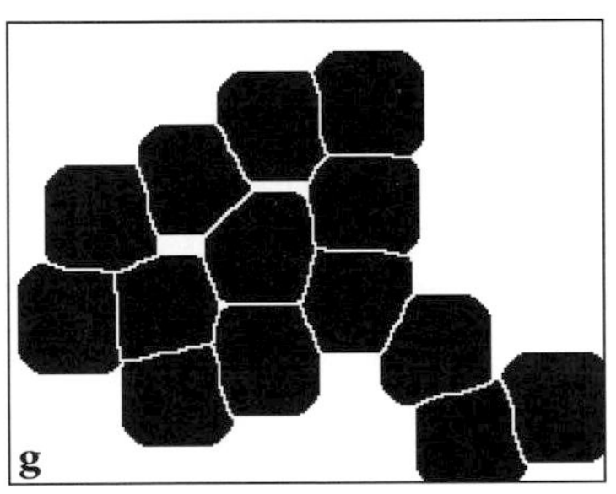
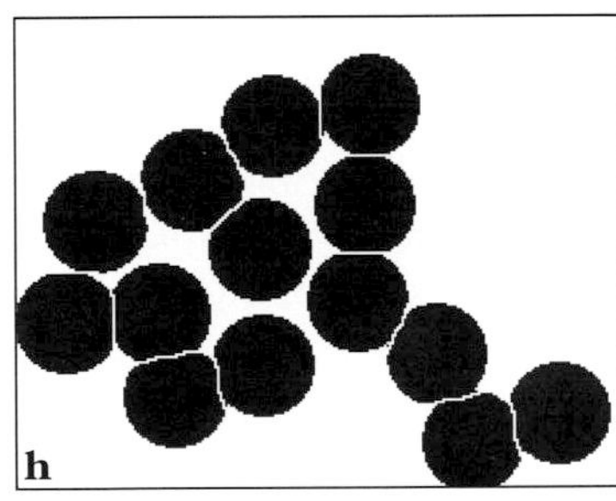

Figure 25. Separation of touching features by erosion/dilation:
a) *original test image;*
b) *after two cycles of erosion, alternating coefficient 0 and 1;*
c) *after four cycles;*
d) *after seven cycles (features are now all fully separated);*
e) *four cycles of dilation applied to image d (features will merge on next cycle);*
f) *seven cycles of dilation using logic to prevent merging of features;*
g) *nine cycles of non-merging dilation (features are larger than original);*
h) *dilated image ANDed with original to restore feature boundaries.*

example. Because of its ability to close up breaks in features, this combination is called a closing. The dilation and erosion operations are usually balanced in closings, as they are in openings.

Figure 27 shows an example of a closing used to connect together the parts of the cracked fibers shown in cross section. The cracks are all narrow, so dilation causes the pixels from either

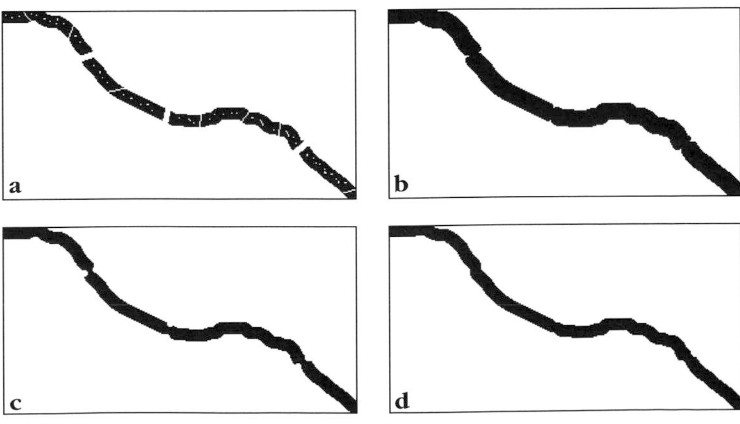

Figure 26. Using closing to connect parts of a broken feature:
a) *original test image;*
b) *application of two cycles of dilation, alternating coefficient 0 and 1;*
c) *application of two cycles of erosion (same coefficients) to image b;*
d) *the result of erosion and dilation with a depth of four cycles, showing more uniform width for the reconstructed line.*

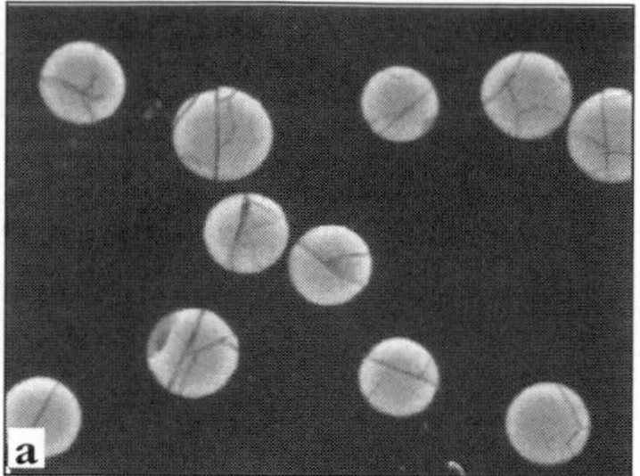
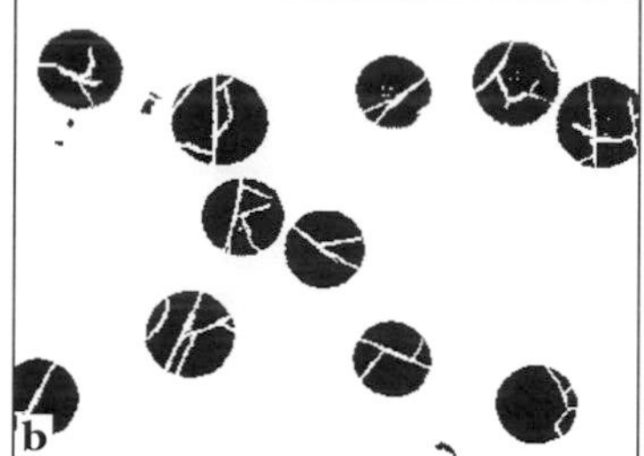
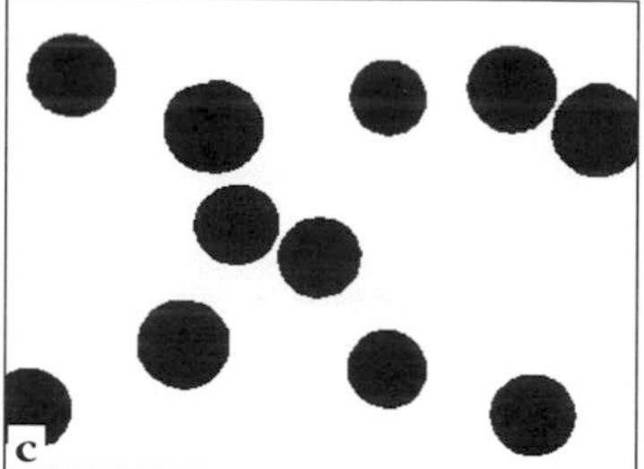

Figure 27. Joining parts of features with a closing:
a) *original image, cross section of cracked glass fibers;*
b) *brightness thresholding, showing divisions within the fibers;*
c) *after application of a closing.*

side to spread across the gap. The increase in fiber diameter is then corrected by an erosion, but the cracks do not reappear, since there are no OFF pixels there.

The classical erosion and dilation operations illustrated above turn a pixel ON or OFF if it touches any pixel in the opposite state. Usually, touching in this context includes any of the adjacent 8 pixels, although some systems deal only with the 4 edge-sharing neighbors. (These operations would also be much simpler and more isotropic on a hexagonal pixel array, but again, practical considerations lead to the general use of a grid of square pixels.)

A wide variety of other rules are possible. One approach is to count the number of neighbor pixels in the opposite state, compare this number to some threshold value, and only change the state of the central pixel if that test coefficient is exceeded. In this method, classic erosion would use a coefficient of zero. One effect of different coefficient values is to alter the rate at which features grow or shrink and to some extent to control the isotropy of the result. This will be illustrated below.

It is also possible to choose a large coefficient, from 5 to 7, to select only the isolated noise pixels and leave most features alone.

Figure 28. Removal of debris from an image:
a) *original image of a pigment cell;*
b) *brightness thresholding shows the pigment granules plus other, small and irregular features;*
c) *erosion (coefficient = 5) leaves the large and regular granules.*

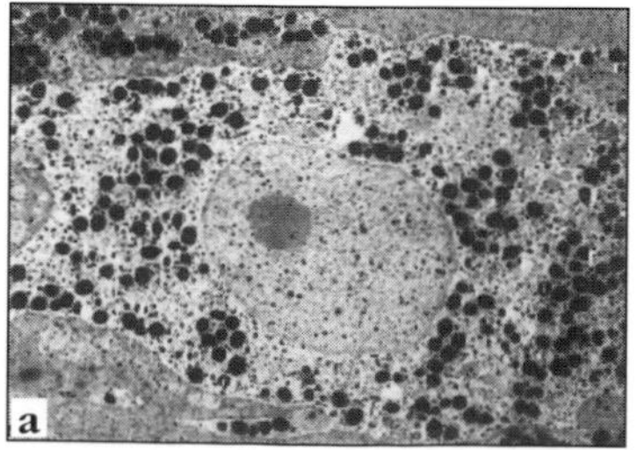
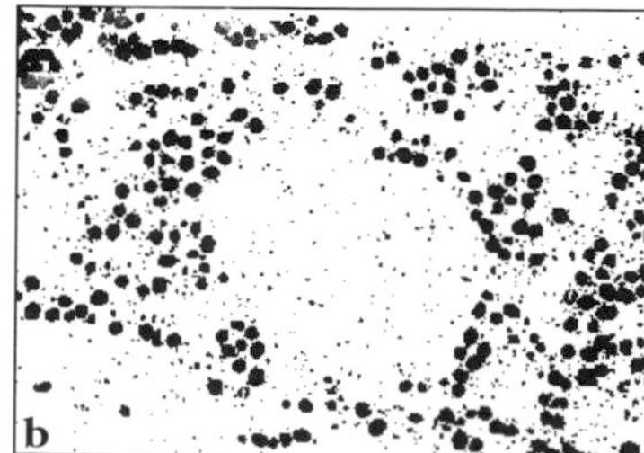
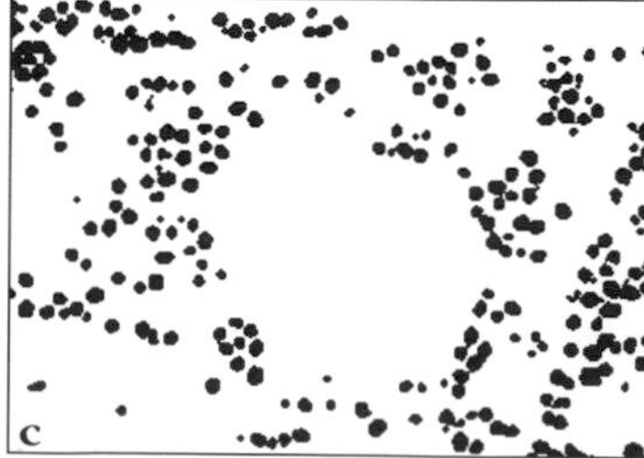

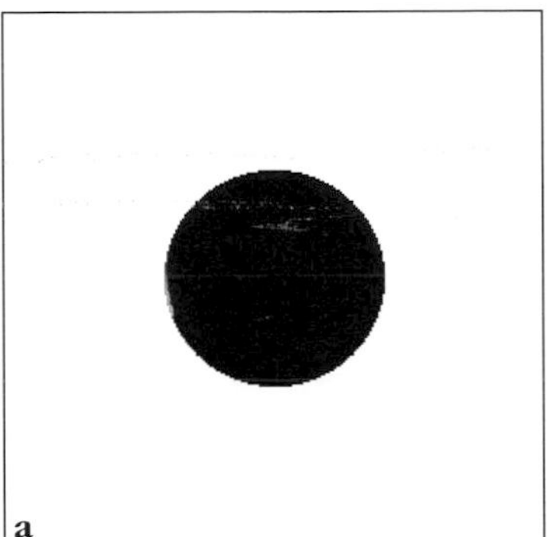

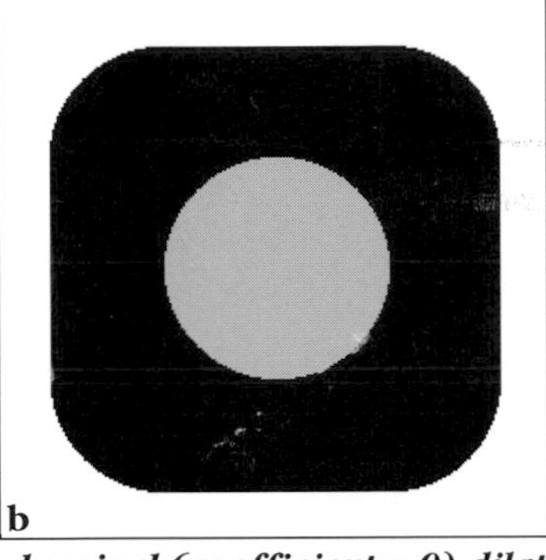

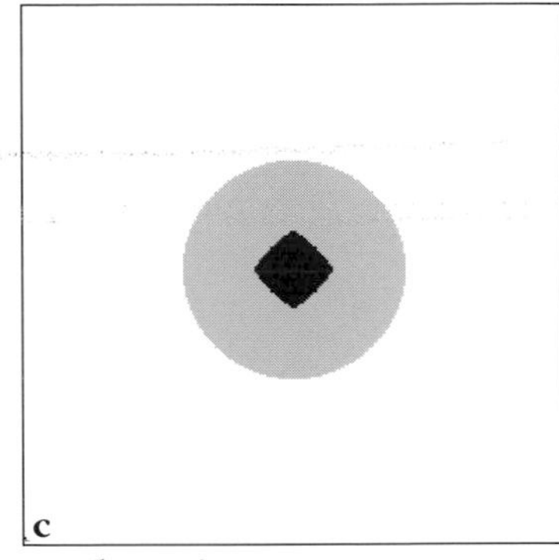

Figure 29. Testing the isotropy of classical (coefficient = 0) dilation and erosion:
***a)** original circle; **b)** after 50 repetitions of dilation; **c)** after 25 repetitions of erosion.*

For example, choosing a coefficient of 7 will cause only single isolated pixels to be reversed (removed or set to OFF in an erosion, vice versa for a dilation). Coefficient values of 5 or 6 may be able to remove lines of pixels (such as those straddling a boundary) without affecting anything else.

An example of this method is shown in **Figure 28**. Thresholding the original image of the pigment cell produces a binary image showing the features of interest and it creates many smaller and irregular groups of pixels. Performing a conventional opening to remove them would also cause the shapes of the larger features to change and some of them to merge. Applying erosion with a coefficient of 5 removes the small and irregular pixel groups, without affecting the larger and more rounded features, as shown. The erosion is repeated until no further changes take place (the number of ON pixels in the binary image does not change). This works because a corner pixel in a square has exactly 5 touching background neighbors and is not removed, while more irregular clusters have pixels with 6 or more background neighbors.

Isotropy

It is not possible for a small 3×3 neighborhood to define a really isotropic neighbor pattern. Classic erosion applied to a circle will not shrink the circle uniformly, but will proceed at a faster rate in the 45° diagonal directions because the pixel spacing is greater in those directions. As a result, a circle will erode toward a diamond shape, as shown in **Figure 29.** Once the feature reaches this shape, it will continue to erode uniformly, preserving the shape. However, in most cases, features are not really diamond shaped, which represents a potentially serious distortion.

Likewise, classic dilation applied to a circle also proceeds faster in the 45° diagonal directions, so that the shape dilates toward a square (also shown in **Figure 29**). Again, square shapes are stable in dilation, but the distortion of real images toward a block

Figure 30. Isotropy tests using a coefficient of 1:
a) the circle after 50 repetitions of dilation;
b) the circle after 25 iterations of erosion.

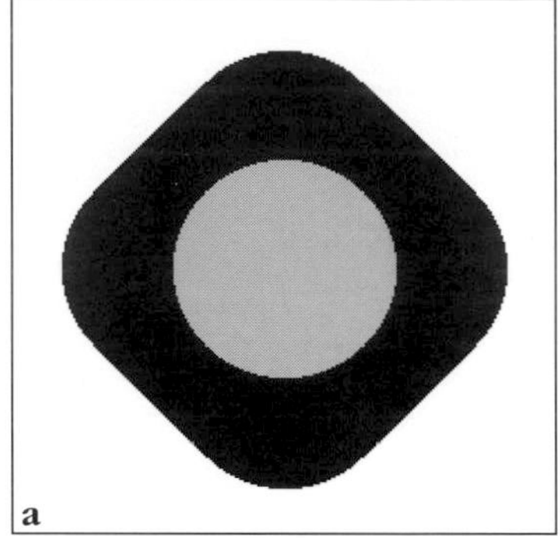

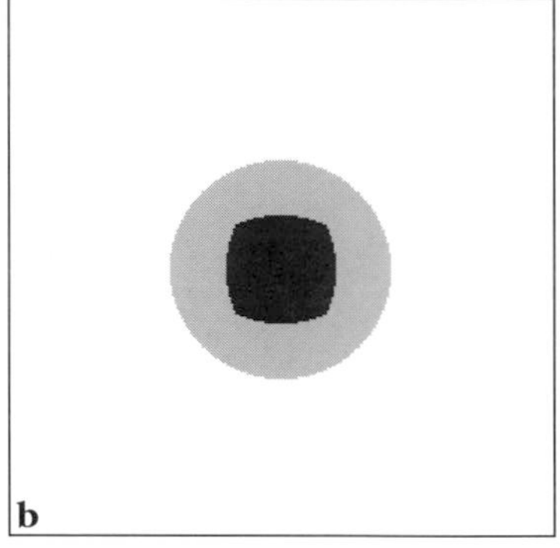

appearance in dilation can present a problem for further interpretation.

Interestingly, a coefficient of 1 instead of 0 produces a very different result. For dilation, a background pixel that touches more than 1 foreground pixel (i.e., 2 or more out of the possible 8 neighbor positions) will be turned ON and vice versa for erosion. Eroding a circle with this procedure tends toward a square and dilation tends toward a circle, just the reverse of using a coefficient of 0. This is shown in **Figure 30.**

There is no possible intermediate value between 0 and 1, since the pixels are counted as either ON or OFF. If the corner pixels were counted as 2 and the edge-touching pixels as 3, it would be possible to design a coefficient that better approximated an isotropic circle. This would produce a ratio of $3/2 = 1.5$, which is a reasonable approximation to $\sqrt{2}$, the distance ratio to the pixels. In practice, this is rarely done because of the convenience of dealing with pixels in binary images as a simple 0 or 1 value.

Another approach that is much more commonly used for achieving an intermediate result between the coefficients of 0 and 1 with their directional bias is to alternate the two tests. As shown in **Figure 31,** this produces a much better circular shape in both erosion and dilation. This raises the idea that erosion or dilation need not be performed only once. The number of repetitions, also called the depth of the operation, corresponds roughly to

Figure 31. Improved isotropy using alternating test coefficients of 0 and 1:
a) the circle after 50 repetitions of dilation;
b) after 25 repetitions of erosion.

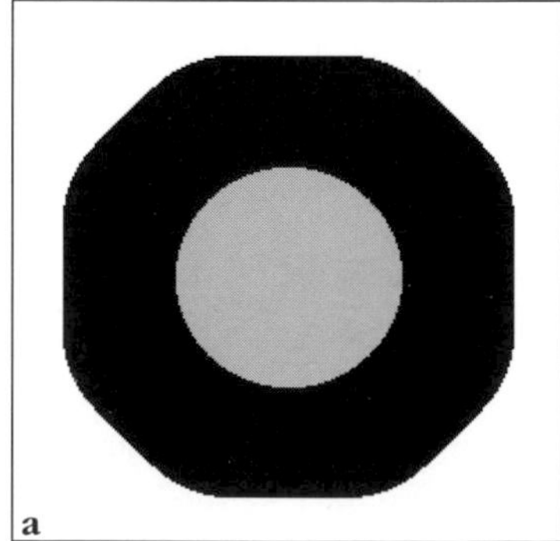

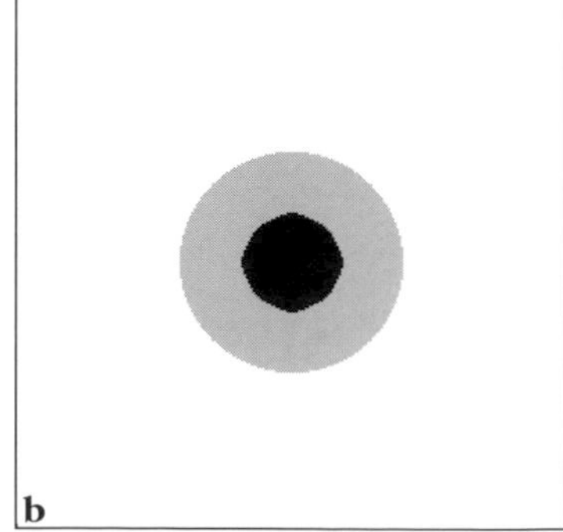

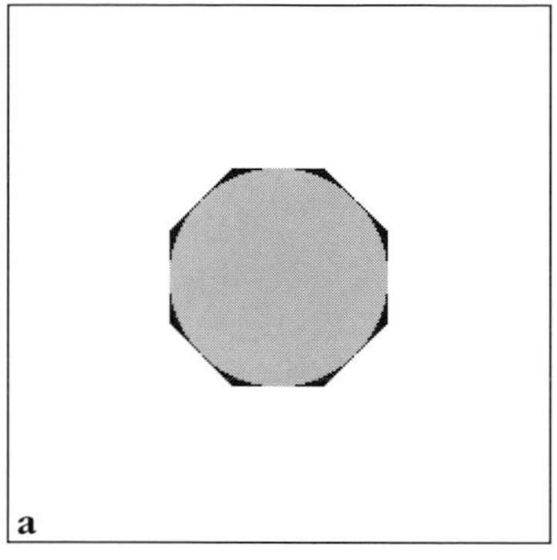

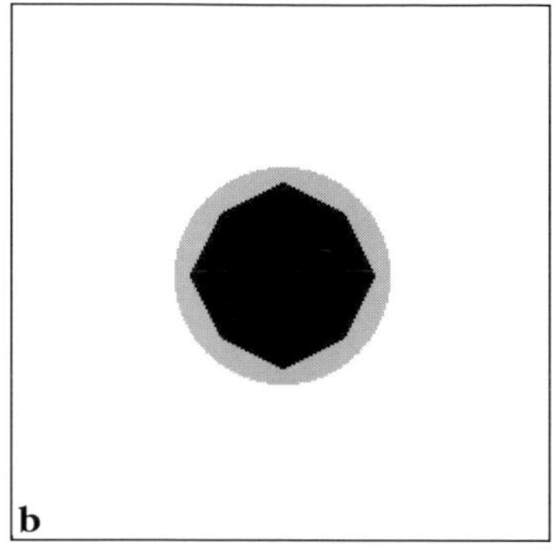

Figure 32. Octagonal shape and slow rate of addition or removal using a coefficient of 3:
a) *original circle after 50 repetitions of dilation (no further changes occur);*
b) *circle after 25 repetitions of erosion.*

the distance that boundaries will grow or shrink radially. It may be expressed in pixels or converted to the corresponding scale dimension.

Each neighbor pattern or coefficient has its own characteristic anisotropy. **Figure 32** shows the rather interesting results using a coefficient of 3. Like an alternating 0,1 pattern, this produces an 8-sided polygon. However, the rate of erosion is much lower, and in dilation the figure grows to the bounding octagon and then becomes stable, with no further pixels being added. This is sometimes used to construct bounding or convex polygons around features.

Measurements using erosion and dilation

Erosion performed n times (using either a coefficient of 0 or 1, or alternating them) will cause features to shrink radially by about n pixels (somewhat depending on the shape of the original feature). This will cause features whose smallest dimension is less than $2n$ pixels to disappear altogether. Counting the features that have disappeared (or subtracting the number that remain from the original) gives an estimate of the number of features smaller than that size. This means that erosion and counting can be used to get an estimate of size distributions without actually performing feature measurements (Ehrlich et al., 1984).

For irregularly shaped and concave features, the erosion process may cause a feature to subdivide into parts. Simply counting the number of features as a function of the number of iterations of erosion is therefore not a good way to determine the size distribution. One approach to this problem is to follow erosion by a dilation with the same coefficient(s) and number of steps. This will merge together many (but not necessarily all) of the separated parts and give a better estimate of their number. However, there is still considerable sensitivity to the shape of the original features. A dumbbell-shaped object will separate into two parts when the handle between the two main parts erodes; they will not merge. This may be desirable, if indeed the purpose is to count the two main parts.

A second method is to use Feature-AND, discussed above. After each iteration of erosion, the remaining features are used to select only those original features that touch them. The count of original features then gives the correct number. This is functionally equivalent to keeping feature labels on each pixel in the image and counting the number of different labels present in the image after each cycle of erosion. This method of estimating size distributions without actually measuring features, using either of these correction techniques, has been particularly applied to measurements in geology, such as mineral particle sizes or sediments.

The opposite operation, performing dilations and counting the number of separate features as a function of the number of steps, seems to be less common. It provides an estimate of the distribution of the nearest distances between features in the image. When this is done by conventional feature measurement, the x,y location of each feature is determined; then sorting in the resulting data file is used to determine the nearest neighbor and its distance. When the features are significantly large compared to their spacing or when their shapes are important, it can be more interesting to characterize the distances between their boundaries. This dilation method can provide that information directly and with less effort.

Instead of counting the number of features that disappear at each iteration of erosion, it is much easier simply to count the number of ON pixels remaining. This provides some information about the shape of the boundaries. Smooth Euclidean boundaries erode at a constant rate. Irregular and especially fractal boundaries do not, since many more pixels are exposed and touch opposite neighbors. This effect has been used to estimate fractal dimensions, although several more accurate methods are available with only a little extra work (one comes from the Euclidean distance map, discussed below).

Fractal dimensions and the description of a boundary as fractal based on a self-similar roughness is a fairly new idea that is finding many applications in science and art (Mandelbrot, 1982; Feder, 1988). No description of the rather interesting background and uses of the concept is included here for want of space. The basic idea behind measuring a fractal dimension by erosion and dilation comes from the Minkowski definition of a fractal boundary dimension. By dilating a region and Ex-ORing the result with another image formed by eroding the region, the pixels along the boundary are obtained. For a minimal depth of erosion and dilation, this will be called the custer and is discussed below.

To measure the fractal dimension, the operation is repeated with different depths of erosion and dilation (Flook, 1978), and the effective width (total number of pixels divided by length and number of cycles) of the boundary is plotted vs. the depth on a log-log scale. For a Euclidean boundary, this plot shows no trend; the number of pixels along the boundary selected by the Ex-OR increases linearly with the number of erosion/dilation cycles. However, for a rough boundary with self-similar fine detail, the graph shows a linear variation on log-log axes whose slope gives the fractal dimension of the boundary directly. **Figure 33** shows an example.

It should perhaps be noted here, for lack of a better place, that another more efficient method for determining the boundary fractal dimension is known as box-counting or mosaic amalgamation (Kaye, 1986; Russ, 1990b). This is quite different from the classical structured walk method (Schwarz & Exner, 1980), which would require the boundary to be represented as a polygon instead of as pixels. The number of pixels through which the boundary passes (for boundary representation) are counted as the pixel size is increased by coarsening the image resolution (combining pixels in 2×2, 3×3, 4×4, ... blocks). For a fractal boundary, this also produces a straight line plot on a log-log scale which is interpreted as in the example above, although technically this is a slightly different fractal dimension.

Counting the number of pixels as a function of dilations also provides a rather indirect measure of feature clustering, since as nearby features merge, the amount of boundary is reduced and the region's rate of growth slows. Counting only the pixels and not the features makes it difficult to separate the effects of boundary shape and feature spacing. If all of the features are initially very small or if they are single points, this method can provide a fractal dimension (technically a Sierpinski fractal) for the clustering.

Extension to grey scale images

In Chapter 3, one of the image processing operations described was the use of a ranking operator, which finds the brightest or darkest pixel in a neighborhood and replaces the central pixel with that value. This operation is sometimes described as a grey scale erosion or dilation, depending on whether the use of the brightest or darkest pixel value results in a growth or shrinkage of the visible features.

Just as an estimate of the distribution of feature sizes can be obtained by eroding of features in a binary image, the same technique is also possible using grey scale erosion on a grey scale image. **Figure 34** shows an example. The lipid spheres in this SEM image are partially piled up and obscure one another, which is normally a critical problem for conventional image-measurement techniques. Applying grey scale erosion reduces the feature sizes and counting the bright central points that disappear at each step of repeated erosion provides a size distribution.

The assumption in this approach is that the features will ultimately separate before disappearing. This works for relatively

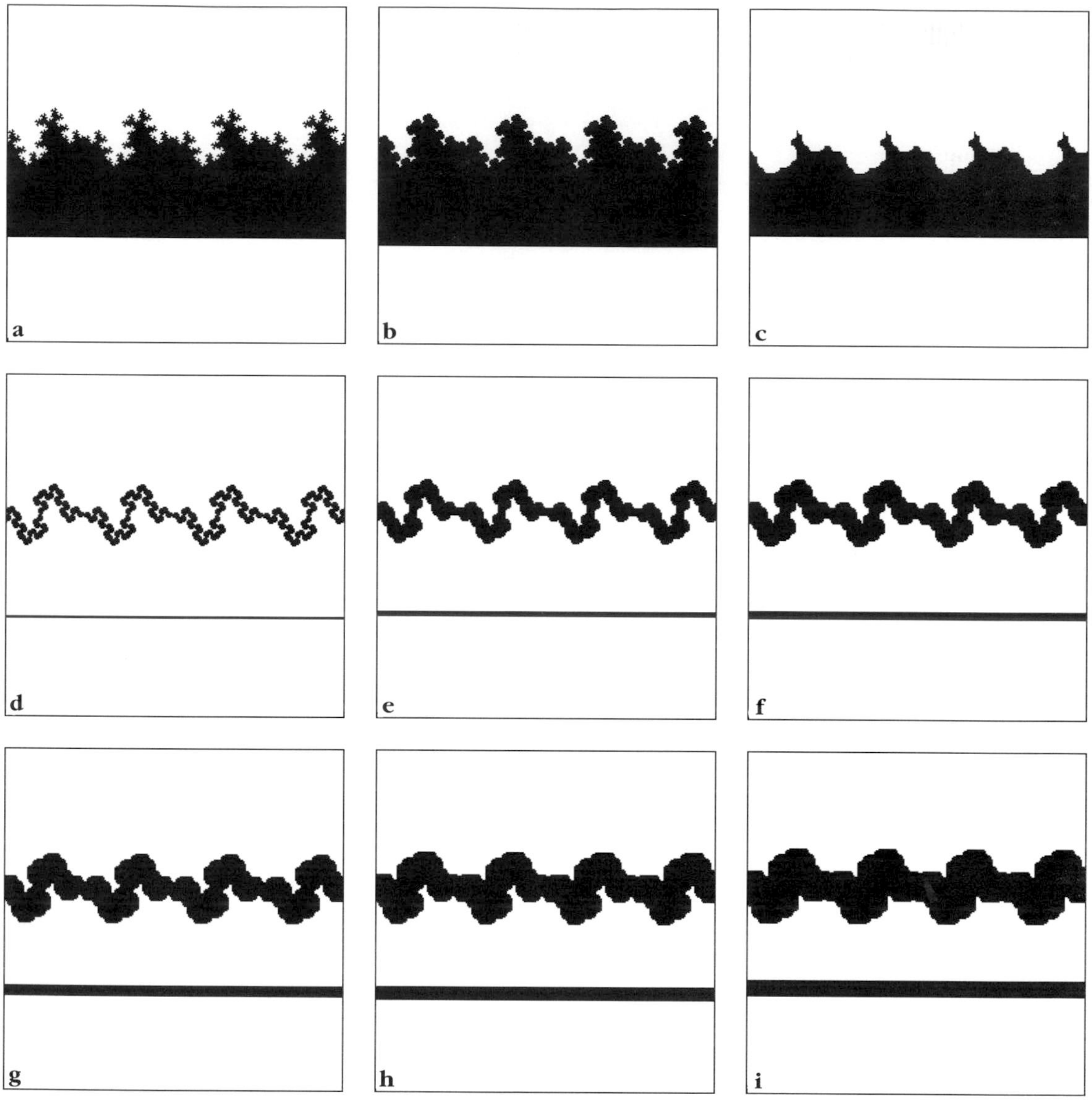

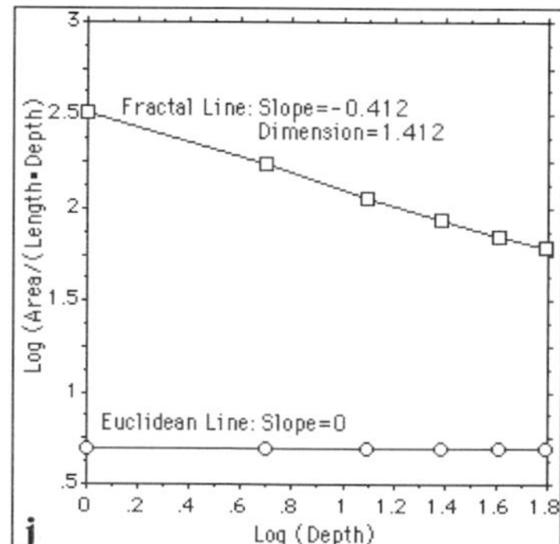

Figure 33. Measurement of Minkowski fractal dimension by erosion/dilation:

a) *test figure with upper boundary a classical Koch fractal and lower boundary a Euclidean straight line;*

b) *dilation of image a (1 cycle, coefficient = 0);*

c) *erosion of image a (1 cycle, coefficient = 0);*

d) *Ex-OR of b and c;*

e) *Ex-OR after 2 cycles;*

f) *Ex-OR after 3 cycles;*

g) *Ex-OR after 4 cycles;*

h) *Ex-OR after 5 cycles;*

i) *Ex-Or after 6 cycles;*

j) *plot of log of effective width (area of Ex-OR divided by length and number of cycles) vs. log of number of cycles.*

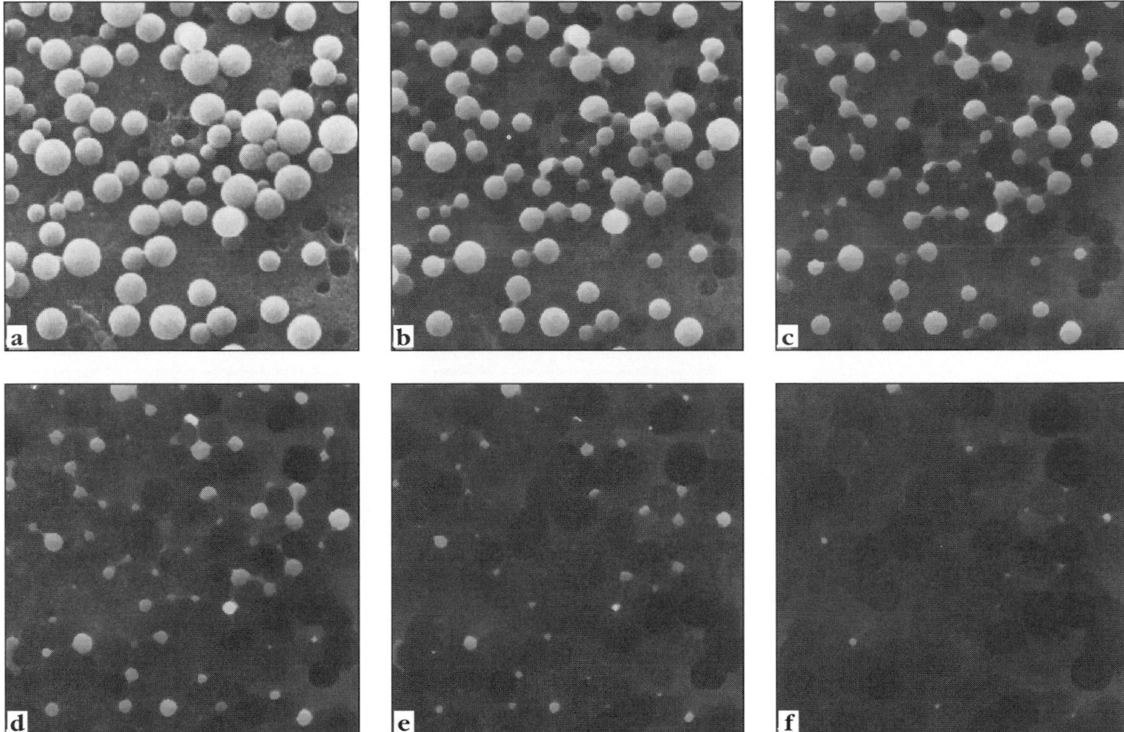

Figure 34. Use of grey scale erosion to estimate size distribution of overlapped spheres:
a) *original SEM image of lipid droplets;*
b) *to* ***f)*** *result of applying 1, 2, 3, 4, and 5 repetitions of grey scale erosion (keeping darkest pixel value in a 5-pixel-wide octagonal neighborhood).*

simple images with well-rounded convex features, none of which are more than about half hidden by others. No direct image processing method can count the number of cannon balls in a pile if the inner ones are hidden. It is possible to estimate the volume of the pile and guess at the maximum number of balls contained, but impossible to know whether they are actually there or whether something else is underneath the topmost layer.

Coefficient and depth parameters

The important parameters for erosion and dilation are the neighborhood comparison test that is used and the number of times the operation is repeated. The use of a simple test coefficient based on the number of neighbors, irrespective of their location in the neighborhood, still provides considerable flexibility in the functioning of the operation. **Figures 35, 36, 37**, and **38** show several examples of erosion, dilation, opening, and closing operations using different coefficients and depths.

Notice that each coefficient produces results having a characteristic shape, which distorts the original features. Also, the greater the depth, or number of iterations in the operation, the greater

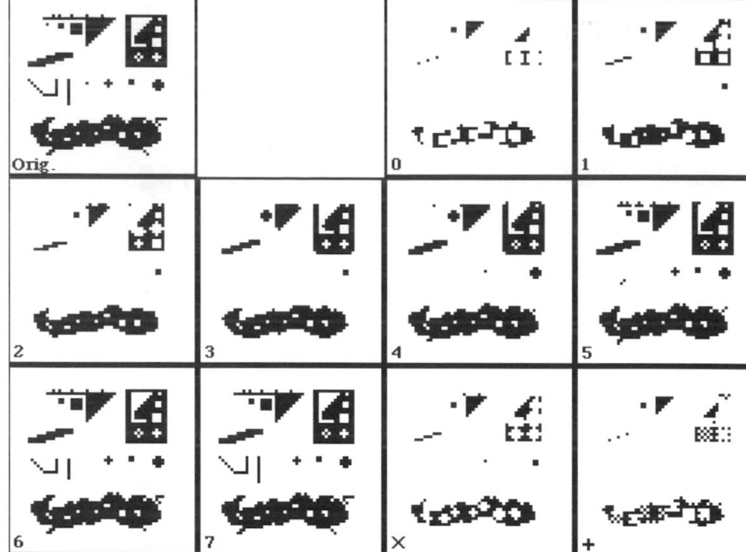

Figure 35. *Effect of changing the neighborhood test in erosion, for coefficient values from 0 (classical erosion) to 7, and matching only to diagonal or orthogonal neighbors. Figure enlarged to show individual pixels.*

this effect, in addition to the changes in the number of features present.

Specific neighbor patterns are also used for erosion and dilation operations. The most common are ones that compare the central pixel to its 4 edge-touching neighbors (usually called a + pattern because of the neighborhood shape) or to the 4 corner-touching neighbors (likewise called an x pattern), changing the central pixel if any of the 4 neighbors is of the opposite type (ON or OFF). They are rarely used alone, but can be employed in an alternating pattern to obtain greater directional uniformity than classical erosion, as discussed above. **Figures 35** to **38** include some representative examples.

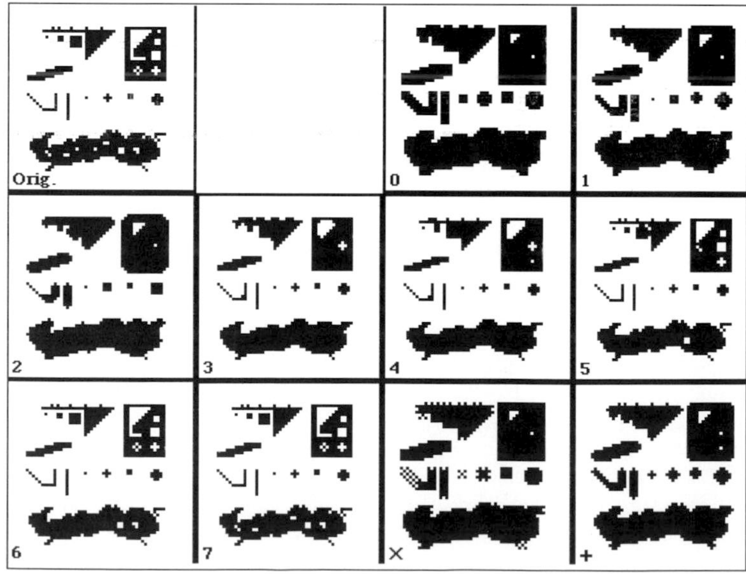

Figure 36. *Effect of changing the neighborhood test in dilation, for coefficient values from 0 (classical dilation) to 7, and matching only to diagonal or orthogonal neighbors. Figure enlarged to show individual pixels.*

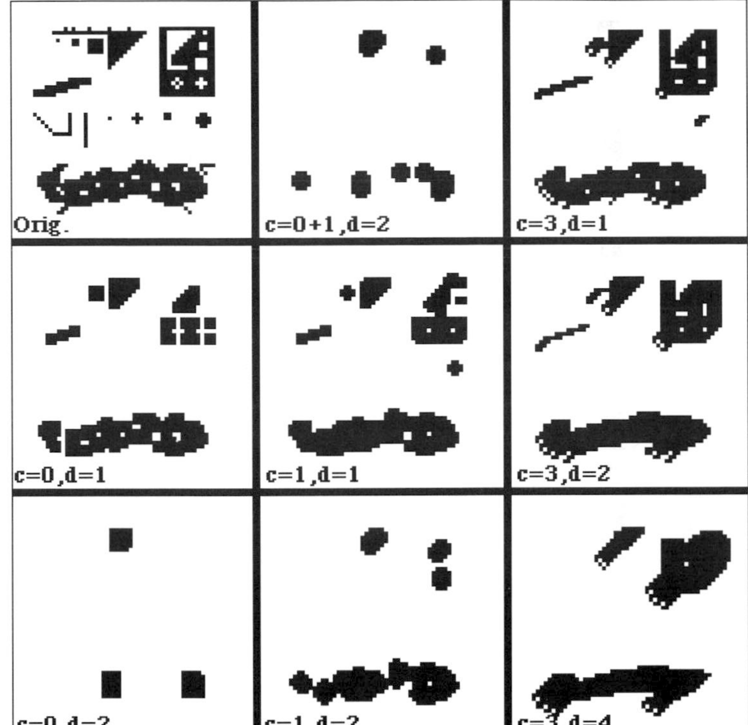

Figure 37. *Effect of changing the parameters in performing an opening: c = test coefficient, d = depth (c = 0 +1 indicates alternating test coefficients). Figure enlarged to show individual pixels.*

Any specific neighbor pattern can be used, of course. It is not even required to restrict the comparison to immediately touching neighbors. As for grey scale operations, larger neighborhoods make it possible to respond to more subtle textures and achieve greater control over directionality. The general case for this type of operation is called the hit-or-miss operator, which specifies any pattern of neighboring pixels divided into three classes:

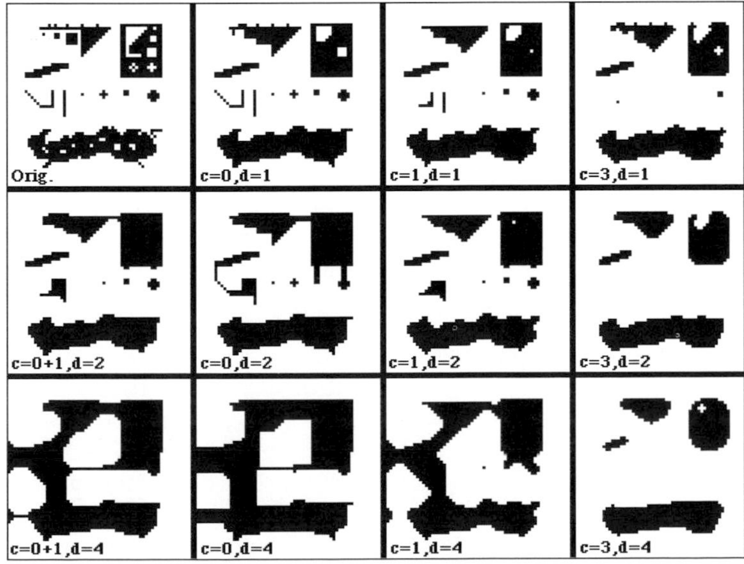

Figure 38. *Effect of changing the parameters in performing a closing: c = test coefficient, d = depth (c = 0 +1 indicates alternating test coefficients). Figure enlarged to show individual pixels.*

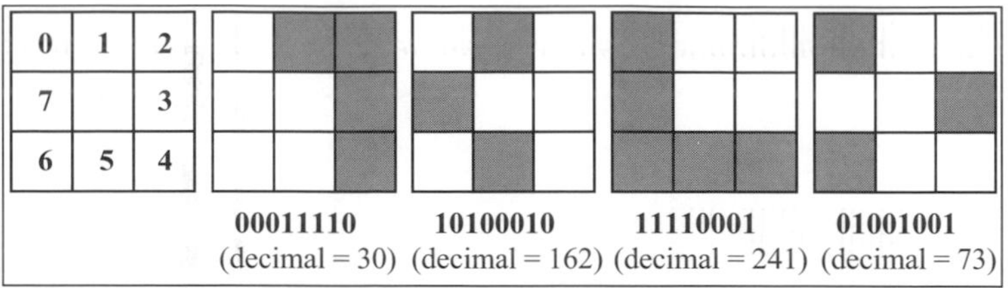

Figure 39. *Constructing an address into a fate table by assigning each neighbor position to a bit value.*

those that must be ON, those that must be OFF, and those that do not matter (are ignored). If the pattern is found, then the pixel is set to the specified state (Serra, 1982; Coster & Chermant, 1985).

This is also called template matching. The same type of operation carried out on grey scale images is called convolution and is a way to search for specific patterns in the image. This is also true for binary images; in fact, template matching with thresholded binary images was one of the earliest methods for optical character reading and is still used for situations in which the character shape, size, and location are tightly controlled (such as the characters at the bottom of bank checks). Much more flexible methods are needed to read more general text, however. In practice, most erosion and dilation is performed using only the 8 nearest-neighbor pixels for comparison.

One method for implementing neighborhood comparison that makes it easy to use any arbitrary pattern of pixels is the fate table. The 8 neighbors in the neighborhood each have a value of 1 or 0, depending on whether the pixel is ON or OFF. Assembling these 8 values into a number produces a single byte, which can have any of 256 possible values. This value is used as an address into a table, which provides the result (i.e., turning the central pixel ON or OFF). **Figure 39** illustrates the relationship between the neighbor pattern and the generated address.

Efficient ways to construct the address by bitwise shifting of values, which takes advantage of the machine-language idiosyncracies of specific computer processors, makes this method very fast. The ability to create several tables of possible fates to deal with different erosion and dilation rules, perhaps saved on disk and loaded as needed, makes the method very flexible. However, it does not generalize well to larger neighborhoods or three-dimensional images (discussed in Chapter 8), because the tables become too large.

There are some applications for highly specific erosion/dilation operations that are not symmetrical or isotropic. These always require some independent knowledge of the image, the desired information, and the selection of operations that will selectively extract it. However, this is not as important a criticism as it may seem, since all image processing is to some extent knowledge-directed. The human observer tries to find operations to extract in-

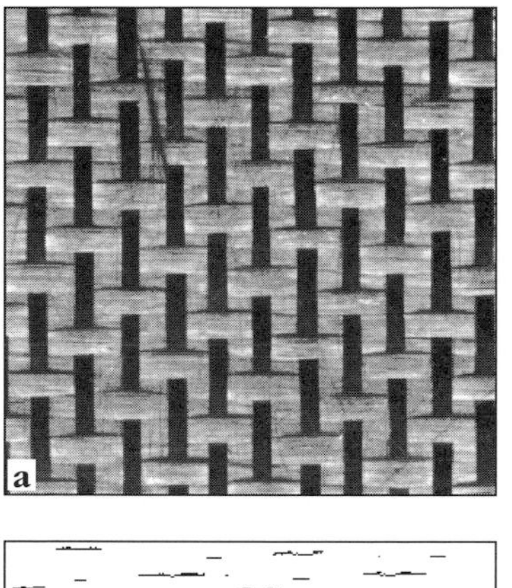

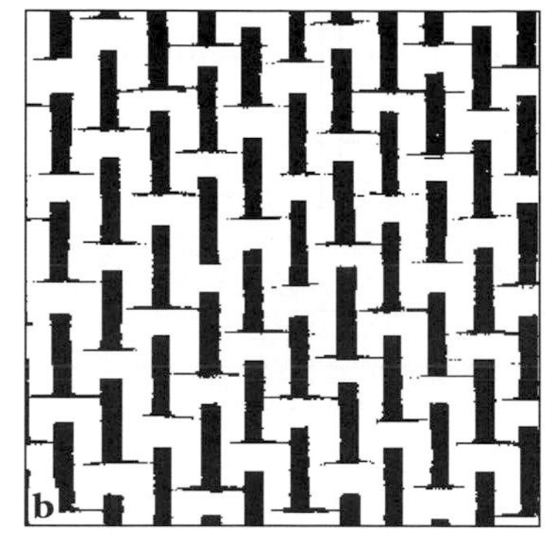

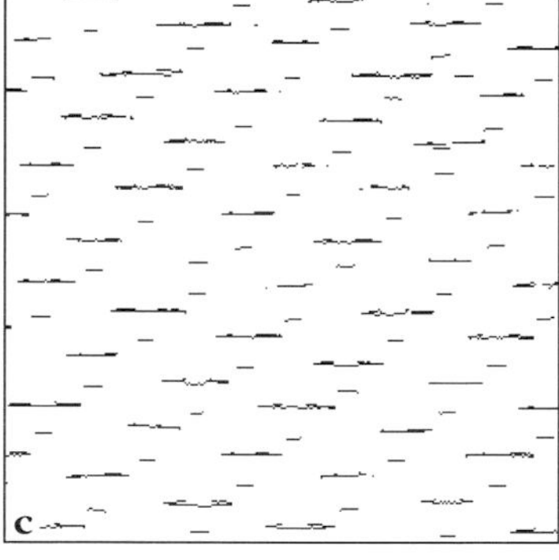

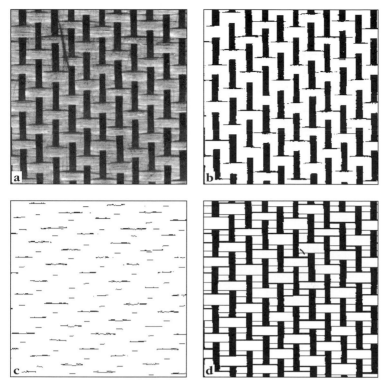

Figure 40. Using directional erosion and dilation to segment an image:
a) *original grey scale image of a woven textile;*
b) *brightness thresholding of image (a);*
c) *end pixels isolated by performing a vertical erosion and Ex-ORing with the original;*
d) *completed operation by repeated horizontal dilation of image (c) and then ORing with the original.*

formation he or she has some reason to know or expect to be present.

Figure 40 shows an example. The horizontal textile fibers vary in width as they weave above and below the vertical ones. Measuring this variation is important to modeling the mechanical properties of the weave, which will be embedded into a composite. The dark vertical fibers can be thresholded based on brightness, but delineating the horizontal fibers is very difficult. The procedure shown in the figure uses the known directionality of the structure.

After thresholding the dark fibers, an erosion is performed to remove only those pixels whose neighbor immediately below or above is part of the background. These pixels, shown in **Figure 40c**, can then be isolated by performing an Ex-OR with the original binary. They include the few points distinguishable between horizontal fibers and the ends of the vertical fibers where they are covered by horizontal ones.

Next, a directional dilation is performed in the horizontal direction. Any background pixel whose left or right touching neighbor is ON is itself set to ON and this operation is repeated enough times to extend the lines across the distance between vertical fibers. Finally, the resulting horizontal lines are ORed with the original binary image to outline all of the individual fibers (**Figure 40d**). Inverting this image produces measurable features.

__Figure 41. X-ray "dot" maps from the SEM:__

a) *backscattered electron image of a gold grid above an aluminum stub;*

b) *secondary electron image;*

c) *gold X-ray dot image;*

d) *aluminum X-ray image (note shadows of grid).*

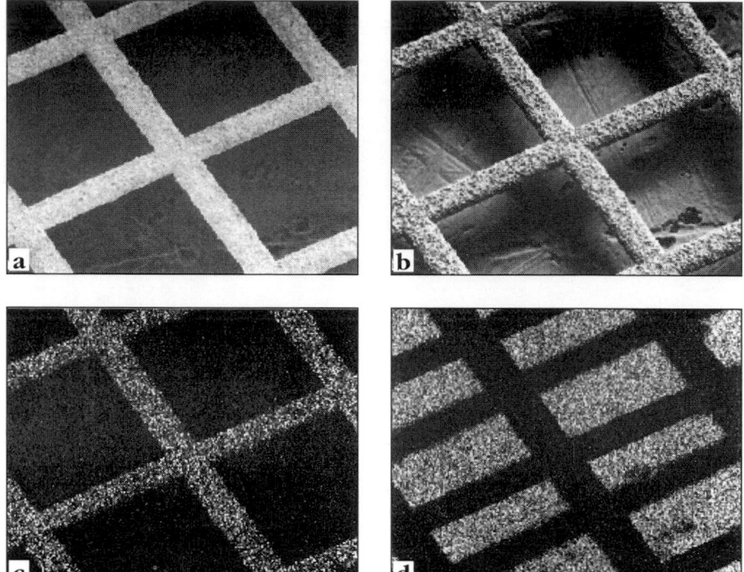

Examples of use

Some additional examples of erosion and dilation operations will illustrate typical applications and methods. One of the major areas of use is for X-ray maps from the SEM. These are usually so sparse that even though they are recorded as grey scale images, they are virtually binary images even before thresholding because most pixels have zero photons and a few pixels have one photon. Regions containing the element of interest are distinguished from those that do not by a difference in the spatial density of dots, which humans are able to interpret by a Gestalt grouping operation. This very noisy and scattered image is difficult to use to locate feature boundaries. Dilation may be able to join points together to produce a more useful representation.

Figure 41 shows a representative X-ray map from an SEM. Notice that the dark bands in the aluminum dot map represent the

__Figure 42. Delineating the gold grid:__

a) *thresholded X-ray map;*

b) *image a after 2 repetitions of closing, alternating 0 and 1 coefficient;*

c) *the backscattered electron image masked to show the boundaries from image b; notice the approximate location of edges.*

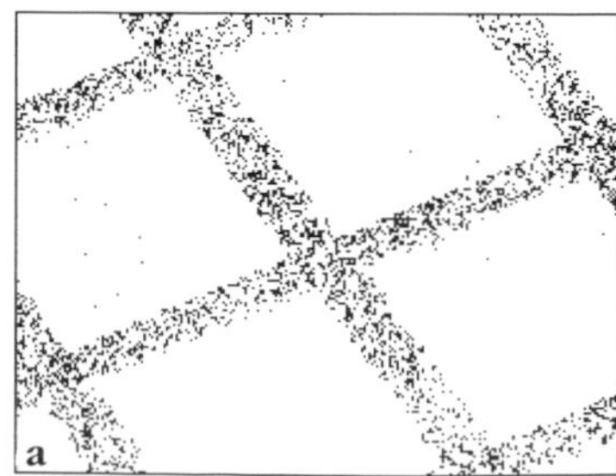

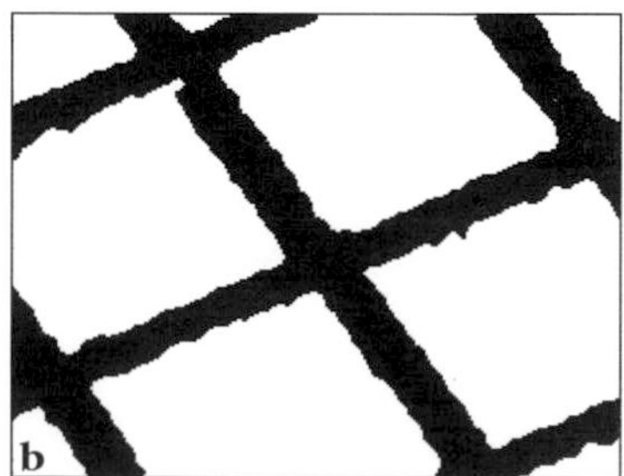

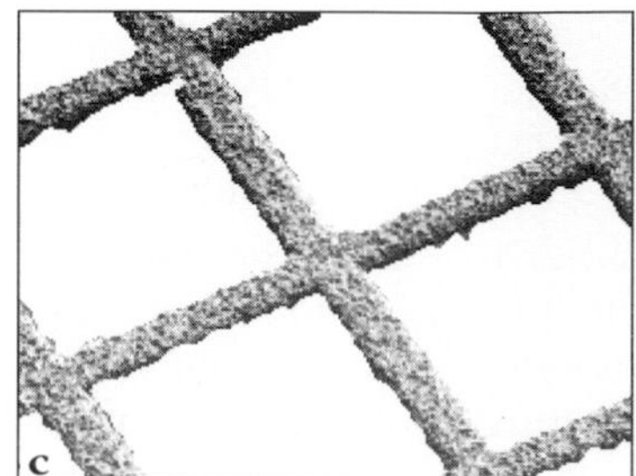

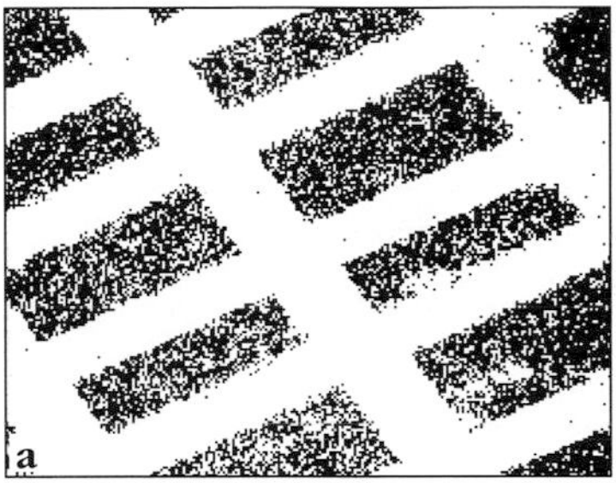

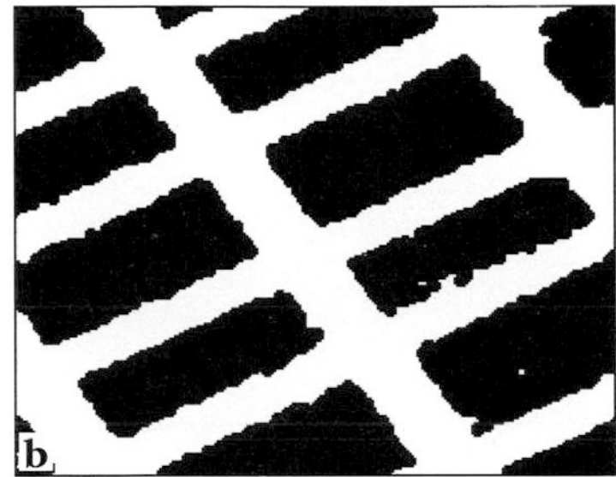

Figure 43. Delineating the aluminum map:
a) *simple thresholding (notice the isolated continuum X-ray pixels within the grids);*
b) *after erosion with a coefficient of 7 to remove the isolated pixels and dilation (2 cycles) with an alternating 0 and 1 coefficient to fill the regions.*

shadows where the gold grid blocks the incident electron beam or the emitted X-rays en route to the detector. **Figure 42** shows the result of thresholding the gold map and applying a closing to merge the individual dots. **Figure 43** illustrates the results for the aluminum map. Because it has more dots, it produces a somewhat better definition of the region edges.

Other images from the light and electron microscope sometimes have the same essentially binary image as well. Examples include ultrathin biological tissue sections stained with heavy metals and viewed in the TEM and chemically etched metallographic specimens. The dark regions are frequently small, corresponding to barely resolved individual particles whose distribution and clustering reveal the desired microstructure (membranes in tissue, eutectic lamellae in metals, etc.) to the eye. As for the case of X-ray dot maps, it is sometimes possible to utilize dilation operations to join such dots to form a well-defined image.

In **Figure 44,** lamellae in a metal are etched and the purpose is to distinguish the regions with and without the lamellae. Dila-

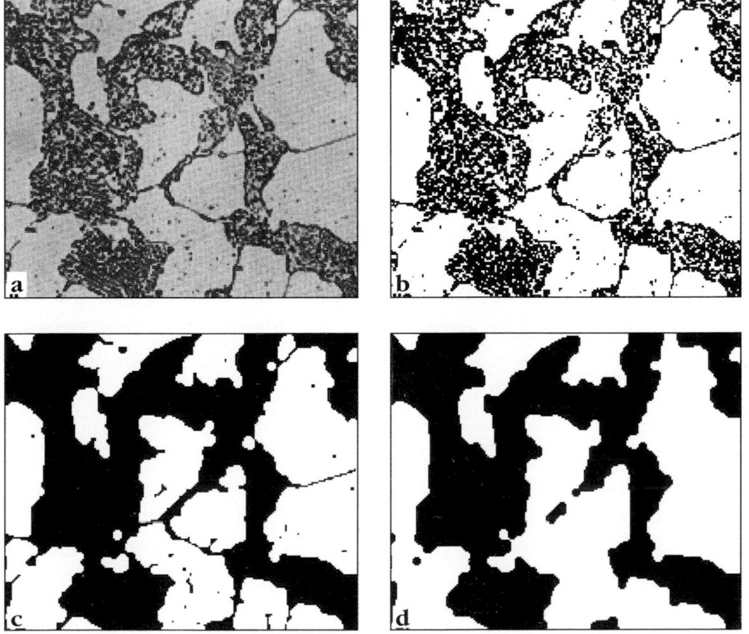

Figure 44. Combined closing and opening to delineate a region:
a) *original grey scale image of chemically etched metallographic specimen;*
b) *brightness threshold applied to image a;*
c) *closing (alternating coefficient 0 and 1, depth = 2) applied to image b;*
d) *opening (same parameters) applied to image c.*

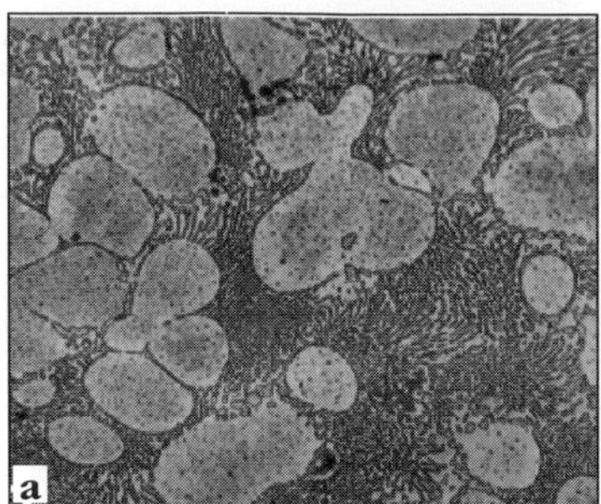

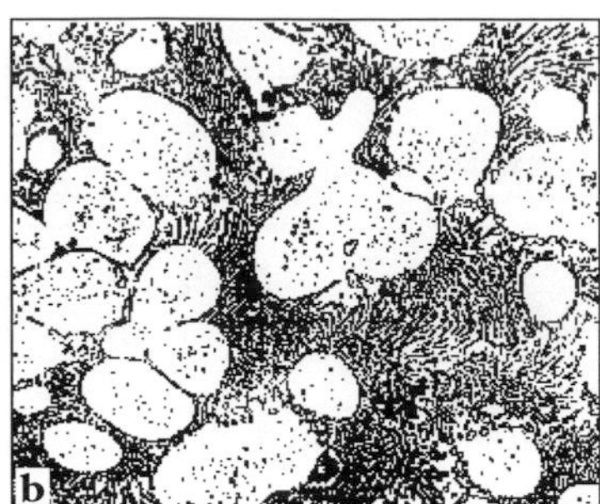

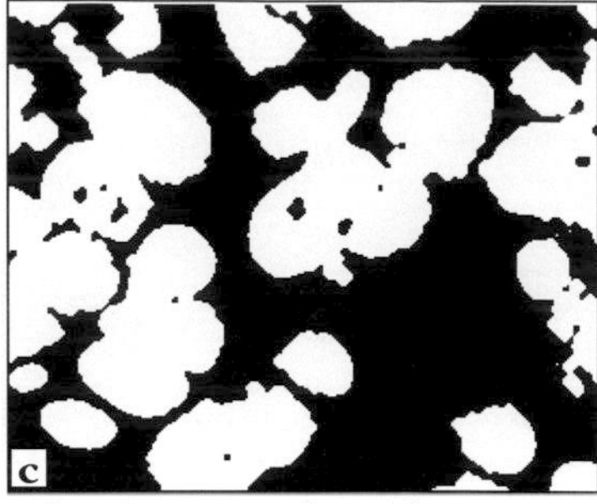

Figure 45. *Another example of combined closing and opening. In this case the closing used an alternating 0,1 coefficient with depth of 2, but the opening used a coefficient of 3 and depth of 4 to remove the small noise spots in the white phase regions.*

tion followed by erosion (a closing) merges together the individual lamellae, but there are also dark regions within the essentially white grains because of the presence of a few dark points in the original image. Following the closing with an opening (for a total sequence of dilation, erosion, erosion, dilation) produces a useful result.

In the example of **Figure 44,** the same coefficients and depths (alternating tests of 0 and 1 neighbors for approximate isotropy and two iterations for each dilation or erosion) were used. There is no fundamental reason for this symmetry. In **Figure 45,** a more difficult image is similarly processed, using different coefficients and depths for the initial closing and the final opening. Of course, the choice of appropriate parameters is largely a matter of experience with a particular type of image and human judgement of the correctness of the final result. In other words, it takes trial and error to produce the image the human saw in the first place.

Notice the basic similarity between using these morphological operations on a thresholded binary image and various texture operators on the original grey scale image. In most cases, equivalent results can be obtained with either approach (provided the available software offers both sets of tools).

Erosion/dilation procedures are often used in combination with Boolean combinations and feature identification and filling. **Figure 46** shows a representative sequence of operations, used in this case to produce a representation of particles in a plasma-sprayed coating. The original grey scale image (**Figure 46a**) shows a polished cross section through a complex, sprayed coating applied to a turbine blade. The dark grey particles with light interiors are hard, wear-resistant materials included to improve coating performance. Thresholding to select dark grey shows the periphery of the particles (**Figure 46b**), but does not include their central cores, which have the same average brightness as the matrix. Some of the particles do not show these cores, because the plane of sectioning has not passed through the core.

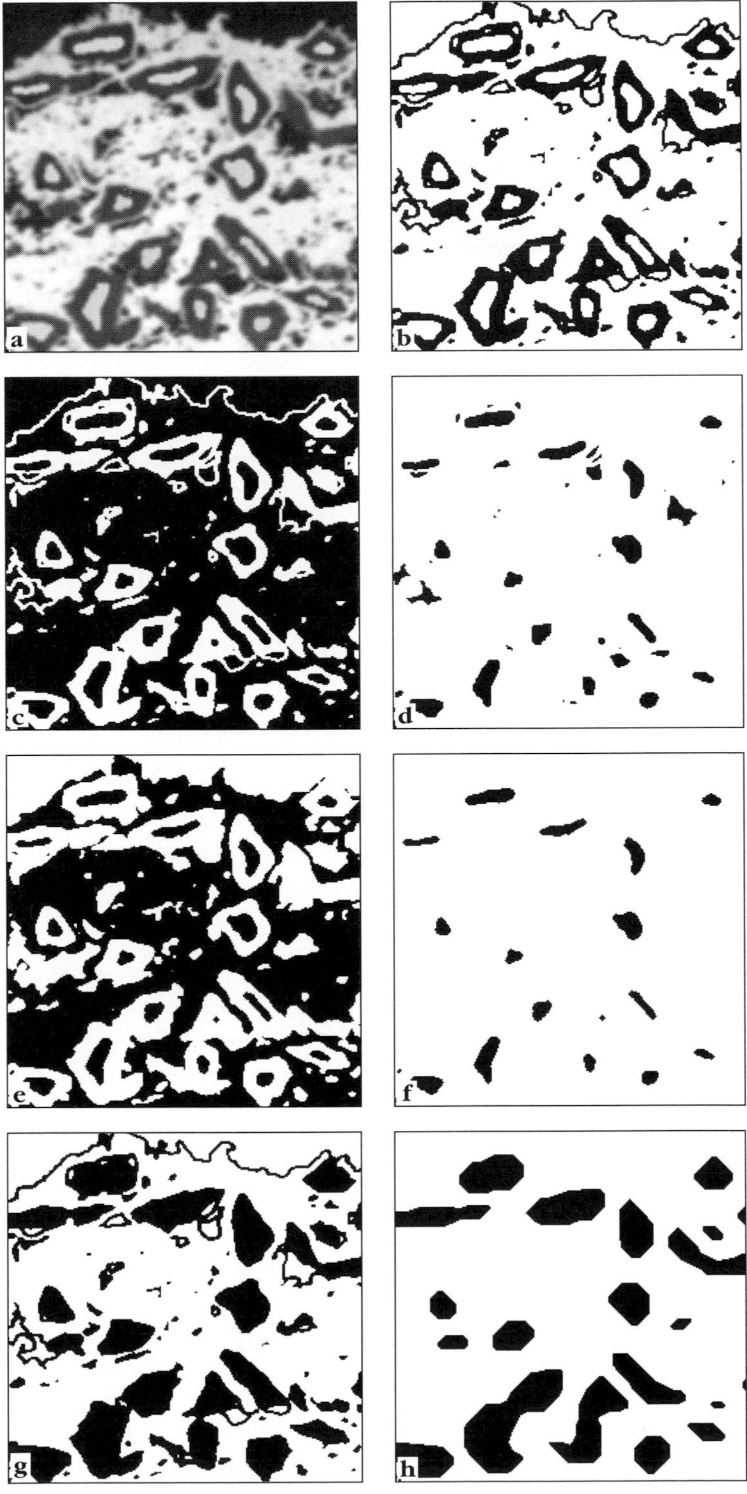

Figure 46. Combined operations to isolate particles in a coating:
a) *original grey scale image;*
b) *thresholded on dark grey showing periphery of particles;*
c) *inversion of image b;*
d) *elimination of edge-touching region to leave features corresponding to particle cores as well as pores;*
e) *thresholding of original image to select light grey characteristic of matrix and cores;*
f) *AND of image e with d to select cores;*
g) *OR of image f with b, to fill holes within particles;*
h) *application of opening (coefficient = 3, depth = 10) to remove boundary-straddling pixels.*

Inverting this image (**Figure 46c**) causes the interior cores to become features that do not touch the edges of the field of view. However, keeping only the features that do not touch the edge (**Figure 46d**) includes pores, as well as cores. The original image

Figure 47. Schematic diagram of forming a custer:
a) *original image;*
b) *erosion of a;*
c) *dilation of a;*
d) *Ex-OR of b and c.*

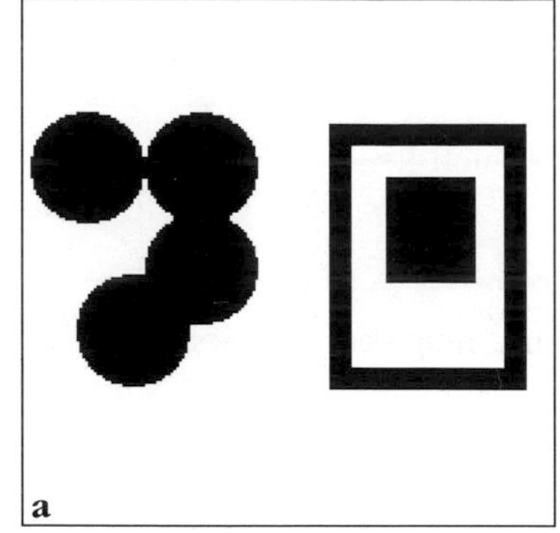

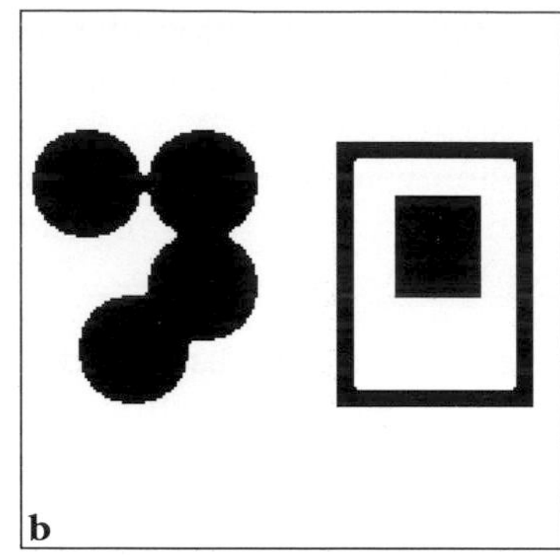

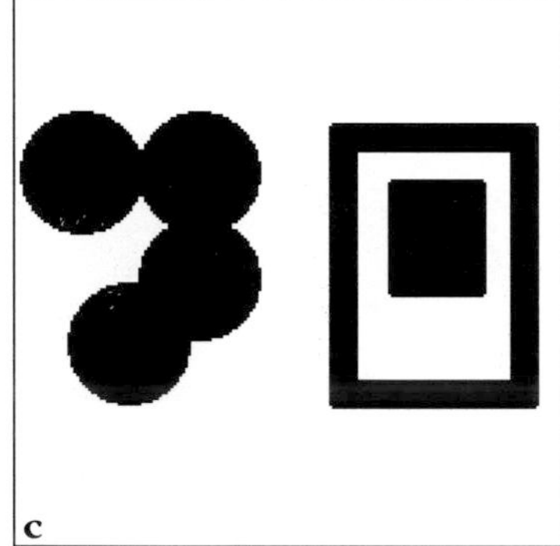

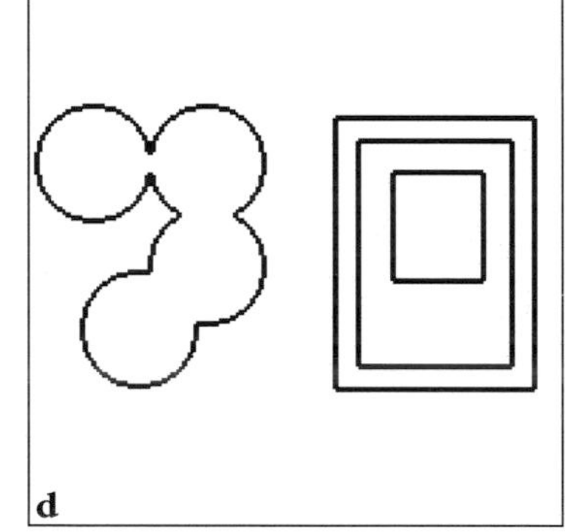

is thresholded again to select the light grey values characteristic of the matrix and the cores (**Figure 46e**), then ANDed with the inverted image to select only the cores (**Figure 46f**). Identified as features in the inverted image, they are bright in the grey scale image, since the pores are dark.

These cores are then ORed with the original binary image of the particle periphery (**Figure 46g**) to fill in the particles (but not the voids). Finally, an opening (coefficient = 3, depth = 10) removes the pixels straddling the boundaries between lighter and darker regions. The final result (**Figure 46h**) is a binary image of the particles suitable for counting or measurement. This may seem like a rather complicated procedure, and indeed it does require some human judgement to determine what characteristics of the desired features can be used to isolate them and how a procedure to perform the necessary operations should be implemented, but the time required is minimal, since all of these operations are individually very simple.

The custer

In the discussion of fractal dimension measurement above, the Ex-OR combination of an erosion and a dilation was used to define the pixels along a boundary. This is called the custer of a feature, apparently in reference to George Herbert Armstrong Custer, who was also surrounded. **Figure 47** shows the erosion/dilation formation of a custer. In some cases, a custer is approximated by Ex-ORing the original binary image with a single erosion or dilation. This can be accomplished by performing an erosion with neighborhood rules, which keep only those pixels with at least one background neighbor (or similar rules for dilation).

The custer can be used to determine neighbor relationships between features or regions. As an example, **Figure 48** shows a three-phase metal alloy imaged in the light microscope. Each of the individual phases can be readily delineated by thresholding (and in the case of the medium grey image, an opening to remove lines of pixels straddling the white-black boundary). Then the custer of each phase can be formed as described.

Combining the custer of each phase with the other phases using an AND keeps only the portion of the custer that is common to the two phases. The result is to mark the boundaries as white-grey, grey-black, or black-white, so that the extent of each type can be determined by simple counting. In other cases, Feature-AND can be used to select the entire features that are adjacent to one region (and hence touch its custer).

Skeletonization

Erosion can be performed with special rules that remove pixels, except when doing so would cause a separation of one region into two. The rule for this is to examine the touching neighbors; if they do not form a continuous group, then the central pixel cannot be removed (Pavlidis, 1980). The definition of this condition is dependent on whether four- or eight-connectedness is used, as shown in **Figure 49**. In either case, the selected patterns can be used in a fate table to conduct the erosion; for the four-connected case, only 2^4 or 16 entries are needed (Russ, 1984).

Figure 50 shows several features with their (eight-connected) skeletons. The skeleton is a powerful shape factor for feature recognition, containing both topological and metric information. The topological values include the number of end points, the number of nodes where branches meet, and the number of internal holes in the feature. The metric values are the mean length of branches (both those internal to the feature and those having a free end) and the angles of the branches. These parameters seem to correspond closely to what human observers see as the significant characteristics of features. Feature 49 shows the nomenclature used.

Locating the nodes and end points in a skeleton is simply a matter of counting neighbors. End points have a single neighbor, while nodes have more than two. Segment length can also be determined by counting, keeping track of the number of pixel

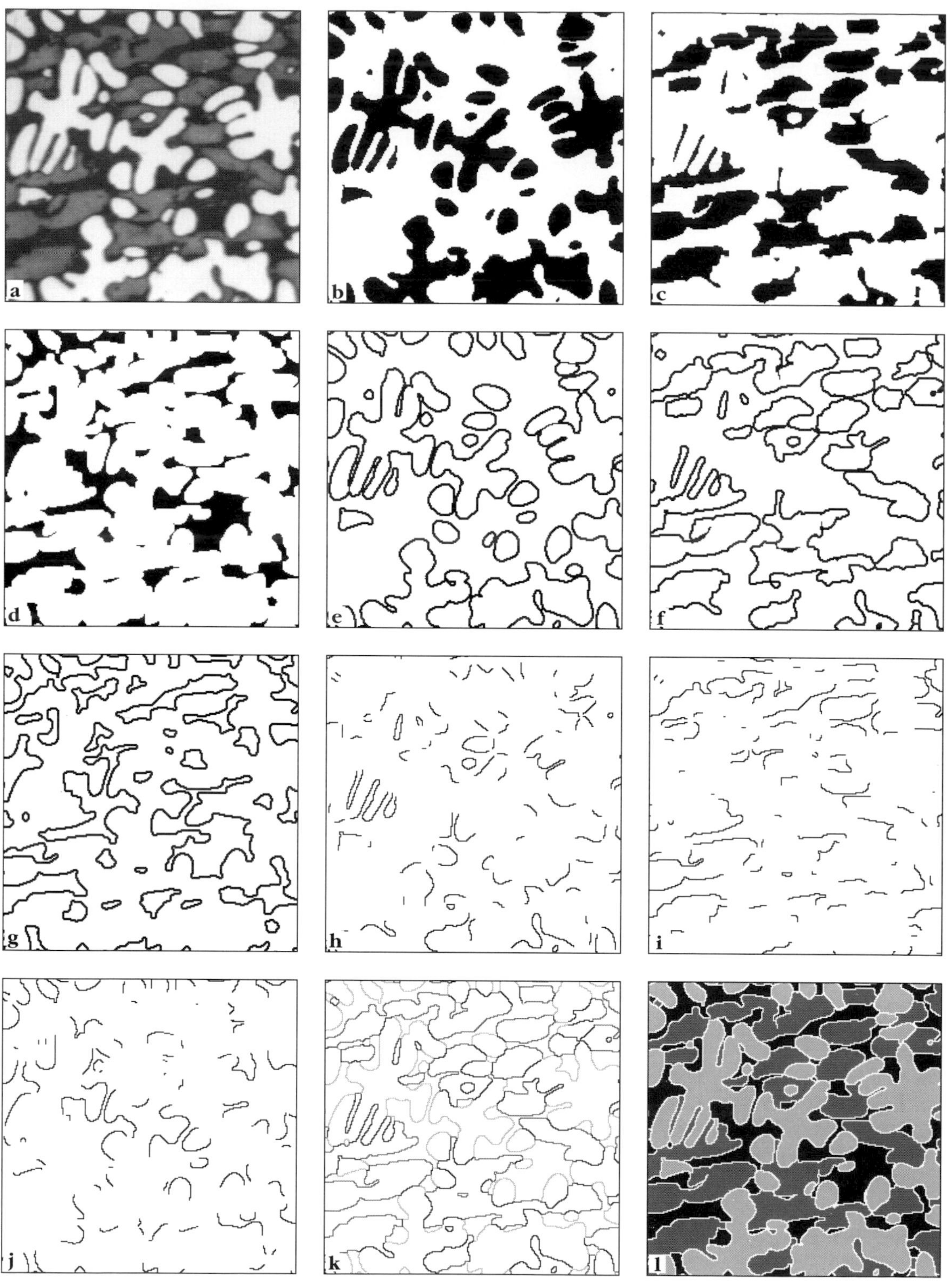
a
b
c
d
e
f
g
h
i
j
k
l

Figure 48. Use of Boolean logic to measure neighbor relationships:
a) *an original light microscope image of a three-phase metal;*
b) *thresholded white phase;*
c) *thresholded grey phase;*
d) *thresholded black phase;*
e) *surrounding outline of white phase produced by dilation and Ex-OR with original;*
f) *surrounding outline of grey phase produced by dilation and Ex-OR with original;*
g) *surrounding outline of black phase produced by dilation and Ex-OR with original;*
h) *AND of white outlines and grey features;*
i) *AND of grey outlines with black features;*
j) *AND of black outlines with white features;*
k) *OR of all ANDed outlines using different grey tones to identify each phase/phase interface;*
l) *outlines filled to show idealized phase regions.*

pairs that are diagonally or orthogonally connected. Counting the number of nodes, ends, loops, and branches defines the topology of the feature. Measuring the distribution of link and branch lengths and their orientation provides metric information.

The problem with skeletonization is its sensitivity to minor changes in the shape of the feature. As shown in **Figure 51,** changing as little as a single pixel on the exterior boundary of a feature can alter the skeleton to add a branch and node. Changing a single pixel within the feature produces a loop and completely alters the topology. Considering the difficulty of obtaining a perfect binary representation of a feature or region and the

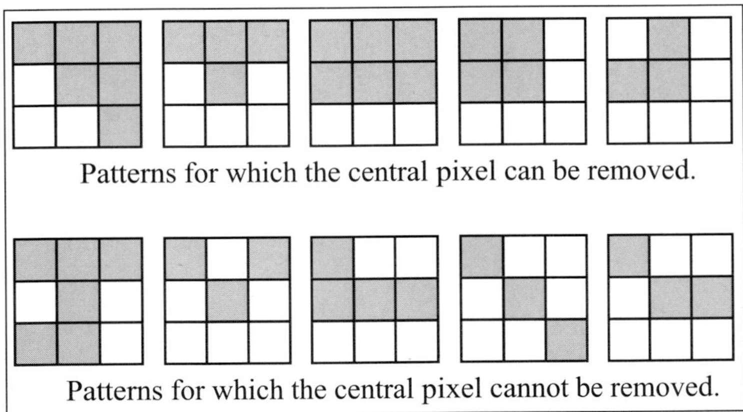

Patterns for which the central pixel can be removed.
Patterns for which the central pixel cannot be removed.

Figure 49. *Representative neighbor patterns which allow and do not allow the central pixel to be removed in skeletonization.*

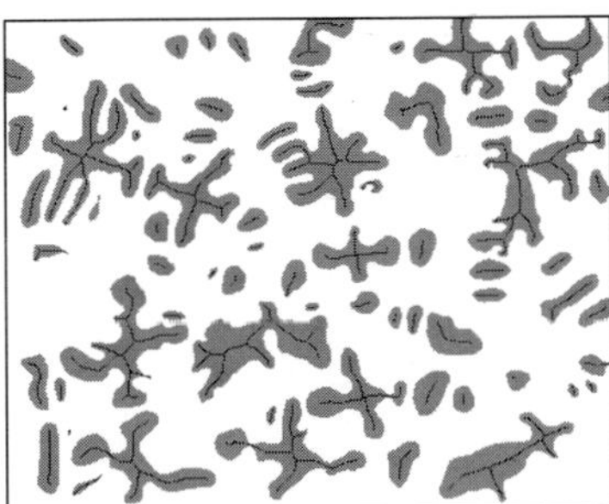

Figure 50. *A binary image containing multiple features, with their skeletons superimposed.*

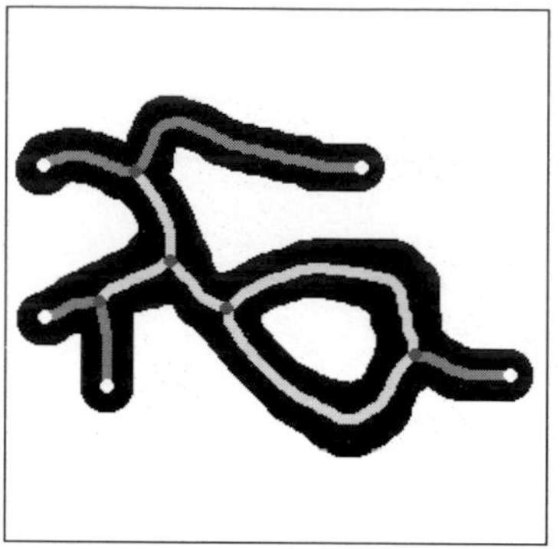

Figure 51. *The skeleton of a feature with 5 end points, 5 nodes, 5 branched, 5 links, and one loop (skeleton has been dilated for visibility).*

need for the various operations discussed so far in this chapter to modify and attempt to correct them, it can be unwise to depend on a technique so sensitive to these variations.

Just as the skeleton of features may be determined in an image, it is also possible to skeletonize the background. This is often called the skiz of the features. **Figure 52** shows an example. Consisting of points equidistant from feature boundaries, it effectively divides the image into regions of influence around each feature (Serra, 1982). It may be desirable to eliminate from the skiz those lines that are equidistant from two portions of the boundary of the same feature. This is easy to do, since the branches have an end; other lines in the skiz are continuous and have no ends, except at the image boundaries. Pruning branches from a skeleton (or skiz) simply requires starting at each end point (points with a single neighbor) and eliminating touching pixels until a node (a point with more than two neighbors) is reached.

Boundary lines and thickening

Another use for skeletonization is to thin down boundaries that may appear broad or of variable thickness in images. This is particularly common in light microscope images of metals whose grain boundaries are revealed by chemical etching. This preferentially attacks the boundaries, but in order to produce dark,

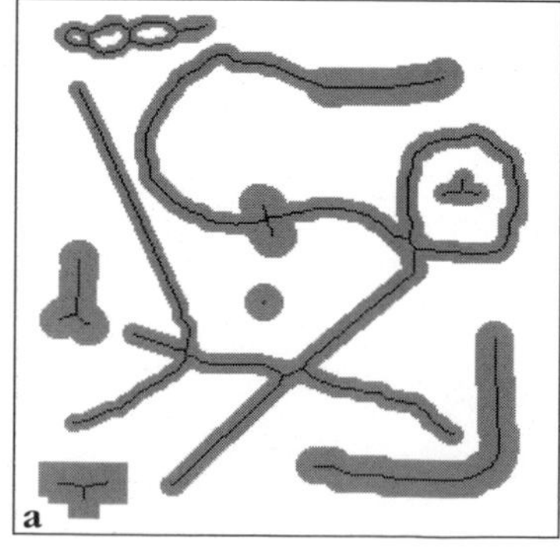

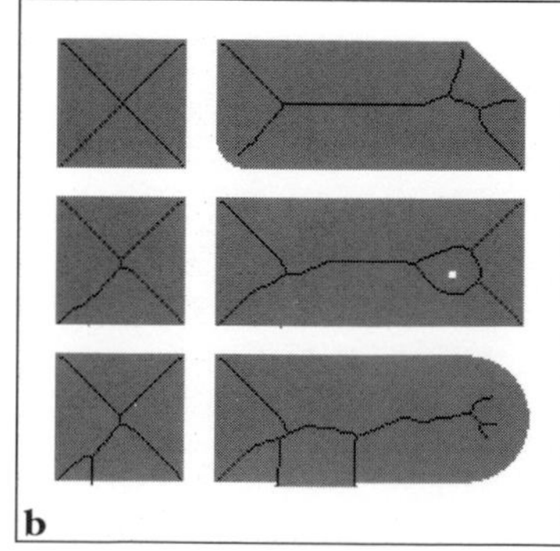

Figure 52. Examples of skeletons superimposed on features:

a) *for long and thin features the skeleton represents ths shape well;*

b) *modifying the original feature by as little as a single pixel on the exterior or interior alters the skeleton by adding branches or loops.*

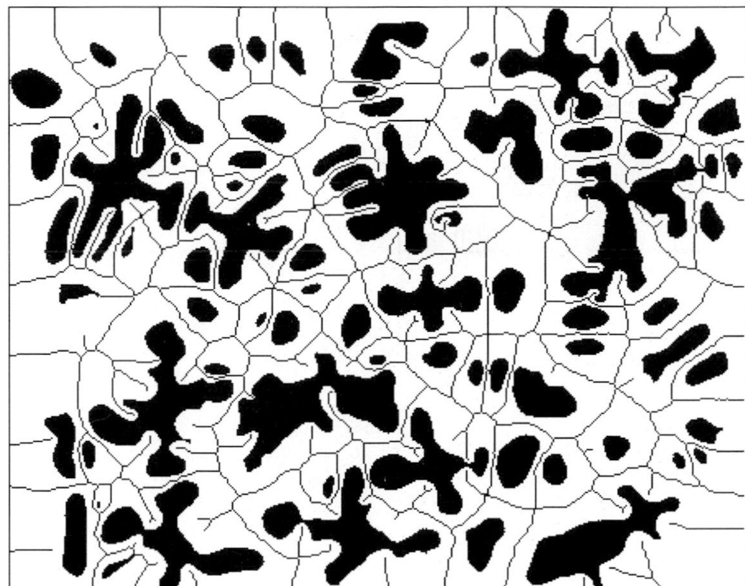

Figure 53. *The skiz of the features in the same image as Figure 50.*

continuous lines, it also broadens them. In order to measure the actual size of grains, the adjacency of different phases, or the length of boundary lines, it is preferable to thin the lines by skeletonization.

Figure 54 shows an example. The original polished and etched metal sample has dark and wide grain boundaries, as well as dark patches corresponding to carbides and pearlite. Thresholding it produces broad lines, which can be skeletonized to reduce them to single-pixel width. Since this is properly a continuous tesselation, it can be cleaned up by removing all branches that have end points, a process referred to as pruning.

The resulting lines delineate the grain boundaries, but because they are eight-connected, they do not separate the grains for individual measurement. Converting the lines to four-connected, called thickening, can be accomplished with a dilation that adds pixels only for a few neighbor patterns corresponding to eight-connected corners (or the skeleton could have been produced using eight-connected rules to begin with). The resulting lines do separate the grains, which can be identified and measured as shown.

Unfortunately, the grain boundary tesselation produced by simple thresholding and skeletonization is incomplete in many cases. Some of the boundaries may fail to etch because the crystallographic mismatch across the boundary is small or the concentration of defects or impurities is low. The result is a tesselation with some missing lines, which would bias subsequent analysis. **Figure 55** shows an example of this situation. The original image (obtained by thresholding and skeletonization) is

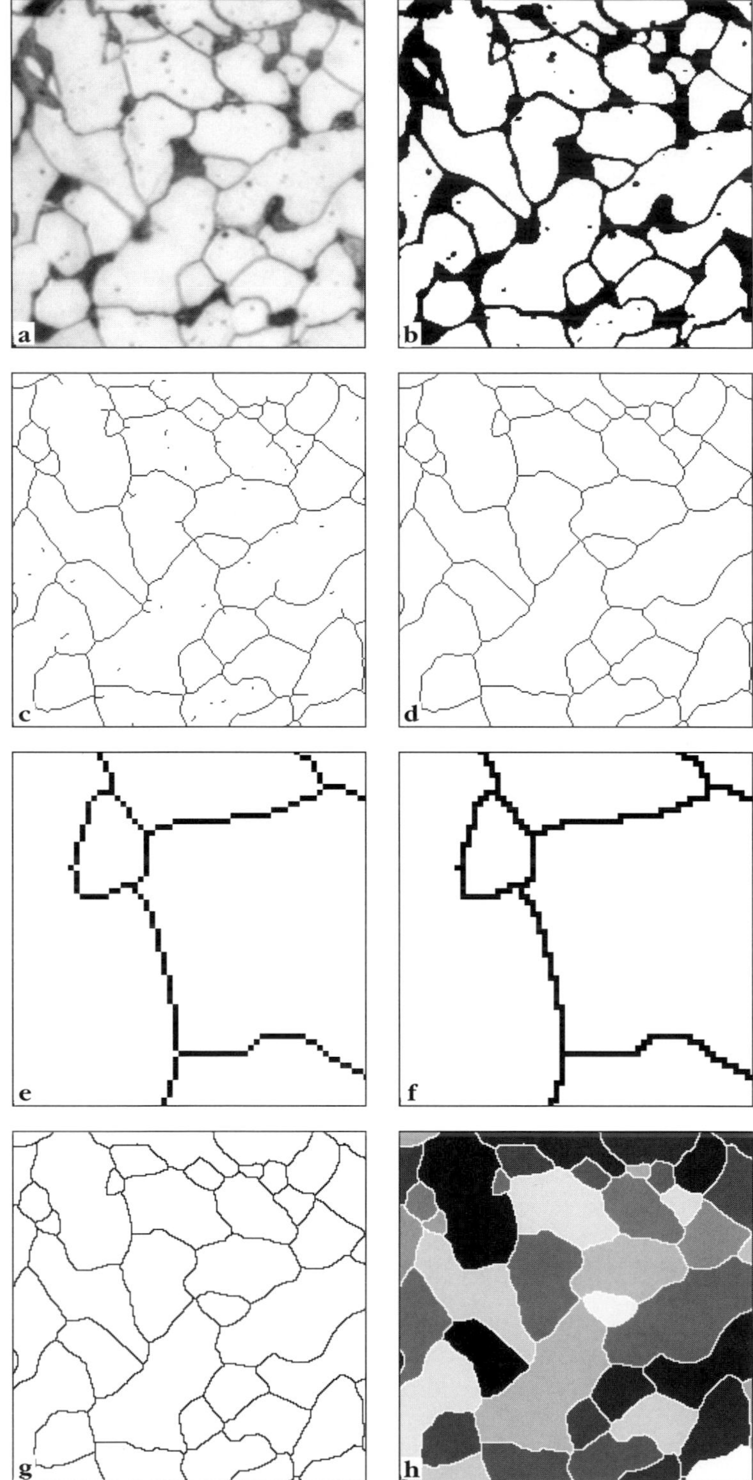

Figure 54. Skeletonization of grain boundaries:
a) *metallographic image of etched 1040 steel;*
b) *thresholded image showing boundaries and dark patches of iron carbide (and pearlite);*
c) *skeletonized from image b;*
d) *pruned from image c;*
e) *enlarged to show eight-connected line;*
f) *converted to four-connected line;*
g) *grains separated by thickened lines;*
h) *identification of individual grains.*

complete, but a portion of the boundaries have been randomly erased. This primarily removes lines, rather than junctions (which tend to etch well).

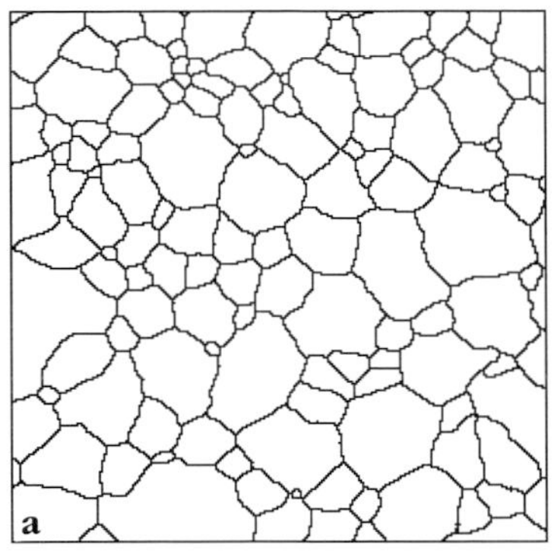

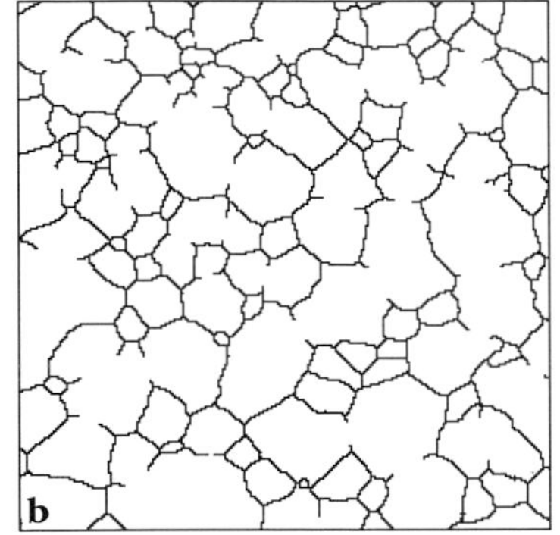

Figure 55: Example of missing grain boundary lines:
a) *original image (beryllium copper alloy) with complete tesselation produced as in Figure 53;*
b) *random removal of boundary lines.*

Figure 56 shows one of the simplest approaches to deal with this situation. Skeletonizing the incomplete network is used to identify the end points (points with a single neighbor). It is reasoned that these points should occur in pairs, so each is dilated by some arbitrarily selected distance which, it is hoped, will span half of the gap in the network. The resulting dilated circles are ORed with the original network and the result is again skeletonized. Wherever the dilation has caused the circles to touch, the result is a line segment that joins the corresponding end points.

This method is imperfect, however. Some of the points may be too far apart for the circles to touch, while in other places, the circles may obscure details by touching several existing lines,

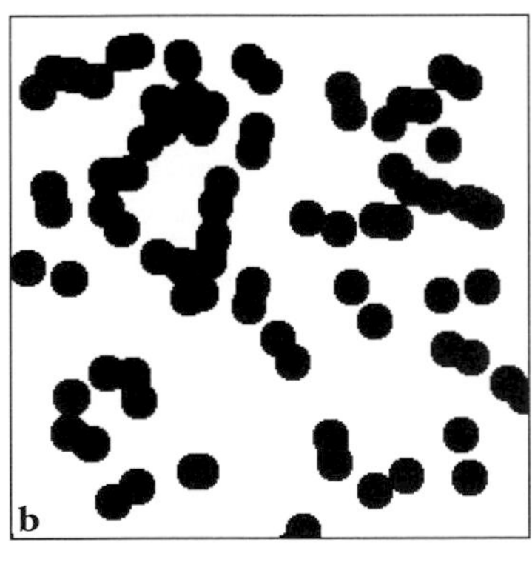

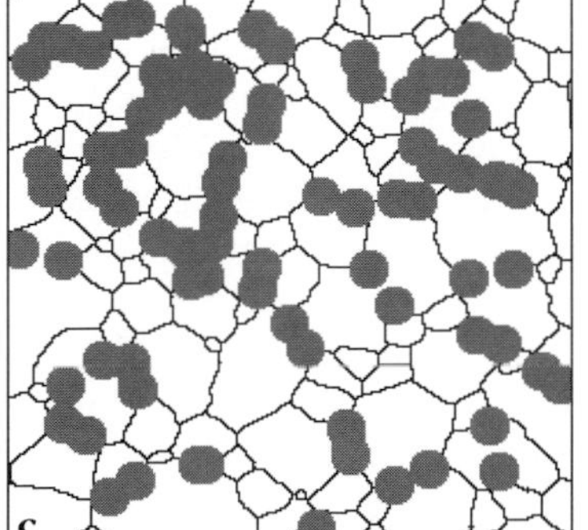

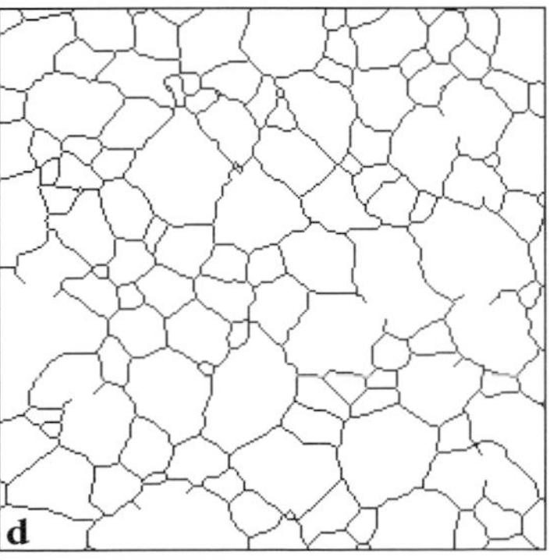

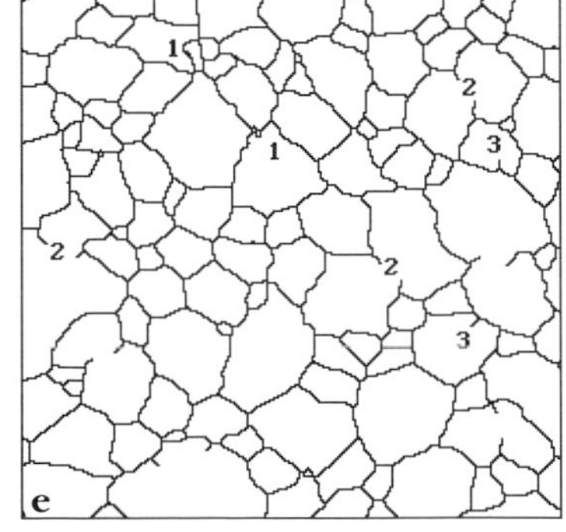

Figure 56. Dilation method for completing grain boundary tesselation:
a) *skeletonized boundaries with end points located;*
b) *dilation of end point by arbitrary radius;*
c) *OR of boundary image with dilated circled;*
d) *re-skeletonization of network;*
e) *result with some typical errors marked: 1 = removal of small grains; 2 = large gaps still not joined; 3 = dangling single ends.*

oversimplifying the resulting network. It is not easy to select an appropriate dilation radius, since the gaps and grains are not all the same size. In addition, unmatched ends or points, due to dirt or particulates within the grains, can cause difficulties.

Other methods are also available. A computationally intensive approach locates all of the end points and uses a relaxation method to pair them up, so that line direction is maintained, lines are not allowed to cross, and closer points are matched first. This suffers some of the same problems as dilation if unmatched end points or noise are present, but at least it deals well with gaps of different sizes. A third approach, though imperfect, is perhaps the most efficient and reasonably accurate method. It is shown below in conjunction with a Euclidean distance map (EDM).

Euclidean distance map

The image processing functions discussed in this and preceding chapters operate either on grey scale images (to produce other grey scale images) or on binary images (to produce other binary images). An EDM is a tool that works on a binary image to produce a grey scale image. The definition is simple enough: each pixel, in either the features or the background or both, is assigned a brightness value equal to its distance from the nearest boundary. This is normally interpreted to mean that the brightness of each point in the image encodes the straight line distance to the nearest point on any boundary. In a continuous image, as opposed to a digitized one containing finite pixels, this is unambiguous. In most pixel images, the distance is taken from each pixel in the feature to the nearest pixel in the background.

Searching through all of the background pixels to find the nearest one to a boundary and calculating the distance in a Pythagorean sense would be an extremely inefficient and time-consuming method of constructing an EDM. Furthermore, since the brightness values of the pixels are quantized, some round-off errors in distance must be accepted. Some researchers have implemented an EDM using distance measured in only a few directions. For a lattice of square pixels, this may be restricted either to the 90° directions, or it may also include the 45° directions (Rosenfeld and Kak, 1982). This is equivalent to deciding to use a 4-neighbor or 8-neighbor convention for considering whether pixels are touching. In either case, the distance from each pixel to one of its 4 or 8 neighbors is taken as 1, regardless of the direction. Consequently, as shown in **Figure 57,** the distance map from a point gives rise to either square or diamond-shaped artefacts and is quite distorted, as compared to the Pythagorean distance. These measuring conventions are sometimes described as city-block models (connections in 4 directions) or chessboard models (8 directions), because of the limited moves available in those situations.

6	5	4	3	4	5	6
5	4	3	2	3	4	5
4	3	2	1	2	3	4
3	2	1	0	1	2	3
4	3	2	1	2	3	4
5	4	3	2	3	4	5
6	5	4	3	4	5	6

3	3	3	3	3	3	3
3	2	2	2	2	2	3
3	2	1	1	1	2	3
3	2	1	0	1	2	3
3	2	1	1	1	2	3
3	2	2	2	2	2	3
3	3	3	3	3	3	3

$\sqrt{18}$	$\sqrt{13}$	$\sqrt{10}$	3.0	3.2	3.6	4.2
$\sqrt{13}$	$\sqrt{8}$	$\sqrt{5}$	2.0	2.2	2.8	3.6
$\sqrt{10}$	$\sqrt{5}$	$\sqrt{2}$	1.0	1.4	2.2	3.2
$\sqrt{9}$	$\sqrt{4}$	$\sqrt{1}$	0	1.0	2.0	3.0
$\sqrt{10}$	$\sqrt{5}$	$\sqrt{2}$	1.0	1.4	2.2	3.2
$\sqrt{13}$	$\sqrt{8}$	$\sqrt{5}$	2.0	2.2	2.8	3.6
$\sqrt{18}$	$\sqrt{13}$	$\sqrt{10}$	3.0	3.2	3.6	4.2

Figure 57. *Arrays of pixels with their distance from the center pixel shown for the cases of 4- and 8-neighbor paths and in Pythagorean units.*

A conceptually straightforward, iterative technique for constructing such a distance map can be programmed as follows.

1. Assign a brightness value of 0 to each pixel in the background.
2. Set a variable *N* equal to 0.
3. For each pixel that touches (in either the 4- or 8-neighbor sense, as described above) a pixel whose brightness value is *N*, assign a brightness value of *N* + 1.
4. Increment *N* and repeat step 3, until all pixels in the image have been assigned.

The time required for this iteration depends on the size of the features (the maximum distance from the background). A more efficient method is available that gives the same result with two passes through the image (Danielsson, 1980). This technique uses the same comparisons, but propagates the values through the image more rapidly.

1. Assign the brightness value of 0 to each pixel in the background and a large positive value (greater than the maximum feature width) to each pixel in a feature.
2. Proceeding from left to right and top to bottom, assign each pixel within a feature a brightness value one greater than the smallest value of any of its neighbors.
3. Repeat step 2, proceeding from right to left and bottom to top.

A further modification provides a better approximation to the Pythagorean distances between pixels (Russ & Russ, 1988b). The diagonally adjacent pixels are neither a distance 1 (8-neighbor rules) or 2 (4-neighbor rules) away, but actually $\sqrt{2} = 1.414...$ pixels. This is an irrational number, but closer approximations than 1.00 or 2.00 are available. For instance, modifying the above rules so that a pixel brightness value must be larger than its 90° neighbors by 2 and greater than its 45° neighbors by 3 is equivalent to using an approximation of 1.5 for the square root of 2.

The disadvantage of this method is that all of the pixel distances are now multiplied by 2, increasing the maximum brightness of

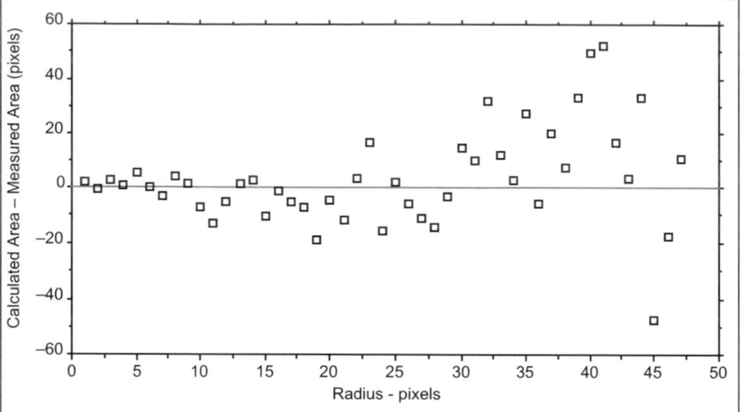

Figure 58. *Difference between theoretical area value (πr^2) and the actual area covered by the EDM as a function of brightness (distance from boundary) shows increasing but still small errors for very large distances.*

the EDM image by this factor. For images capable of storing a maximum grey level of 255, this represents a limitation on the largest features that can be processed in this way. However, if the EDM image is 16 bits deep (and can hold values up to 65,535), this is not a practical limitation. It also opens the way to selecting larger ratios of numbers to approximate √2, getting a correspondingly improved set of values for the distance map. For instance, 7/5 = 1.400 and 58/41 = 1.415.

It takes no longer to compare or add these values than it does any others and they allow dimensions larger than 1,024 pixels. Since this dimension is the half-width, features or background up to 2,048 pixels wide can be processed (1,024 · 41 = 41,984, which is less than $2^{16} - 1$ = 65,535). Of course, the final image can be divided down by the scaling factor (41 in this example) to obtain a result in which pixel brightness values are the actual distance to the boundary (rounded or truncated to integers) and the total brightness range is within the 0 to 255 range that most displays are capable of showing.

The accuracy of an EDM constructed with these rules can be judged by counting the pixels whose brightness values place them within a distance *s*. This is just the same as constructing a cumulative histogram of pixel brightness in the image. **Figure 58** plots the error in the number of pixels vs. integer brightness for a distance map of a circle 99 pixels in diameter; the overall errors are not too large. Even better accuracy for the EDM can be obtained by performing additional comparisons to pixels beyond the first 8 nearest neighbors. Adding a comparison to the 8 neighbors in the 5×5 neighborhood whose Pythagorean distance is √5 produces values having even less directional sensitivity and more accuracy for large distances. If the integer values 58 and 41 mentioned above are used to approximate √2, then the path to these pixels consisting of a “knight’s move” of one 90° and one 45° pixel step would produce a value of 58 + 41 or 99. Substituting a value of 92 gives a close approximation to the Pythagorean distance and produces more isotropic results.

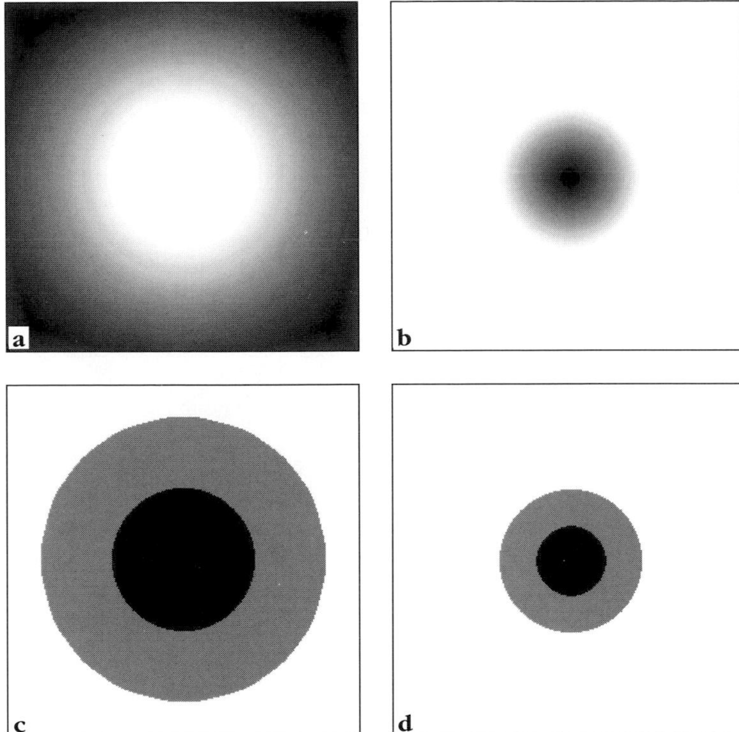

Figure 59. Isotropy achieved by using the Euclidean distance map for dilation and erosion (compare to Figures 29, 30, and 31):
a) *the EDM of the background around the circle;*
b) *the EDM of the circle;*
c) *dilation achieved by thresholding the backgound EDM at a value of 50;*
d) *erosion achieved by thresholding the circle EDM at a value of 25.*

It is interesting to compare each of the erosion methods discussed above to the ideal circular pattern provided by the EDM. Simple thresholding of the distance map can be used to select circles farther from the edge than any desired extent of erosion. Similarly, the distance map of the background can be thresholded to perform a dilation. Both of these operations can be carried out without any iteration. The distance map is constructed non-iteratively as well, so the execution time of the method does not increase with feature size (as do classical erosion methods) and is preferred for large features or depths. **Figure 59** shows the erosion and dilation of a circle using the distance map; compare this to **Figures 29** to **31** for classical erosion and dilation.

When more irregular shapes are eroded, the difference between the iterative methods and thresholding the EDM is less obvious visually. However, the directional bias of the iterative comparisons is still present and can be measured. **Figure 60** shows a binary image containing features with a variety of shapes. The dark pixels are those removed by thresholding the EDM to a depth of 6. Applying the various iterative erosion patterns described above removes some pixels that are at a greater distance than 6 pixels from the boundary or leaves ones which are closer to it.

Figure 61 shows the results in the form of a plot. The uppermost line in the plot shows the number of pixels present as a function of their distance from the boundary. This information comes directly from the brightness histogram of the EDM. Each of the

Figure 60. *Binary test image showing the pixels removed by thresholding the EDM at a depth of 6.*

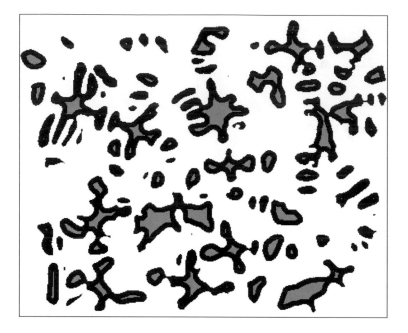

other lines shows how many pixels were removed by various iterative erosion patterns, as a function of the pixel's distance from the boundary. The alternating cross-and-X or square-and-X patterns and the unconditional erosion (coefficient = 0) remove all of the pixels at a distance up to 6 pixels from the boundary, but also remove additional pixels that are farther away. Coefficients of 1 or 2 remove no pixels farther than 6 pixels from the boundary, but do not remove all of the ones within 6 pixels of the boundary. None of the iterative methods accurately duplicates the results obtained by thresholding the EDM.

Figure 61. *Plot of number of pixels removed in 6 cycles of erosion applied to Figure 60 using various iterative patterns, versus their actual distance from the boundary as given by the EDM. The OXOX and Coeff = 0 curves are superimposed exactly.*

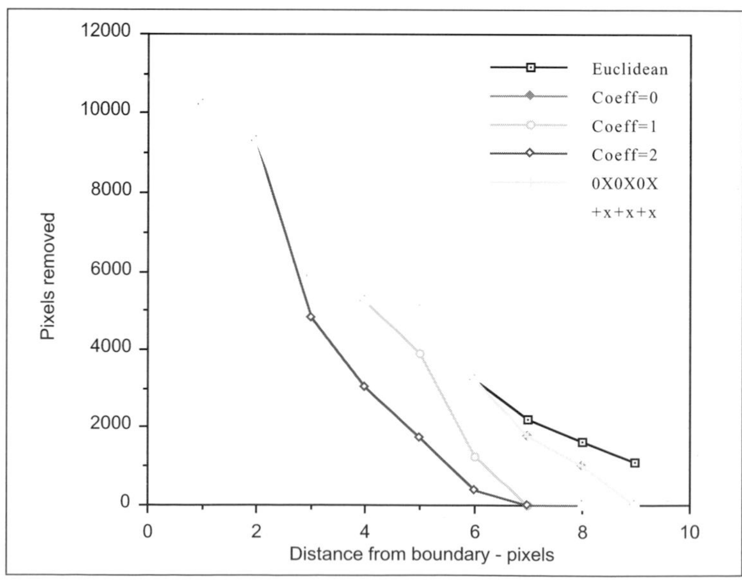

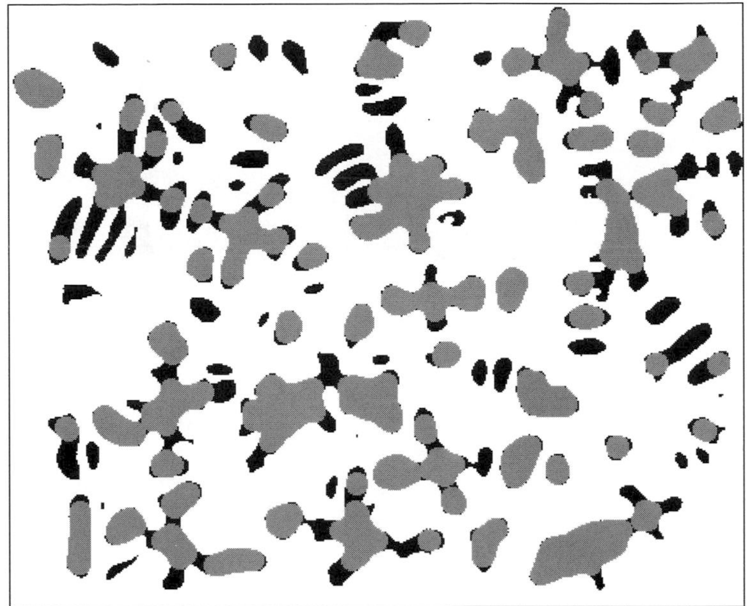

Figure 62. *Opening produced by thresholding the EDM of features (erosion) and then of background (dilation) to a depth of six. Dark pixels are those removed. The image is the same as in Figures 60 amd 63.*

Similar results are obtained when dilations are performed or when combinations of erosions and dilations are carried out. Dilations are performed by first obtaining the EDM of the background. This can be accomplished either by inverting a copy of the image (reversing all of the black and white pixels in the binary image) or by constructing the EDM of the background at the same time as the features, by using complementary logic in the program. **Figures 62** and **63** compare the results of an opening applied to the same image as in **Figure 60.** In **Figure 62,** the opening of depth 6 is applied by thresholding a distance map

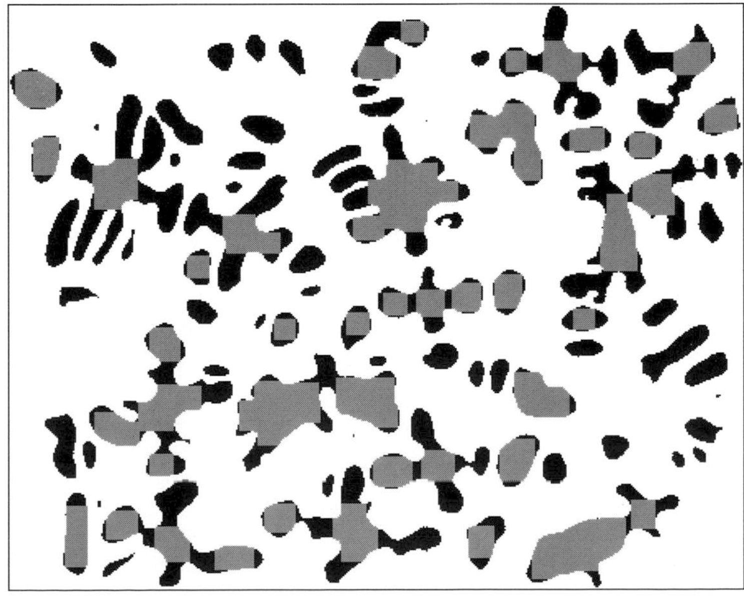

Figure 63. *Opening produced by classic erosion/dilation to a depth of six. Dark pixels are those removed. The image is the same as in Figures 60 and 62.*

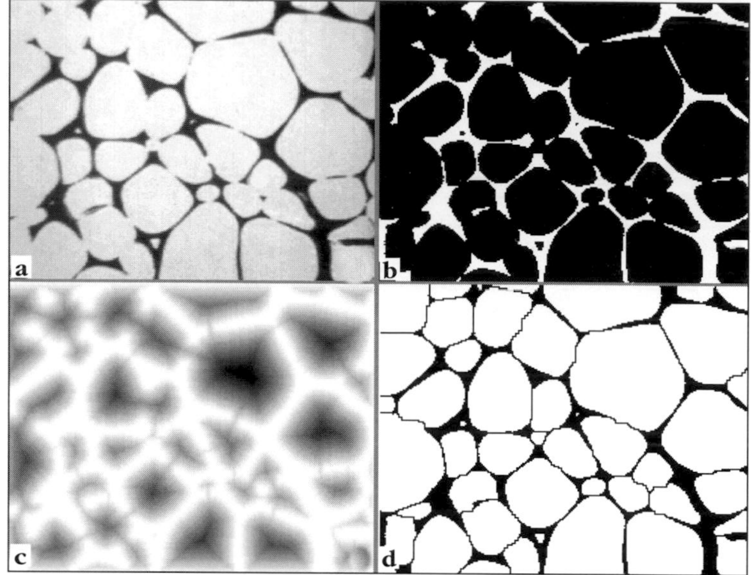

Figure 64. Watershed segmentation applied to a sintered microstructure:
a) *original grey scale image;*
b) *thresholded binary image;*
c) *Euclidean distance map;*
d) *segmentation lines produced by the algorithm.*

of the features and then of the background. In **Figure 63,** the opening is performed using classical erosion and dilation. Notice the rather significant differences in pixels and even features that have been removed and also the resulting different feature shapes.

Watershed segmentation

A common difficulty in measuring images occurs when features touch, and therefore cannot be separately identified, counted, or measured. This situation may arise when examining an image of a thick section in transmission, where actual feature overlap may occur, or when particles resting on a surface tend to agglomerate and touch each other. One method for separating touching, but mostly convex, features in an image is known as watershed segmentation (Beucher & Lantejoul, 1979; Lantejoul & Beucher, 1981). It relies on the fact that eroding the binary image will usually cause touching features to separate before they disappear.

The classical method for accomplishing this separation (Jernot, 1982) is an iterative one. The image is repetitively eroded, and at each step separate features that disappeared from the previous step are designated ultimate eroded points (UEPs) and saved as an image, along with the iteration number. This is necessary because the features will in general be of different sizes and would not all disappear in the same number of iterations, as mentioned above in connection with **Figure 33**. The process continues until the image is erased.

Then, beginning with the final image of UEPs, the image is dilated using classical dilation, but with the added logical constraint that no new pixel may be turned ON if it causes a connection to form between previously separate features or if it was not ON in the original image. At each stage of the dilation, the image of UEPs that corresponds to the equivalent level of erosion is added to the image using a logical OR. This process causes the features to grow back to their original boundaries, except lines of separation appear between the touching features.

The method just described has two practical drawbacks: the iterative process is slow, requiring each pixel in the image to be processed many times, and the amount of storage required for all of the intermediate images is quite large. The same result can be obtained more efficiently using an EDM. Indeed, the name "watershed" comes directly from the EDM. Imagine that the brightness values of each pixel within features in an EDM correspond to a physical elevation. The features then appear as mountain peaks. The ultimate eroded points are the peaks of the mountains, and where features touch the flanks of the mountains intersect. The saddles, or watersheds, of these mountains are the lines selected as boundaries by the segmentation method. The placement of these lines according to the relative height of the mountains (size of the features) gives the best estimate of the separation lines between features.

Implementing the segmentation process using an EDM approach (Russ & Russ, 1988b) is very efficient, both in terms of speed and storage. Only a single distance map image is required, and it is constructed without iteration. The ultimate eroded points are located as a special case of local maxima (there is a further discussion of UEPs below) and the brightness value of each directly corresponds to the iteration number at which it would disappear in the iterative method. Dilating these features is fast, because the distance map supplies a constraint. Starting at the brightest value and iteratively decrementing this to 1 covers all of the brightness levels. At each one, only those pixels at the current brightness level in the distance map need to be considered. Those that do not produce a join between feature pixels are added to the image. The process continues until all of the pixels in the features, except for those along the boundary lines, have been restored.

Figure 64 shows an example of this method, applied to a binary image from a polished section through a sintered metal powder. The original image (**Figure 64a**) shows considerable contact between the individual particles, which must be separated to measure the binary image (**Figure 64b**). The EDM (**Figure 64c**) shows the peaks rising to different heights, depending on the size of the features. Since the features are not perfectly round, the location of the peak (or UEP) within each one is asymmetric and the maximum brightness value corresponds to the shortest distance to the nearest boundary points. After the dilation process, **Figure 64d** shows the features with separation lines.

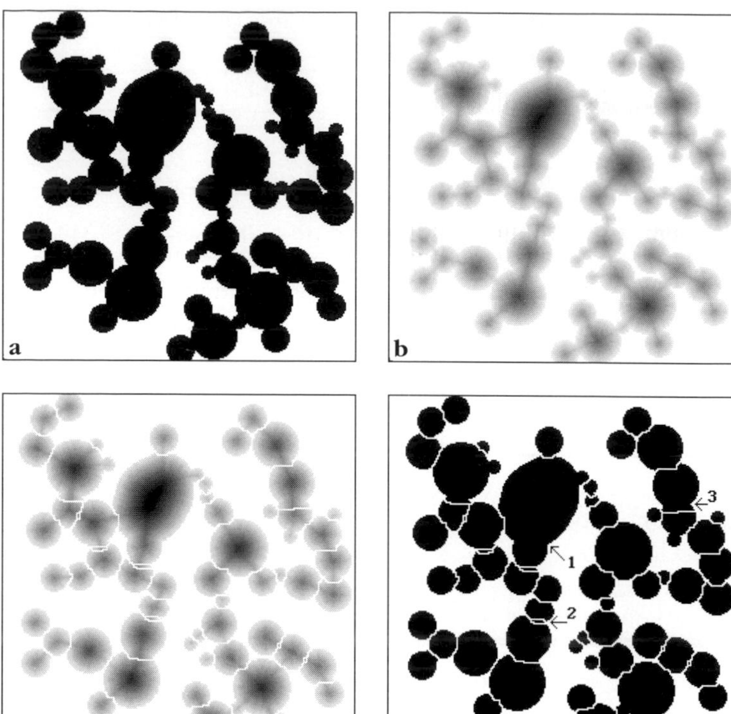

Figure 65. Example of watershed segmentation:
a) *original binary image of an agglomerated soot particle;*
b) *Euclidean distance map of image a;*
c) *watershed segmentation lines superimposed on image c;*
d) *result, showing typical errors: 1 = features not separated because there is no minimum in ridge of EDM; 2 = multiple separation lines where ridge has a long and gradual minimum subject to noise; 3 = displaced separation line due to presence of a third feature.*

Of course, this method is not perfect. **Figure 65** illustrates the most common difficulties. The original image is an agglomerated soot particle. Watershed segmentation does not separate particles whose contact is broad enough that the ridge in the EDM has no minimum. Also, it produces multiple separation lines when the minimum is so gradual that minor variations or noise in the edge shape can cause fluctuations in the ridge value. The presence of a third feature may shift the location of the minimum, thereby shifting the separation line. All of these problems arise because finding the minimum is a local process and hence is susceptible to local noise.

Watershed segmentation also provides another tool to complete grain boundary tesselations, discussed above. **Figure 66** shows the same test image as **Figure 55.** Inverting the image so that the grains are features rather than the boundaries and then performing watershed segmentation reconstructs most of the boundaries. As shown in the image, it misses some boundaries and adds others, depending on the shape of the grains.

Ultimate eroded points

The UEPs described in the watershed segmentation technique can be used as a measurement tool in their own right. The number of points gives the number of separable features in the image, while the brightness of each point gives a measure of their

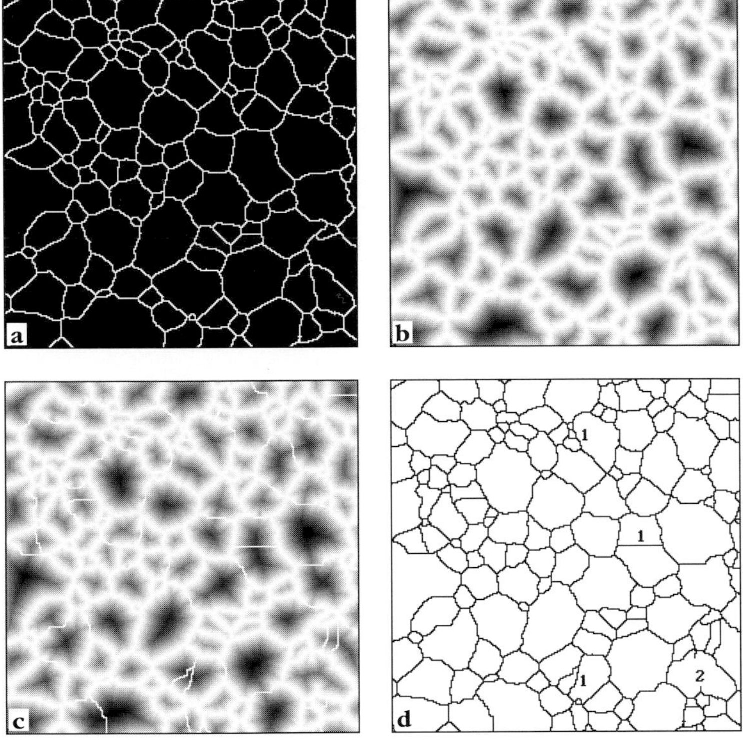

Figure 66. Watershed segmentation method for separating grains, using the same image as in Figure 55:
a) *inverted image showing complete network;*
b) *Euclidean distance map of Figure 55b;*
c) *automatic segmentation of image b;*
d) *resulting network with some typical errors marked:*
1 = extra lines drawn across grains of non-convex shape;
2 = missing lines for pairs of squat grains.

sizes. In addition, the location of each point can be used as a location for the feature if clustering or gradients are to be investigated.

The formal definition of a UEP in a continuous, rather than pixel-based, image is simply a local maximum of brightness. When the image is subdivided into finite pixels, the definition must take into account the possibility that more than one pixel may have equal brightness, forming a plateau. The operating definition for finding these pixels is recursive.

$$\{U: \quad \forall\, U_j \text{ neighbors of } U_i,\ |U_j| \le |U_i| \\ \text{AND} \\ \forall\, U_j \text{ neighbors of } U_i \text{ such that } |U_j| = |U_i|,\ U_i \in U\}$$

In other words, the set of pixels which are UEPs must be as bright or brighter than all neighbors; if the neighbors are equal in brightness, then they must also be part of the set.

The brightness of each pixel in the distance map is the distance to the nearest boundary. For a UEP, this must be a point that is equidistant from at least three boundary locations. Consequently, the brightness is the radius of the feature's inscribed circle. **Figure 67** applies this to the measurement of latex spheres, in a thin section imaged in a TEM. Each feature is shown marked with the location of the UEP. The figure shows a histogram of particle size as determined by the brightness of the UEPs. This is much faster than convex segmentation, since the iterative dilation

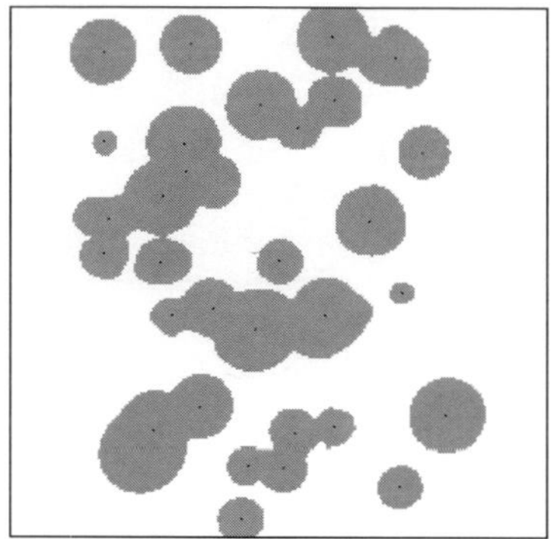

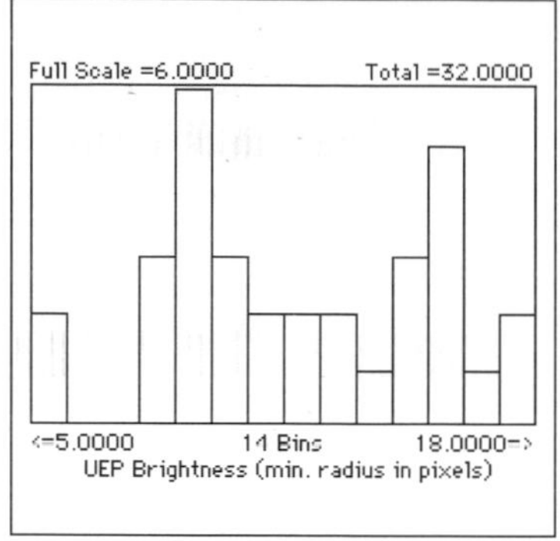

Figure 67. Ultimate eroded points in a binary image of partially overlapped latex spheres, and the histogram of the brightness of the points which gives a direct measure of particle sizes.

is bypassed, and much faster than measurement, since no feature identification or pixel counting is required.

Fractal dimension measurement

The method described above for determining a fractal dimension from successive erosion and dilation operations has two shortcomings: it is slow and has orientational bias because of the anisotropy of the operations. The EDM offers a simple way to obtain the same information (Russ, 1988). For example, **Figure 68** shows an image containing four irregular features (paint pigment particles from an SEM image). The EDM is shown in **Figure 69.** Thresholding this image at different brightness levels selects bands of pixels having any distance from the original boundary (now defined as a line between pixels). The perimeter defined

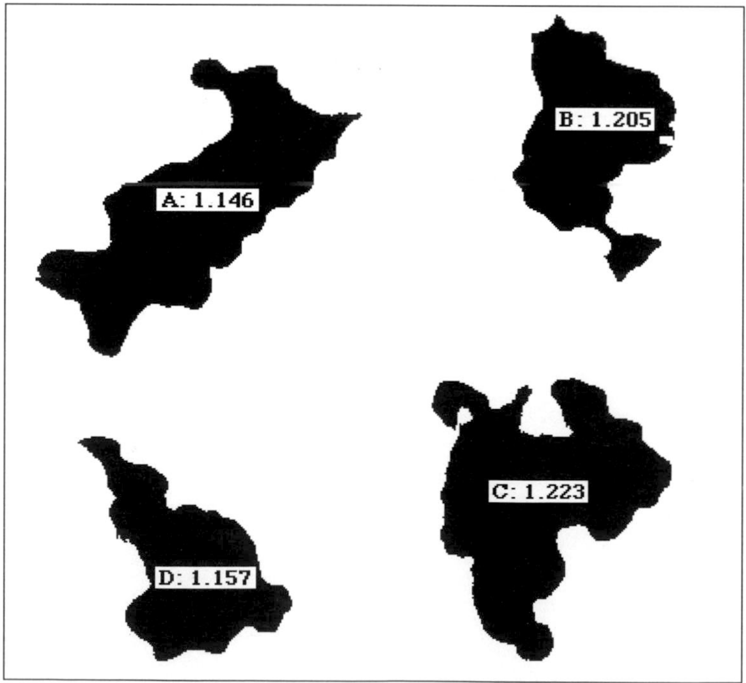

Figure 68. Binary image of four paint pigment particles, each marked with its fractal dimension.

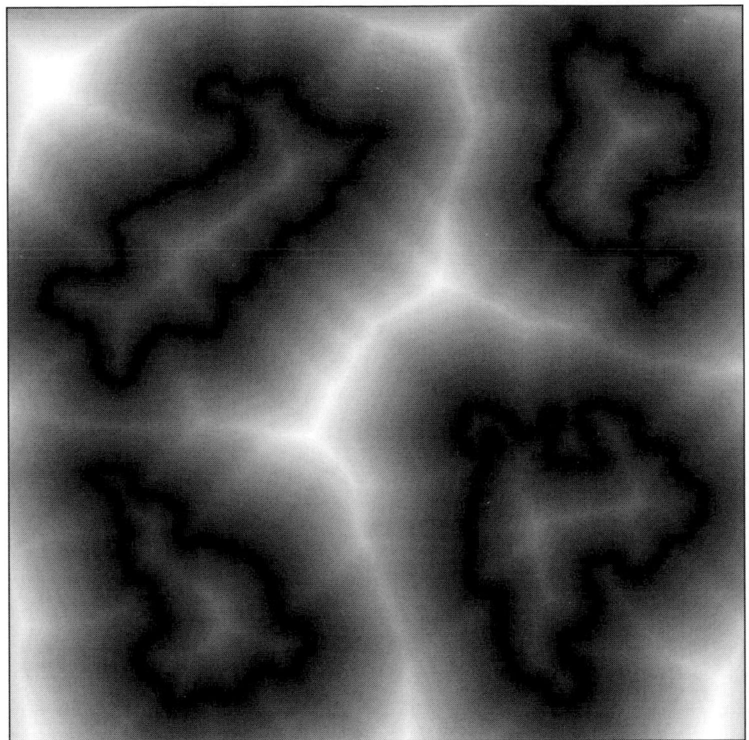

Figure 69. *Euclidean distance map of both the features and the background in Figure 68. (Plotted with inverted grey scale to show boundaries.)*

by this band is simply the area (number of pixels) in the band divided by its mean width (the number of brightness levels included in the band). **Figure 70** shows examples of the bands of

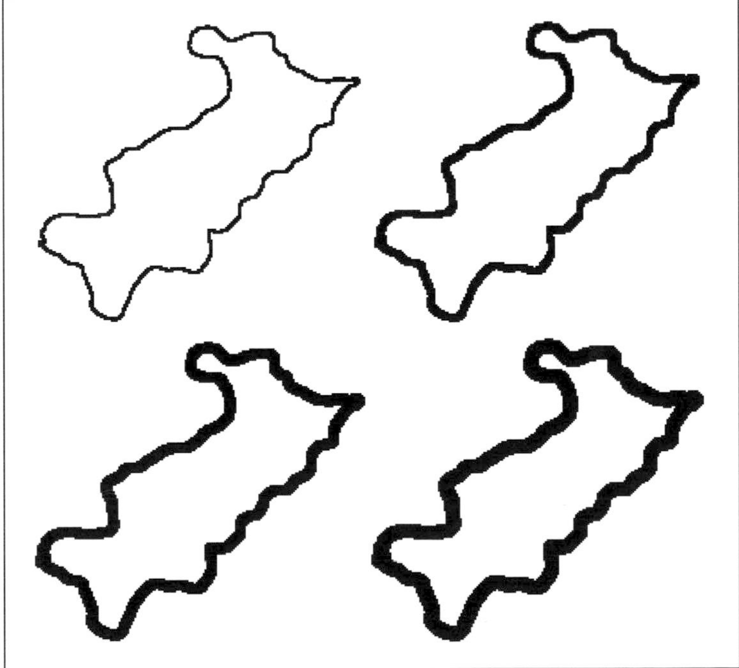

Figure 70. *The results of progessively thresholding the EDM of feature A in Figure 69 at different values, to obtain the pixels within varying distances of the boundary.*

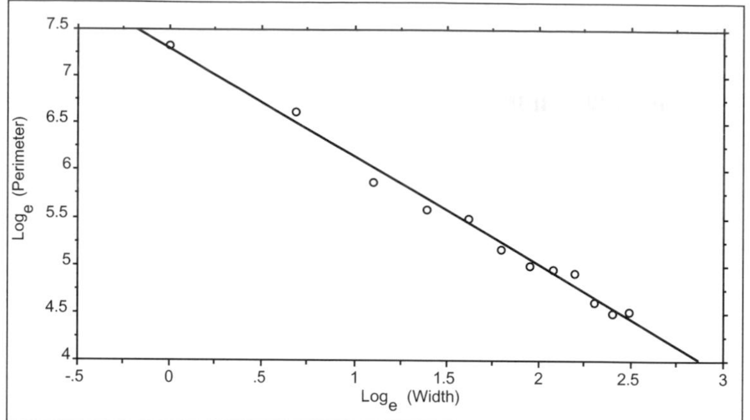

Figure 71. *Richardson plot of perimeter (area of the thresholded band divided by width) vs. width for feature A in Figure 68. The slope of the plot is −0.146, giving a fractal dimension of 1.146. The area can be determined directly from the histogram of the EDM, without creating the thresholded images in Figure 70.*

pixels along the boundary (called Minkowski sausages) obtained by thresholding the distance map.

Plotting this perimeter vs. the width of the sausage on a log-log Richardson plot produces slopes giving the feature fractal dimension, as illustrated in **Figure 71.** The resulting fractal dimensions for the four features are shown in **Figure 68**. The method is fast and robust, and the values vary less with feature size, position, or orientation than any of the other methods described. In fact, it is not even necessary to perform the various thresholding operations to obtain the thickened boundary lines. Instead, the brightness histogram of the distance map directly gives the number of pixels at each distance, which can be used to form the regression plot.

Medial axis transform

The skeletonization discussed above uses an iterative erosion that removes pixels from the outside edges, provided that they do not cause a disconnection that would separate a feature into

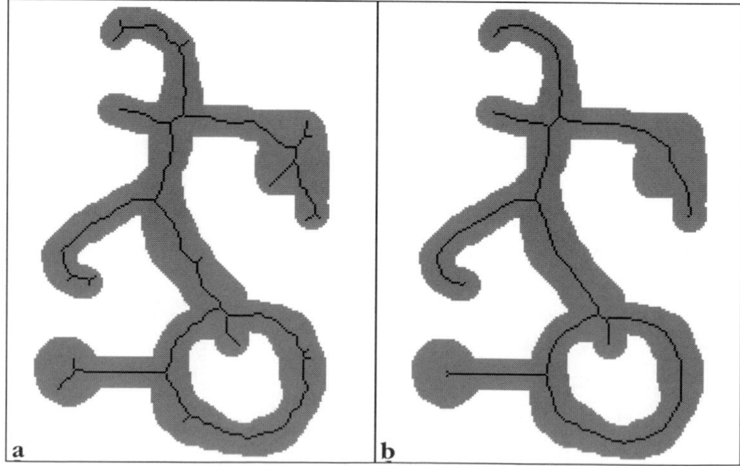

Figure 72. *Comparison of the skeleton (a) and medial axis transform (b) of the same feature. The skeleton is much more sensitive to irregularities along the feature periphery.*

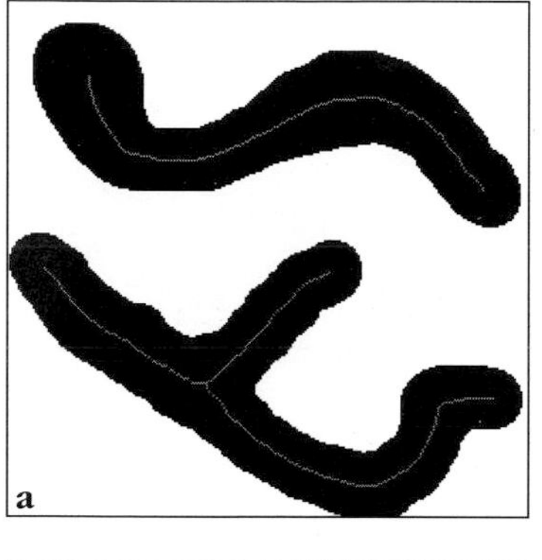

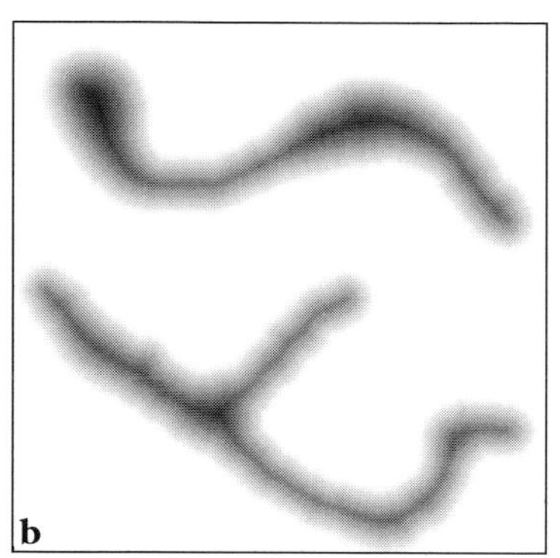

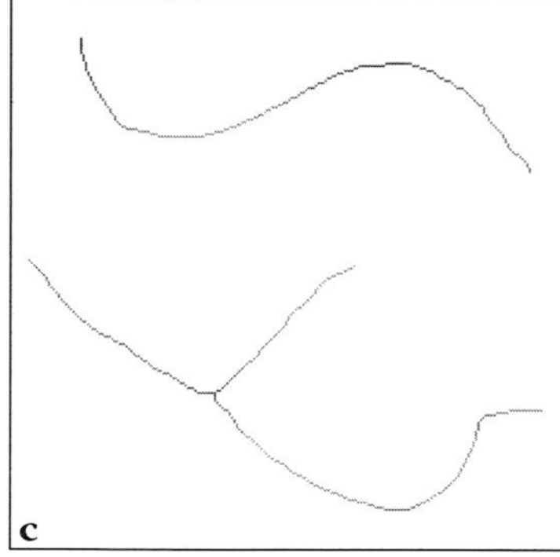

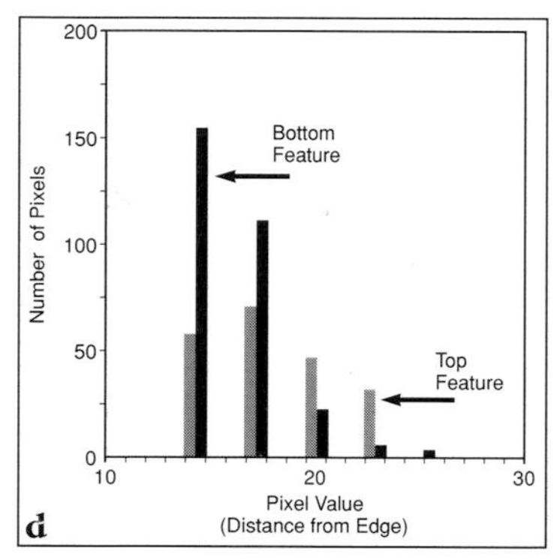

Figure 73. Use of the Euclidean distance map to measure feature width:
a) *test image consisting of two features of variable width, one with a branch point, and the skeleton of each shown superimposed;*
b) *Euclidean distance map of the features;*
c) *using the skeleton to select only the points in the distance map which lie along the axis, but retaining their grey values;*
d) *histogram of the values of the points in image c for each pixel, which characterizes the mean and variation in feature width.*

two (or more) parts. The number of iterations required is proportional to the largest dimension of any feature in the image. As is usual with erosion operations, there may be directional bias.

Very similar information can be obtained much more quickly from the distance map. The ridge of locally brightest values in the EDM contains those points that are equidistant from at least two points on the boundaries of the feature. This ridge constitutes the medial axis transform (MAT). As for the UEPs, the MAT is precisely defined for a continuous image but only approximately defined for an image composed of finite pixels (Mott-Smith, 1970).

In most cases, the MAT corresponds rather closely to the skeleton obtained by sequential erosion. Since it is less directionally sensitive than any erosion pattern and because of the pixel limitations in representing a line, it may differ slightly in some cases. The uses of the MAT are the same as the skeleton. End points and nodes can be counted and the branches and links measured. Because it comes from the EDM, which is constructed without iteration, the MAT can be faster to obtain. **Figure 72** shows a comparison of the skeleton and MAT of an irregular feature. The skeleton is more sensitive to minor irregularities along the feature periphery, which can produce additional branches.

A combined use of the MAT and EDM is shown in **Figure 73.** The values along the MAT represent the distance to the edge of the feature and can be used to find the maximum and minimum

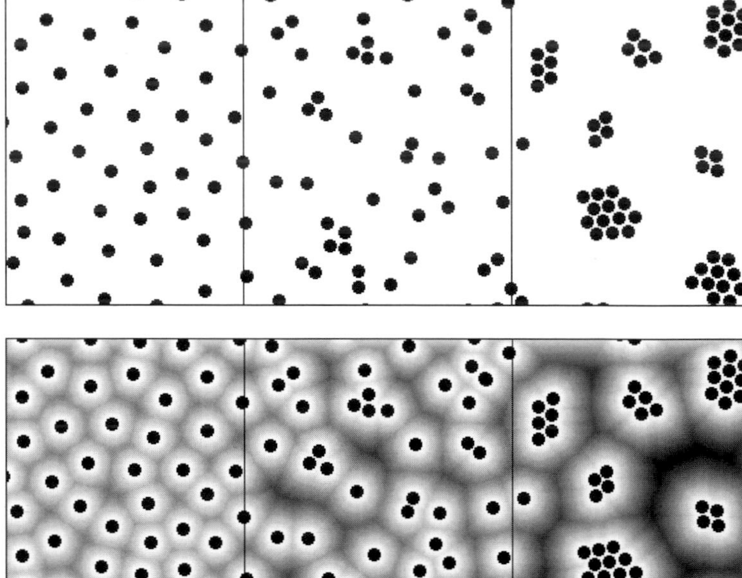

Figure 74. Example distributions of features:
TOP: left) *uniformly spaced;* ***center)*** *randomly arranged;* ***right)*** *clustered;*
BOTTOM: *Euclidean distance map of the background around features.*

widths. A histogram of these values gives the variation in width. Interpretating these values is complicated for a feature with branch points, however.

Cluster analysis

The spatial distribution of features in an image is often interesting, but it is not simple to characterize. One method of characterization (Schwarz & Exner, 1983) uses the spatial coordinates of the centroids of features, sorts through them to locate the nearest-neighbor feature for each feature present, and then constructs a distribution plot of the frequency of nearest-neighbor distances. This requires measuring individual features. It is also based on center-to-center distances, and not the distance between feature boundaries. The histogram of brightness values for the EDM of the background between features also contains information on clustering features.

Figure 74 shows an example of distributions that are clustered, spaced, and random, with the EDM of the background surrounding them. The cumulative histograms of these images are shown in **Figure 75**; the curves are significantly different for the three cases. For tightly clustered feature distributions, the curve rises steeply because there are few points far from a feature boundary. Conversely, for a well-spaced arrangement of features, the curve rises slowly. The slopes, fitted to the straight line portions of the data in the central 80% of the values, are shown.

The axes of these plots are area fraction of the background ver-

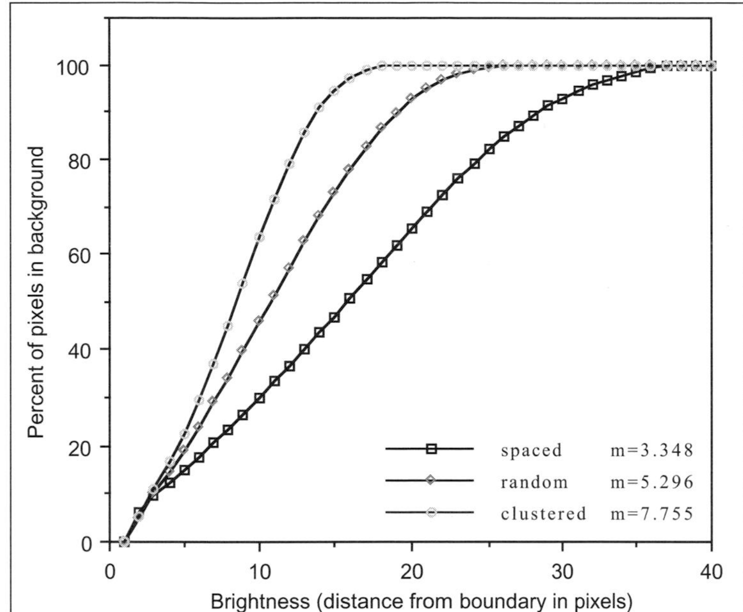

Figure 75. *Cumulative brightness histograms for the EDM of the background pixels in each region of Figure 74, with the least-squares slope for the central 80% of each distribution.*

tically and brightness horizontally. Brightness values are just distances from the nearest feature boundary, so the slopes of the lines have units of 1/length. The length characterized by these slopes is a measure of how far from a feature boundary a randomly placed point on the image is expected to lie. This method can be applied to images without measuring individual features. It is sensitive to the clustering of etch pits marking dislocations in silicon; to inclusions in metals, oxides, or other defects in coatings; etc.

Edge effects are present for the center-to-center method (since it cannot be known if the nearest feature to one near the edge is actually within the field of view). To overcome this problem, the distance map can be constructed with brightness values that increase toward the edge of the image, so that the edge will form a ridge. This is equivalent to surrounding the image with repetitions of the same distribution, with each of the four sides forming a mirror image as shown schematically in **Figure 76**. This approximation will be satisfactory if the region covered by the image is a statistically representative sample of the complete population of features, the usual requirement for stereological measurements.

A different approach to detecting clusters is shown in **Figure 77.** The figure could represent the clustering of cell nuclei in tumors or of pores in a ceramic, for example. The skeleton of the background surrounding the points, or the skiz, is obtained first. Then an EDM of the regions inside the skiz lines is calculated and the original points used as a mask. This assigns the values from the distance map to the points. These are not distances from any physical feature in the original specimen, such as cell walls or

Figure 76. *Features in an image with mirror reflections on all four sides, with their EDM showing the straight ridges formed at the image boundary lines.*

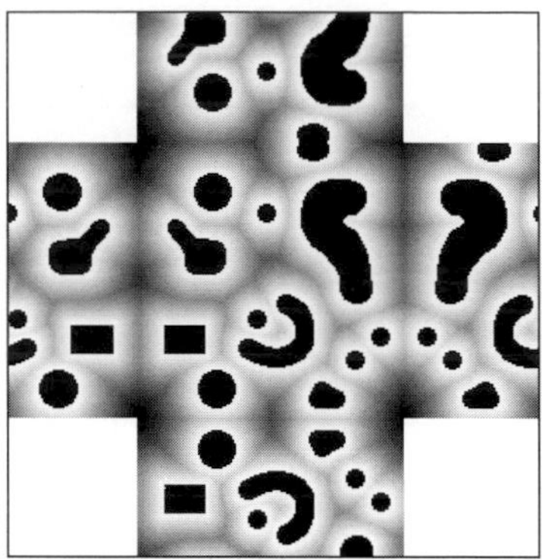

grain boundaries, but simply distances from the lines in the skiz. However, the skiz represents the loci of points equidistant from the points, so the brightness values are proportional to the distance from each point to its nearest neighbor. This allows the points that are clustered together to be selected by simple brightness thresholding.

Figure 77. *Measurement of clustering using the skiz and EDM:*
a) *diagram of features;*
b) *skiz (skeleton of the background);*
c) *Euclidean distance map of the regions delineated by the skiz;*
d) *values from the EDM assigned to the original features (using it as a mask). The clustered features can now be selected by thresholding.*

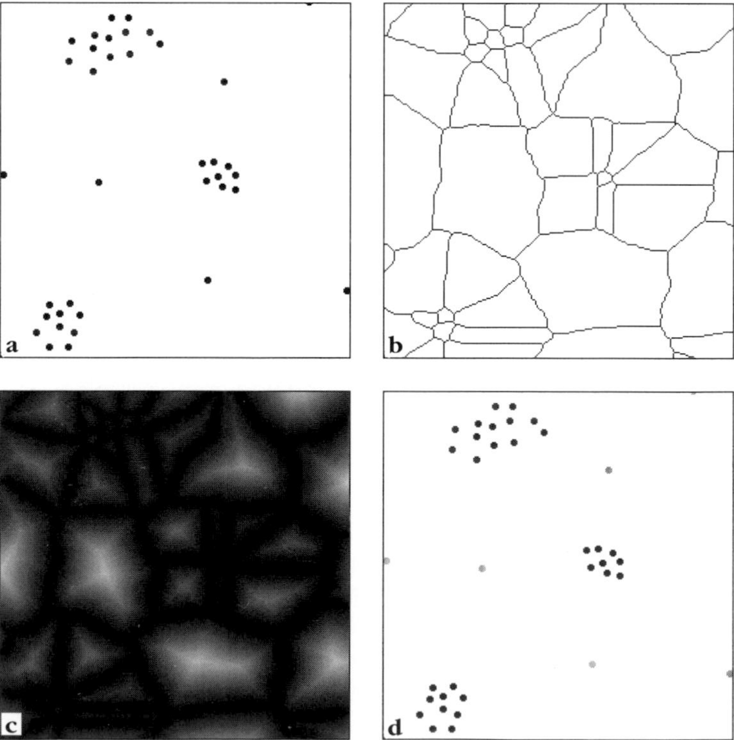

7

Tomography

Basics of reconstruction

Images produced by Computer Assisted Tomography (CAT scans) and similar methods using magnetic resonance, sound waves, isotope emission, X-ray scattering or electron beams deserve special attention. They are formed by computer processing many individual pieces of projection information obtained nondestructively through the body of an object, which must be unfolded to see the internal structure. The mathematical description of the process presented here is that of X-ray absorption tomography, the first and still one of the most widely used applications, both in medicine and in industrial testing (Herman, 1980; Kak & Slaney, 1988). Similar sets of equations apply to the other signal modalities.

As X-rays pass through material, some are absorbed along the way according to the composition and density they encounter. The intensity (number of photons per second) is reduced according to a linear attenuation coefficient μ, which for an interesting specimen is not uniform but has some spatial variation, so that we can write $\mu(x,y,z)$, or, for a two-dimensional plane through the object, $\mu(x,y)$. The linear attenuation coefficient is the product of the mass absorption coefficient, which depends on the local elemental composition and the density. In medical tomography, the composition varies only slightly and it is primarily variations in density which produce images. For industrial applications, significant variations in composition are also usually

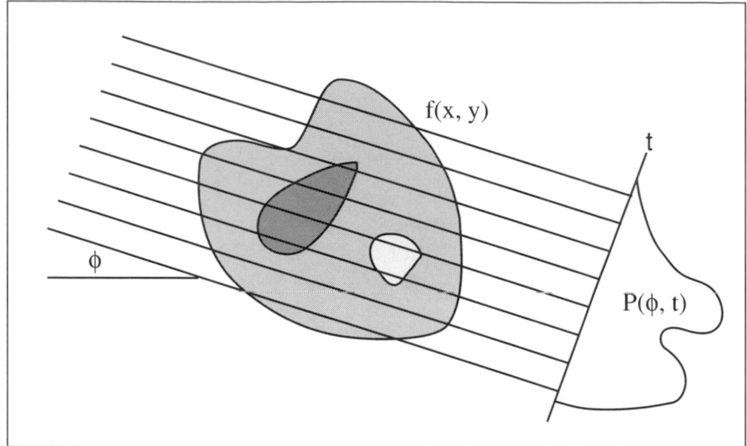

Figure 1. Illustration of a set of projections through an object at a viewing angle φ forming the function P.

present. The measured intensity along a straight line path through this distribution is given by

$$\int \mu(x,y)\,dS = \log_e \frac{I_o}{I_d}$$

where I_o is the incident intensity (from an X-ray tube or radioisotope), which is known and generally held constant, and I_d is the detected intensity. This is called the ray integral equation and describes the result along one projection through the object.

If a series of parallel lines are measured, either one at a time by scanning the source and detector or all at once using many detectors, a profile of intensity is obtained which is called a view. As shown schematically in **Figure 1**, this function is usually plotted as the inverse of the intensity, or the summation of absorption along each of the lines. The function is written as $P(\phi,t)$, to indicate that it varies with position along the direction t as rays

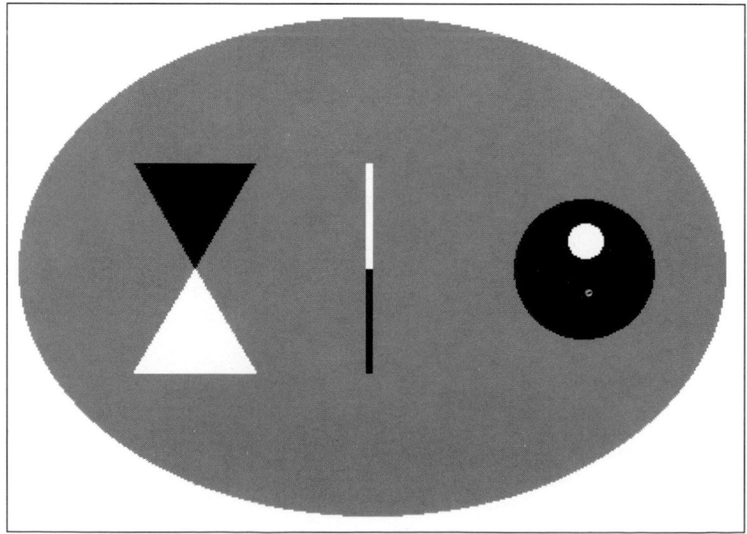

Figure 2. A phantom (test object with geometrical shapes of known density).

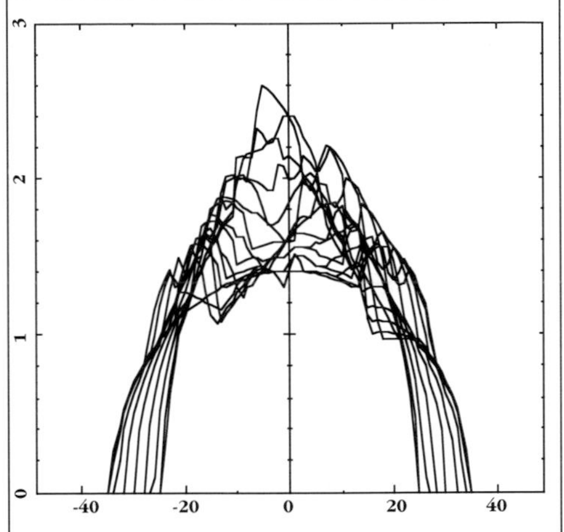

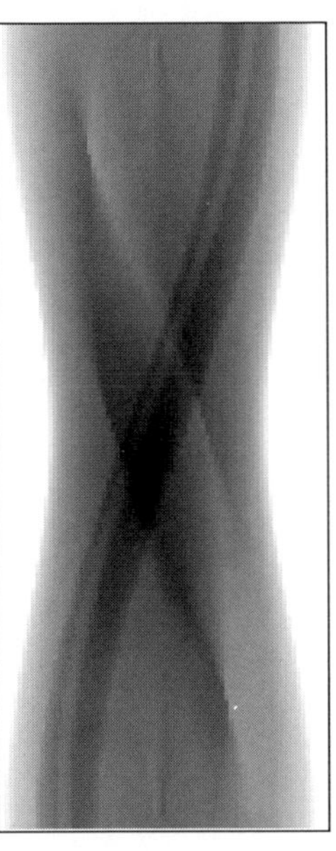

Figure 3. *Sixteen attenuation profiles for the phantom in Figure 2, and the sinogram or Radon transform produced by plotting 180 such profiles (each as one horizontal line).*

sample different portions of the object, and also with angle ϕ, as the mechanism is rotated around the object to view it from different directions (or equivalently as the object is rotated).

Each of the views is a one-dimensional profile of measured attenuation as a function of position, corresponding to a particular angle. The collection of many such views can be presented as a two-dimensional plot or image in which one axis is position t and the other is angle ϕ. This is called a sinogram or the Radon transform of the two-dimensional slice. **Figures 2** and **3** show a simple example. The construction of a planar figure as shown is called a phantom and may used to evaluate the important variables and different methods for reconstructing the object slice from the projection information. The individual projection profiles shown in **Figure 3** show some variation as the angle is changed, but this is difficult to interpret. The sinogram in **Figure 3** organizes the data so that it can be examined more readily.

The name sinogram comes from the sinusoidal variation of projection positions through the various structures within the phantom as a function of rotation, which is evident in the example. The name Radon transform acknowledges the fact that the principles of this method of imaging were published in 1917 by Radon. As we will see, however, the equations that he presented did not provide a practical way to implement a reconstruction, since they required a continuous array of projections, and it was not until Hounsfield and Cormack developed a practical reconstruction algorithm and hardware that CAT scans became a routine medical possibility. A.M. Cormack developed a mathematically manageable reconstruction method at Tufts University in 1963-64 and G.N. Hounsfield designed a working instrument at EMI, Ltd. in England in 1972. They shared the Nobel prize in 1979.

Figure 4. Reconstruction in frequency space. The (complex) one-dimensional Fourier transforms of projection sets or views at different angles are plotted into a two-dimensional frequency domain image, which is then reconstructed:
a) *8 views in frequency space;*
b) *180 views in frequency space;*
c) *reconstruction from image a;*
d) *reconstruction from image b.*

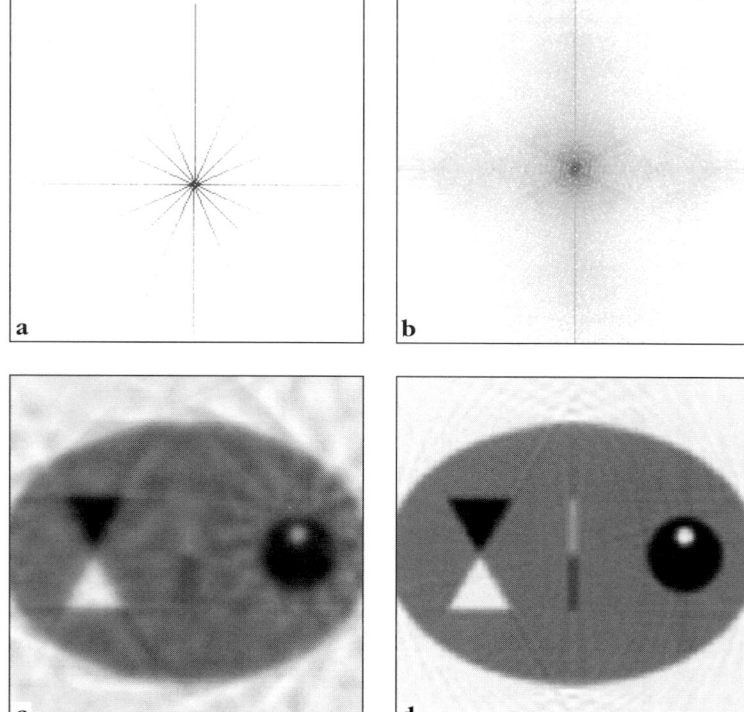

The Fourier transform of the set of projection data in one view direction can be written as

$$S(\phi\varpi) = \int P(\phi,t)\, e^{-j2\pi\varpi t} dt$$

Radon showed that this could also be written as

$$S(\phi\varpi) = \iint f(x,y)\, e^{-j2\pi\varpi(x\cos\phi + y\sin\phi)} dx dy$$

which is simply the two-dimensional Fourier transform $F(u,v)$ for the function $f(x,y)$ with the constraints that $u = \omega \cos \phi$ and $v = \omega \sin \phi$, which is simply the equation of the line for the projection.

What this means is that starting with the original image of the phantom, forming its two-dimensional Fourier transform as discussed in Chapter 4, and then looking at the information in that image along a radial direction from the origin normal to the direction ϕ would give the function S, which is just the one-dimensional Fourier transform of the projection data in direction ϕ in real space. The way this is useful in practice is to measure the projections P in many directions, calculate the one-dimensional transforms S, plot the complex coefficients of S into a two-dimensional transform image in the corresponding direction, and, after enough directions have been measured, perform an inverse two-dimensional Fourier transform to recover the spatial-domain image for the slice. This permits a reconstruction of the slice image from the projection data, so that a non-destructive internal image can be obtained. This is the principle behind tomographic imaging.

Figure 4 shows an example. Eight views or sets of projections are taken at equal angle steps and the Fourier transform of each is calculated and plotted into a two-dimensional complex image, which is then reconstructed. The image quality is only fair, because of the limited number of views. When 180 views at 1-degree intervals are used, the result is quite good. The artefacts that are still present arise because of the gaps in the frequency-space image. This missing information is especially evident at high frequencies (far from the origin), where the lines from the individual views become more widely spaced. All tomographic reconstruction procedures are sensitive to the number of views, as we will see.

By collecting enough views and proceeding in this way, it is possible to perform true tomographic imaging. In practice, few systems actually work this way. An exactly equivalent procedure that requires less computation is also available, known as filtered backprojection. This is the method used in most medical scanners and in some industrial applications.

The principle behind backprojection is simple to demonstrate. The attenuation plotted in each projection in a view is due to the structure of the sample along the individual lines, or ray integrals. It is not possible to know from one projection just where along the line the attenuation occurs, but it is possible to evenly distribute the measured attenuation along the line. If this is done for only a single view, the result is not very interesting. But if it is done along projections from several views, the superposition of the density or attenuation values should correspond to the features present in the structure.

Figure 5 illustrates this for the same phantom. It is possible to see the dense (dark) cylinder with its hollow (light) core in the projections. Data from several views overlap to delineate the cylinder in the reconstructed image. There is a problem with this result, however. The attenuation, or density, of uniform regions in the original phantom is not constant but increases toward the center of the section. Also, edges are blurred.

The cause of this problem can be described in several different but equivalent ways. The projections from all of the views contribute too much to the center of the image, where all projections overlap. The effect is the same as if the image was viewed through an out-of-focus optical system, whose blur, or point-

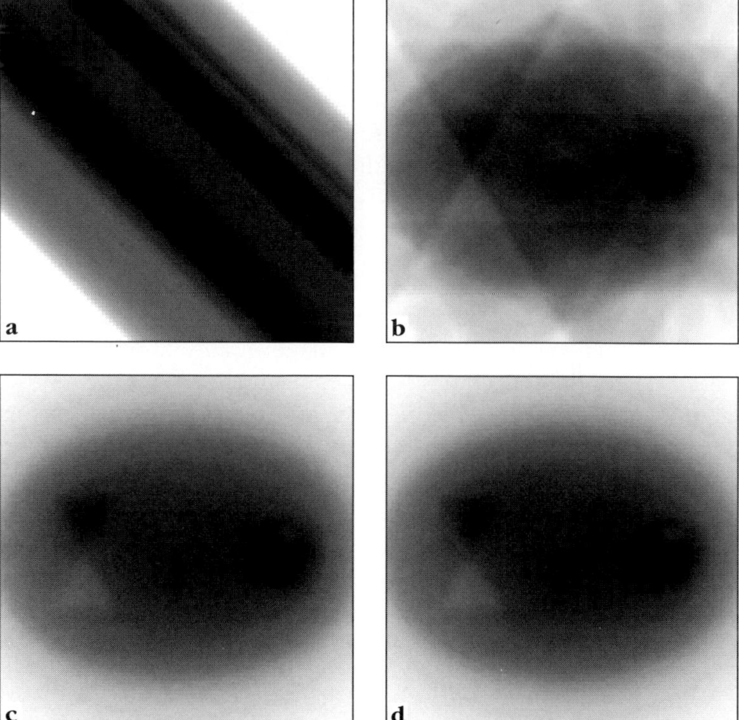

Figure 5. Back projection in the spatial domain. The attenuation values in each view are projected back through the object space along each projection line. Adding together the data from many view directions does show the major features, but the image is blurred:
a) *1 view;*
b) *6 views;*
c) *30 views;*
d) *180 views.*

spread function, is proportional to $1/r$, where r is the frequency, or the distance from the center of the frequency transform.

We saw in Chapter 4 how to remove a known blur from an image: multiply the frequency-space transform by the inverse function before retransforming. Based on the Fourier approach and writing the reverse transformation in terms of polar coordinates this gives

$$f(x,y) = \int_{0}^{\pi}\int_{-\infty}^{\infty} S(\phi\varpi)\ |\varpi|\ e^{j2\pi\varpi t} d\varpi d\phi$$

or, in terms of x and y,

$$f(x,y) = \int_{0}^{\pi}\int_{-\infty}^{\infty} Q_{\phi}(x\cos\phi + y\sin\phi) d\phi$$

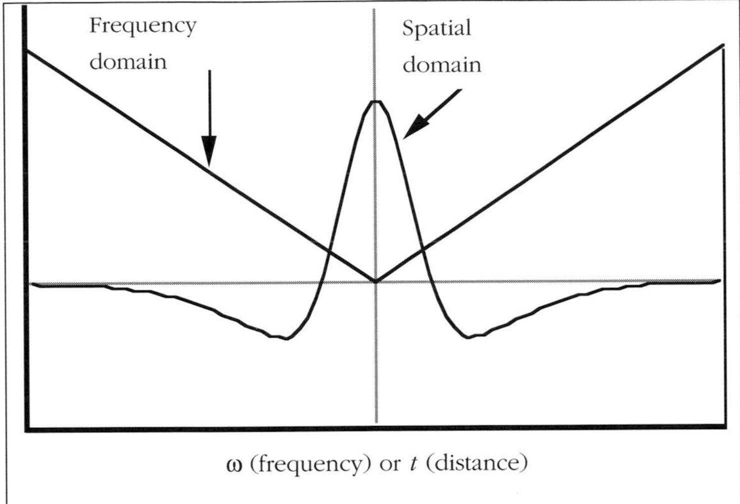

Figure 6. *An ideal inverse filter, which selectively removes low frequencies, and its spatial domain equivalent kernel.*

where

$$Q_\phi = \int_{-\infty}^{+\infty} S(\phi,\varpi)\,|\varpi|\; e^{j2\pi\varpi t} d\varpi$$

This is just the convolution of *S*, the Fourier transform of the projection, by $|\omega|$, the absolute value of frequency. In frequency space, this is an ideal inverse filter, which is shaped as shown in **Figure 6**. As was pointed out in Chapter 4, convolutions can also be applied in the spatial domain. The inverse transform of this ideal filter is also shown in **Figure 6**. Note its similarity to the shape of a Laplacian or difference of Gaussians, as discussed in Chapter 3.

As a one-dimensional kernel or set of weights, this function can be multiplied by the projection *P* just as kernels were applied to two-dimensional images in Chapters 2 and 3. The weights are multiplied by the values and the sum is saved as one point in the filtered projection. This is repeated for each line in the projection set, or view. **Figure 7** shows the result for the projection data, presented in the form of a sinogram. Edges (high frequencies) are strongly enhanced and low-frequency information is suppressed.

The filtered data are then projected back and the blurring is eliminated, as shown in **Figure 8**. Filtered backprojection using an ideal or inverse filter produces results identical to the inverse Fourier transform method described above. The practical implementation of filtered backprojection is easier, because the projection data from each view can be filtered by convolution (a one-dimensional operation) and the data spread back across the image as it is acquired, with no need for storing the complex (i.e., real and imaginary values) frequency space image needed for the Fourier method or retransforming it afterwards.

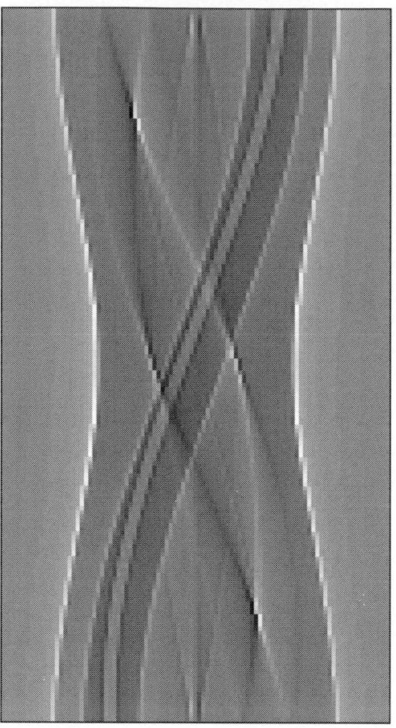

Figure 7. *The filtered projection data from Figure 2, shown as a sinogram.*

Notice in **Figure 8** that the quality of the image and the effect of number of views on the artefacts is identical to that shown for the frequency-space method in **Figure 3**. In the absence of noise in the data and other effects which will be discussed below, these two methods are exactly equivalent.

Algebraic reconstruction methods

The problem of solving for the density (actually, for the linear attenuation coefficient) of each location in the image can also be viewed as a set of simultaneous equations. Each ray integral (or summation, in the finite case we are dealing with here) provides one equation. The sum of the attenuation coefficients for the pixels along the ray, each multiplied by a weighting factor that takes into account the actual path length of that ray through the pixel, is equal to the measured absorption. **Figure 9** illustrates the relationship between the pixels and the ray integral equations.

The number of unknowns in this set of equations is the number of pixels in the image of the slice through the specimen. The number of equations is equivalent to the number of ray integrals, which is generally the number of detectors used along each projection profile times the number of view angles. This is a very large number of equations, but fortunately many of the weights are zero (most pixels are not involved in any one particular ray integral equation). Furthermore, the number of equations rarely equals the number of unknowns. There are a number of practical and well-tested computer methods for solving such sets of sparse equations when they are under- or overdetermined.

It is not our purpose here to compare the various solution meth-

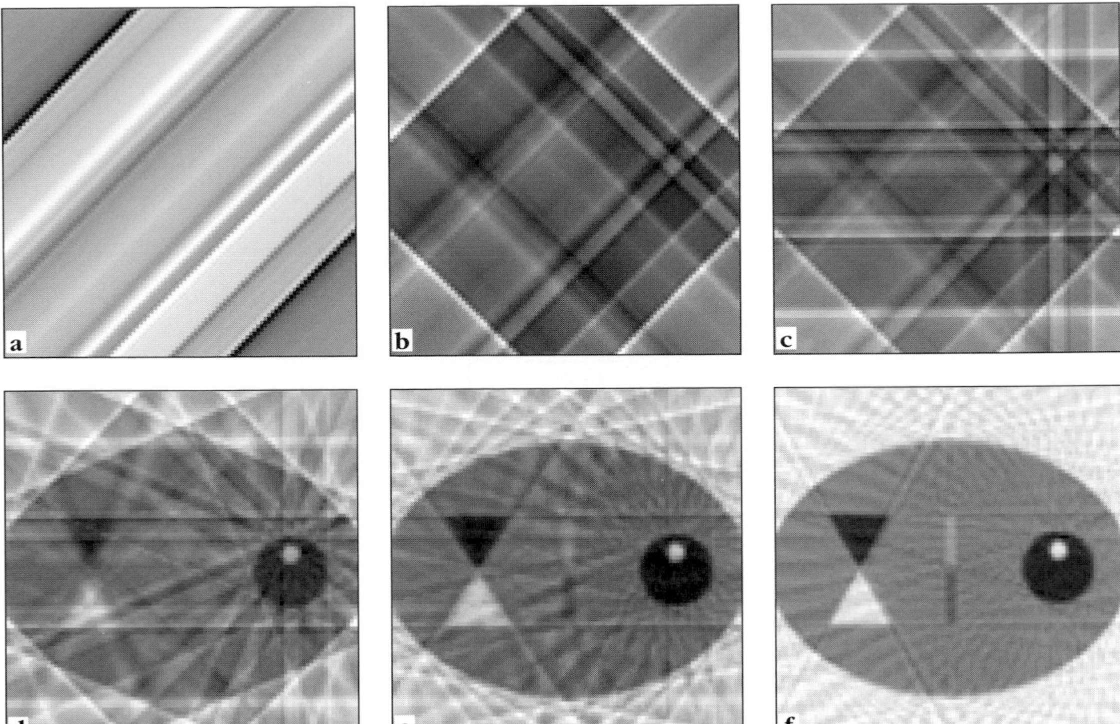

g

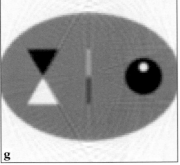

Figure 8. ***Filtered backprojection. The method is the same as in Figure 5, except that the values for each view have been filtered by convolution with the function in Figure 6:***
a) *1 view;*
b) *2 views;*
c) *4 views;*
d) *8 views;*
e) *16 views;*
f) *32 views;*
g) *180 views.*

ods. A suitable understanding can be attained using the simplest of the methods, known as algebraic reconstruction (Gordon, 1974). In this approach, the equations are solved iteratively. The set of equations can be written as

$$A^{m \cdot n} x^{n} = b^{m}$$

where n is the number of voxels, m is the number of projections, and A is the matrix of weights corresponding to the contribution of each voxel to each ray path. The voxel values are the x values and the projection measurements are the b values. The classic ART method calculates each iterative set of x values from the preceding ones as

$$x^{k+1} = x^{k} + A_i (b_i - A_i^{\lambda} x^{k}) \|A_i\|^2$$

Figure 9. *Schematic drawing of pixels (or voxels, since they have depth) in a plane section of the specimen, and the ray integral equations which sum up the attenuation.*

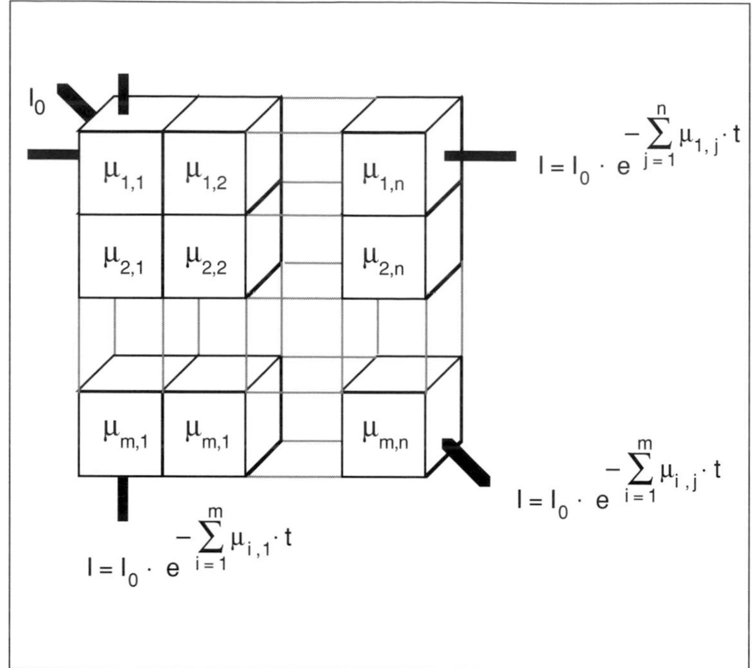

The value of λ, the relaxation coefficient, generally lies between 0 and 2 and controls the speed of convergence. When λ is very small, this becomes equivalent to a conventional least-squares solution. Practical considerations, including the order in which the various equations are applied, are dealt with in detail in the literature (Censor, 1983, 1984).

Figure 10 shows a simple example of this approach. The 16×16 array of voxels has been given density values from 0 to 20, as shown in **Figure 10b**, and three projection sets at view angles of 0, 90, and 180 degrees calculated for the "fan beam" geometry shown in **Figure 10a**. For an array of 25 detectors, this gives a total of 75 equations in 256 unknowns. Starting with an initial guess of uniform voxels (with density 10), the results after 1, 5, and 50 iterations are shown. The void areas and internal square appear rather quickly and the definition of boundaries gradually improves. The errors, particularly in the corners of the image, where fewer ray equations contain any information, and at the corners of the internal dense square, where the attenuation value changes abruptly, are evident. Still, considering the extent to which the system is underdetermined, the results are rather good.

Kacmarz' method for this solution is illustrated in **Figure 11** for the very modest case of three equations, two unknowns, and λ = 1. Beginning at some initial guess, for instance that all of the pixels have the same attenuation value, one of the equations is applied. This is equivalent to moving perpendicular to the line representing the equation. This new point is then used as a starting point to apply the next equation, and so on. Since in the real case the equations do not all meet in a perfect point, because of finite precision in the various measurements, counting statistics, machine variation, etc., there is no single point that represents a stable answer. Instead, the solution converges toward a region that is mostly within the region between the various lines, oscillating there. However, in a high-dimensionality space with some noisy equations, it is possible for the solution to leave this region and wander away after many iterations.

In actual cases having many dimensions, the convergence may not be very fast. The greatest difficulty for the iterative algebraic technique is deciding when to stop. Logically, we would like to continue until the answer is as good as it can get, but without knowing the "truth" this is not possible to judge exactly. Some methods examine the change in the calculated image after each iteration, attempting to judge by that when to stop (for instance, when the normalized total variation in pixel values falls below some arbitrary limit or when it increases from the previous iteration). This method is prone to serious errors in some cases, but it is used nonetheless. It should be noted that the penalty for continuing the iteration is not simply the computational cost but also the possibility that for some sets of data, the answer may start to diverge (leave the bounded region near the cross-over point). This is, of course, highly undesirable.

Given the drawbacks to the algebraic approach and the relative simplicity and straightforward approach of the filtered backprojection method, why would we use this method? There are several potential advantages of algebraic methods such as ART. First, the filtered backprojection method, and the Fourier-transform method that it embodies, requires that the number of views be rather large and that they be equally spaced, so that frequency space is well-filled with data. Missing angles or entire sets of angles that may be unattainable due to physical limitations present problems for filtered backprojection and introduce significant artefacts. ART methods can still produce an acceptable reconstruction. There may still be lack of detail in portions of the reconstructed image that are undersampled by the projections, but the artefacts do not spread throughout the entire image. In fact, acceptable reconstructions are often obtained with only a very few views, as shown in **Figure 10**.

Another advantage to ART is the ability to apply constraints. For instance, it is possible in a filtered backprojection or Fourier transform method to calculate negative values of density (attenuation) for some voxels, because of the finite measurement precision. Such values have no physical meaning. In the iterative algebraic method, any such values can be restricted to zero. In the schematic diagram of **Figure 11**, this amounts to restricting the solution to the quadrant of the graph with positive values.

In fact, any other prior knowledge can also be applied. If it is known that the only possible values of density and attenuation in

Figure 10. Example of the application of an iterative solution. Three projection sets were calculated for an array of 25 detectors, with view directions of 0, 90, and 180° (a). The simulated specimen (b) contains a 16×16 array of voxels. The calculation results after
c) *one,*
d) *five, and*
e) *fifty iterations are shown.*

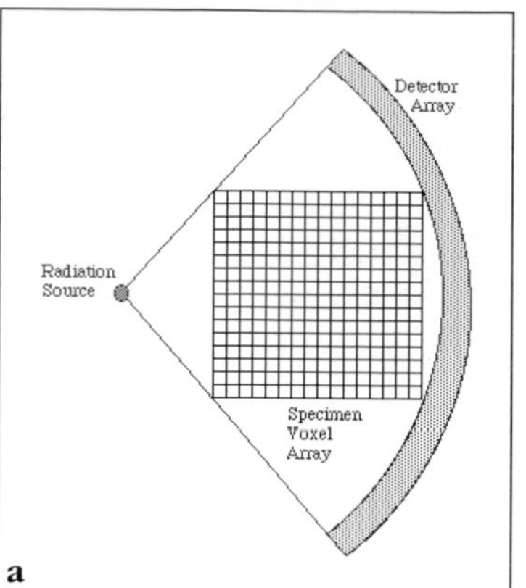

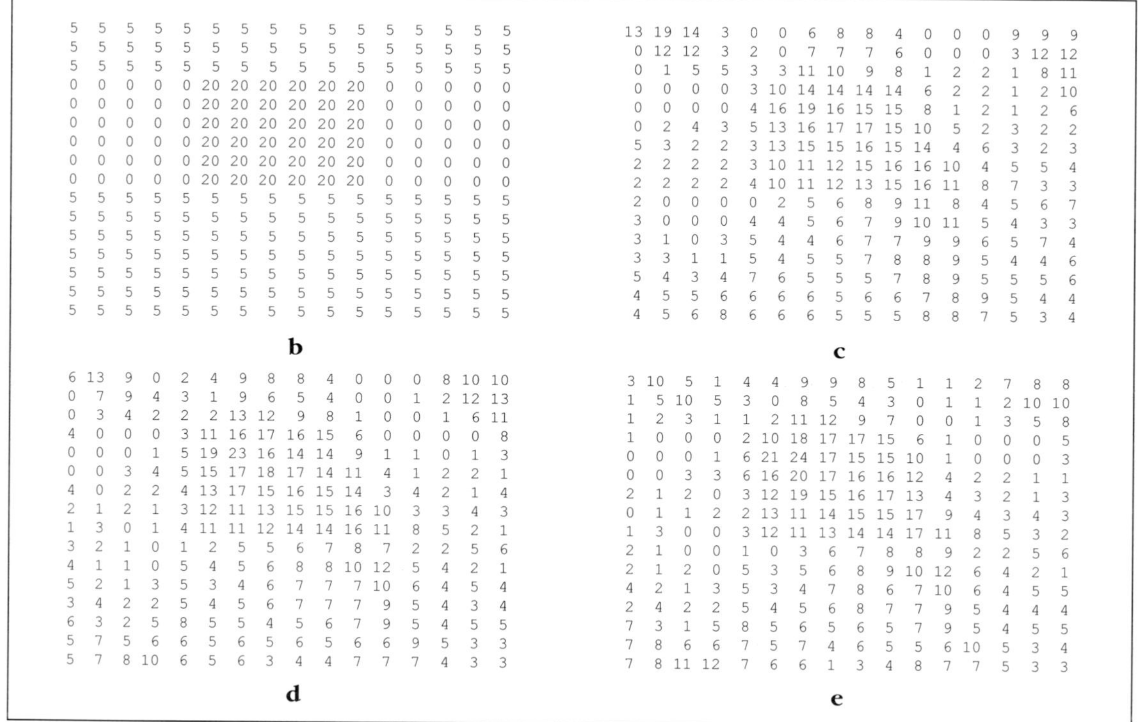

5	5	5	5	5	5	5	5	5	5	5	5	5	5	5	5
5	5	5	5	5	5	5	5	5	5	5	5	5	5	5	5
5	5	5	5	5	5	5	5	5	5	5	5	5	5	5	5
0	0	0	0	0	20	20	20	20	20	20	0	0	0	0	0
0	0	0	0	0	20	20	20	20	20	20	0	0	0	0	0
0	0	0	0	0	20	20	20	20	20	20	0	0	0	0	0
0	0	0	0	0	20	20	20	20	20	20	0	0	0	0	0
0	0	0	0	0	20	20	20	20	20	20	0	0	0	0	0
0	0	0	0	0	20	20	20	20	20	20	0	0	0	0	0
5	5	5	5	5	5	5	5	5	5	5	5	5	5	5	5
5	5	5	5	5	5	5	5	5	5	5	5	5	5	5	5
5	5	5	5	5	5	5	5	5	5	5	5	5	5	5	5
5	5	5	5	5	5	5	5	5	5	5	5	5	5	5	5
5	5	5	5	5	5	5	5	5	5	5	5	5	5	5	5
5	5	5	5	5	5	5	5	5	5	5	5	5	5	5	5
5	5	5	5	5	5	5	5	5	5	5	5	5	5	5	5

b

13	19	14	3	0	0	6	8	8	4	0	0	0	9	9	9
0	12	12	3	2	0	7	7	7	6	0	0	0	3	12	12
0	1	5	5	3	3	11	10	9	8	1	2	2	1	8	11
0	0	0	0	3	10	14	14	14	14	6	2	2	1	2	10
0	0	0	0	4	16	19	16	15	15	8	1	2	1	2	6
0	2	4	3	5	13	16	17	17	15	10	5	2	3	2	2
5	3	2	2	3	13	15	15	16	15	14	4	6	3	2	3
2	2	2	2	3	10	11	12	15	16	16	10	4	5	5	4
2	2	2	2	4	10	11	12	13	15	16	11	8	7	3	3
2	0	0	0	0	2	5	6	8	9	11	8	4	5	6	7
3	0	0	0	4	4	5	6	7	9	10	11	5	4	3	3
3	1	0	3	5	4	4	6	7	7	9	9	6	5	7	4
3	3	1	1	5	4	5	5	7	8	8	9	5	4	4	6
5	4	3	4	7	6	5	5	5	7	8	9	5	5	5	6
4	5	5	6	6	6	6	5	6	6	7	8	9	5	4	4
4	5	6	8	6	6	6	5	5	5	8	8	7	5	3	4

c

6	13	9	0	2	4	9	8	8	4	0	0	0	8	10	10
0	7	9	4	3	1	9	6	5	4	0	0	1	2	12	13
0	3	4	2	2	2	13	12	9	8	1	0	0	1	6	11
4	0	0	0	3	11	16	17	16	15	6	0	0	0	0	8
0	0	0	1	5	19	23	16	14	14	9	1	1	0	1	3
0	0	3	4	5	15	17	18	17	14	11	4	1	2	2	1
4	0	2	2	4	13	17	15	16	15	14	3	4	2	1	4
2	1	2	1	3	12	11	13	15	15	16	10	3	3	4	3
1	3	0	1	4	11	11	12	14	14	16	11	8	5	2	1
3	2	1	0	1	2	5	5	6	7	8	7	2	2	5	6
4	1	1	0	5	4	5	6	8	8	10	12	5	4	2	1
5	2	1	3	5	3	4	6	7	7	7	10	6	4	5	4
3	4	2	2	5	4	5	6	7	7	7	9	5	4	3	4
6	3	2	5	8	5	5	4	5	6	7	9	5	4	5	5
5	7	5	6	6	5	6	5	6	5	6	6	9	5	3	3
5	7	8	10	6	5	6	3	4	4	7	7	7	4	3	3

d

3	10	5	1	4	4	9	9	8	5	1	1	2	7	8	8
1	5	10	5	3	0	8	5	4	3	0	1	1	2	10	10
1	2	3	1	1	2	11	12	9	7	0	0	1	3	5	8
1	0	0	0	2	10	18	17	17	15	6	1	0	0	0	5
0	0	0	1	6	21	24	17	15	15	10	1	0	0	0	3
0	0	3	3	6	16	20	17	16	16	12	4	2	2	1	1
2	1	2	0	3	12	19	15	16	17	13	4	3	2	1	3
0	1	1	2	2	13	11	14	15	15	17	9	4	3	4	3
1	3	0	0	3	12	11	13	14	14	17	11	8	5	3	2
2	1	0	0	1	0	3	6	7	8	8	9	2	2	5	6
2	1	2	0	5	3	5	6	8	9	10	12	6	4	2	1
4	2	1	3	5	3	4	7	8	6	7	10	6	4	5	5
2	4	2	2	5	4	5	6	8	7	7	9	5	4	4	4
7	3	1	5	8	5	6	5	6	5	7	9	5	4	5	5
7	8	6	6	7	5	7	4	6	5	5	6	10	5	3	4
7	8	11	12	7	6	6	1	3	4	8	7	7	5	3	3

e

the specimen correspond to specific materials, then the values can be easily constrained to correspond. Any geometric information, such as the outside dimensions of the object, can also be included (in this case, by forcing the voxels outside the object boundaries to zero).

It is even possible to set up a grid of voxels that are not all the same size and spacing. This might allow, for instance, the use of fine voxel spacing in the interior of an object, where great detail is desired, but a much coarser grid outside. This would still allow the calculation of the contribution of the outside material to the ray integrals but would reduce the number of unknowns to produce a better solution for any given number of views and projections. Sets of non-square voxels can also be used, to conform to specific object shapes and symmetries, when necessary.

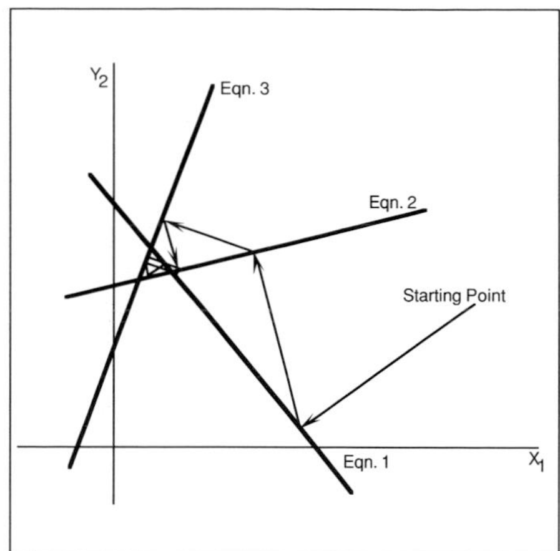

Figure 11. *Schematic diagram of Kacmarz' method for iteratively solving a set of equations, shown here for the case of two unknowns.*

The flexibility of the algebraic method and its particular abilities to use *a priori* information often available in an industrial tomography setting compensates for its slowness and requirements for large amounts of computation. The calculation of voxel weights (the *A* matrix) can be tedious, especially for fan beam or other complex geometries, but no more so than backprojection in such cases, and it is a one-time calculation. Using solution methods other than the iterative approach described here can provide improved stability and convergence.

Maximum entropy

There are other ways to solve these huge sets of sparse equations. One is the so-called maximum entropy approach. Maximum entropy was mentioned in Chapter 2 as an image processing tool to remove noise from a two-dimensional image. Bayes' theorem is the cornerstone for the maximum entropy approach, given that we have relevant prior information that can be used as constraints. In the case where no prior information is available but noise is a dominant factor, Bayes' theorem leads to the classical or "least-squares" approximation method. It is the use of prior information that permits a different approach.

The philosophical justification for the maximum entropy approach comes from Bayesian statistics and information theory. It has also been derived from Gibbs' concept of statistical thermodynamics (Jaynes, 1985). For the nonspecialist, it can be described as follows: find the result (distribution of brightnesses in image pixels, distribution of density values in a voxel array, or practically anything else) that is feasible (consistent with the known constraints, such as the total number of photons, the non-negativity of brightness or density at any point, the physics involved in the detector or measurement process, etc.) and has the configuration of values that is most probable.

This probability is defined as being able to be formed in the most ways. For an image formed by photons, all photons are considered indistinguishable. The order in which they arrive is unimportant, so the distribution of photons to the various pixels can be carried out in many ways. For some brightness patterns (images), the number of ways to form the pattern is much greater than others. We say that these images with greater multiplicity have a higher entropy. Nature can form them in more ways, so they are more likely. The entropy is defined as $S = -\sum p_i \log p_i$, where p_i is the fraction of pixels with brightness value i.

The most likely image (from a simply statistical point of view) is for all of the pixels to receive the same average number of photons, producing a uniformly grey scene. However, this may not be permitted by our constraints, one of which is the measured brightness pattern actually recorded. The difference between the calculated scene and the measured one can only be allowed to have a set upper limit, usually based on the estimated noise characteristics of the detector, the number of photons, etc. Finding the feasible scene having the highest multiplicity is the maximum entropy method.

In solving for the tomographic reconstruction of an object from the set of ray integral equations obtained from various view angles, for example, we have a large set of simultaneous equations in many unknowns. Instead of formally solving the set of simultaneous equations, for instance by a traditional Gauss-Jordan elimination scheme, which would take far too many steps to be practical, the maximum entropy approach recasts the problem. Start with any initial guess (the quality of that guess matters little in the end result) and then iteratively, starting at that point, find another solution (within the class of feasible solutions, as defined by the constraints) that has a higher entropy. Deciding which way to move in the space defined by the parameters (the values of all the voxels) is usually done with LaGrange multipliers by taking partial derivatives and trying always to move "uphill", where the objective function used to evaluate each set of values is the entropy.

It is usually found that the solution having the maximum feasible entropy (i.e., permitted by the constraints) is hard against the boundary formed by those constraints–and if they were relaxed, the solution would move higher (to a more uniform image). For the noise-removal problem discussed in Chapter 2, the constraint is commonly the chi-squared value of the smoothed image compared to the measured one. This is generally assumed to be due to classical noise, so it should have an upper limit and a known distribution.

For tomographic reconstruction, the constraints are based on satisfying the ray integral equations. These are not all consistent, so a weighting scheme must be imposed on the error; linear weighting is the simplest and most often used. It turns out that in most cases, the cluster of solutions with high entropies, all permitted by the constraints, are virtually indistinguishable. In other words,

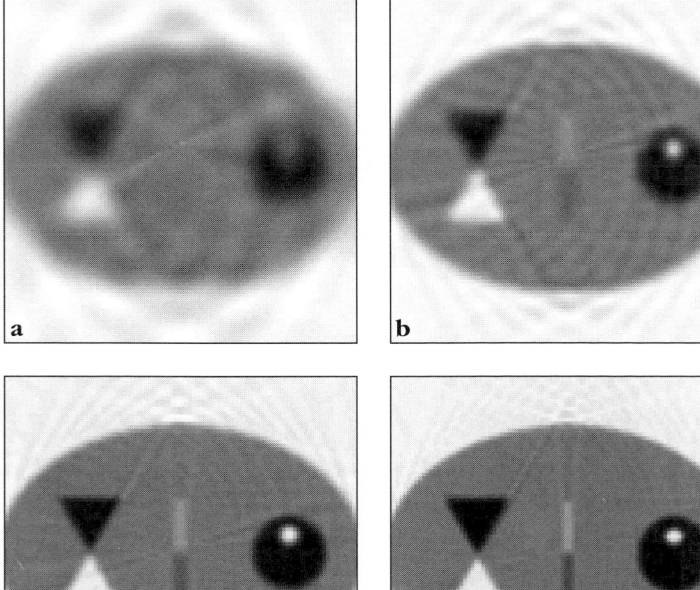

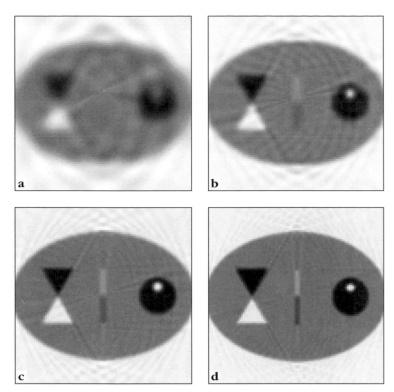

Figure 12. Effect of number of ray integrals in projection set on reconstructed image quality. Each image is reconstructed with 100 × 100 pixels and is calculated from 180 view angles. The images show the use of

a) *25,*
b) *49,*
c) *75,*
d) *99 ray projections, respectively.*

the maximum entropy method does lead to a useful and robust solution. While the solution is still iterative, the method is quite efficient compared to other solution techniques.

Defects in reconstructed images

The reconstructed example shown above was calculated using simulated projection data with no noise or other defects. In real tomography, a variety of defects may be present in the projection sets, which propagates errors back into the reconstructed image. Using the same phantom, several of the more common defects can be demonstrated.

Ideally, a large number of view angles and detector positions along each projection set will be used to provide enough information for the reconstruction. In the event that fewer projections in a set or fewer views are used, the image has more reconstruction artefacts and poorer resolution, boundary definition, and precision and uniformity of voxel values. **Figure 12** shows the effect of fewer projections in each set but nevertheless uses 180 view angles. The reconstructed images are displayed with 100×100 pixels. This ideally requires a number of ray integrals in each projection set equal to at least $\sqrt{2}$ times the width, or 141 pixels. With fewer integrals, the resolution of the reconstruction degrades.

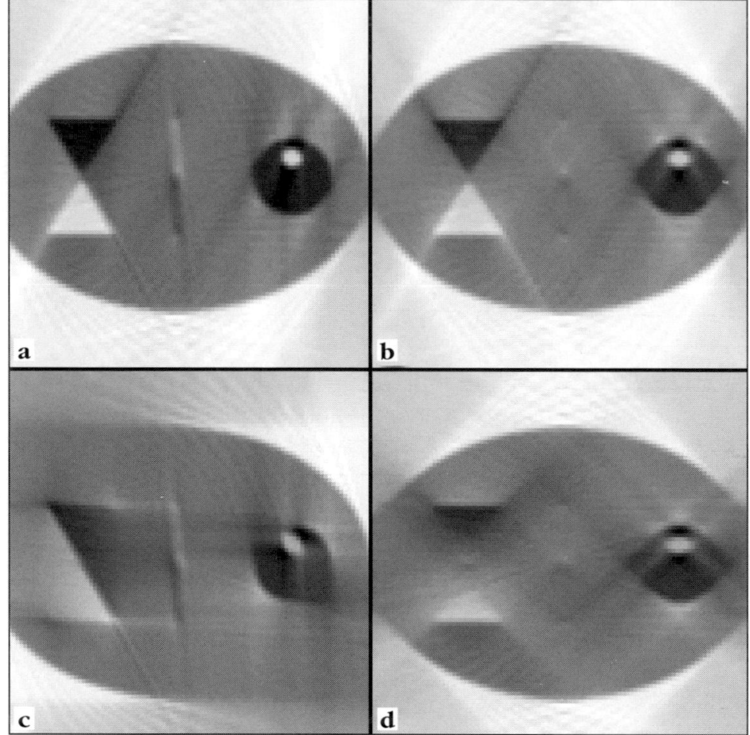

Figure 13. Effect of using a set of view angles which do not uniformly fill the angular range:
a) *150° coverage;*
b) *120° coverage;*
c) *90° coverage;*
d) *a different 90° range.*

If fewer view angles are used (but the angular spacing is still uniform), the artefacts in the reconstruction increase, as was shown above in **Figure 8**. If the view angles are not uniformly spaced, the results are much worse, as shown in **Figure 13**.

In actual images, the number of X-ray photons detected at each point in the projection set is subject to fluctuations due to counting statistics. In both medical and industrial tomography, the number of photons is often limited. In medical applications, this is to limit the total exposure to the subject. In industrial applications, it is due to the finite source strength of either the X-ray tube or radioisotope source and the need to acquire as many views as possible within a reasonable time. In either case, the variation in the number of detected X-rays varies in a Gaussian or normal distribution whose standard deviation is the square root of the number counted. Counting an average of 100 X-rays produces a variation whose standard deviation is 10% ($\sqrt{100} = 10$), while an average of 10,000 X-rays is needed to reduce the variation to 1% ($\sqrt{10^4} = 10^2$).

The process of reconstruction amplifies the effect of noise in the projections, filtering suppresses the low frequencies and keeps the high frequencies, and the counting fluctuations vary randomly from point to point and so are represented in the highest-frequency data. **Figure 14** shows the result. Adding a statistical or counting fluctuation of a few percent to the simulated projection data produces a much greater noise in the reconstructed im-

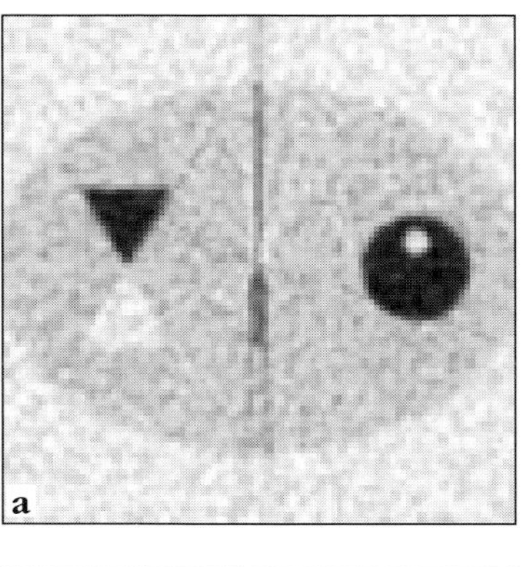

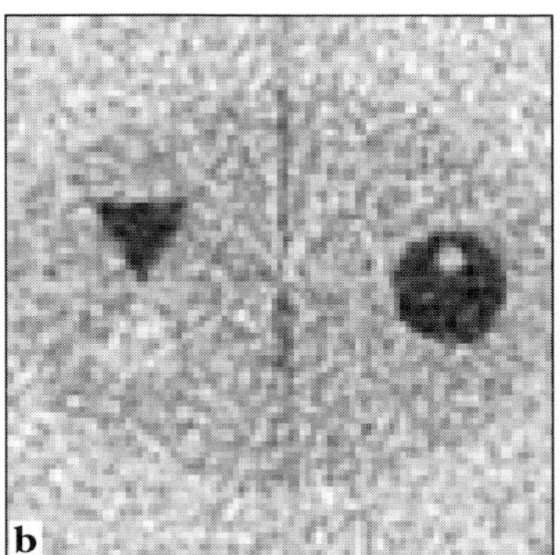

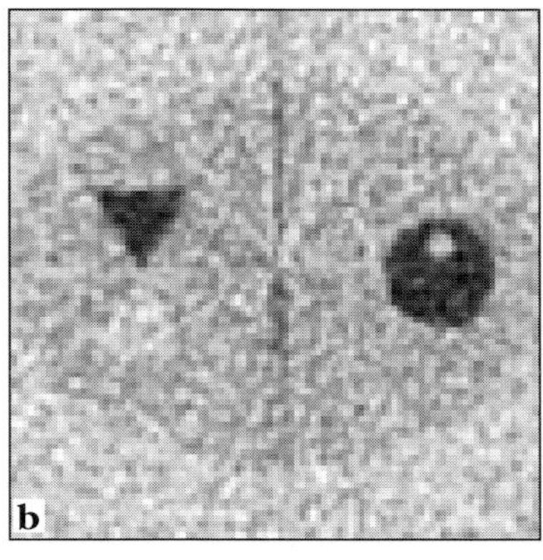

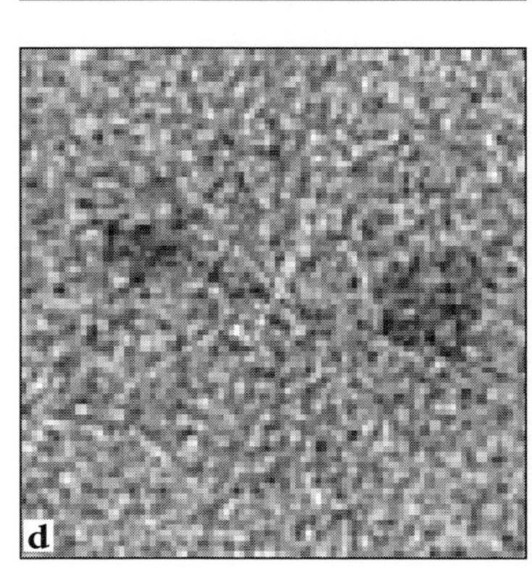

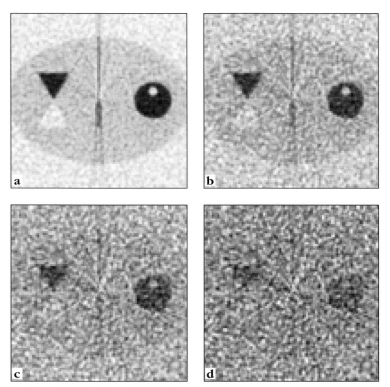

Figure 14. Effect of counting statistics on reconstruction. The images were reconstructed from simulated projection data to which Gaussian random fluctuations were added:
a) *2%;*
b) *5%;*
c) *10%;*
d) *20%.*

age. Although the density differences in the three regions of the phantom vary by 100%, some of the regions disappear altogether when 10% or 20% noise is added to the projection data.

Suppressing high-frequency noise in the projection data by the filtering process can somewhat reduce the effect of noise, as shown in **Figure 15**. Notice that the noise variations in the reconstructed images are reduced, but the high-frequency data needed to produce sharp edges and reveal the smaller structures is gone as well.

Several different filter shapes are used for this purpose. **Figure 16** shows representative examples, in comparison to the shape of the ideal inverse filter discussed above. The plots are in terms of frequency. All of the filters reduce the low-frequency values, which is required in order to prevent blurring, and all of the noise-reduction filters also attenuate the high frequencies in order to suppress noise.

Another important source of errors in the reconstruction of images is imprecise knowledge of the location of the center of rotation, or variation in that center due to imperfect mechanical mechanisms (Barnes et al., 1990). As shown in **Figure 17**, this also produces a magnified effect in the reconstructed image. The characteristic U-shaped arcs result from an off-center rotation because view angles in a range of 180° were used. If 360° rotation is used, a complete circular arc is present (**Figure 18**) which also distorts the reconstruction but is more difficult to recognize. Note

Figure 15. *Reconstructions from the same projection data with superimposed counting statistics variations as in Figure 14, but using a Hann filter instead of an ideal inverse filter to reduce the high-frequency noise.*

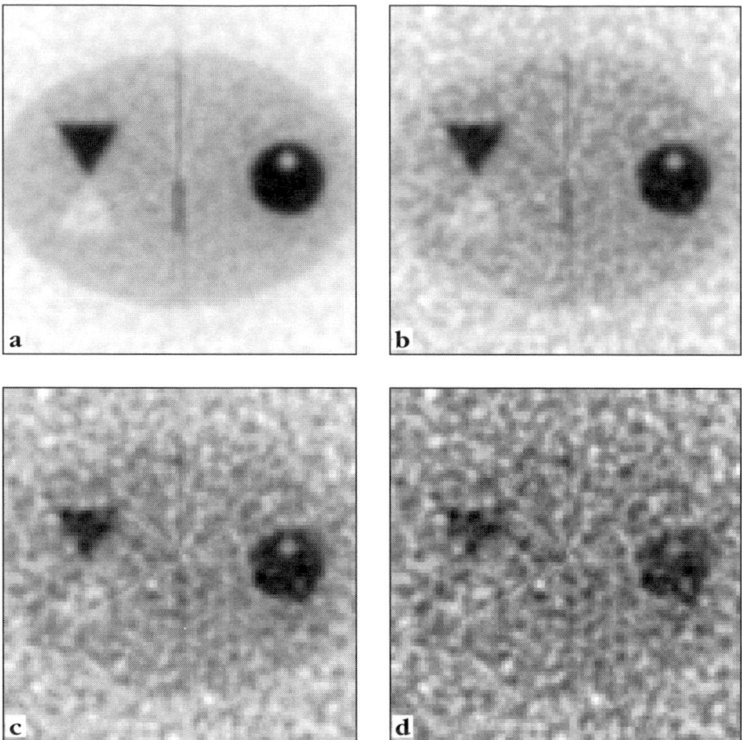

that it is not common to collect data over a complete 360° set of angles, because in the absence of off-center rotation or beam hardening the second half of the data are redundant. The effect of a variable center is equal in magnitude with 360° rotation, but it is harder to recognize. In general, it is required that the location of the center of rotation and its constancy must be less than about one-tenth of the expected spatial resolution in the reconstructed images.

Beam hardening is the name used to describe the effect in which the lower energy or softer, X-rays from a polychromatic source

Figure 16. Filter profiles for noise reduction in filtered backprojection:
Ideal inverse: Weight = $|f|$
Hann: Weight = $|f| \cdot \{0.5 + 0.5 \cos [(\pi/2)(f/f_m)]\}$
Hamming: Weight = $|f| \cdot \{0.54 + 0.46 \cos (\pi f/f_m)\}$
Butterworth ($n = 3$): Weight = $|f| \cdot 1/(1+(f/2f_m)^{2n})$

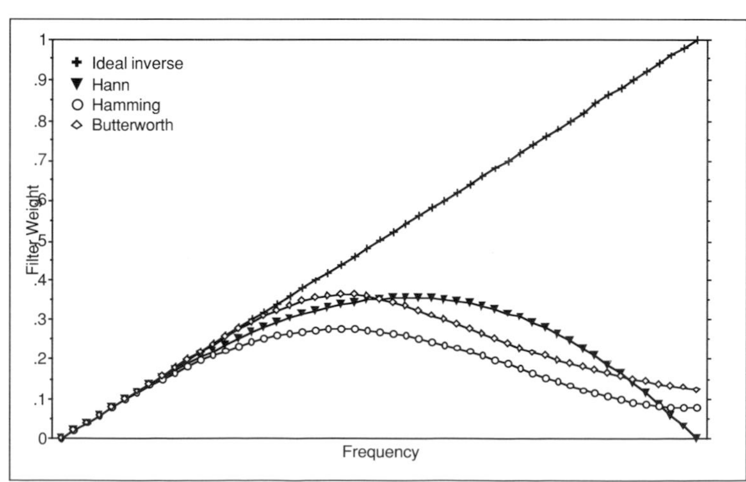

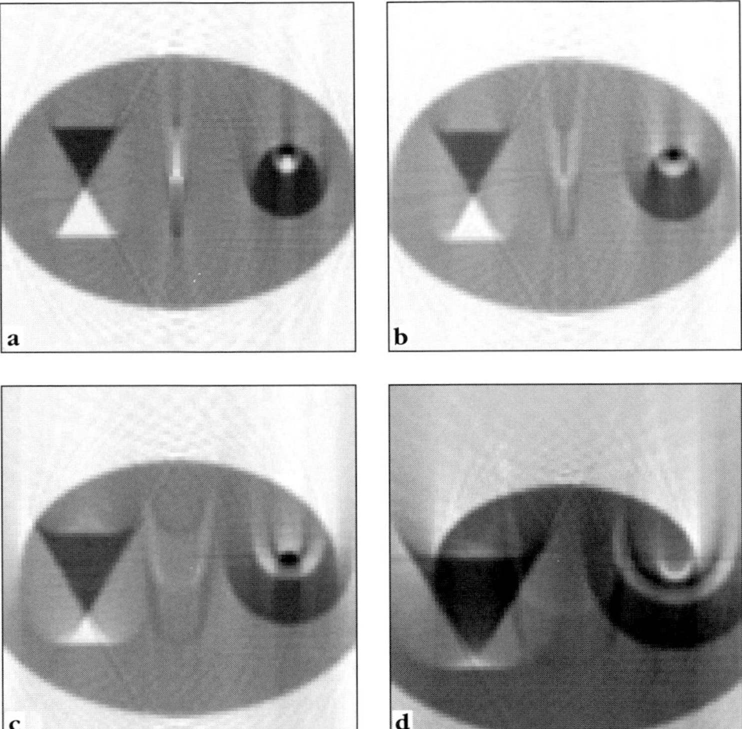

Figure 17. Effect of errors in the center of rotation on the reconstructed image. In each of these images, the center is consistent, but displaced from the location assumed in the rotation by a fraction of the image width:
a) *0.5%;*
b) *1.0%,*
c) *2.5%;*
d) *5.0%*

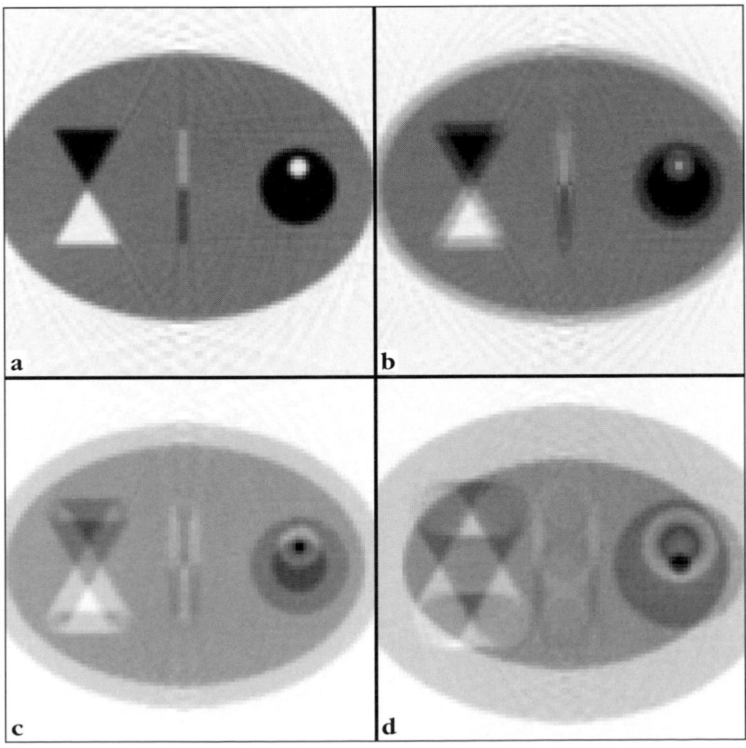

Figure 18. Repeating the reconstructions of Figure 17 using the same number of views (180) but spread over 360° instead of 180°, with the center of rotation displaced from the assumed location by a fraction of the image width:
a) *0.5%;*
b) *1.0%,*
c) *2.5%;*
d) *5.0%*

Figure 19. *Schematic diagram of beam hardening. The energy spectrum of X-rays from an X-ray tube is shown at the beginning, middle, and end of the path through the specimen. As the lower energy X-rays are absorbed, the attenuation coefficient of the sample changes independent of any actual change in composition or density.*

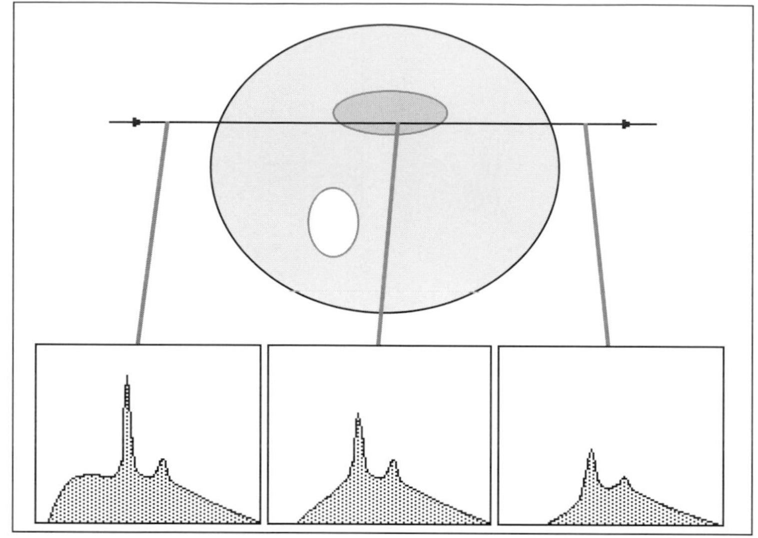

(such as a conventional X-ray tube) are preferentially absorbed in a sample. Consequently, the effective attenuation coefficient of a voxel is different, depending on whether it is on the side of the specimen near the source or farther away. This is indicated schematically in **Figure 19**. Beam hardening is not a major problem in medical tomography because the variation in composition of the various parts of the human body is only slight. The body is mostly water with some addition of carbon, a trace of other elements, and some calcium in bones. The reconstructed image shows a variation in density, but the range of variation is

Figure 20. *Example of beam hardening effect on the sinogram or Radon transform (a) and the inverse filtered data (b). Notice that the contrast of each feature changes according to where it lies within the rotated object.*

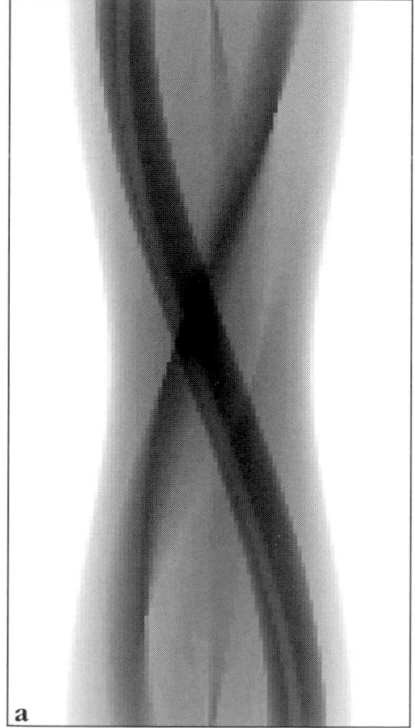

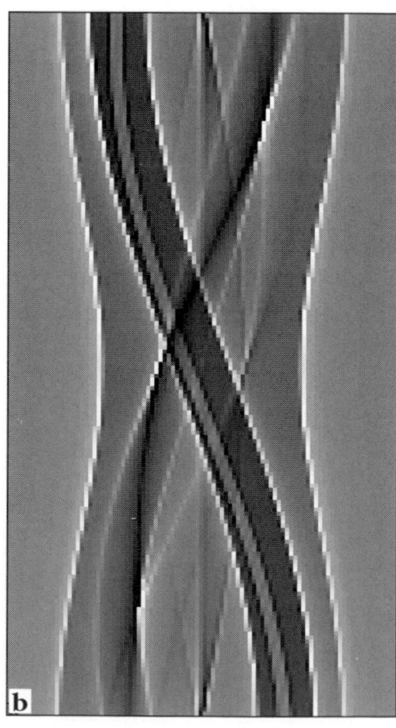

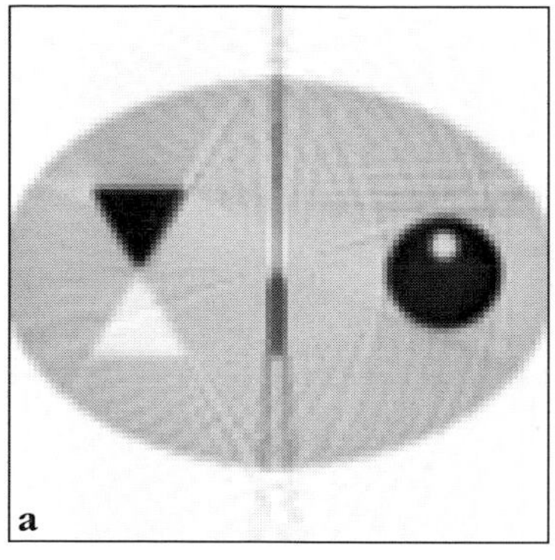

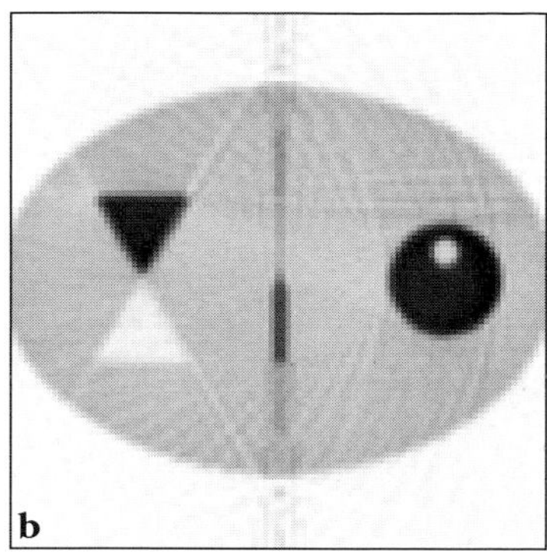

Figure 21. Reconstruction of the beam hardened data:
a) *180 views covering 180°;*
b) *180 views covering 360°.*

small. This makes X-ray tubes an acceptable source and simple backprojection a suitable reconstruction method.

Industrial applications commonly encounter samples with a much greater variation in composition, ranging across the entire periodic table and with physical densities varying from zero (voids) to more than ten times the density of biological tissue. This makes beam hardening an important problem. One solution is to use a monochromatic source, such as a radioisotope or a filtered X-ray tube. Another is to use two different energies (Schneberk et al., 1991) or a combination of absorption and X-ray scattering data (Prettyman et al., 1991), using the two projection sets to correct for the change in composition in the reconstruction process. However, this increases the complexity significantly and requires an algebraic method rather than backprojection or Fourier techniques.

Figure 20 shows a representative example of the beam hardening effect in the same phantom used above. In this case, the sample composition is specified as void (the lightest region and the surroundings), titanium (the medium-grey region of the elliptical object), and iron (the dark region). The total width is 1 cm and the X-ray tube is assumed to be operating at 100 kV. This is in fact a very modest amount of beam hardening. A larger specimen, lower tube voltage, elements with a higher atomic number, or a greater variation in atomic number or density would produce a much larger effect.

Figure 21 shows reconstructions of the image using view angles covering 180° and 360°, respectively. In most tomography, 180° is adequate, since the projections are expected to be the same regardless of the direction along a ray path. This is not true in the case of beam hardening (as it was not for the case of off-center rotation), so better results are obtained with a full 360° of data. Notice, though, that artefacts are still present. This is particularly true of the central feature, in which the narrow void is hardly visible. **Figure 22** shows the same phantom with no beam hardening, produced by specifying a monochromatic X-ray source.

Figure 22. Reconstruction of the same phantom as in Figure 20 but using a monochromatic 50-kV X-ray source. Notice particularly the void in the center of the object, which is not visible in Figure 21.

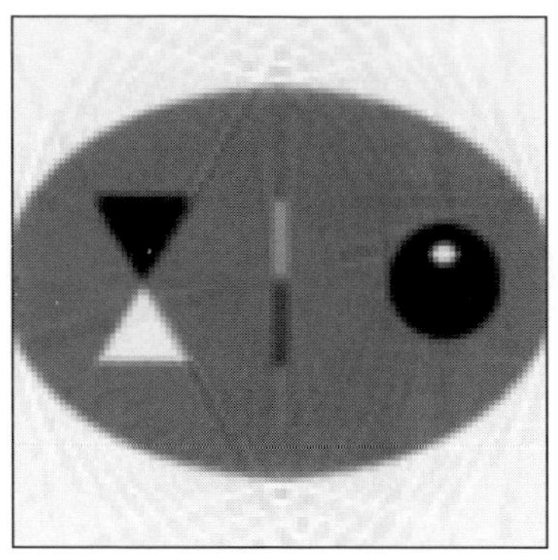

When X-rays pass through material, the attenuation coefficient that reduces the transmitted intensity consists of two principal parts: absorption of the X-rays by the excitation of a bound electron and X-ray scattering, either coherently or incoherently, into a different direction. In either case, the photons are lost from the direct ray path and measured intensity decreases. However, in the case of scattering, X-rays may be redirected to another location in the detector array (see the discussion of the geometries of various generations of instrument designs, below). When this happens, the measured projection profiles contain additional background on which the attenuation data is superimposed. The presence of the background also produces artefacts in the reconstruction, as shown in **Figure 23**. The effect is visually similar to those produced by beam hardening.

Figure 23. Reconstruction of the phantom in Figure 22 when the measured projection sets include scattered background radiation of
a) *5,*
b) *10,*
c) *20, and*
d) *40% of the average intensity. The effect on the image is similar to beam hardening. Small features are obscured by artefacts, and the overall contrast changes.*

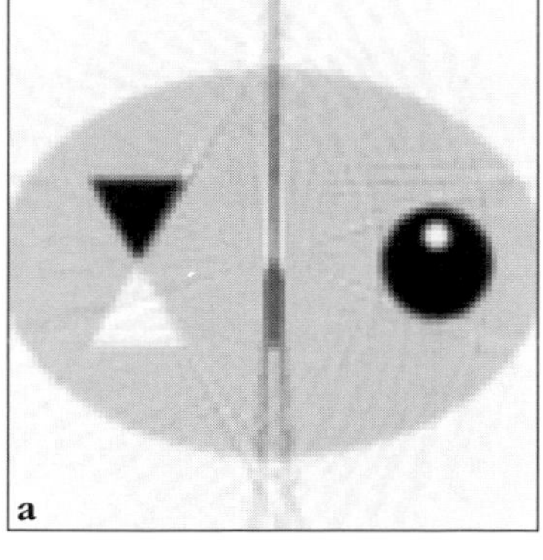

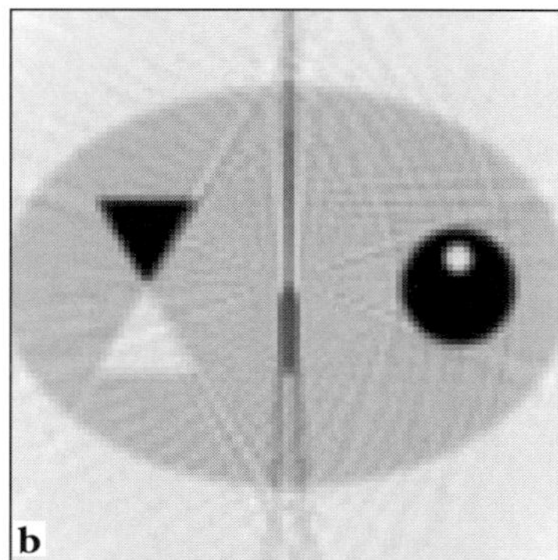

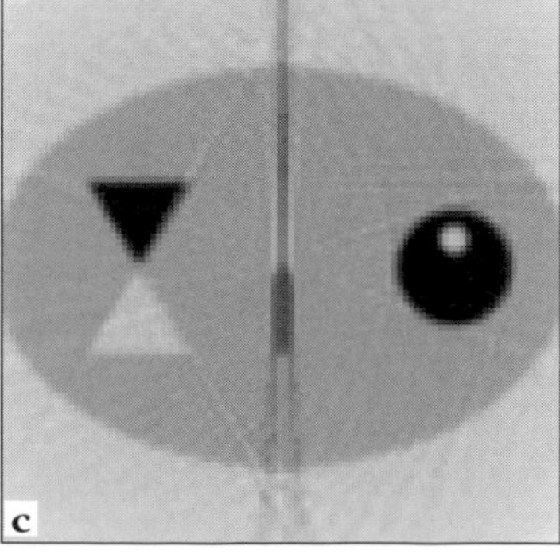

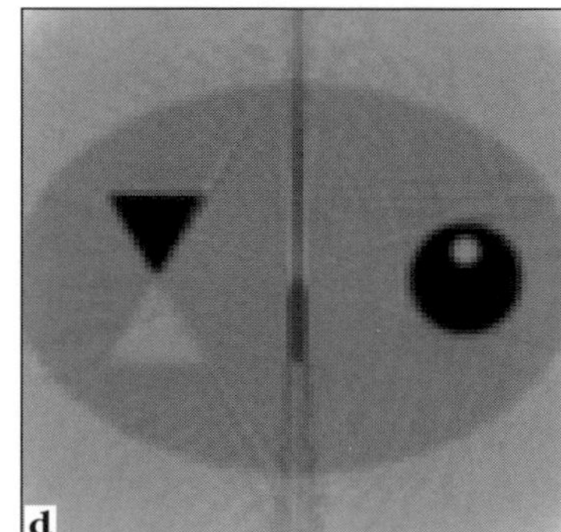

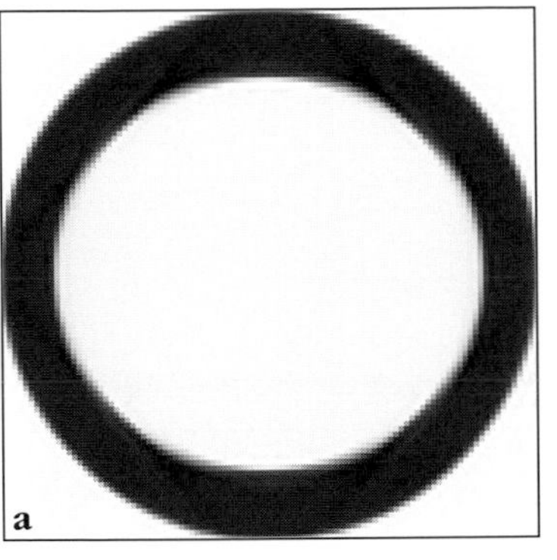

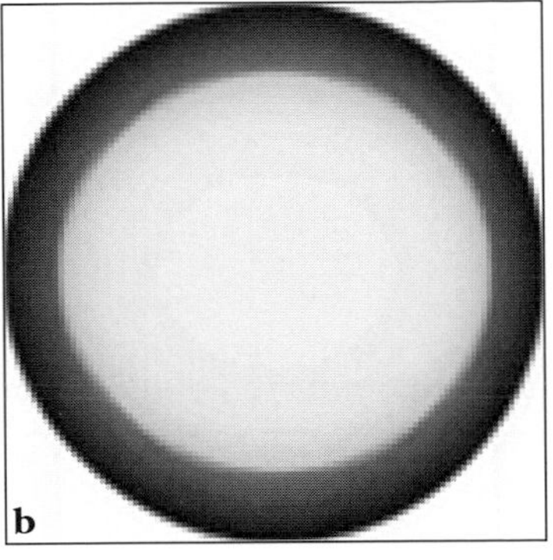

Figure 24. Reconstruction of a simple annulus with outer composition of calcium carbonate (an approximation to bone) and an inner composition of water (an approximation to tissue):
***a)** no scattered background;*
***b)** 10% scattered background in projection data.*

In addition, uniform regions in the object are reconstructed with a variable density due to the background. **Figure 24** shows this for a simple annular object and **Figure 25** shows plots across the center of the reconstructions. The deviation from a uniform density in the reconstruction is called "cupping." Note that this example uses materials similar to those in the human body. However, medical tomography is not usually used to produce a quantitatively accurate measure of density, but rather to show the location of internal structures. Industrial tomography is often called upon to accurately measure densities in order to quantify gradients in parts due to processing; this source of error is, therefore, of concern.

Although medical applications rarely need to measure densities exactly, they do require the ability to show small variations in density. A test phantom often used to demonstrate and evaluate performance in this category is the Shepp and Logan (1974) head phantom. Composed of ellipses with densities close to 1.0, it mimics in simplified form the human head, surrounded by a much denser skull and containing regions that are slightly lower or higher in density, which model the presence of tumors. The ability to image these areas is critical to detecting anomalies in actual head scans.

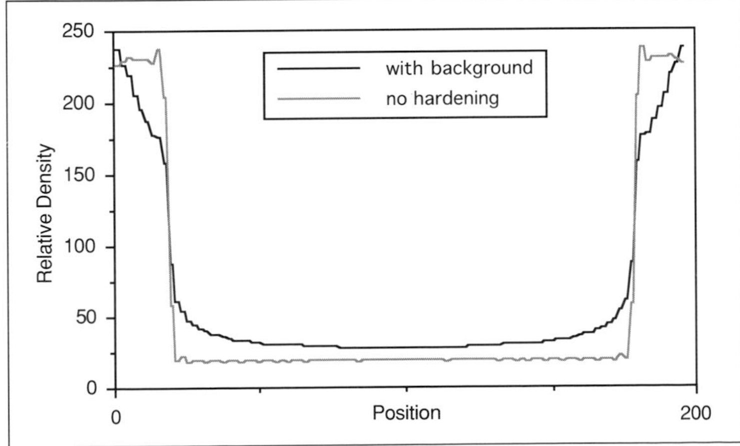

Figure 25. *Line profiles of the density in the images in Figure 24.*

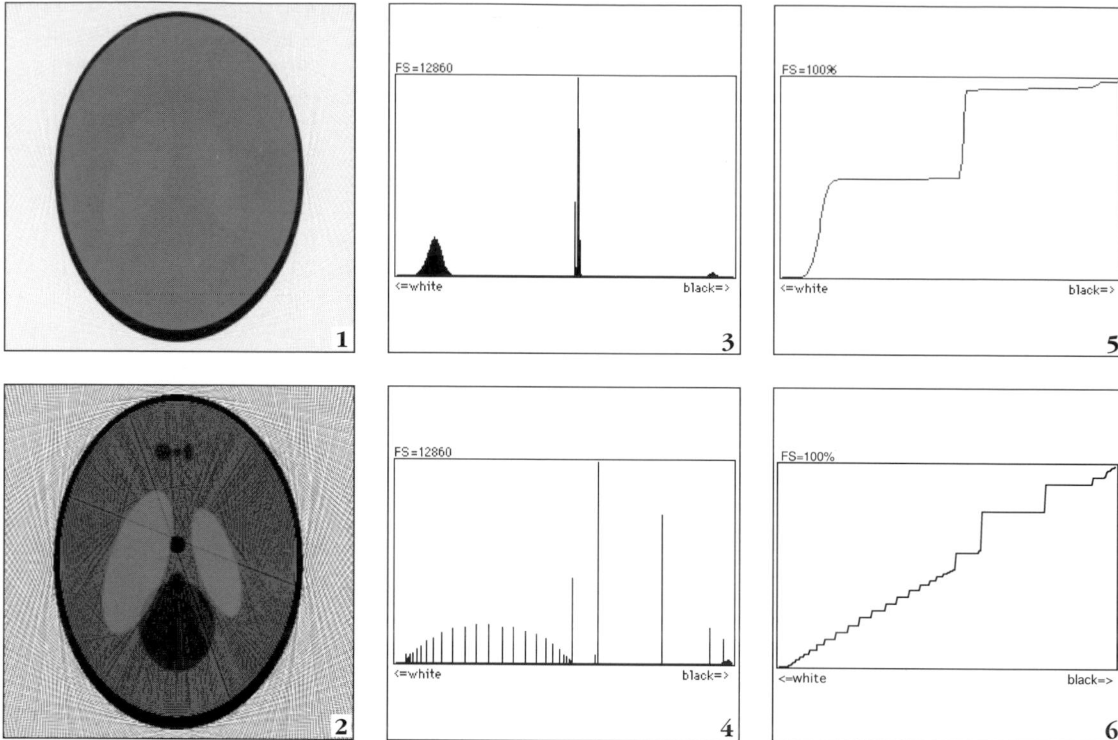

Figure 26. *Shepp and Logan phantom, intended to represent the difficulty of visualizing a tumor inside the human head. The regions of varying density inside the "brain" range in relative densities from 1.0 to 1.04, while the "skull" has a density of 2.0. They are not visible in the reconstructed image unless some contrast expansion is used. Here, histogram equalization (bottom) is used to spread the grey scale nonlinearly to show the various ellipses and their overlaps (and also to increase the visibility of artefacts in the reconstruction). The graphs show the brightness histograms and their cumulative plots. In the latter, the effect of the equalization is especially evident.*

Figure 26 shows a reconstruction of this phantom. Linearly using the full dynamic range of the display (values from 0 to 255) to represent the image does not reveal the internal detail within the phantom. Applying histogram equalization (as discussed in Chapter 3) expands the contrast in the center of the histogram so that the different regions become visible. The figure shows the cumulative histograms of display brightness for the original and histogram-equalized images. In the former, the steps show the principal density values; after equalization, the values more closely approximate a straight line and the steps show the distinction between similar regions. A profile plot across the central region shows the different regions with quite uniform density values (**Figure 27**).

Tomography can be performed using modalities other than X-ray absorption. One is emission tomography, in which a radioactive isotope placed inside the object reveals its location by emitting gamma ray photons. Detectors around the object specify the lines along which the source of the photons lie, produc-

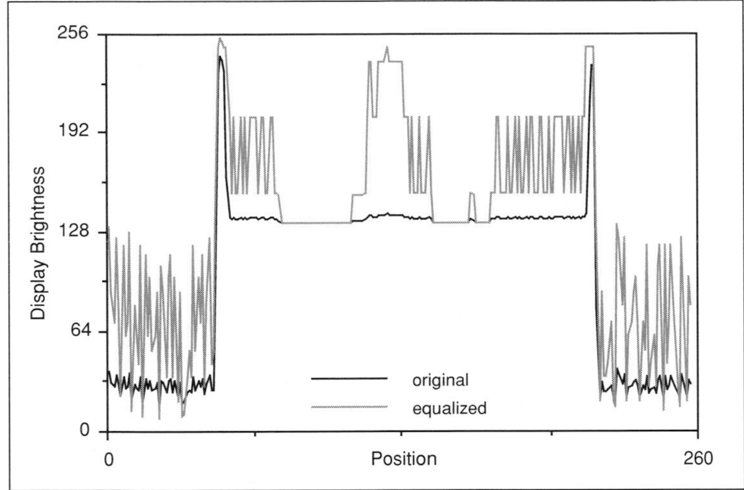

Figure 27. *Brightness profiles across the images in Figure 26, showing the uniformity and sharpness of transitions for the regions and the effect of histogram equalization.*

ing data functionally equivalent to the attenuation profiles of the conventional case. **Figure 28** shows an example of emission tomography using actual data, in which another artefact is evident.

The bright areas in the reconstruction are cavities within a machined part containing a radioactive isotope. The sinogram shows the detected emission profiles as a function of view angle. Notice that the width of the regions varies with angle. This is due to the finite width of the collimators on the detectors, which cover a wider dimension on the far side of the object, as indicated schematically in **Figure 29**. This effect is also present in X-ray absorption tomography, due to the finite aperture size of the source and the detectors. If the angle of the collimators is known, this effect can be included in the reconstruction, either by progressively spreading the data as the filtered profile is spread back across the voxel array, or by adjusting the voxel weights in the algebraic reconstruction technique.

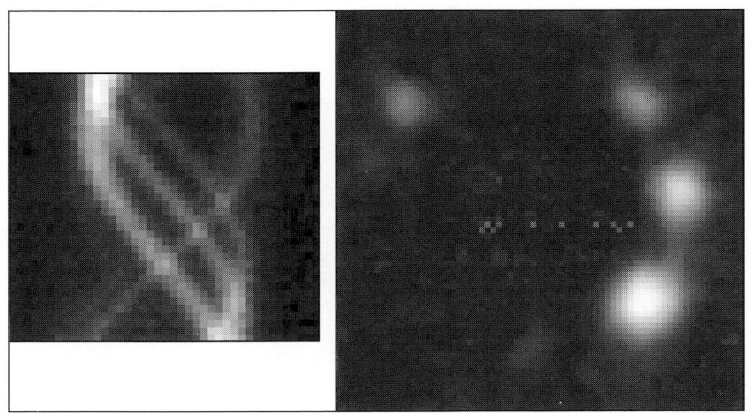

Figure 28. *Emission tomography. The sample is a block of aluminum containing several cylindrical cavities containing cobalt. The detector collects a series of intensity profiles as a function of rotation, shown in the form of a sinogram at the left. Note that the width of the trace for the single isolated cylinder varies as the sample is rotated, due to the finite angle of the entrance collimator to the detector. The reconstruction of the cross-section is shown at the right.*

Figure 29. *Schematic diagram showing the effect of a finite collimator angle on the dimensions and voxels covered in different parts of the object.*

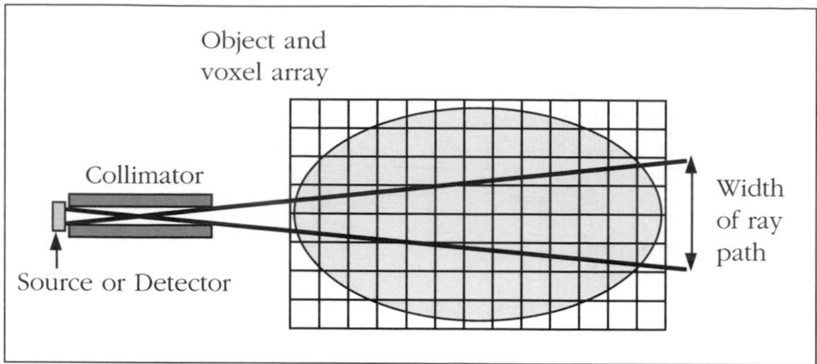

Imaging geometries

First-generation tomographic systems collected projection sets at a variety of view angles by moving a source and detector, as shown in **Figure 1**. **Figure 30** shows the procedure used to collect a complete set of projection data. This is called a pencil-beam geometry, in which each ray integral is parallel and the projection set can be directly backprojected. It is not very efficient, since only a small solid angle of the generated X-rays and only a single detector are in use.

Second-generation instruments added a set of detectors, so that a fan beam of X-rays could be detected and attenuation measured along several lines at the same time, as shown in **Figure 31**. Fewer view angles are required to collect the same amount of data, but the attenuation measurements from each detector correspond to different angles, so some reordering of the data is necessary before it can be used.

A fan-beam geometry is appealing in its efficiency. Therefore, the next logical step in third-generation instruments used for

Figure 30. *First-generation geometry. The detector and source move together to collect each projection set, and rotate to many view angles to collect all of the required data.*

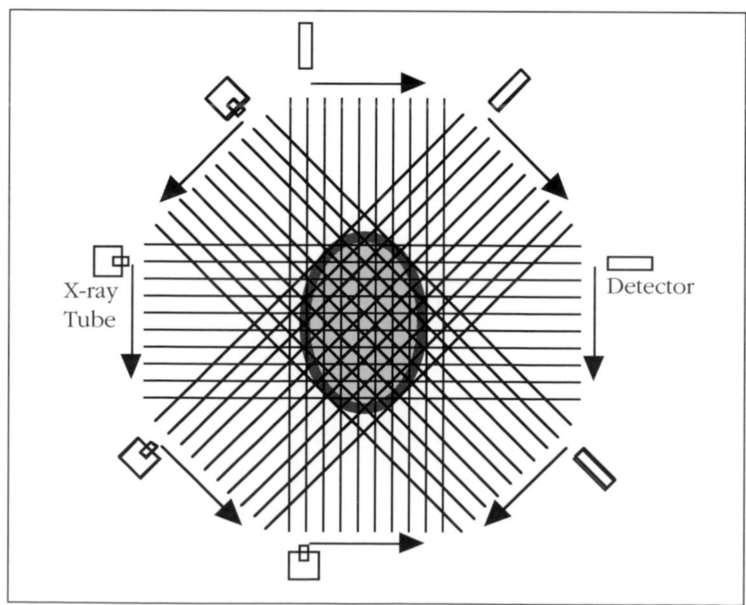

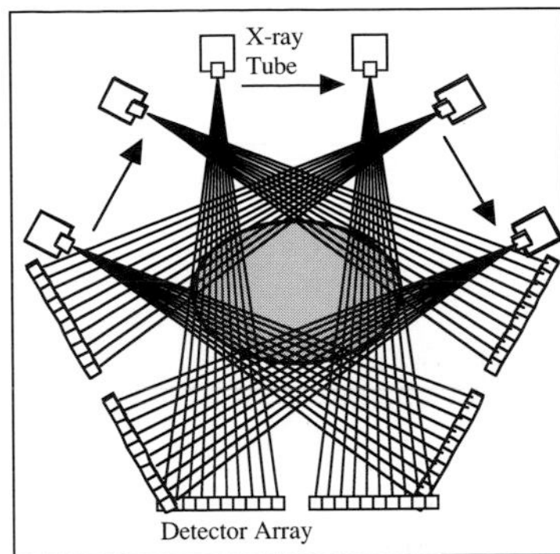

Figure 31. *Second-generation geometry. The detector array simultaneously measures attenuations in a fan beam, requiring fewer view angles than first-generation systems to collect the data.*

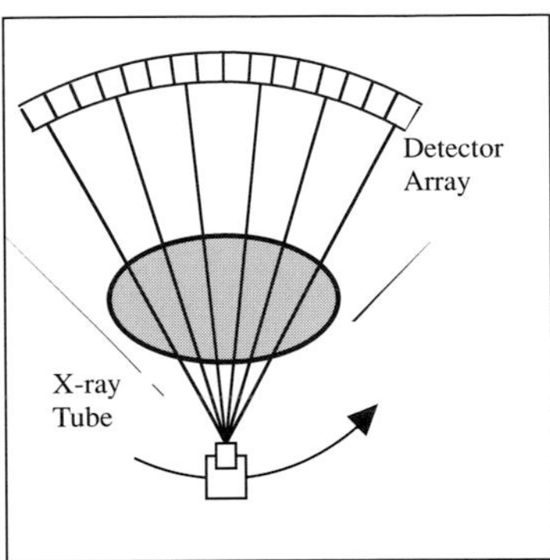

Figure 32. *Third-generation geometry. The X-ray tube and detector array rotate together around the object being imaged, as the tube is rapidly pulsed to produce each view.*

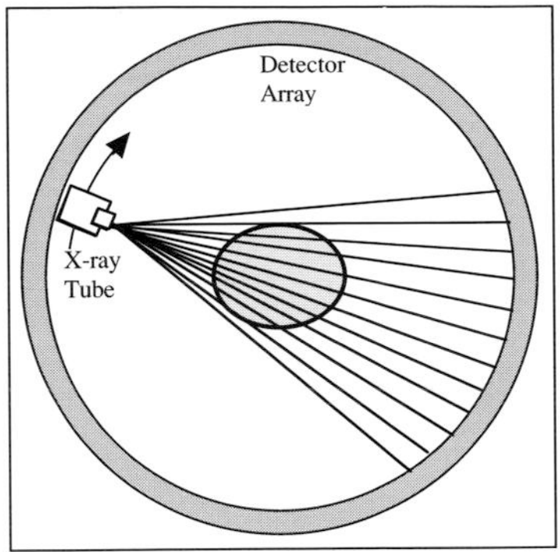

Figure 33. *Fourth-generation geometry. The detector array forms a complete ring and is fixed. The X-ray tube rotates around the object and is pulsed. Data from the detectors are sorted out to produce the projection sets.*

medical imaging was to use a larger array of detectors (and to arrange them in an arc, so that each one covered the same solid angle and had normal X-ray incidence) and a single X-ray tube. Rotating them together about the object as the X-ray tube was pulsed produced the series of views (**Figure 32**). In fourth-generation systems, a complete ring of detectors is installed and only the source rotates (**Figure 33**). Notice that the X-rays are no longer normally incident on the detectors in this case. There is a fifth-generation design in which even less hardware motion is required: the X-rays are generated by magnetically deflecting an electron beam against a fixed target ring and rotating the source of X-rays, producing the same effective geometry as in fourth-generation systems.

These latter types of geometry are less common in industrial tomography, since they are primarily designed for rapid medical imaging to minimize exposure and acquire all of the projections before anything can move in the person being imaged. First- or second-generation (pencil or fan beam) methods collecting a series of discrete views provide greater flexibility in dealing with industrial problems.

All of these methods are equivalent, however, if the various ray integrals using individual detectors in the fan-beam geometry are sorted out according to angle and either backprojected, used in a Fourier-transform method, or used to calculate an algebraic reconstruction with appropriate weights.

Three-dimensional tomography

While the most common application of tomography is to form images of planar sections through objects without physical sectioning, the method can be directly extended to generate complete three-dimensional images. Chapter 8 shows several examples of three-dimensional displays of volume data. Most of these, including most of the tomographic images, are actually serial section images. Whether formed by physical sectioning, optical sectioning (for instance, using the CSLM), or conventional tomographic reconstruction, these methods are not true three-dimensional data sets.

The distinction is that the pixels in each image plane are square, but do not become cubes as they are extended into the third dimension as voxels. The distance between the planes, or the depth resolution, is not inherently the same as the pixel size or resolution within the plane. In fact, few of these methods have depth resolution that is even close to the lateral resolution. Some techniques, such as physical or optical sectioning, have much poorer depth resolution. Others, such as the secondary ion mass spectrometer, have depth resolution that is far better than the lateral resolution of images. This has profound effects for three-dimensional image presentation, image processing, and especially for three-dimensional structural measurement.

True three-dimensional imaging is possible with tomographic reconstruction. The object is represented by a three-dimensional array of cubic voxels and the individual projection sets become two-dimensional arrays (projection images). The set of view directions must include orientations that move out of the plane and into three dimensions, described by two polar angles. This does not necessarily require rotating the object with two different polar angles, since using a cone-beam imaging geometry provides different angles for the projection lines, just as a fan-beam geometry does in two dimensions. However, the best reconstructions are obtained with a series of view angles that covers the three-dimensional orientations as uniformly as possible.

The reconstruction can be performed by any of the methods used in two dimensions. For Fourier inversion, the frequency space is also a three-dimensional array, and the two-dimensional images produced by each projection are transformed and the complex values plotted on planes in the array. As for the two-dimensional case, filling the space as completely and uniformly as possible is desirable. The Fourier inversion is performed in three dimensions but this is a direct extension of methods in lower dimensions. In fact, the inversion can be performed in one dimension at a time (successively along rows in the u, v, and w directions).

Backprojection can also be used for three-dimensional reconstruction. As in the two-dimensional case, it is simply an implementation of the Fourier transform mathematics. Filtering the two-dimensional images must be performed with a two-dimensional convolution, which can be carried out either by kernel operation in the spatial domain or by multiplication in the Fourier domain. The principal difficulty with the backprojection method

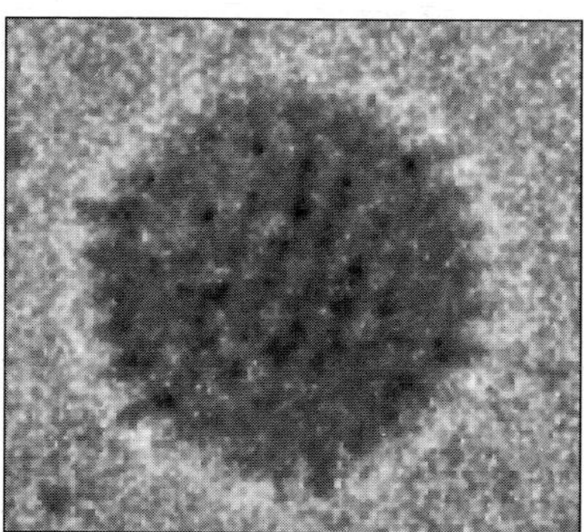

Figure 34. Transmission electron microscope image of single adenovirus particle.

is that calculating the matrix of weights can be quite tricky. These values represent the attenuation path length along each of the ray integrals through each of the voxels.

Algebraic reconstruction methods are also applicable to voxel arrays. The difficulty in obtaining a uniform set of view angles, particularly the case for electron microscopy, can make this approach particularly attractive. This raises the point that tomographic reconstruction is by no means limited to X-rays. Examples of medical imaging using nuclear magnetic resonance (MRI) are shown in Chapter 8.

In the SEM, contrast is produced by attenuation and a series of views at different angles can be reconstructed to show three-dimensional structure. This is difficult for materials specimens because of electron diffraction from planes of atoms in the crystal structure. This source of contrast is not easily modeled by the usual attenuation calculation, since one voxel may have quite different values in different directions. However, for noncrystaline materials, such as biological specimens, reconstruction is straightforward (Engel & Massalski, 1984; Hegerl, 1989).

Even more efficient than collecting a series of different views using multiple orientations of a single specimen is using images of identical specimens having different orientations. **Figure 34** shows an example. The two-dimensional image is an electron micrograph of a single virus particle. The specimen is an adenovirus, which causes respiratory ailments.

The low dose of electrons required to prevent damage to the specimen makes the image very noisy. In a typical specimen there are many such particles, each in a different, essentially random orientation. Collecting the various images, indexing the orientation of each one by referring to the location of the triangular facets on the virus surface, and performing a reconstruction produces a three-dimensional reconstruction of the particle in which each voxel value is the electron density. Modeling the surface of the outer protein coat of the virus, as discussed in Chapter 8, produces the surface-rendered image shown in **Figure 35** (Stewart & Burnett, 1991).

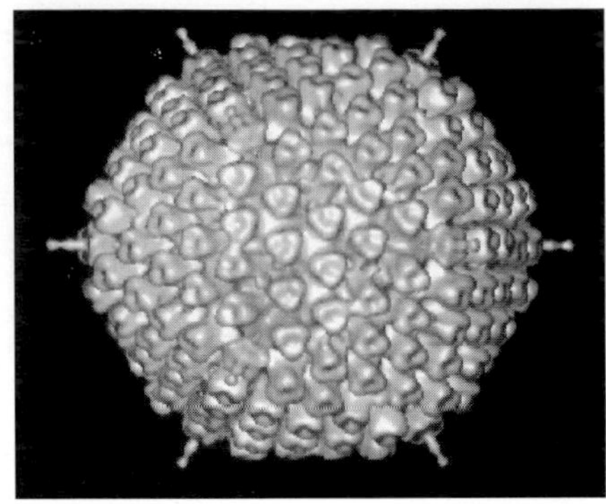

Figure 35. Reconstruction of the adenovirus particle from many transmission images.

At a very different scale, tomography has also been performed on the earth itself, using seismography. Seismic waves are created by earthquakes or large explosions, such as nuclear weapons tests. They generate two types of waves that propagate through the earth to receivers (seismographs) at many different locations. P-waves (pressure waves) are compressional pulses that can penetrate through every part of the earth's interior, while S-waves (shear waves) are transverse deformations that cannot propagate through the liquid outer core. In fact, the presence of a liquid core was deduced in 1906 by the British seismologist R. D. Oldham by the shadow cast by the core in seismic S-wave patterns.

The paths of seismic waves are not straight (**Figure 36**), but bend because of the variations in temperature, pressure, and composition within the earth, which affects the speed of transmission–just as the index of refraction of glass affects light and causes it to bend. Also like light, the seismic waves may reflect at interfaces, where the speed of propagation varies abruptly. This happens at the core-mantle boundary and the surface of the inner core. The propagation velocities of the P- and S-waves are different and respond differently to composition.

Collecting many seismograms from different events creates a set of ray paths that do not uniformly cover the earth; rather, they depend on the chance (and nonuniform) distribution of earthquakes and the distribution of seismographs. Nevertheless, ana-

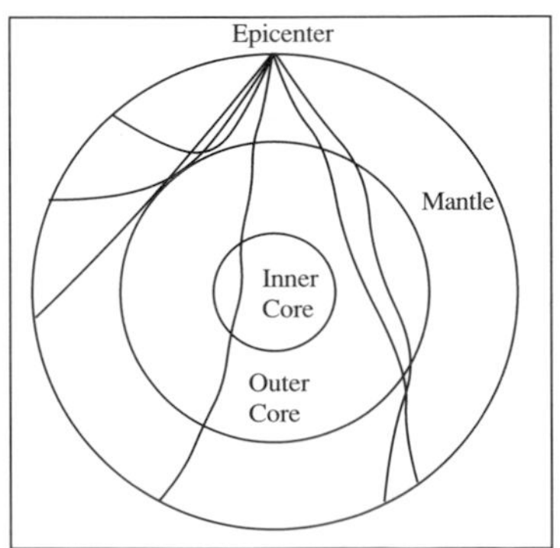

Figure 36. Diagram of paths taken by pressure and shear waves from earthquakes, which reveal information about the density along the paths through the core and mantle, and the location of discontinuities.

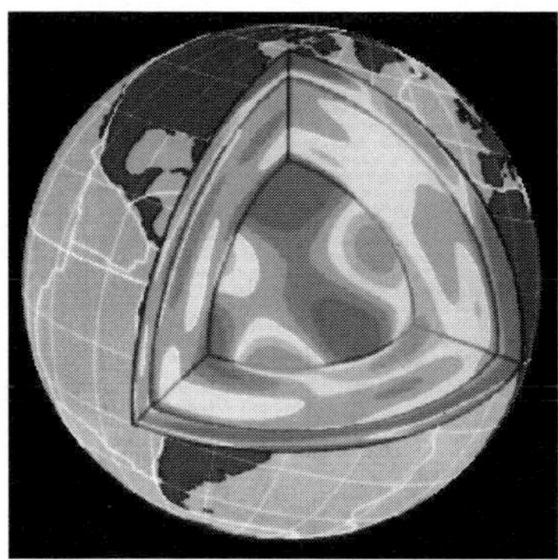

Figure 37. Computed tomogram of the mantle, showing rock densities (light shades are hot, light rocks which are rising, and conversely).

lyzing the travel times of waves that have taken different paths through the earth permits the formation of a tomographic reconstruction. The density of the material (shown by shading in **Figure 37**) indicates the temperature and the direction of motion (cool, dense material is sinking through the mantle toward the core, while hot, light material is rising). Convection in the mantle is the driving force behind volcanism and continental drift.

Also of great utility are waves that have reflected (one or more times) from the various surfaces. For instance, the difference in travel times of S-waves that arrive directly vs. those which have reflected from the core-mantle boundary permits the elevation of that boundary to be mapped with a resolution better than 1 kilometer, revealing that the boundary is not a smooth, spherical surface. Since the relatively viscous mantle is floating on a low-velocity liquid core and it is the relatively fast motion of the latter that produces the earth's magnetic field, the study of this interface is important in understanding the earth's dynamics.

Global tomographic reconstruction is generally insensitive to small details of structure, such as faults, but another current program to perform high-resolution tomography under the state of California (where there are plenty of faults of more than casual interest to surface-dwelling humans) employs an array of high-sensitivity seismographs. Reflections produced by the very frequent minor earthquakes map out the faults.

High-resolution tomography

Medical tomography has a typical resolution of about 1 mm, which is adequate for its purpose, and radiologists generally feel comfortable with a series of planar-section images. However, there is considerable interest in applying truly three-dimensional tomographic imaging to study the microstructure of various materials, including metals, ceramics, composites, and polymers. Some of microstructural features cannot be determined from the conventional two-dimensional microscopy of cross-section surfaces. This includes determining the number of particles of arbitrary or variable shape in a volume and the topology of networks

Figure 38. *Diagram of the use of balanced absorption edge filters to isolate a single energy band. The plots show the absorption coefficient as a function of energy for two different filters containing the elements chromium and nickel. Elements in the sample with absorption edges between these two energies, such as manganese, iron, and cobalt, will be imaged in the ratio of the two intensities.*

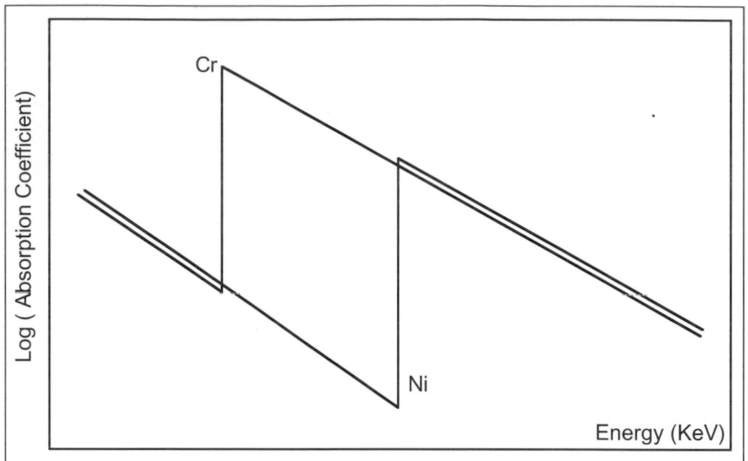

or pore structures, which controls the permeability of materials to fluids.

This information can only be determined by having the full three-dimensional data set, with adequate resolution and, ideally, with cubic voxels. Resolution on the order of 1 μm has been demonstrated using a synchrotron as a very bright point-source of X-rays. Resolution of about 10 μm is possible using more readily available sources, such as microfocus X-ray tubes.

Such a source is not monochromatic, which would cause significant beam-hardening effects for many specimens. Absorption filters can be used to select just a single band of energies. For each view angle, two projection images are collected using filters whose absorption edge energies are different. The ratio of the two images yields the attenuation information for the elements whose absorption edges lie between the two filter energies, as indicated in **Figure 38**. A series of such image pairs can provide separate information on the spatial distribution of many elements.

Figure 39. *Diagram of a cone-beam imaging system. The projection image magnification is the ratio of b:a. The attainable resolution is limited by the spot size of the X-ray source.*

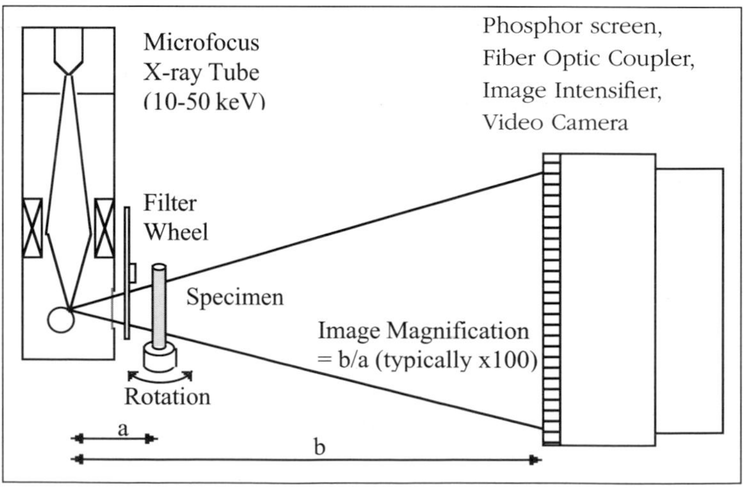

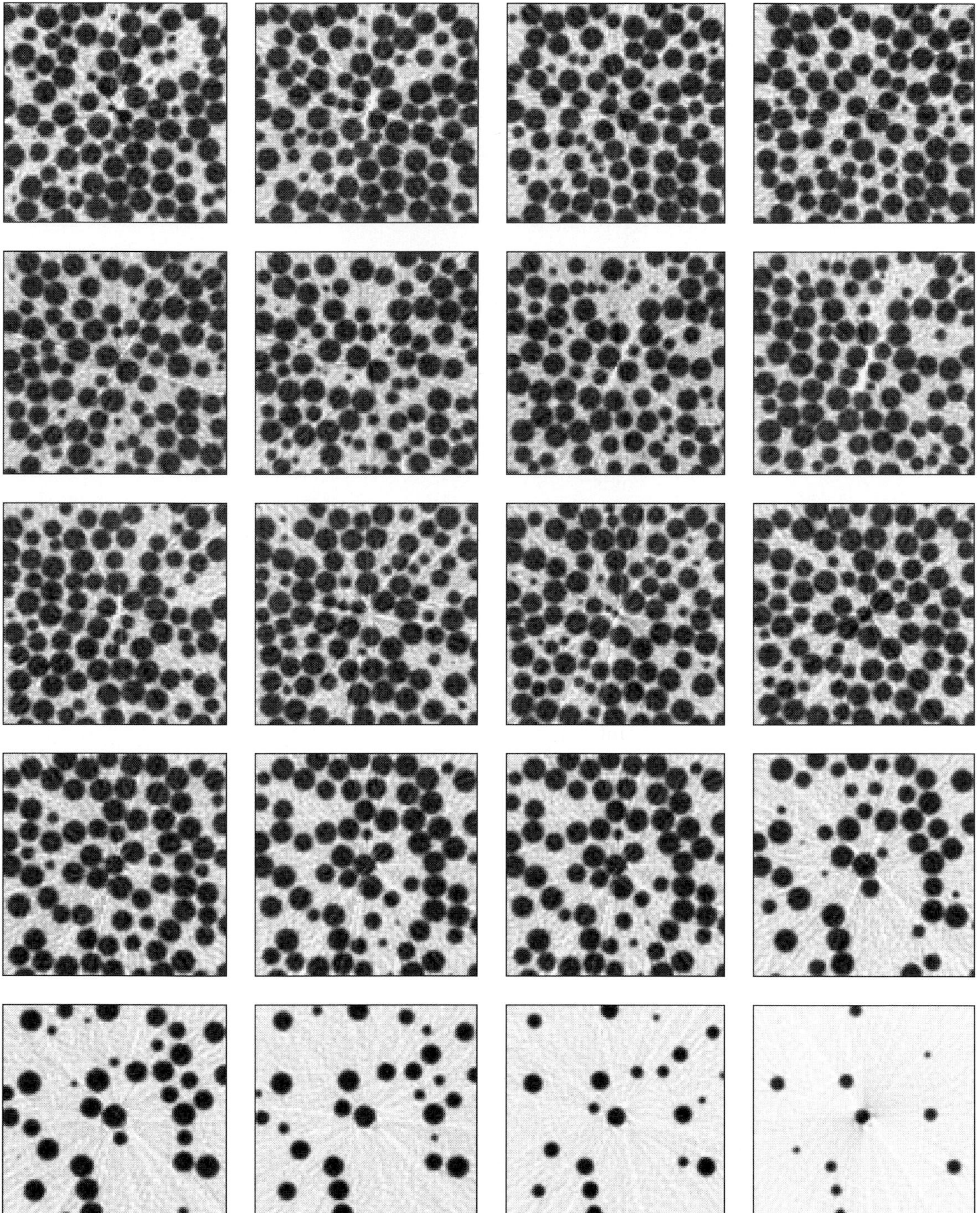

Figure 40. *Twenty individual planes of reconstructed voxels showing a sintered alumina ceramic consisting of 100-μm-diameter spheres.*

Cone-beam geometry is well-suited to this type of microstructural imaging, since it magnifies the structure (Johnson et al., 1986; Russ, 1988; Kinney et al., 1989, 1990; Deckman, 1989). **Figure 39** shows this schematically. The magnification is strictly

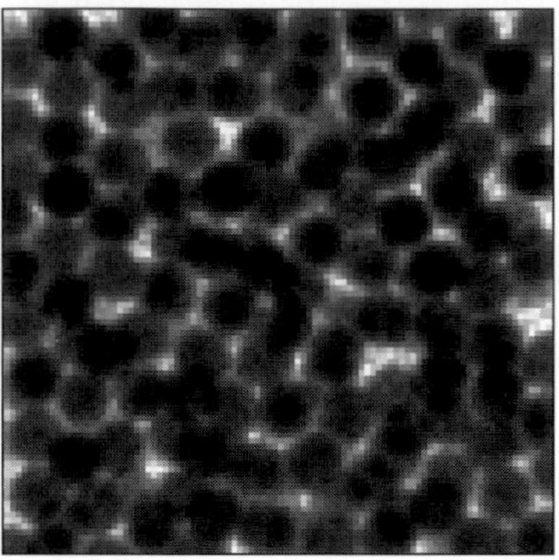

Figure 41. *A single two-dimensional projection set through the structure shown in Figure 40.*

geometric, since X-rays are not refracted by lenses, but it can amount to as much as 100:1. The projected images can be collected using conventional video technology, after conversion to visible light by a phosphor or channel plate and suitable intensification. Since the intensity of conventional small-spot X-ray sources is very low, the use of high-brightness sources (such as a synchrotron) is particularly desirable for high-resolution imaging.

As discussed in Chapter 8, three-dimensional imaging requires many voxels and the reconstruction process is very computer-intensive. The time required to perform the reconstruction is, however, still shorter than that required to collect the various projection images. These are generally photon-limited and generate considerable noise, which affects the reconstruction as indicated above. In order to collect reasonable-quality projections from a finite intensity source, the number of view angles is limited. Angles are arranged to optimally cover the polar angles in three-dimensional space. This of course places demands on the quality of the mechanism used to perform the rotations and tilts, because the center of rotation must be constant and located within a few micrometers to preserve the image quality, as discussed above.

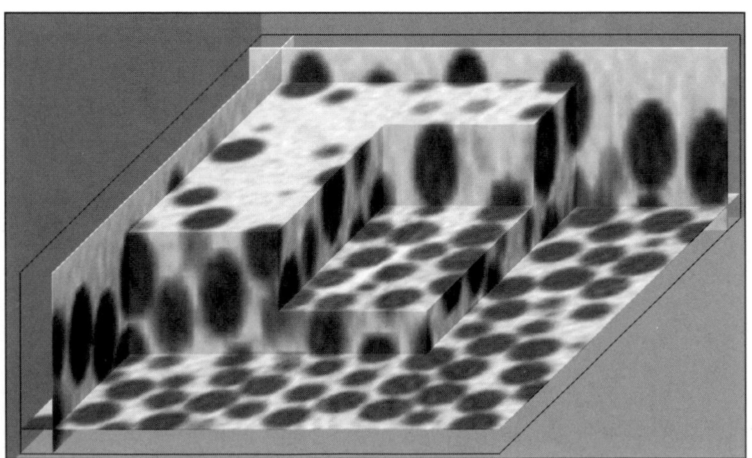

Figure 42. *Three-dimensional presentation of the data from Figure 40.*

Presenting three-dimensional information requires the extensive use of computer graphics methods (discussed in Chapter 8). **Figure 40** shows a simple series of voxel planes from a three-dimensional tomographic reconstruction of a porous alumina ceramic. The individual particles are approximately 100-μm-diameter spheres that fill about 60% of the volume of the sample. The voxels are 10-μm cubes. **Figure 41** shows one of the projection sets through this specimen, a two-dimensional image in which the spherical particles overlap along the lines of sight and are partially transparent. A three-dimensional presentation of these data is shown in **Figure 42**.

Three-Dimensional Imaging

Many of the two-dimensional images used in the preceding chapters have been sections through three-dimensional structures. This is especially true in the various types of microscopy, where either polished flat planes or cut thin sections are needed in order to form the images in the first place. But the specimens thus sampled are three-dimensional and the goal of the microscopist is to understand the three-dimensional structure.

There are quantitative, extremely powerful and useful tools that convert measurements of two-dimensional (2D) images to three-dimensional (3D) values (Underwood, 1970; Weibel, 1979; Russ, 1986). They enable the measurement of volume fraction of phases, surface area of interfaces, mean thickness of membranes, and even the size distribution of particles seen only in random section. Valuable as such measurement data may be, however, they cannot provide the typical viewer with a real sense of the structure. As pointed out in the first chapter, we are overwhelmingly visual creatures–we need to *see* the 3D structure.

Furthermore, our world is 3D. We are accustomed to looking at external surfaces or occasionally through transparent media, not at thin sections or polished, cut surfaces. Try to imagine (again the need to resort to a word with its connotation of vision) standing by a busy street in which you can see only through an imaginary plane that exists transverse to traffic flow. What do cars and people look like as they pass through that plane?

If you have a well-developed geometric sense or experience as a radiologist or draftsman, you may be able to accurately visualize the appearance of the plane as portions of torsos, engine blocks, even simple shapes, such as tires, are cut by the plane. Most people will have difficulty imagining such collections of sections and when asked to sketch the sections of even simple shapes will produce wildly inaccurate results.

Few people can make the transition in the opposite direction: given a collection of section data, reconstruct in the mind a correct representation of the 3D structure. This is true even for those who feel quite comfortable with the 2D images themselves. Within the world of the 2D images, recognition and understanding can be learned as a separate knowledge base that need not relate to the 3D world. Observing the characteristic appearance of dendrites in polished metal samples or of mitochondria in thin SEM sections of cells does not necessarily mean that the complex 3D shapes of these objects becomes familiar.

Because of this difficulty in using 2D images to study 3D structure, there is an interest in 3D imaging. It may be performed directly, as in the previous chapter, by actually collecting a 3D set of information all at once or indirectly, by gathering a sequence of 2D (slice) images and then combining them. There are a variety of ways to acquire the data needed for 3D imaging and an even greater variety of ways to present the information to the user. Many are discussed in this chapter. The large number of approaches suggests that no one way is best, either for most viewers or for most applications.

Sources of 3D data

Chapter 7 described 3D imaging by tomographic reconstruction. This is perhaps the premier method for measuring the density and even, in some cases, the elemental composition of solid specimens. It can produce a set of cubic voxels (the 3D analog of the pixels that represent the digitization of 2D images). This is not the only, or even the most common, way that tomography is presently used. Most medical and industrial applications produce one or a series of 2D section planes, which are spaced farther apart than the pixel resolution within the plane (Baba et al., 1984, 1989; Briarty & Jenkins, 1984; Johnson & Capowski, 1985).

A radiologist viewing an array of 2D images is expected to combine them in the mind to see the 3D structures present. Only a few current-generation systems use the techniques discussed in this chapter to present 3D views directly. In industrial tomography, the greater diversity of structure (and correspondingly less ability to predict what is expected) and the greater amount of time available for study and interpretation has encouraged the use of computer graphics, but they are still the exception, rather than the rule.

Tomography can be performed using a variety of different signals. This includes seismic waves, ultrasound, magnetic resonance, conventional X-rays, gamma rays, neutron beams, and electron microscopy, as well as other even less-familiar methods. Resolution may vary from kilometers (seismic tomography) to centimeters (most conventional medical scans), millimeters (typical industrial applications), micrometers (current experimental work with synchrotron sources), and even nanometers (SEM reconstruction of viruses and atomic lattices). The same basic presentation tools are available regardless of the imaging modality or the dimensional scale.

The most important variable in tomographic imaging, as for all of the other 3D methods discussed here, is whether the data set is planes of pixels or true voxels. As discussed in Chapter 7, it is possible to set up an array of cubic voxels, collect projection data from a series of views in three dimensions, and solve (either algebraically or by backprojection) for the density of each voxel. However, the most common way to perform tomography is to define one plane at a time as an array of square pixels, collect a series of views in two dimensions, solve for the densities in that plane, and then proceed to the next plane. When used in this way, tomography shares many similarities (and problems) with other essentially 2D imaging methods, which we will collectively define as serial imaging or serial section techniques.

Serial sections

The name serial section comes from light-microscopy imaging of biological tissue, in which blocks of tissue embedded in resin are cut by a microtome into a series of individual slices. Collecting these slices (or at least some of them) for microscopic viewing enables researchers to assemble a set of photographs that can then be used to reconstruct the 3D structure.

This technique illustrates most of the problems that may be encountered with any 3D imaging method based on a series of individual slices. First, the individual images must be aligned. The microtomed slices are collected on slides and viewed in arbitrary orientations. Even if the same structures can be located in the different sections (not always an easy task, since some variation in structure with depth must be present or there would be no incentive to do this kind of work), the pictures do not line up.

Using the details of structure visible in each section provides only a coarse guide to alignment. As shown in **Figure**s **1, 2,** and **3,** shifting or rotating each image to visually align structures in one section with those in the next can completely alter the reconstructed 3D structure. It is generally assumed that given enough image detail, some kind of average alignment will avoid these major errors. However, it is far from certain that a best visual alignment is the correct one or that automated methods that overlap sequential images will produce the proper alignment.

Figure 1. Alignment of serial sections with translation: sections through an inclined circular cylinder may be misconstrued as a vertical elliptical cylinder.

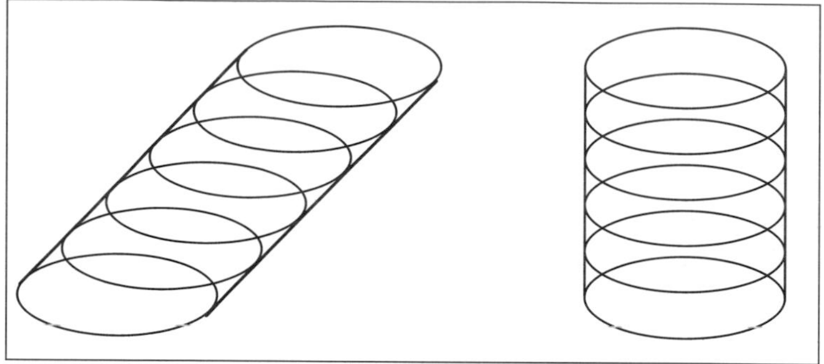

Automatic methods generally seek to minimize the mismatch between sections either by aligning the centroids of features in the planes, so that the sum of squares of distances is minimized, or by overlaying binary images from the two sections and shifting or rotating to minimize the area resulting from combining them with an Ex-OR operation, discussed in Chapter 6. This is illustrated in

Figure 2. Alignment of serial sections with rotation:
a) *actual outlines in 3D serial section stack;*
b) *surface modeling applied to outlines, showing twisted structure;*
c) *erroneous result without twist when outlines are aligned to each other.*

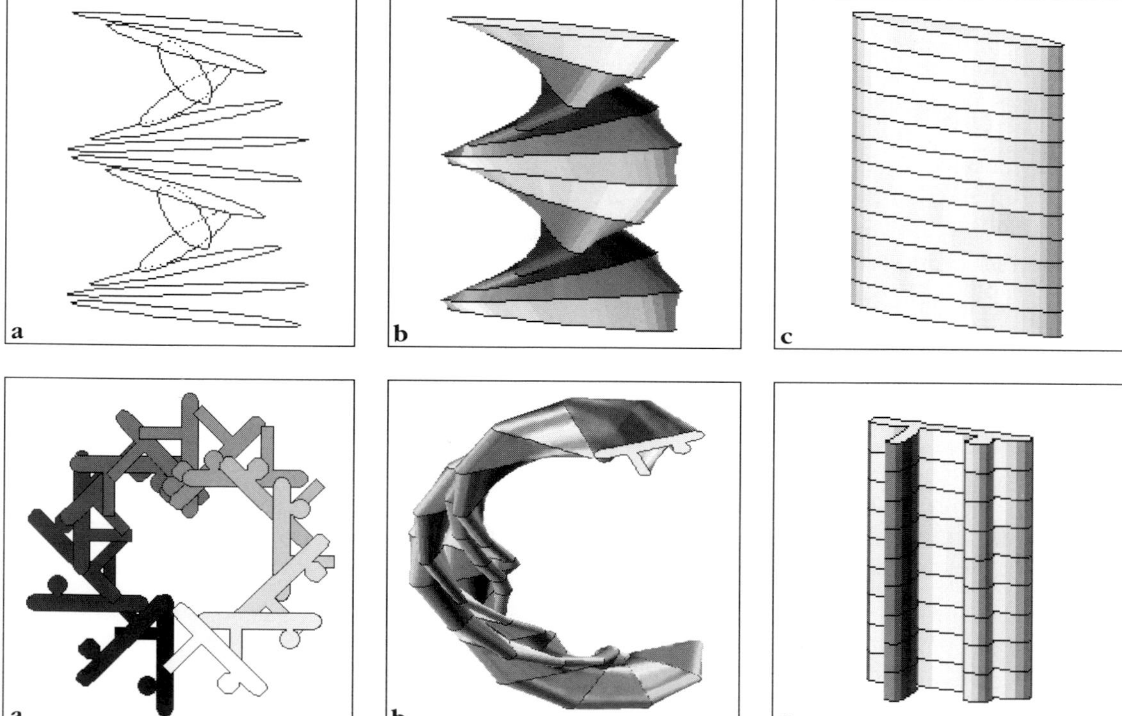

Figure 3. Loss of combined rotation and translation by aligning serial sections:
a) *example data viewed normally, using shading to mark slices at different depths;*
b) *surface modeling of data from image a;*
c) *incorrect result if sequential slices are aligned for best match with each other.*

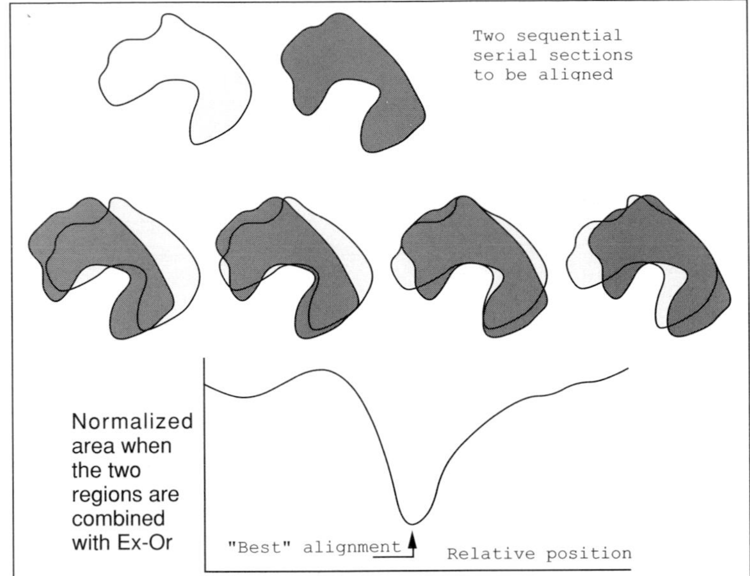

Figure 4. *Alignment of serial sections by "best fit" of features seeks to minimize mismatched area, measured by Ex-OR function, as a function of translation and rotation.*

Figure 4. There are two problems with this approach: solving for the minimum in either quantity as a function of three variables (x and y shift and angular orientation) is difficult and must usually proceed iteratively and slowly and there is no reason to expect the minimum point to really represent the true alignment, as discussed above.

One approach that improves on the use of internal image detail for alignment incorporates fiducial marks in the block before sectioning. This could take the form of holes drilled by a laser, threads or fibers placed in the resin before it hardens, etc. By using several such marks, which can reasonably be expected to maintain their shape from section to section, and continuing in some known direction through the stack of images, much better alignment is possible. Placing and finding fiducial marks in the close vicinity of the structures of interest is often difficult. In practice, there may still be difficulties if the sections are not contiguous and alignment errors may propagate through the stack of images.

Once the alignment points are identified (either from fiducial marks or internal image detail), rotating and translating of one image to line up with the next is performed, as discussed in Chapter 2. Resampling the pixel array and interpolating to prevent aliasing produces a new image. This takes some computational time, but it is minor compared to the difficulty of obtaining the images in the first place.

Unfortunately, for classical serial sectioning the result of this rotation and translation is not a true representation of the original 3D structure. The act of sectioning using a microtome generally produces some distortion in the block. This 5% to 20% compression in one direction is the same for all sections (since they

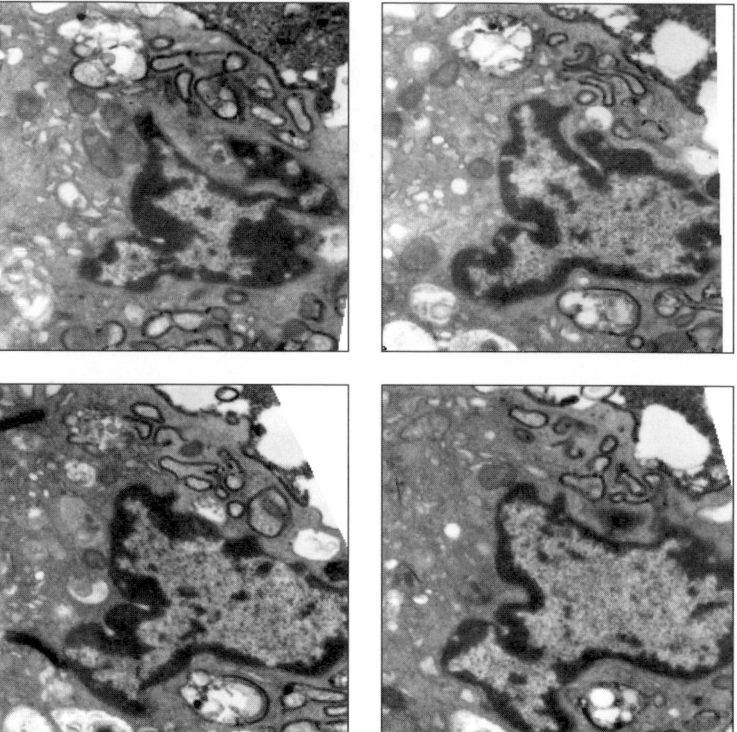

Figure 5. *Four serial section images from a stack (courtesy Dr. C. D. Bucana, Univ. of Texas M. D. Anderson Cancer Center, Houston, TX), which have already been rotated for alignment. The membranes at the upper left corner of the images are thresholded and displayed for the entire stack of images in Figure 6.*

are cut in the same direction). If the fiducial marks have known absolute coordinates, then it is possible to stretch the images to correct for the distortion.

Otherwise, it may be possible to use internal information to estimate the distortion. For example, if there is no reason to expect cell nuclei to be elongated in any preferred direction in the tissue, then the dimensions of many nuclei may be measured to determine an average amount of compression. Obviously, this approach includes some assumptions and can only be used in particular circumstances.

Another difficulty with serial sections is calibrating dimension in the depth direction. The thickness of the individual sections is known only approximately (for example, by judging the color of light produced by interference from the top and bottom surfaces). It may vary from section to section and even from place to place within the section, depending on the local hardness of the material being cut. Constructing an accurate depth scale is quite difficult; dimensions in the depth direction will be much less accurate than those measured within one section plane.

If only some sections are used, such as every second or fifth, then this error becomes much worse. It also becomes difficult to confidently follow structures from one image to the next. However, before computer reconstruction methods became common, this kind of skipping was often necessary simply to reduce the

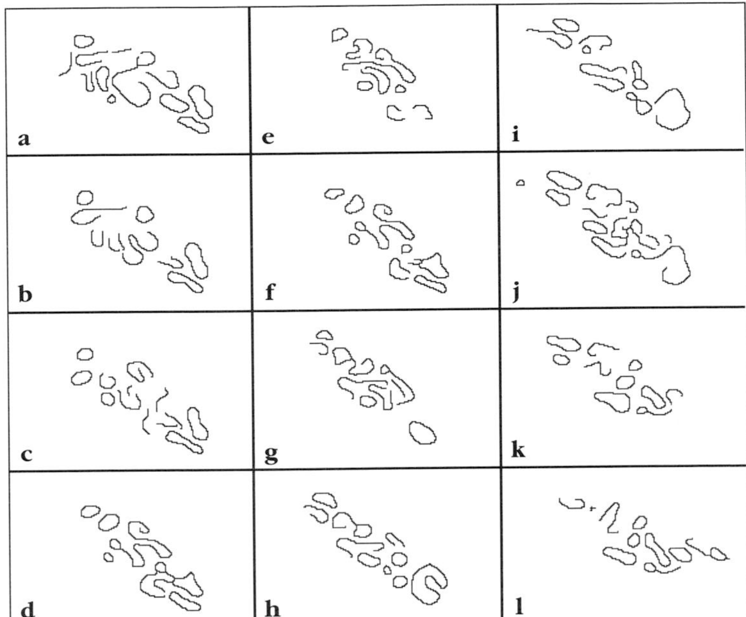

Figure 6. Membranes from the sequential images illustrated in Figure 5, showing the changes from section to section. Because of the separation distance between the planes, these variations are too great to model the shape of the surfaces in 3D.

amount of data which the human observer had to juggle and interpret.

This is particularly true when ultra-thin sections are cut for viewing in a TEM instead of a light microscope. As the sections become thinner, they increase in number and are more prone to distortion. Some may be lost (for instance due to folding) or intentionally skipped. Portions of each section are obscured by the support grid, which also prevents some from being used. At higher magnification, the fiducial marks become larger, less precisely defined, and–above all–more widely spaced, so that they may not be in close proximity to the structure of interest.

Figure 5 shows a portion of a series of TEM images of tissue, in which the 3D configuration of the membranes (dark stained lines) is of interest. The details of the edges of cells and organelles have been used to approximately align pairs of sections through the stack, but different details must be used for different pairs, as there is no continuity of detail through the entire stack. The membranes can be isolated in these images by thresholding (**Figure 6**), but the sections are too far apart to link the lines together to reconstruct the 3D shape of the surface. This is a common problem with conventional serial section images

Optical sectioning

The difficulties just described for the classical serial sectioning of biological tissue have greatly increased interest in other serial imaging methods that avoid some of the problems. A new development in light microscopy, the CSLM, makes practical the idea of optical sectioning. Chapter 3, **Figure 55** showed the prin-

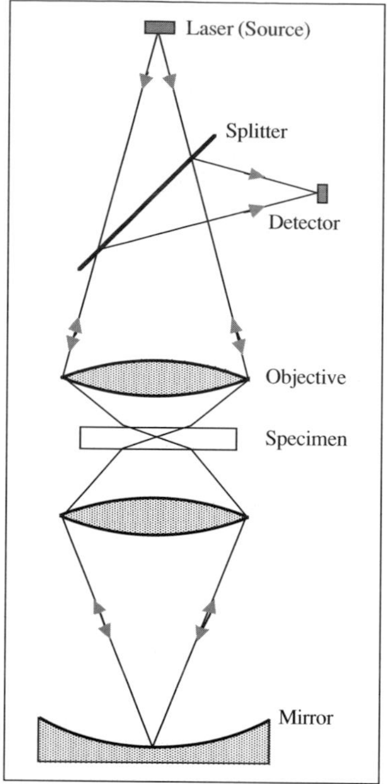

Figure 7. *Transmission confocal scanning light microscopy can be performed by passing the light through the specimen twice. Light is not imaged from points away from the in-focus point, which gives good lateral and excellent depth resolution compared to a conventional light microscope. (Figure 61, Chapter 3 shows the more common reflected light confocal microscope.)*

ciple of the CSLM. Light from a point source (often a laser) is focused on a single point in the specimen, collected by an identical set of optics, and reaches a pinhole detector.

Any portion of the specimen away from the focal point, and particularly out of the focal plane, cannot scatter light to interfere with the formation of the image. Scanning the beam with respect to the specimen (by moving the light source, the specimen, or using scanning elements in the optical path) builds up a complete image of the focal plane. If the numerical aperture of the lenses is high, the depth of field of this microscope is very small, though still several times the lateral resolution within individual image planes. Even more important, the portion of the specimen away from the focal plane contributes very little to the image. This makes it possible to image a plane within a bulk specimen, even one that would ordinarily be considered translucent because of light scattering.

This method of isolating a single plane within a bulk sample, called optical sectioning, works because the CSLM has a very shallow depth of field. Translating the specimen in the z direction and collecting a series of images makes it possible to build up a 3D data set for viewing, using the methods shown further on in this chapter.

Several imaging modalities are possible with the CSLM. The most common is reflected light, in which the light reflected back from the sample returns through the same objective lens used to focus

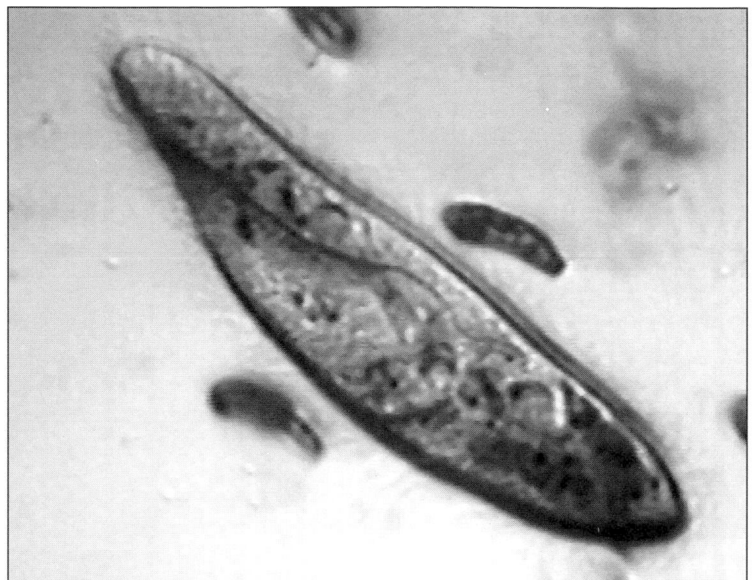

Figure 8. *CSLM image showing a 1/30 second image of a paramecium swimming in a droplet of water, as it passed through the focal plane of the microscope.*

the incident light and is then diverted by a mirror to a detector. This geometry is shown in **Figure 7**. It permits the acquisition of transmitted-light images for focal-plane sectioning bulk translucent or transparent materials. **Figure 8** shows an example of a transmitted-light focal-plane section.

Both transmitted- and reflected-light images of focal-plane sections can be used for 3D imaging for different types of specimens. The characteristic of reflected-light confocal images is that the intensity of light reflected to the detector drops off very rapidly as points are shifted above or below the focal plane. This means that in a transparent medium, only the surfaces of structures will reflect light. For any single image plane, only the portion of the field of view where some structure passes through the plane will appear bright; the rest of the image will be dark. This permits some rather straightforward reconstruction algorithms, which will be shown.

Another widely used imaging method for the CSLM is emission, or fluorescence, in which the wavelength of the incident light causes excitation of a dye or other fluorescing probe introduced to the specimen. The lower-energy (longer wavelength) light emitted by this probe is separated from the incident light, for instance by a dichroic mirror, and used to form an image in which the location of the probe or dye appears bright. Building up a series of images in depth allows the structure labeled by the probe to be reconstructed.

The transmitted light mode, while it is the most straightforward in terms of optical sectioning, is actually little-used as yet. This is partly due to the difficulties in constructing the microscope with matched optics above and below the specimen, compared to the reflection and emission modes in which the optics are only above it. However, the use of a lens and mirror beneath the specimen (shown in **Figure 7**) to return the light to the same detector present in the more standard microscope design can produce most of the same imaging advantages (some light intensity is lost passing through the specimen twice).

The principal advantages of optical sectioning are avoiding physical specimen distortion due to cutting and having image alignment from the various imaging planes. Depth resolution, while inferior to the lateral resolution in each plane by about a factor of two to three times, is still useful for many applications. However, this difference in resolution raises some difficulties for 3D image processing, even if the distance between planes is made smaller than the resolution so that the stored voxels are cubic (which is by no means common).

Sequential removal

Many materials are opaque and therefore cannot be imaged by any transmission method. This prevents any type of optical sectioning. Indeed, metals, composites, and ceramics are usually examined in a reflected light microscope. It may still be possible to collect a series of depth images for 3D reconstruction by sequentially polishing such materials.

The means of removing material from the surface depends strongly on the hardness of the material. For some soft metals, polymers, and textiles, a microtome can be used just as it was for the block of biological material, except that instead of examining the slice of material removed, the surface left behind is imaged. This still avoids most problems of alignment and distortion, especially if the cutting can be done *in situ* without removing the specimen from the viewing position in the microscope. It is still difficult to determine the precise thickness of material removed in each cut and to assure its uniformity.

For harder materials, the grinding or polishing operations used to produce conventional sections for 2D images can be employed. This generally requires removing and replacing the specimen, so fiducial marks are again needed to locate the same region. Probably the most common approach is the use of hardness indentations. Several pyramid-shaped impressions are made in the surface of the specimen so that after additional abrasion or polishing, the deepest parts of the indentations are still visible. These can be accurately aligned with the marks in the original image. In addition, the reduction in size of the impression, whose shape is known, gives a measure of the depth of polish and therefore of the spacing between the two images. With several such indentations, the overall uniformity of polish can also be judged, although local variations due to the hardness of particular phases may be present.

For still harder materials or ones in which conventional polishing might cause surface damage, other methods may be used. Electrolytic, or chemical, etching is generally difficult to control and is little used. Ion beam erosion is slow, but is already in use in many laboratories for the thinning of TEM specimens. Controlling the erosion to obtain uniformity and avoid surface roughening presents challenges for many specimens.

In situ ion beam erosion is used in SEM and scanning Auger microscopes, for instance to allow surface contamination to be removed. This capability can be used to produce a series of images in depth since these microscopes generally have resolution far better than that of the light microscope. The time involved in performing the erosion may be quite long (hence costly), while the uniformity of eroding through complex structures (the most interesting kind for imaging) may be poor.

One kind of microscope performs this type of erosion automatically as part of its imaging process. The ion microscope, or secondary ion mass spectrometer (SIMS), uses a beam of heavy ions to erode a layer of atoms from the specimen surface, which are then separated according to element in a mass spectrometer and recorded, for example, using a channel plate multiplier and more-or-less conventional video camera to form an image of one plane in the specimen for one element at a time. The depth of erosion is usually calibrated for these instruments by measuring the signal profile of a known standard, such as may be found in the same methods used to produce modern microelectronics.

The rate of surface removal is highly controllable (if somewhat slow) and capable of essentially atomic resolution in depth. The lateral resolution, by contrast, is about the same level as a conventional light microscope. In this case, instead of having voxels (which are high in resolution in the plane but poorer in the depth direction), the situation is reversed. This still creates processing and measurement problems, as compared to true cubic voxels.

Furthermore, the erosion rate for ion beam bombardment in the SIMS may vary from place to place in the specimen as a function of composition, structure, or even crystallographic orientation. This does not necessarily show up in the reconstruction, since each set of data is assumed to represent a plane, but can cause significant distortion in the final interpretation. In principle, stretching the data in 3D can be performed just as images can be corrected for deformation in 2D. However, without fiducial marks or accurate quantitative data on local erosion rates, it is difficult to see how to accomplish this in actual data.

The ability to image many different elements with the SIMS creates a rich data set for 3D display. True-color 2D images have three bands (whether it is saved as RGB or HSI, as discussed in Chapter 1) and satellite 2D images may have as many as seven

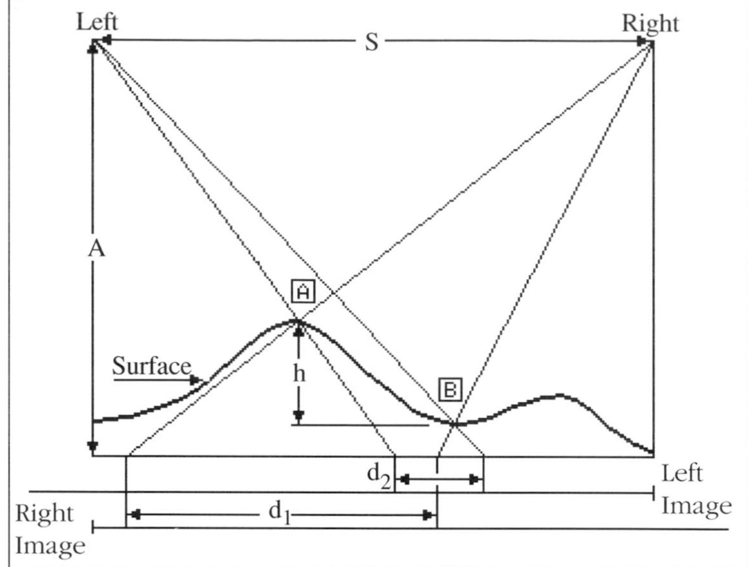

Figure 9. *Diagram of stereo viewing of two points on a surface. The parallax (difference between d_1 and d_2) in the two images gives the relative elevation* $h = A \cdot (d_1 - d_2)/S$.

bands, including infrared. The SIMS may have practically any number of bands; four or more are quite common. The ability of the instrument to detect trace levels (typically parts per million or better) of every element in the periodic table means that for even relatively simple specimens, the multiband data will present a challenge to store, display, and interpret.

Stereo

There remains another way to see 3D structures. It is the same way that humans see depth in some real-world situations. Having two eyes that face forward so that their fields of view overlap permits us to use stereoscopic vision to judge the relative distance to objects. In humans, this is done point by point, by moving our eyes in their sockets to bring each subject to the fovea, the portion of the retina with the densest packing of cones. The muscles, in turn, tell the brain what motion was needed to achieve convergence, so we know whether one object is closer or farther than another.

We will see stereo vision used below as a means to transmit 3D data to the human viewer. It would be wrong to think that all human depth perception relies on stereoscopy. In fact, much of our judgement about the 3D world around us comes from other cues–shading, relative size, precedence, and so on–that work just fine with one eye and are used in some computer-based measurement methods (Roberts, 1965; Horn, 1970; Carlsen, 1985; Pentland, 1986). For the moment, however, let us see how stereoscopy can be used to determine depth to put information into a 3D computer database.

The light microscope has a rather shallow depth of field, which diminishes even more in the CSLM, discussed above. This means that looking at a specimen with deep relief is not very satisfactory. However, the SEM has lenses with very small aperture angles and consequently has very great depth of field. This is most commonly used with the SEM to produce in-focus images of rough surfaces. Tilting the specimen or electromagnetically deflecting the scanning beam can produce a pair of images from different points of view which form a stereo pair. Looking at one picture with each eye fools the brain into seeing the original rough surface.

Measuring the relief of surfaces from such images is the same in principle (and in practice) as using stereo pair images taken from aircraft or satellites to measure the elevation of topographic features on the earth or another planet. The richer detail in the satellite photos makes it easier to find matching points practically anywhere in the images. By the same token, however, it requires more matching points to define the surface than the simpler geometry of typical specimens observed in the SEM. The mathematical relationship between the measured parallax (the apparent displacement of points in the left- and right-eye image) and the relative elevation of the two points on the surface is given in **Figure 9.**

Automatically matching points from stereo pairs is a difficult task for computer-based image analysis (Marr & Poggio, 1976; Medioni & Nevatia, 1985; Kayaalp & Jain, 1987). It is usually performed by using the pattern of brightness values in one image, say the left one, as a template to search for the most nearly identical pattern in the right image. The area of search is restricted by the possible displacement, which depends on the angle between the two views and the maximum roughness of the surface. Some points will not be matched by this process, because they may not be visible in both images. Other points will match poorly, because the local pattern of brightness values in the pixels includes some noise and several parts of the image may have similar noise levels.

Matching many points produces a new image, in which each pixel can be given a value based on the parallax or surface elevation. This range image will contain many false matches, but operations such as a median filter usually do a good job of removing the outlier points to produce an overall range image of the surface. We will see later on in this chapter how range images can be displayed.

A second approach to matching stereo pairs is based on the realization that many of the points in each image will not match well, because they are just part of the overall surface or structure and are not the interesting points where surfaces meet or other discontinuities are present. This is presumably related to human vision, which usually spends most of its time on only a few points in each scene where discontinuities are found. Locating

Figure 10. Drawing contour lines (isoelevation lines) on the triangular facets joining an arbitrary arrangement of points whose elevations have been determined by stereoscopy.

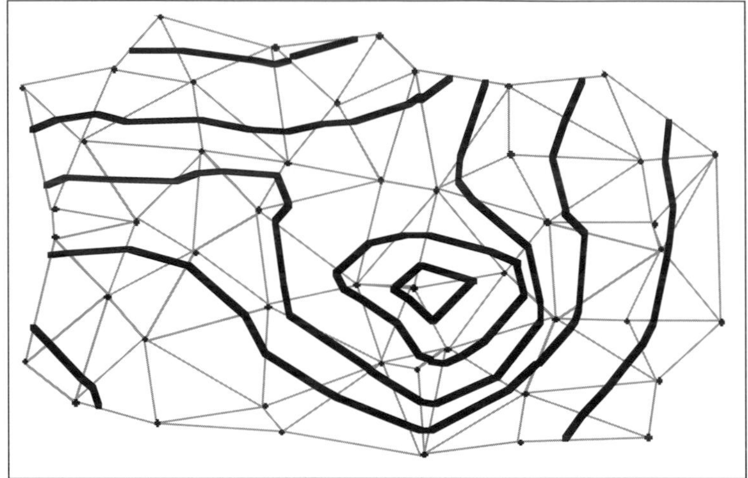

these interesting points based on some local property, such as the variance, produces a comparatively short list of points to be matched between the two images (Moravec, 1977; Quam & Hannah, 1974). A typical case may have only thousands of points, compared to the million or so pixels in the original images.

These points are then matched in the same way as above, by correlating their neighborhood brightness patterns. There is the additional information that for most surfaces, the order of points is preserved. This, along with the limits on possible parallax for a given pair of images, reduces the typical candidate list for matching to ten or less and produces a list of surface points and their elevations. It is then assumed that the surface between these points is "well behaved": usually, that it consists of planar facets. If the facets are small enough, it is still possible to generate a contour map of the surface, as shown in **Figure 10.** A complete display of elevation, called a range image, can be produced by interpolation, as shown in **Figure 11.** Other displays of these surfaces are shown below.

The TEM also has a very large depth of field. In most cases, the specimens observed in the TEM are very thin (in order to permit electron penetration); this is unimportant. However, with the newest generation of high-voltage microscopes, comparatively thick samples (of the order of one micrometer) may be imaged. This is enough to contain a considerable amount of 3D structure at the resolution of the TEM (of the order of a few nanometers). Therefore, using the same approach of tilting the specimen to acquire stereo pair images, it is possible to obtain information about the depth of points and the 3D structure.

Presenting the images to a human viewer's eyes so that the two pictures, acquired at different times, can be fused in the mind and examined in depth is not difficult. Accomplished for years photographically, it is now often done with a modest tradeoff in lateral resolution using a computer to record and display the im-

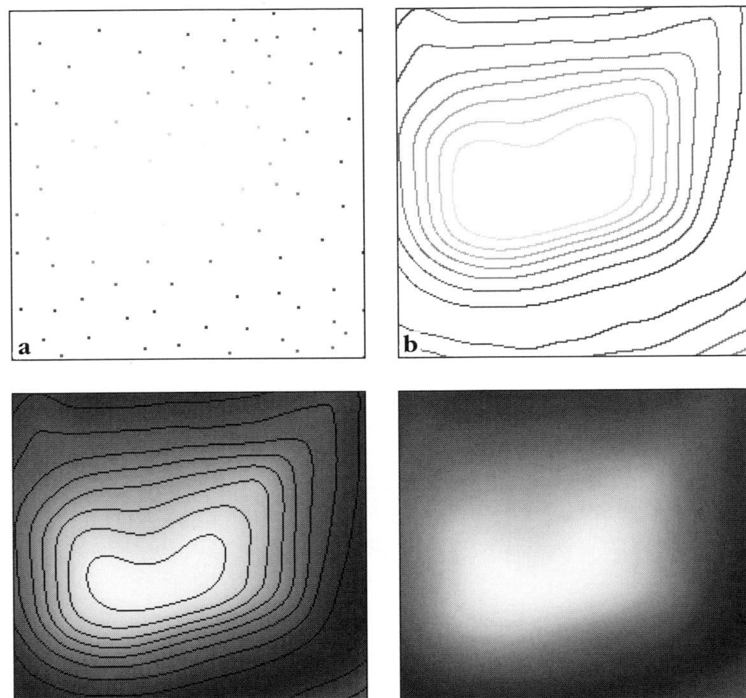

Figure 11. Interpolation of a range image:
a) *isolated, randomly arranged points with measured elevation;*
b) *contour lines drawn through the tesselation;*
c) *smooth interpolation between contour lines;*
d) *the constructed range image.*

ages. The methods discussed below for using stereo pair displays to communicate 3D information from generated images are equally applicable here.

It is far more difficult to have the computer determine the depth of features in the structure and construct a 3D database of points and their relationship to each other. Part of the problem is that there is so much background detail from the (mostly) transparent medium surrounding the features of interest, which may dominate the local pixel brightnesses so that matching becomes impossible. Another part of the problem is that it is no longer possible to assume that points maintain their order. In a 3D structure, points may change their order as they pass in front or in back of each other.

The consequence of these limitations has been that automatically fusing stereo pair images from the TEM has been attempted in only a very few, highly idealized cases. The problem can be simplified using very high-contrast markers, such as small gold particles bound to selected surfaces using antibodies or some other highly selective stain. In this case, only the markers are considered. There are only a few dozen, and like the interesting points mentioned above for mapping surfaces, they are easily detected (they are usually far darker than anything else in the image) and only a few could possibly match.

Even with these markers, it still may require a human to identify the matches. Given the matching points in the two images, the

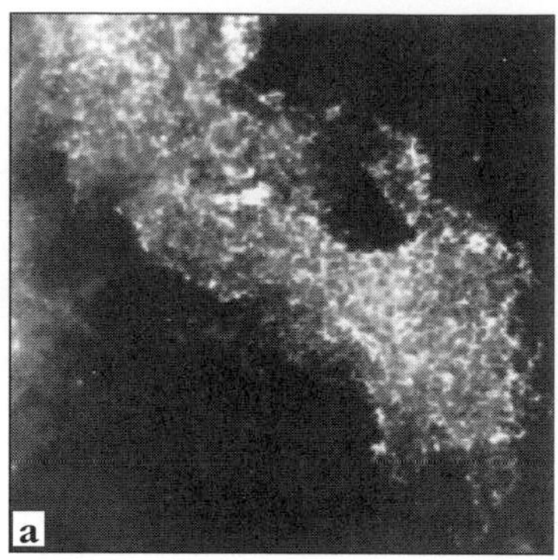

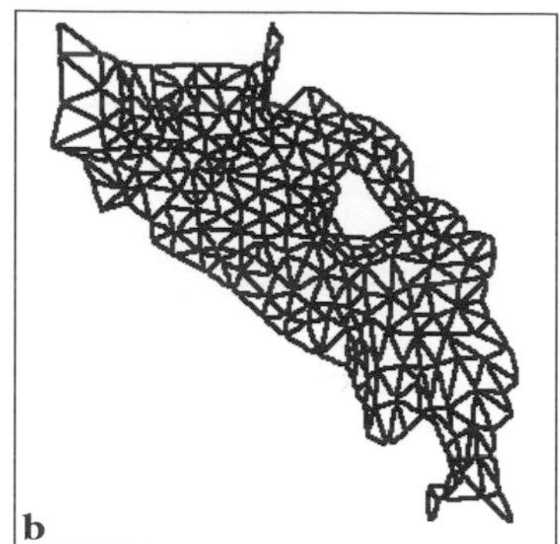

Figure 12. *Example of decorating a surface with metal particles (Golgi stain) shown in this transmission electron micrograph (a) whose elevations are measured stereoscopically to form a network describing the surface (b). (Peachey & Heath, 1989.)*

computer can construct a series of lines describing the surface the markers define, but this may be only a small part of the total structure. **Figure 12** shows an example of this method, in which human matching was performed. Similar methods can be applied to stained networks, the distribution of precipitate particles in materials, etc.

3D data sets

In the case of matching of points between two stereo pair images, the database is a list of a few dozen or perhaps hundreds of coordinates, which usually define either a surface or nodes in a network structure. If these points are to be used for measurement, their coordinates and perhaps some information on which points are connected is all that is required. If image reconstruction is intended, it will be necessary to interpolate additional points in-between to complete a display. This is somewhat parallel to the use of boundary representation in two dimensions. It may offer a very compact record of the essential (or at least of the selected) information in the image. However, it requires expansion to be visually useful to the human observer.

The most common way to store 3D data sets is as a series of 2D images. Each single image, which we have previously described as an array of pixels, is now seen to have depth. This is either because it is truly an average over some depth of the sample, such as in looking through a thin section in the light microscope, or it is based on the spacing between one plane and the next, for instance a series of polished planes observed by reflected light. Because of the depth associated with the planes, we refer to the individual elements as voxels rather than pixels.

Ideally, for viewing, processing, and measurement the voxels will be regular and uniformly spaced. This is often accomplished with a cubic array of voxels, which is easiest to address in computer memory and corresponds to the way that many image acquisition devices function. Other arrangements of voxels in space offer some advantages. In a simple cubic arrangement, the neighboring voxels are at different distances from the central voxel, so

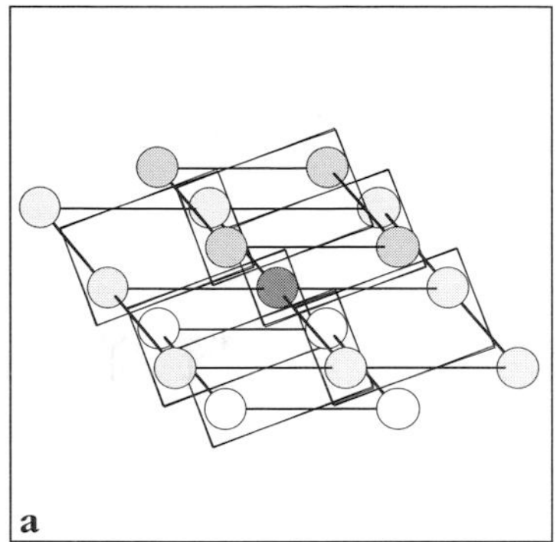

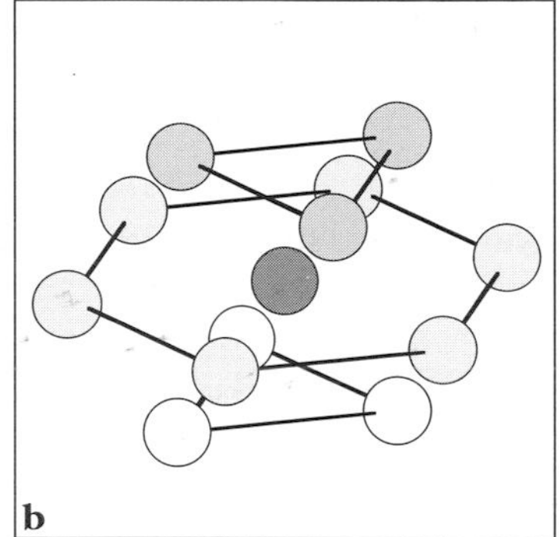

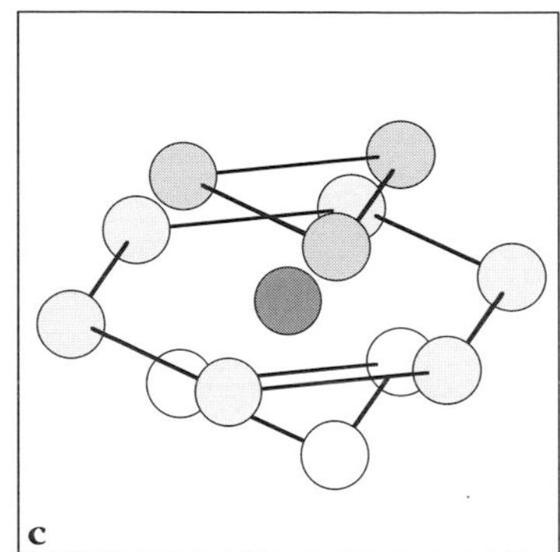

Figure 13. Lattice arrangements of atoms or voxels in which all neighbors are equidistant: ***a)*** *body-centered cubic (BCC);* ***b)*** *face-centered cubic (FCC);* ***c)*** *hexagonal close-packed (HCP). Lines join the uniformly shaded points which lie in each plane.*

more symmetrical arrangements are possible. Atoms in metal crystals typically occupy sites in one of three lattice configurations: body-centered cubic (BCC), face-centered cubic (FCC), or hexagonal close-packed (HCP). The first of these surrounds each atom (or voxel) with 8 touching neighbors at the same distance, while the other two have 12 equidistant neighbors. **Figure 13** shows these arrangements, drawn to emphasize the planes of lattice points.

The advantage of these voxel stacking arrangements is that image processing can treat each of the neighbors identically and measurements are less biased as a function of direction. Of course, in order to fill space, the shapes of the voxels in these cases are not simple. Storing and addressing the voxel array is difficult, as is acquiring or displaying the images. Usually, the acquired image must be resampled by interpolation to obtain voxels in one of these patterns and a reverse interpolation is needed for display. For most purposes, these disadvantages outweigh the theoretical advantages, just as the use of a hexagonal pixel array is rarely used for 2D images. Cubic arrays are the most common 3D arrangement of voxels.

If the voxels are not cubic, because the spacing between planes is different from the resolution within each plane, it may be possible to make adjustments so that they are cubic. In the discussion that follows, we will assume that the depth spacing is greater than the spacing within the plane, but an analogous situation could be described for the reverse case. This adjustment could be made by interpolating additional planes of voxels between those that have been measured. Unfortunately, this will not help much with image processing operations, since the assumption is that all of the neighbors are equal in importance, because with interpolation, neighbors are clearly redundant.

The alternative approach is to reduce the resolution within the plane by sampling every *n*th pixel or by averaging pixels together in blocks, so that a new image is formed with cubic voxels. This also reduces the amount of storage that will be required, since many fewer voxels remain. Though it seems unnatural to give up resolution, it occurs in a few cases where cubic voxels are required for analysis.

A variety of different formats are available to store 3D data sets either as a stack of individual images, or effectively as an array of voxel values with x,y,z indices. Such arrays become very large and very fast. A 512×512 or 640×480 pixel 2D image, which represents a very common size for digitizing video images, occupies 250 or 300 kilobytes of storage using one byte per pixel (256 grey values). This is easily handled in the memory of a desktop computer or recorded on a floppy disk. A 512×512×512 3D image would occupy 128 megabytes of memory! This is too much for any but a few computers and presents difficulties merely in storing or transmitting the image from place to place, let alone processing it. Most of the data sets in this chapter are much smaller, for instance 256×256×50 (3.2 Meg). The same operations shown here can be used for larger data sets, given time, computer power, or both.

It is possible to compress the size of the storage requirements. Individual 2D images can be compressed either by using run-length encoding (especially useful for binary images) or by the JPEG (Joint Photographers Expert Group) compression algorithms, which are based on a discrete cosine transform, discussed in Chapter 1. A standardized algorithm does not yet extend to 3D images, but there are emerging standards for time sequences of images. One, the MPEG (Moving Pictures Expert Group) approach, is based on the fact that most of the pixels do not change much in successive frames in a time series of images. Similar assumptions have been used to transmit video conferences over telephone lines; only the changing pixels must be transmitted for each frame. This high correlation from frame to frame should also be true for a series of 3D planes and may lead to standardized algorithms for compacting such images. They will still require unpacking for display, processing, and measurement, however.

It is instructive to compare this situation to that of computer-aided drafting. Man-made objects with comparatively simple surfaces require only a tiny number of point coordinates to define the entire 3D structure. This kind of boundary representation is very compact, but it often takes many minutes to render a drawing with realistic surfaces from such a data set. For a voxel image, the storage requirements are great but information is immediately available without computation for each location. The various display images shown in this chapter can usually be produced very quickly (sometimes even at interactive speeds) by modest computers.

Given a series of surfaces defined by boundary representation or a few coordinates, for example, display generation may proceed by first constructing all of the points for one plane, calculating the local angles of the plane with respect to the viewer and light source and using them to determine a brightness value, and then plotting that value on the screen. At the same time, another image memory is used to store the actual depth (z value) of the surface at that point. After one plane is complete, the next one is similarly drawn, except that the depth value is compared point by point to the values in the z buffer to determine whether the plane is in front of or behind the previous values. Of course, it is drawn only if it lies in front. This permits multiple intersecting planes to be drawn on the screen correctly. (For more information on graphically presentating 3D data, see Foley & Van Dam, 1984; or Hearn & Baker, 1986.)

Additional logic is needed to clip the edges of the planes to the stored boundaries, change the reflectivity rules used to calculate brightness depending on surface characteristics, and so forth. Standard texts on computer graphics describe algorithms for accomplishing these tasks and devote considerable space to the relative efficiency of various methods (because the time involved can be significant). By comparison, looking up the value in a large array or even running through a column in the array to add densities or find the maximum value is very fast.

Slicing the data set

Since most 3D image data sets are actually stored as a series of 2D images, it is very easy to access any of the individual image planes, which are usually called slices. Playing the series of slices back in order to create an animation, or "movie," is perhaps the most common tool available to let the user view the data. It is often quite effective in letting the viewer perform the 3D integration and since it recapitulates the way the images may have been acquired (but with a much-compressed time base), most viewers can understand them presented in this way. A simple user interface need only allow the viewer to vary the speed of the animation, change direction, stop at a chosen slice, etc.

One problem with presenting original images as slices of data is that the orientation of some features in the 3D structure may not show up very well in the slices. It is useful to be able to change the slice orientation to look at any plane through the data, either in still or animated playback. This is quite easy to do as long as the orientation of the slices is parallel to the x, y, or z axes in the data set. If the depth direction is understood as the z axis, then the x and y axes are the horizontal and vertical edges of the individual images. If the data are stored as discrete voxels, then accessing the data to form an image on planes parallel to these directions is just a matter of calculating the addresses of voxels, using offsets to the start of each row and column in the array. This can be done at real-time speeds if the data are held in memory, but is somewhat slower if the data are stored on a disk

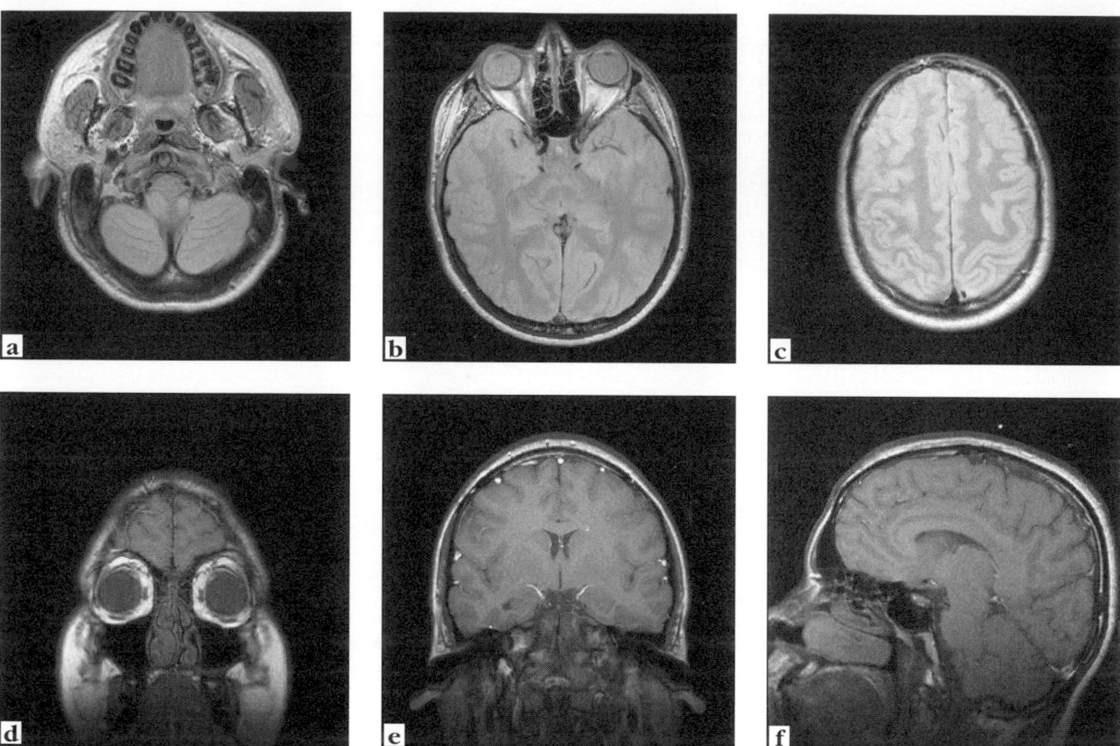

Figure 14. *A few slices from a complete set of MRI head scan data. Images a through c show transaxial sections (3 from a set of 46), images d and e are coronal sections (2 from a set of 42), and f is a sagittal section (1 from a set of 30).*

drive. Voxels that are adjacent along scan lines in the original slice images stored contiguously on disk can be read as a group in a single pass, but when a different orientation is required, the voxels must be located at widely separated places in the file and it takes time to move the head and wait for the disk to rotate.

Displaying an image in planes parallel to the x, y, and z axes was shown in Figure 42 of Chapter 7, while Figure 40 showed the individual slice images (x,y planes) through the data set. **Figure 14** shows an example of orthogonal slices. The images are magnetic resonance images (MRI) of a human head. The views are generally described as transaxial (perpendicular to the subject's spine), sagittal (parallel to the spine and to the major axis of symmetry), and coronal (parallel to the spine and perpendicular to the "straight ahead" line of sight). Several individual sections are shown in each orientation, which can include planes parallel to those passing through the center of the object.

Actually it is not very common to perform this kind of resectioning with MRI data (or most other kinds of medical images) because the spacing of the planes is greater than the resolution in the plane, resulting in a visible loss of resolution in one direction in the resectioned slices due to interpolation in the z direction. The alternative to interpolation is to extend the voxels in

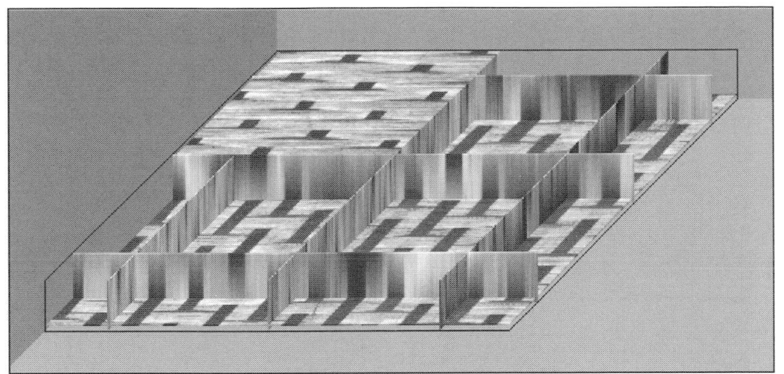

Figure 15. Interpolation in a 3D array. In this example, only two images of the top and bottom of a woven fabric are used. The points between the two surfaces are linearly interpolated and bear no relationship to the actual 3D structure of the textile.

space; in most cases, this is even more distracting to the eye. **Figure 15** shows an example of interpolation that creates an impression of structure not actually present.

In Figure 42 in Chapter 7, this is not a problem, because the data were obtained with cubic voxels. In several of the figures later in this chapter, much greater loss of resolution in the z direction will be evident when plane images are reconstructed by sampling and interpolating the original data. In the case of **Figure 14,** the MRI images were actually obtained as three complete sets of parallel slice images in each of the three directions.

Combining several views at once using orthogonal planes adds to the feeling of three-dimensionality of the data. **Figure 16** shows several examples of this using the same MRI head data based on plane images obtained in the transaxial direction. The poorer resolution in the z direction is evident, but the overall impression of 3D structure is still quite good. These views can also be animated, by moving one (or several) of the planes through the data set while keeping the other orthogonal planes fixed to act as a visual reference.

Unfortunately, there is no good way to demonstrate this time-based animation in a print medium. Children's cartoon books once used a "flip" mode in which animation printed on a series of pages which the viewer could literally flip or riffle at a rapid-enough rate to cause flicker fusion in the eye and see motion. It takes a lot of pages and is only practical for very simple images, such as cartoons. It is unlikely to appeal to the publishers of

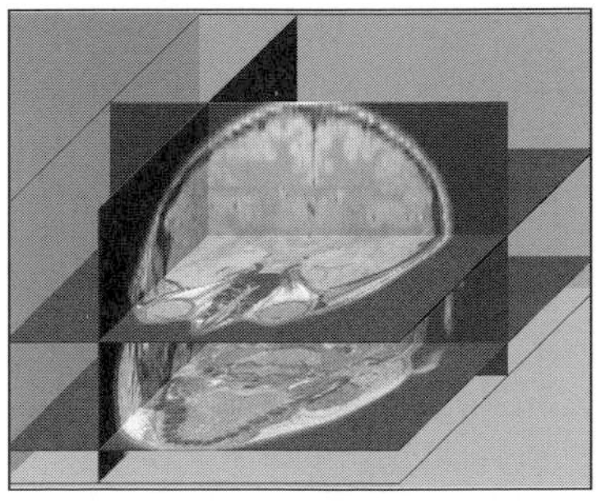

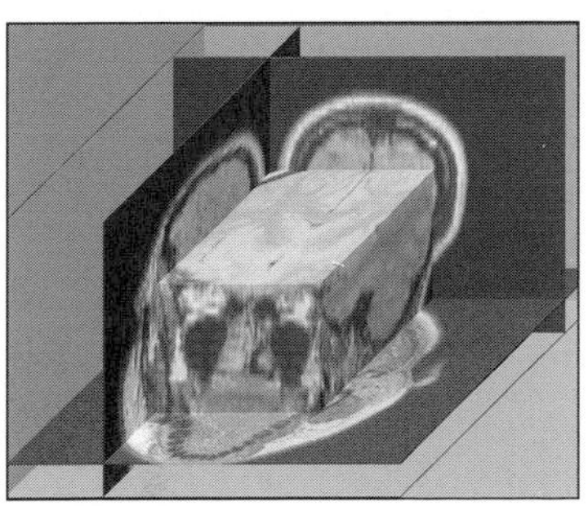

Figure 16. Several views of the MRI head data from Figure 14 along section planes normal to the axes of the voxel array. The voxels were taken from the trans-axial slices, and so the resolution is poorer in the direction normal to the planes than in the planes.

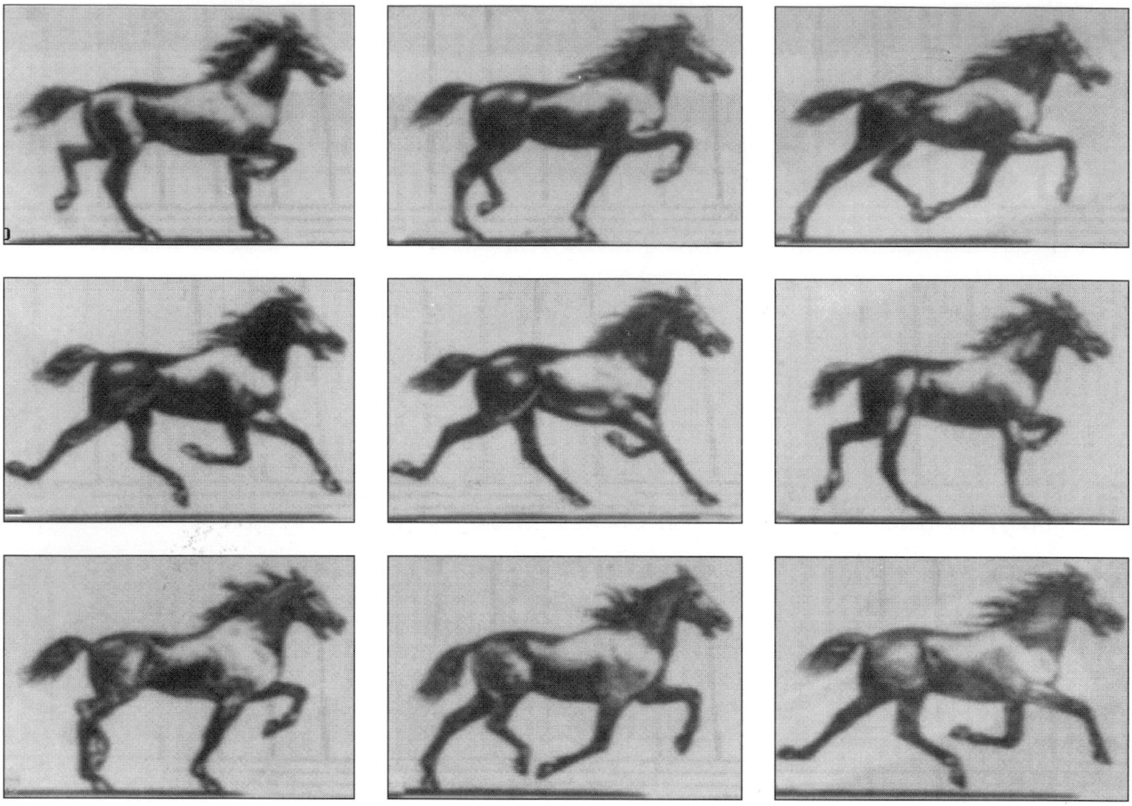

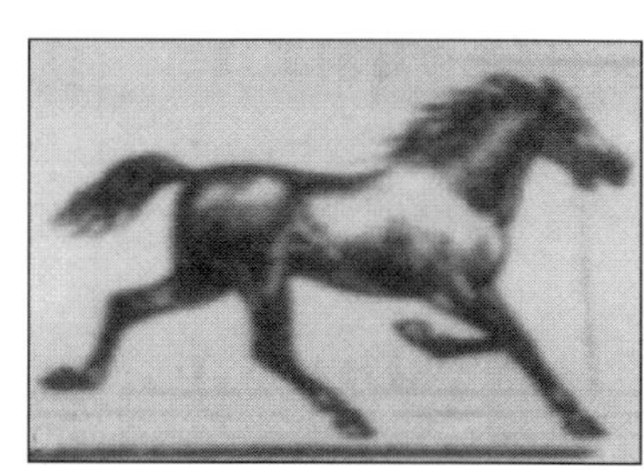

Figure 17. *A few of the series of historic photographs taken by Eadweard Muybridge to show the motion of a running horse. Viewed rapidly in succession, these create the illusion of continuous motion.*

books and technical journals. All that can really be done here is to show a few of the still images from such a sequence, appealing to the reader's imagination to supply a necessarily weak impression of the effect of a live animation.

Figure 17 shows a series of images that can be used to show moving pictures of this kind. They are a portion of the series Eadweard Muybridge recorded of a running horse by setting up a row of cameras that were tripped in order as the moving horse broke threads attached to the shutter release. Muybridge's purpose was to show that the horse's feet were not always in contact with the ground (in order to win a wager for Leland Stanford, Jr.). Once it was realized that such images could be viewed to recreate the impression of smooth motion, our modern motion picture industry (as well as television) became possible.

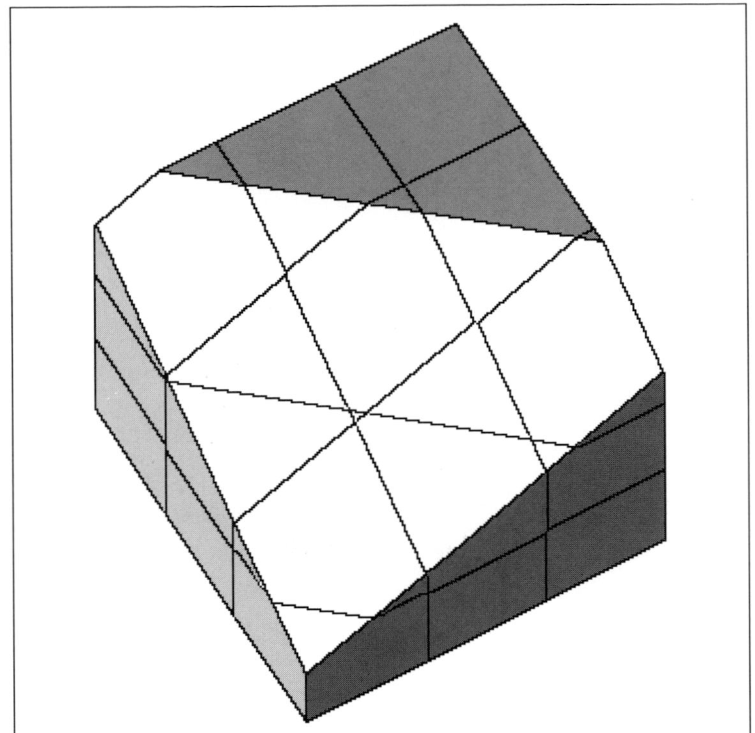

Figure 18. *Intersection of a plane with an array of cubic voxels. The plane is viewed perpendicularly, showing the different areas and shapes of the intersection regions.*

It is difficult to show motion using printed images in books. There is current interest in the use of videotape or compact disk (CD-ROM) formats for the distribution of technical papers, which will perhaps offer a medium that can substitute time for a spatial axis and show 3D structure through motion. The possibilities will be mentioned again in connection with rotation and other time-based display methods.

Arbitrary section planes

Restricting the section planes to those perpendicular to the x, y, or z axes is obviously limiting for the viewer. It is done to conveniently access the voxels in storage and create the display. If some arbitrary planar orientation is selected, the voxels must be found that lie closest to the plane. As for the case of image warping, stretching, and rotating discussed in Chapter 2, these voxels will not generally lie exactly in the plane, nor will they have a regular grid-like spacing that lends itself to forming an image. **Figure 18** shows an example of a plane section through an array of cubic voxels, in which portions of various size and shape are revealed. This complicates displaying the voxel contents on the plane.

The available solutions are either to use the voxels that are closest to the section plane, plot them where they land, and spread them out to fill any gaps that develop, or to establish a grid of points in the section plane and then interpolate values from the

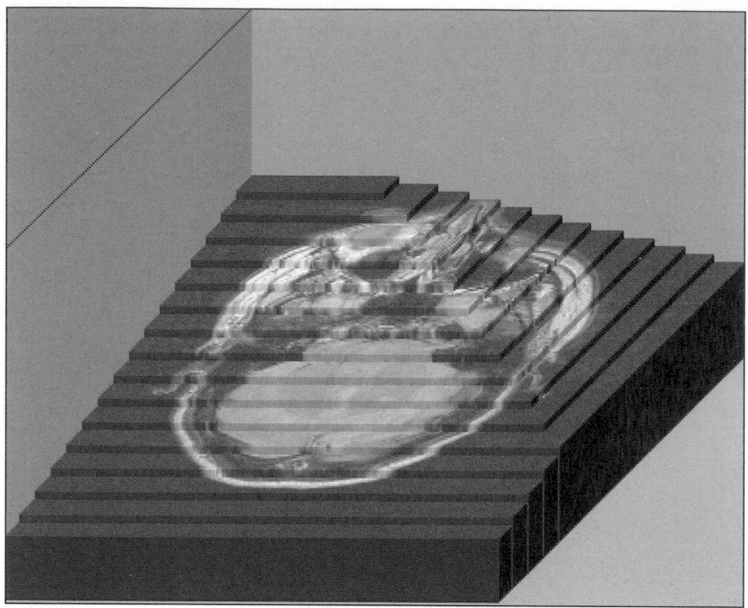

Figure 19. Sampling voxels along inclined planes in a 3D array. Showing the entire voxel is visually distracting and does not produce a smooth image.

nearest voxels, which may be as high as 8 in number. In the case of rotating and stretching, these two solutions have different shortcomings. Using the nearest voxel preserves brightness values (or whatever the voxel value represents) but may distort boundaries and produce stair-stepping or aliasing. Interpolation makes the boundaries appear straight and smooth, but it also smooths the brightness values by averaging, which blurs the steps. It is also slower, because more voxels must be located in the array and the interpolation performed.

Producing an animation by continuously moving a section plane at an arbitrary orientation requires a significant amount of computation, even if it is essentially a simple calculation of addresses and linear interpolation of values. Instead of calculating in real time, many systems instead create new images of each of the plane positions, store them, and then create the animation by playing them back. This is fine for demonstrating something that the user has already found, but because of the time delay is not a particularly good tool for exploring the 3D data set to discover the unexpected.

The ultimate use of planar resectioning would be to change the location and orientation of the section plane dynamically, in real time. This would allow instant response to the scene. Chapter 1 pointed out that humans study things by turning them over, either in the hand or in the mind. This kind of turning over is a natural way to study objects, but requires a fairly large computer memory (to hold all of the voxel data), a fairly speedy processor and display, and a user interface that provides the required number of degrees of freedom.

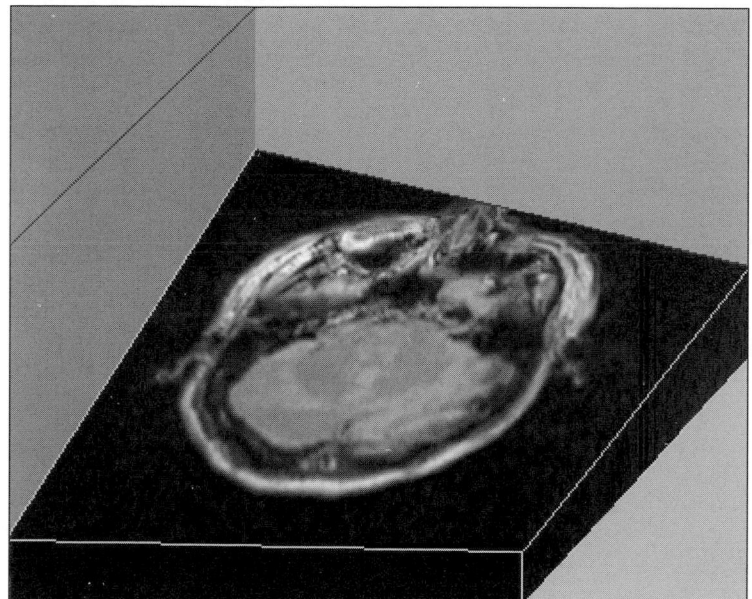

Figure 20. *Smooth interpolation of image pixels as an arbitrary plane is positioned in a voxel array by dragging the corners.*

Positioning an arbitrary plane can be done in two different ways, each of which produces the same results but feels quite different to the user. One is to move the plane with respect to a fixed 3D voxel array. This can be done, for example, by dragging the corners of the plane along the x, y, z axes. A different method is to keep the section plane fixed perpendicularly to the direction of view while allowing the data set to be rotated in space. Combined with the ability to shift the section plane toward or away from the viewer (or equivalently to shift the data set), this allows exactly the same information to be obtained.

The principal difference between these approaches is that in the latter case, the image is seen with perspective or foreshortening so that size comparisons or measurements can be made. This may be important in some applications. On the other hand, keeping the data set fixed and moving the section plane seems to aid the user in maintaining orientation within the structure.

Figure 19 shows the voxels revealed by an arbitrary section plane through the 3D data set from the MRI image series. The appearance of the voxels as a series of steps is rather distracting, so it is more common to show the value of the nearest voxels to the plane, as shown in **Figure 20.** An alternative method, when the size of the voxels is large and the resulting image appears blocky, is to interpolate among the voxels to obtain brightness values for each point on the plane.

Also useful is the ability to make some of the pixels in section planes transparent. This allows other planes to be viewed behind the first and makes the 3D structure of the data more apparent. **Figure 21** shows an example of this for the spherical

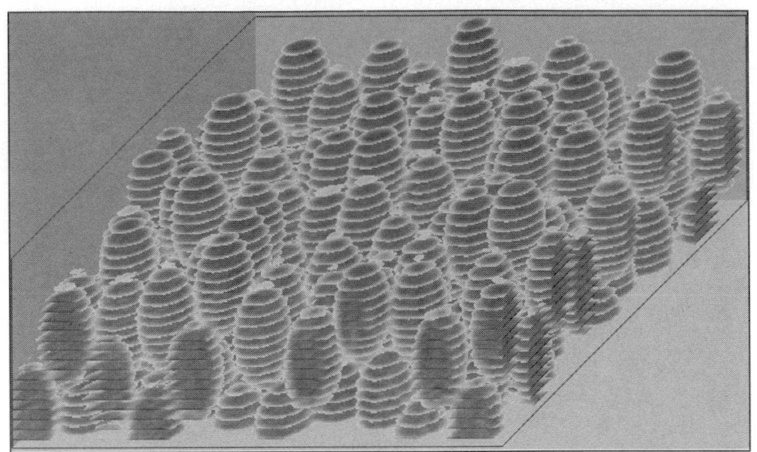

Figure 21. *"Exploded" view of voxel layers in the tomographic reconstruction of spherical particles (Chapter 7, Figure 40). The low-density region surrounding the particles is shown as transparent.*

particle data shown in Chapter 7 (Figures 40 to 42). The series of parallel slices are not contiguous planes of voxels; the separation of the planes has been increased by a factor of two in the z direction. Voxels whose density falls below a threshold roughly corresponding to that of the particles have been made transparent. This allows voxels to be seen which are part of particles in other section planes behind the first.

Figure 22 shows a similar treatment for the MRI data set of the human head. The threshold for choosing which voxels to make transparent is more arbitrary than for the spheres, since there are void and low-density regions inside as well as outside the head. However, the overall impression of 3D structure is clearly enhanced by this treatment.

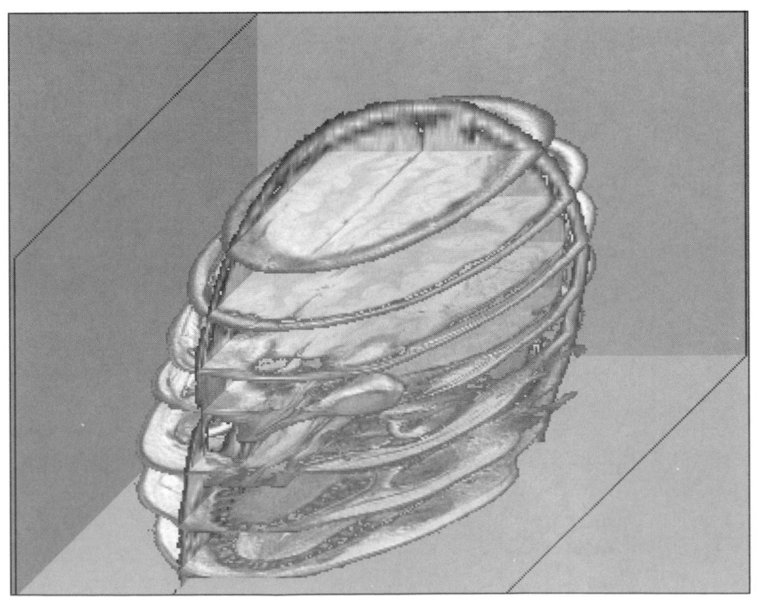

Figure 22. *View of several orthogonal slices of the MRI head data with transparency for the low-density regions in the planes.*

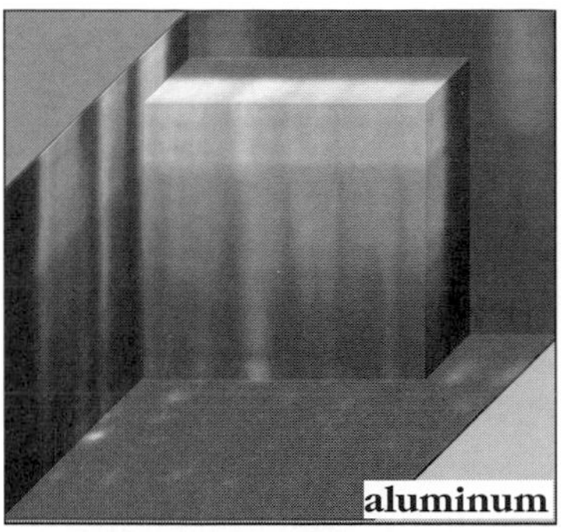

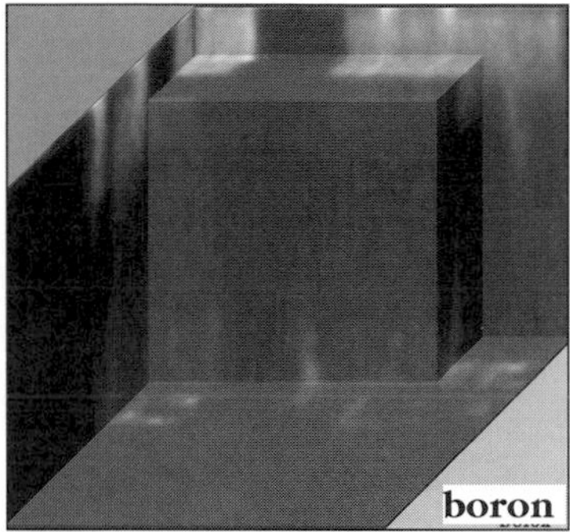

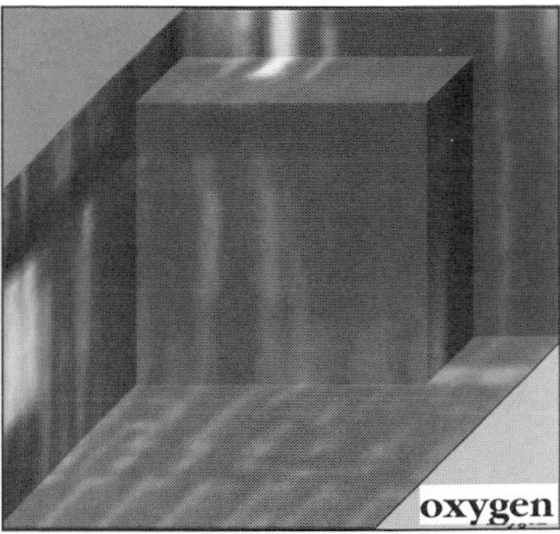

Figure 23. *Views of plane sections for the elements aluminum, boron, and oxygen in a silicon wafer, imaged by secondary ion mass spectrometry. Plate 12 shows a full color image of all three elements on another orthogonal set of planes.*

The use of color

Assigning pseudo-colors to grey scale 2D images was discussed in earlier chapters. It sometimes permits subtle variations to be distinguished which are imperceptible in brightness in the original. As noted before, however, it more often breaks up the overall continuity and *gestalt* of the image so that the image is more difficult to interpret. Of course, the same display tricks can be used with 3D sets of images, with the same consequences.

A subtle use of color is to apply slightly different shading to different planar orientations (shown in **Figure 16**) to increase the impression of three-dimensionality. These images are printed here in monochrome, so only a grey scale difference between the x, y, and z orientations is evident. With color reproduction, light tints of red, green, and blue can be used, as well.

It is more useful to employ different color scales to distinguish different structures. This was also demonstrated for 2D images. It requires separate processing or measurement operations to distinguish the different structures. When applied to 3D data sets, the colored scales assist in seeing the continuity from one image to another, while providing ranges of brightness values for each object.

One of the most common ways that multiple colors can be used to advantage in 3D image data is to code multiband data, such as the elemental concentrations measured from the SIMS. This is analogous to similar coding in 2D images, very frequently used for X-ray maps from the SEM and for remotely sensed satellite images, in which the colors may either be true or used to represent colors beyond the range of human vision (particularly infrared). Of course, the other tools for working with multiband images in 2D, such as calculating ratios, can also be applied in 3D.

Figure 23 shows example images of a SIMS depth imaging of elements implanted in a silicon wafer. Comparing the spatial location of the different elements is made easier by superimposing the separate images and using colors to distinguish the elements. This is done by assigning red, green, and blue to each of three elements and then combining the image planes; the result is shown in **Plate 12.**

Volumetric display

Sectioning the data set, even if some regions are made transparent, obscures much of the voxel array. Only the selected planes are seen and much of the information in the data set is not used. The volumetric display method shows all of the 3D voxel information. For simple structures this can be an advantage, while for very complex ones the overlapping features and boundaries can become confusing.

A volumetric display is produced by ray tracing. In the simplest model used, a uniform light source is placed behind the voxel array. For each straight line ray from the light source to a point on the display screen, the density value of each voxel that lies along the path is used to calculate a reduction in light intensity following the usual absorption rule: $I/Io = \exp(-\Sigma\rho)$. Performing this calculation for rays reaching each point on the display generates an image. The total contrast range may be adjusted to the range of the display by introducing an arbitrary scaling constant. This can be important, because the calculated intensities may be quite small for large voxel arrays.

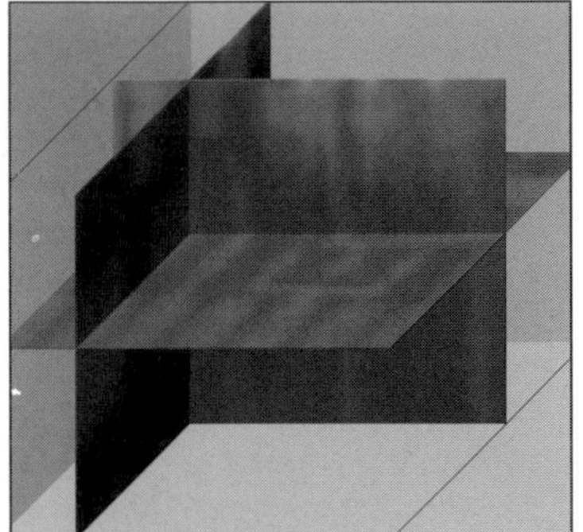

Plate 12. *See color plate, page VI. Color plates appear following page 246.*

Notice that this model assumes that the voxel values actually correspond to density or to some other property that may be adequately modeled by the absorption of light. The image shown in Chapter 7, Figure 41, in fact corresponds closely to this, since it shows the projected view through a specimen using X-rays. In fact, X-ray tomographic reconstruction, discussed in the preceding chapter, proceeds from such views to a calculation of the voxel array. Having the array of voxel values then permits the generation of many kinds of displays to examine the data. It seems counter-productive to calculate the projection view again, and indeed in such a view as shown in the figure, the ability to distinguish the individual particles and see their relationship is poor.

One of the advantages of this mode is that the direction of view can be changed rather easily. For each, it is necessary to calculate the addresses of voxels that lie along each ray. When the view direction is not parallel to one of the axes, this can be done efficiently using integer arithmetic to approximate the sine/cosine values. Also, in this case, an improved display quality is obtained by calculating the length of the line segment along each ray through each pixel. The absorption rule then becomes $I/Io = \exp(-\Sigma\rho t)$.

This method is far short of a complete ray tracing, although it is

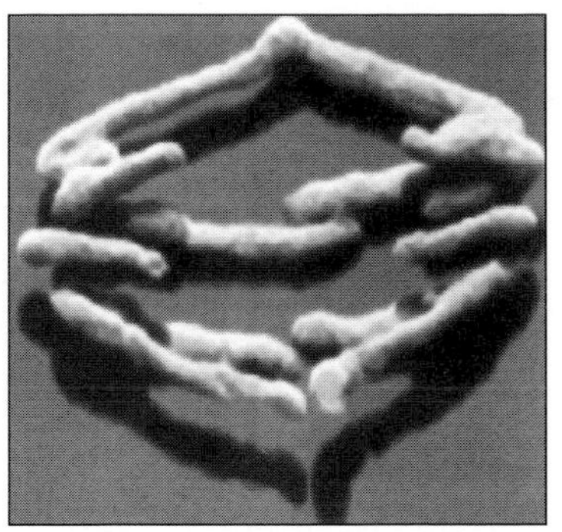

Figure 24. *Reconstruction of chromosomes in a dividing cell from CSLM 3D data. The chromosomes are opaque and the matrix around them transparent, and shadows have been ray cast on the rear plane to enhance the 3D appearance.*

sometimes described as one. In a true ray-traced image, refraction and reflection of the light is included along with the absorption. **Figure 24** shows an example in which the inclusion of shadows greatly increases the 3D impression. More complex shading, in which features cast shadows on themselves and each other, requires calculations that are simply too time-consuming for routine use in this application. With the simple absorption-only method, it is possible to achieve display speeds capable of rotating the array (change the view direction) interactively with high-end desktop computers.

Of course, it is always possible to generate and save a series of projection images that can then be played back as an animation or movie. However, these are primarily useful for communicating information already known to another viewer, while interactive displays may assist in discovering structural relationships in the first place.

These types of volumetric displays are practically always isometric rather than perspective corrected. In other words, the dimension of a voxel or feature does not change with distance. This is equivalent to looking at the scene through a long focal-length lens and, given the inherent strangeness of data in most 3D image sets, does not generally cause significant discomfort to viewers. True perspective correction requires that x, y dimensions on the screen be adjusted for depth. Particularly for rotated views, this adds a significant amount of computation.

Much faster projection image generation is possible if the addressing can be simplified and the variation in distance through different voxels can be ignored. **Figure 25** shows an approximation that facilitates this process. Each plane of voxels is shifted laterally by an integral number of voxel spaces, which makes the address calculation particularly simple. The planes remain normal to the view direction so that all distances through pixels are the same. This kind of shifting can give an impression of rotation for small angles. Beyond about 25 to 30°, the distortion of the 3D structure due to stretching may become visually objectionable. However, this method provides a fast way to cause some relative feature displacement to better understand the structure.

Figure 25. Schematic diagram of shifting image planes laterally to create illusion of rotation or to produce stereo pair images for viewing.

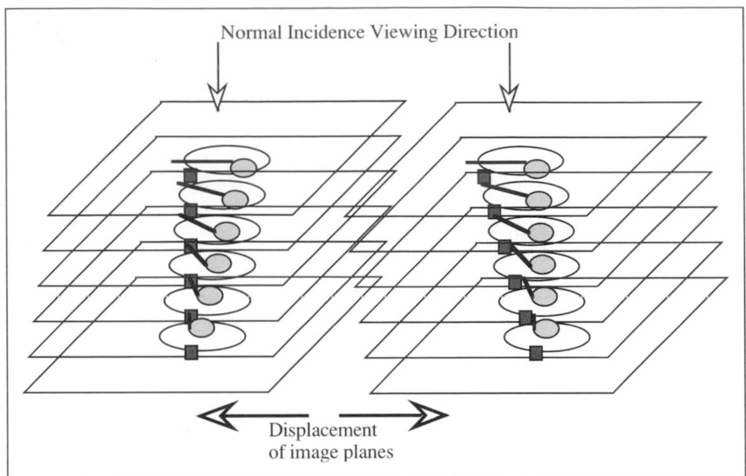

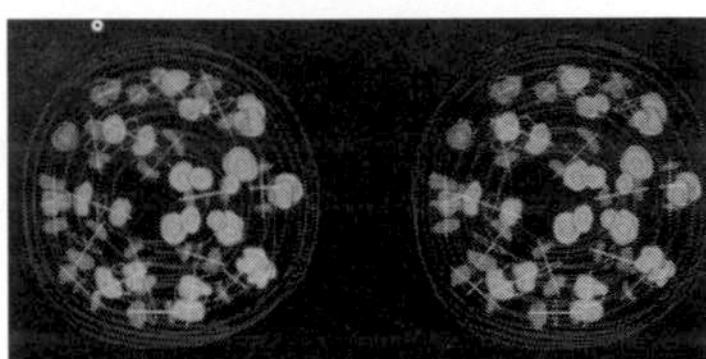

Plate 13. *See color plate, page VI.*

Figure 26 shows such a view through a joint in the leg of a head louse. The original series of images were obtained with a transmission confocal light microscope (TCFLM) with nearly cubic voxels (the spacing between sequential focal planes was 0.2 μm in depth). The individual muscle fibers are visible, but overlapped. Shifting the stack to approximate rotation gives the view the ability to distinguish the various muscle groups. Again, a time sequence (difficult to show in print media) is used as a third dimension to display 3D data as the planes are shifted. Since no complex arithmetic is needed, it is practical to create such animations in a small computer.

Stereo viewing

In many of the images in this chapter, two adjacent images in a rotation or pseudo-rotation sequence can be viewed as a stereo

Figure 26. Volumetric projection image through a stack of 60 CSLM images of a joint in the leg of a head louse. Each plane is displaced by one voxel dimension to produce a view at 45°.

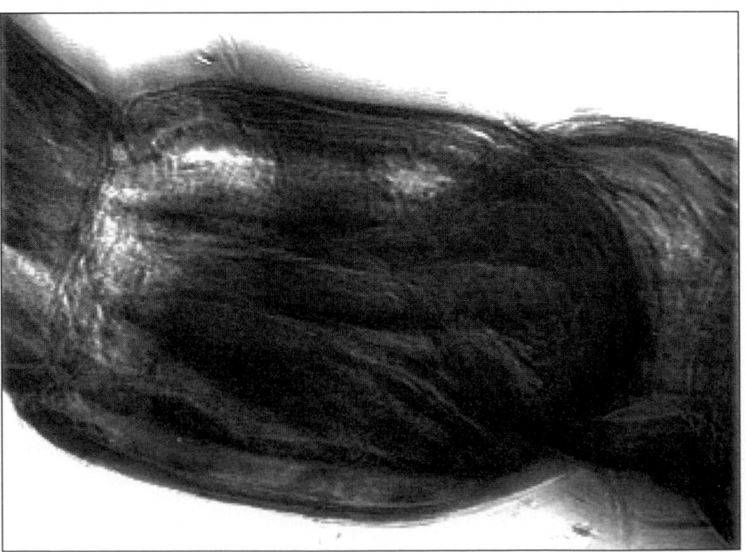

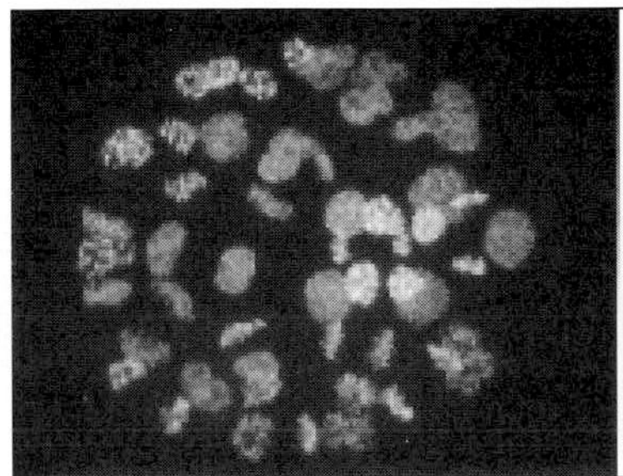

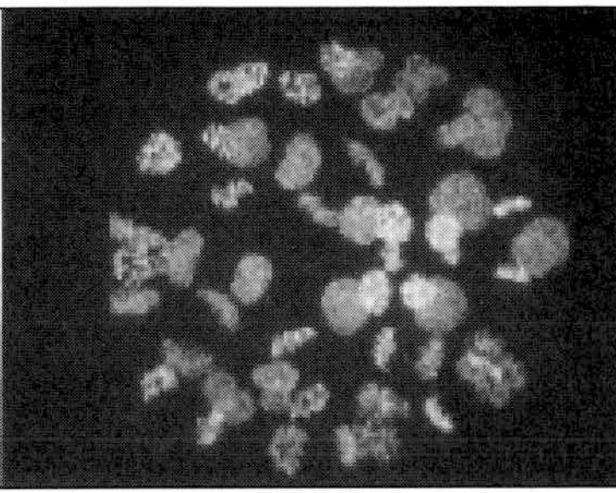

Figure 27. Stereo pair presentation of Feulgen-stained DNA in a sea urchin embryo. The cells form a hollow sphere, evident in the stereo images, with some cells in the act of cell division. This image shows a volumetric image that is "ray cast" or "ray traced," using an emission model, with different offsets for the individual optical sections to produce a stereo effect. See also Plate 13 for a surface image of the same data. (Image courtesy R. G. Summers.)

pair. For some readers, this will require an inexpensive viewer that allows one to focus on the separate images while keeping the eyes looking straight ahead (which the brain expects to correspond to objects at a great distance). Other readers may have mastered the trick of fusing such printed stereo views without assistance. Some, unfortunately, will not be able to see them at all. A significant portion of the population seems not to actually use stereo vision, due (for instance) to uncorrected amblyopia ("lazy eye") in childhood.

Stereo views are so useful to a reasonable fraction of people that it may be useful to display them directly on the viewing screen. Of course, with a large screen, it is possible to draw the two views side by side. **Figure 27** and **Plate 13** show examples of stereo pair presentation of 3D images, using both the volumetric display method discussed above and the surface rendered method discussed below, for the same specimen (derived from CSLM images of a sea urchin embryo). **Figure 28** shows another stereo pair presentation of skeletonized data (skeletonization is also discussed below) obtained from neurons imaged in the CSLM. For many people, this mode requires a viewer and presents some problems of alignment.

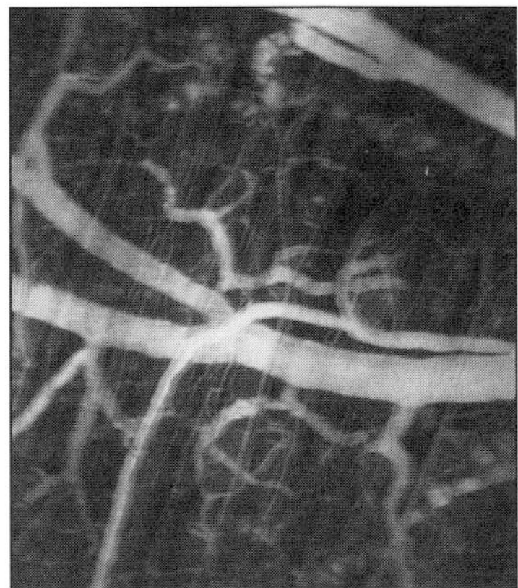

Plate 14. See color plate, page VII.

A more direct stereo display method uses different-colored planes in the display for the left- and right-eye views. For instance, **Figure 29** shows a stereo pair of blood vessels in the skin of a hamster, imaged live using a CSLM in fluorescence mode. The 3D reconstruction method used pseudo-rotation by shifting the focal section planes using the emission rules discussed below. Combining these images using red and green to display two views of the same 3D data set is shown in **Plate 14.**

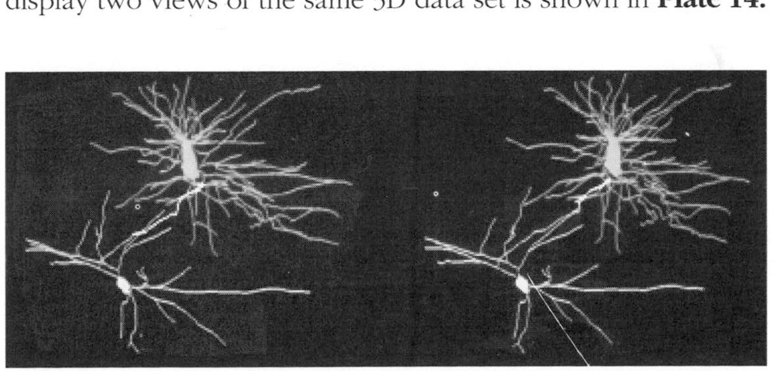

Figure 28. Stereo images of skeletonized lines (manually entered from serial section data) from two neurons in hippocampus of 10-day-old rat, showing branching and 3-D relationships (Turner et al., 1991).

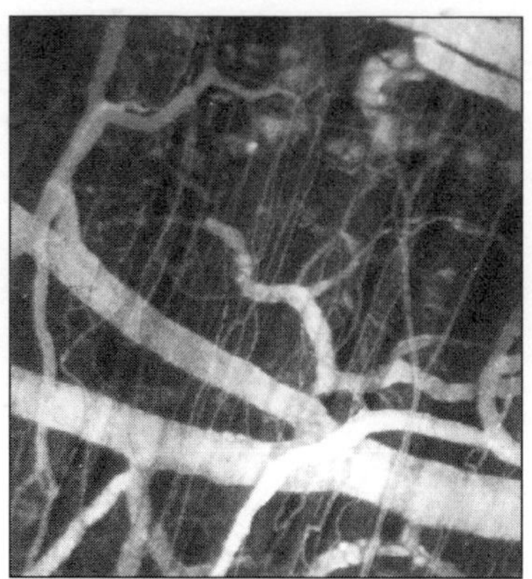 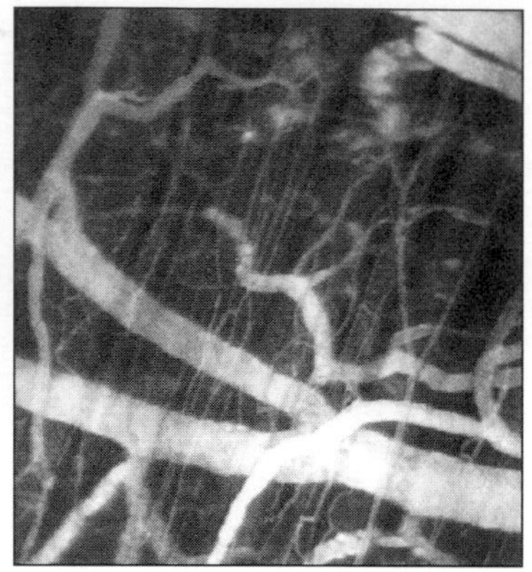

Figure 29. *Stereo view of multiple focal plane images from a CFLM showing light emitted from fluorescent dye injected into the vasculature of a hamster and viewed live in the skin. This image is also shown in Plate 14.*

The images are overlapped and the viewer (equipped with glasses having appropriate red and green filters) can easily look at it. Of course, this method cannot be used for color images, as discussed below.

To project stereo pair images, it is possible to use two slide projectors equipped with polarizing filters, which orient the light polarization at right angles (usually 45 degrees to the right and left of vertical). Viewers wearing polarized glasses can then see the stereo effect and color can still be used. This requires special specular projection screens that reflect light without losing the polarization and works best for viewers in the center of the screen. However, it has become a rather popular method of displaying 3D data. Of course, it is not as practical for interactively exploring a data set, since it is necessary to make photographic slides. Polarization can also be used with live computer displays, as discussed below.

Special display hardware

It is appropriate to mention other specialized display hardware for 3D image analysis. Holography offers the promise of realistic 3D display that can be viewed from different directions, etc. (Blackie et al., 1987). Attempts to generate such displays by calculating the holograms have been experimentally successful, although they are too slow for interactive use. At present, the best holograms are displayed using coherent light from a laser and high-resolution film. In order to produce live displays from a computer, a screen such as an LCD can be used in place of the film. However, the resolution and control of the light modulation (relative intensity) is not really adequate.

Another custom approach is called a varifocal mirror (Fuchs et al., 1982). Each plane of voxels in the 3D array is drawn one at a time on the display CRT. This is not viewed directly by the user, but is reflected from a mirror. The mirror is mounted on a speaker voice coil so that it can be moved. As each different plane of voxels is drawn, the mirror is displaced slightly, as

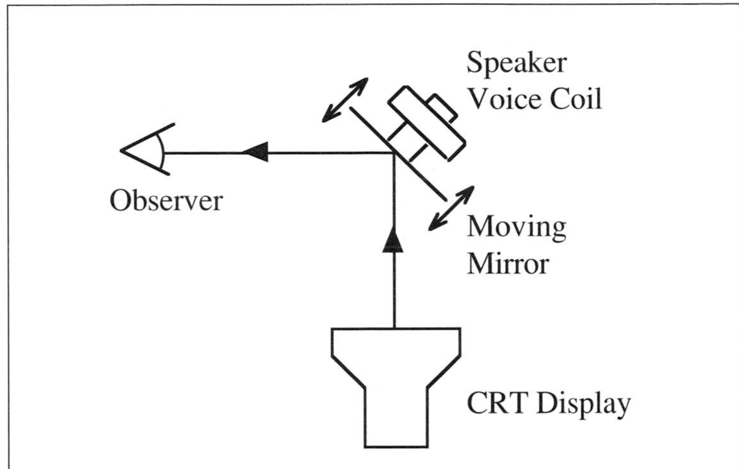

Figure 30. *Diagram of the operation of a varifocal mirror to show depth in images. The speaker voice coil rapidly varies the position of the mirror, which changes the distance from the viewer's eye to the cathode ray tube display as it draws information from different depths in the data set.*

shown schematically in **Figure 30.** This changes the distance from the viewer's eye to the screen, giving the impression of depth. In order to achieve high drawing speeds (so that the entire set of planes can be redrawn at least 30 times per second), this technique is usually restricted to simple outline drawings, rather than the entire voxel data set.

The mirror technique also suffers from a slowdown if the planes are not normal to the x, y, z axes so that trigonometric calculations are required to access the data. The alternative approach is to continue to draw outlines in the major orthogonal planes, but to move the mirror to correspond to the tilting of the plane. This requires a much higher and more complex frequency response from the mechanical devices used to control the mirror.

Another more recent development for viewing of 3D computer graphics displays in real time uses stereo images. The computer calculates two display images for slightly different orientations of the data set or viewing positions. These are displayed alternately using high-speed hardware, which typically shows 120 images per second. Special hardware is then used to allow each eye to see only the correct images at a rate of 60 times per second, fast enough to eliminate flicker (the minimum rate for flicker fusion is usually at least 16 frames per second; commercial moving pictures typically use 24 frames and television uses 25 in European and 30 in U.S. systems).

Visual switching may be done by installing an LCD on the display monitor that can rapidly switch the polarization direction of the transmitted light, so that viewers can wear glasses containing polarizing film. A second approach is to wear special glasses containing active LCDs that can rapidly turn clear or opaque. Synchronizing pulses from the computer cause the glasses to switch as the images are displayed, so that each eye sees the proper view.

Such devices have been used primarily for graphics design, in which substantial computer resources are used to model 3D objects, generate rendered surface views, and allow the user to freely rotate and zoom. With the number of disciplines interested in using 3D computer graphics, it seems assured that new hardware (and the required corresponding software) will continue to evolve for this purpose. These tools will surely be adapted to the display of 3D image data and used at scales ranging from nanometers (electron and ion microscopy) to kilometers (seismic exploration). It is possible to imagine using senses other than visual to deal with multiband data (e.g., sound that changes pitch and volume to reveal density and composition as you move a cursor over the display of a voxel array). However, since vision is our primary sense, it seems likely that most methods will be primarily visual and the researcher who is color-blind or cannot see stereo will remain disadvantaged.

There is also no consensus on the best input and control devices for complex computer graphics displays. Rotating or shifting the viewpoint in response to horizontal or vertical motion of the now ubiquitous mouse gives a rather crude control. For moving points, lines, and planes in 3D, some more flexible device will be required. Simply locating a specific voxel location in the array can be done in several different ways. One is to use an *x,y* input device (mouse, trackball, etc.) for two axes and periodically shift to a different control, which may be a scroll bar on the screen, to adjust the distance along the third axis. Another is to move two cursors, one on an *x-y* projection and one on an *x-z* projection, for example. Such approaches usually feel rather clumsy, because of the need to move back and forth between two areas of the screen and two modalities of interaction. Appropriate cursor color-coding to report depth can help.

Three-axis joysticks and sonic digitizers that allow the operator to point in space (multiple sensors triangulate the position) exist, but are hardly standard. The dataglove, an instrumented glove or framework that fits on the hand and reports joint motions to the computer, has been used to move molecules around each other to study enzyme action. Supplemented by force feedback, this gives the researcher rich information about the ways that molecules can best fit together. Perhaps the ultimate "virtual reality" is to use such gloves while wearing a helmet that reports head position and has built-in displays for each eye, so that the computer can create appropriate stereo displays as you move around inside your data set. However, such tools remain inaccessible to typical users of image analysis computers at the time of this writing.

Ray tracing

The example of volumetric display shown in **Figure 26** performed a simplified ray tracing to sum the density values of voxels and calculate a brightness based on light being absorbed as it propagated from back to front through the 3D data set. While this corresponds to some imaging situations, such as the TCFLM or SEM and tomography, there are many other situations in which different rules are appropriate.

In the process of traversing a voxel array, following a particular line of sight that will end in one pixel of a ray-traced image, the variables which are available include:

a) The brightness and (perhaps) color of the original light source placed behind the array. This will control the contribution that transmission makes to the final image.
b) The location of the first and/or last voxels with a density above some arbitrary threshold taken to represent transparency. These will define surfaces that can be rendered using reflected light. Additional rules for surface reflectivity, the location and brightness of the light sources, etc. must be added.
c) The location of the maximum or minimum values, which may define the location of some internal surface for rendering.
d) The rule for combining voxel values along a path. This may be the multiplication of fractional values, which models simple absorption according to Beer's law for photons, provided that the voxel values are linear absorption values. In some cases, density is proportional to attenuation and so can produce interpretable images. There are other convolution rules available as well, including linear summation, retention of maximum or minimum values, etc. While these may also correspond to some physical situations, their greatest value is that they produce images that can delineate internal structure.
e) The relationship between the voxel values and the intensity (and perhaps color) of light originating in each voxel, which represents fluorescence or other emission processes.

The combining rules mentioned briefly in part d) correspond to the various image processing tools described in Chapters 2 and 3 for combining pixels from two or more images. They include arithmetic (multiplication, addition), rank ordering (minimum or maximum value) and Boolean logic. It is also possible to include lateral scattering, so that point sources of light spread or blur as they pass through the voxel array, or even to combine several modes. This approach to realism through computation is rarely justified, since the measured voxel values are generally not directly related to light transmission or scattering.

A software package for 3D visualization may make any or all of these parameters accessible to the user, as well as additional ones. For example, we will see that controlling the surface reflectivity and roughness and the location of the incident light source(s) affects the appearance of rendered surfaces. In per-

Figure 31. *Volumetric imaging of the MRI head data from Figure 14. Varying the relationship between voxel values and the opacity used to absorb light transmitted along each ray through the structure allows selection of which structures are revealed.*

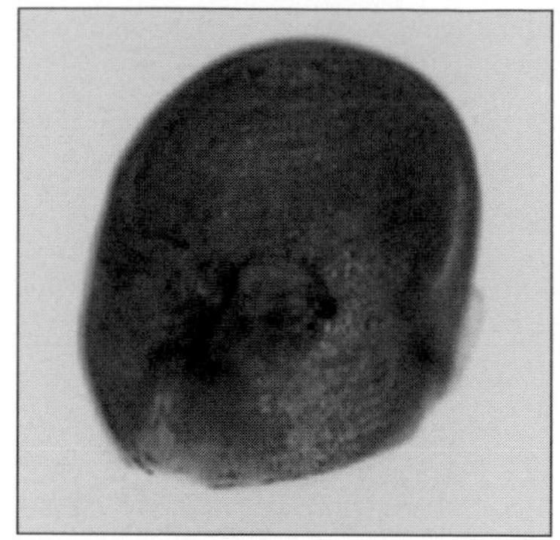
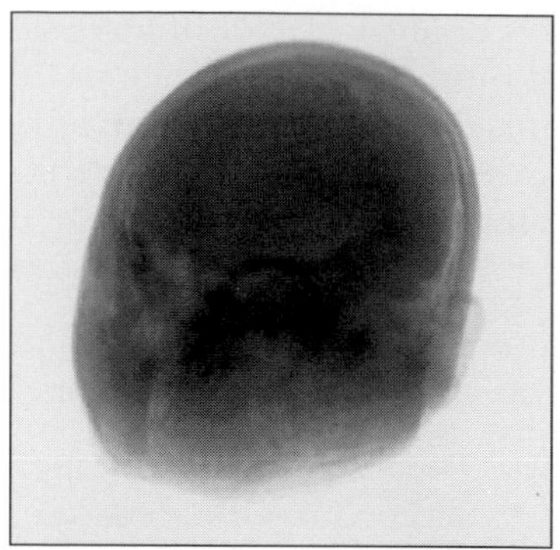
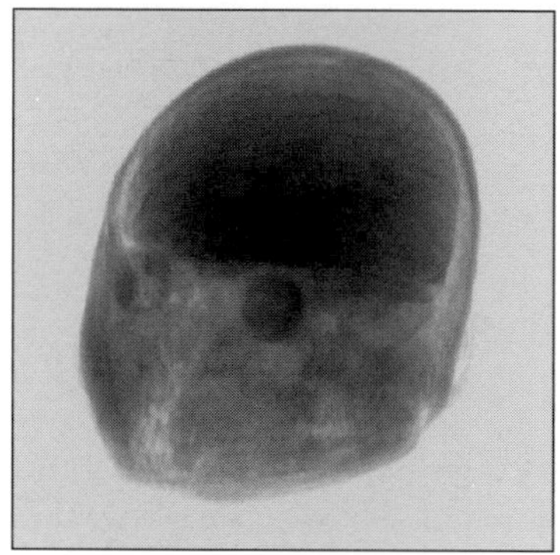
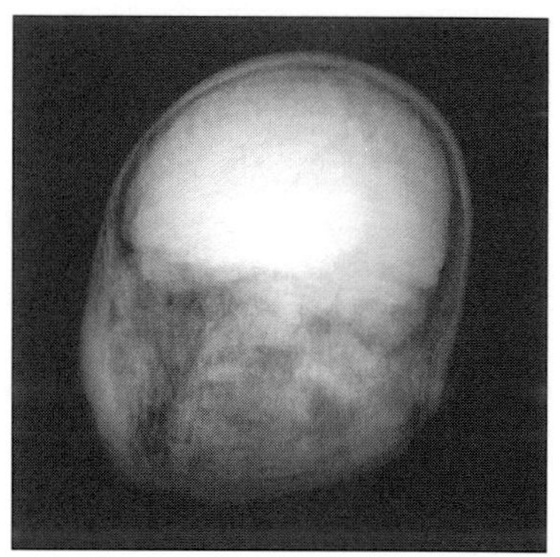

forming a convolution of transmitted light along ray paths from a light source behind the voxel array, the relationship between the voxel values and the absorption of the light is another parameter that offers control. By varying the relationship between voxel value and opacity (linear attenuation coefficient), it is possible to make structures appear or to remove them, allowing others to be seen.

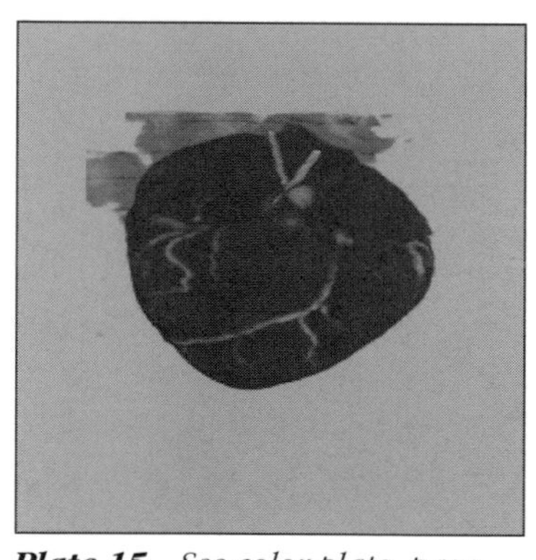

Plate 15. *See color plate, page VII.*

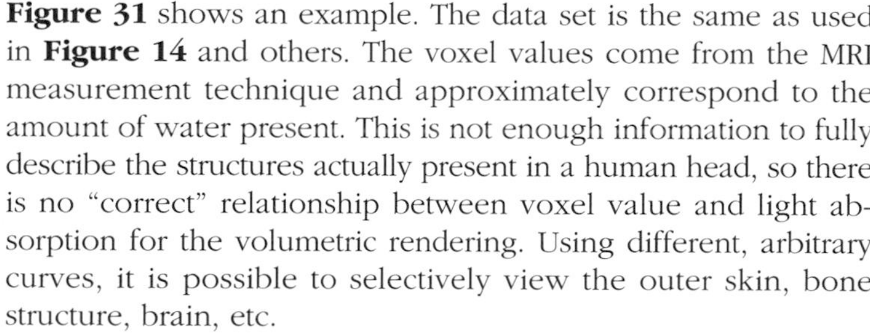

Figure 31 shows an example. The data set is the same as used in **Figure 14** and others. The voxel values come from the MRI measurement technique and approximately correspond to the amount of water present. This is not enough information to fully describe the structures actually present in a human head, so there is no "correct" relationship between voxel value and light absorption for the volumetric rendering. Using different, arbitrary curves, it is possible to selectively view the outer skin, bone structure, brain, etc.

Color permits even more distinctions to be made. **Plate 15** shows images of a hog heart, reconstructed using different relationships for opacity vs. voxel value, which emphasize the heart muscle or the blood vessels. In this example, each voxel is assumed both to absorb the light from the source placed behind the voxel array and to contribute its own light along the ray, in proportion to its value and with color taken from an arbitrary table. The result allows structures with different measured values to appear in different colors.

With only a single value for each voxel, it is not possible to separately model absorption and emission. By performing dual-energy tomography, in which the average atomic number and average density are both determined, or multi-energy tomography, in which the concentrations of various elements in each voxel are measured, such techniques become possible. They represent straightforward implementation of several of the multiband and color imaging methods discussed in earlier chapters, but are not yet common, since neither the imaging instrumentation nor the computer routines are yet widely available. Consequently, it is usually necessary to adopt some arbitrary relationship between the single measured set of voxel values and the displayed rendering, which corresponds to the major voxel property measured by the original imaging process.

In fluorescence light microscopy, X-ray images from the SEM, or ion microscopy (as shown in **Figure 23**), for example, the voxel value is a measure of emitted brightness that is generally proportional to elemental concentration. These 3D data sets can also be shown volumetrically by a simplified ray tracing. Instead of absorbing light from an external light source, the rule is to sum the voxel values as brightnesses along each path.

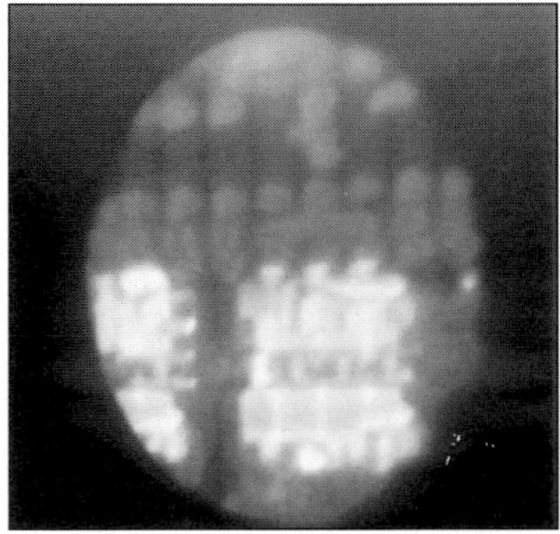

Plate 16. *See color plate, page VIII.*

Figure 29 showed an application using the fluorescence CSLM. A dye injected into the blood vessel of a hamster was excited by the incident light from the microscope. The emitted light was collected to form a series of 2D images at different focal depths, which were then arranged in a stack to produce a 3D data set. In this case, the spacing between the planes is much greater than the resolution within each image plane. Sliding the image stack laterally, as discussed above, produces an approximation of rotation and an impression of depth. The brightness values for each voxel are then summed along vertical columns to produce each image.

This emission model is very easy to calculate but does not take into account any possible absorption of the emitted light intensity by other voxels along the ray path. Generally, simple 3D data sets have only one piece of data per voxel and there is no separate information on density and emission brightness, so no such correction is even possible. Sometimes, a simple reduction in intensity in proportion to the total number of voxels traversed, known as a distance fade, may be used to approximate this absorption effect. Usually, it is assumed that the emission intensity is sufficiently high and the structure sufficiently transparent that no such correction is needed, or that it would not change the interpretation of the structure.

When multiband data are available, as for instance in the SIMS data set used in **Figure 23** and **Plate 12,** emission rules can be used assigning different colors (at least up to three) to different signals. **Figure 32** and **Plate 16** show a volumetric view of this data using emission rules, presented as a stereo pair. The figure

Figure 32. *Stereo pair display of emission rule volumetric images of boron concentration in a silicon wafer, imaged by a secondary ion mass spectrometer.*

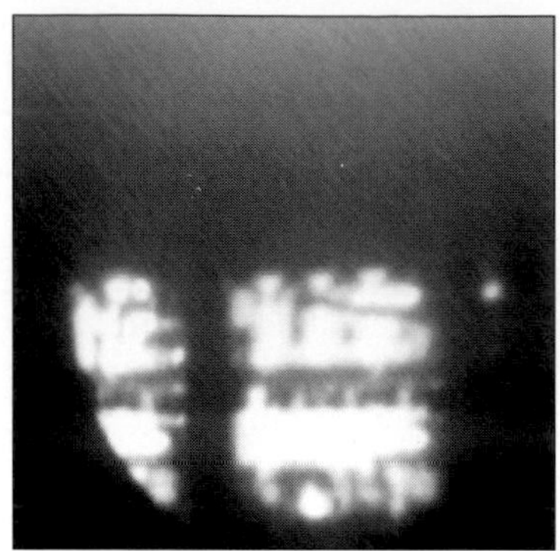
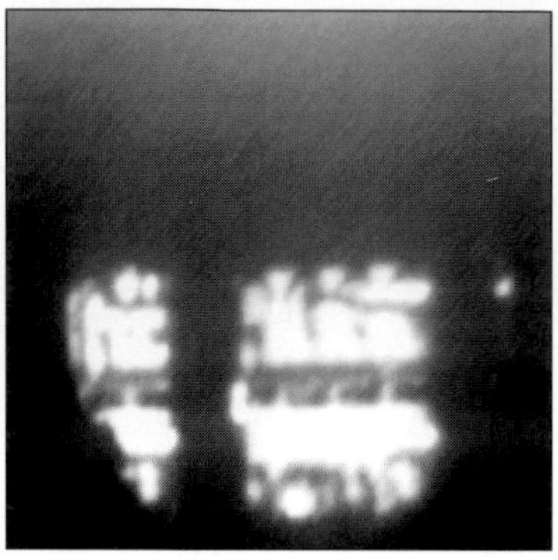

shows a single element (boron), while in the color plate, multiple elements are combined. Using color in the images forces the use of two side-by-side images for viewing. The density of information in the images, resulting from overlaying the 8-bit (256 grey level) values from each element at every point, makes it quite difficult to fuse these images for satisfactory stereo viewing.

Using the same data set, it is possible to define the location of an internal boundary, using the location of the frontmost voxel along each line of sight whose value is above an arbitrary threshold. If the resulting surface is then rendered as a solid surface with incident reflected light, another representation of the data is obtained, as shown in **Figure 33.**

Reflection

Another important imaging modality is reflection. The conventional CSLM, seismic reflection mapping, acoustic microscopy, etc. acquire a 3D image set whose voxel values record the reflection of the signal from that location. This is generally used to locate boundaries where strong reflections occur, within a matrix that may be otherwise opaque. In the CSLM, the matrix is transparent (either air or liquid) and the strongest reflection at each x, y point is where the specimen surface is in focus. This means that recording a set of images as a 3D data array makes it possible to locate the surface in three dimensions.

Figure 33. *Surface-rendered display of the same data as in Figure 32. The internal surface of the boron-rich region is determined by arbitrary thresholding, and then rendered using an arbitrarily placed light source.*

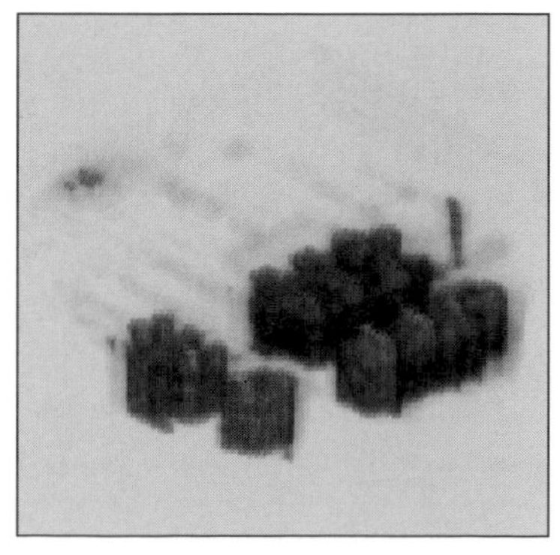

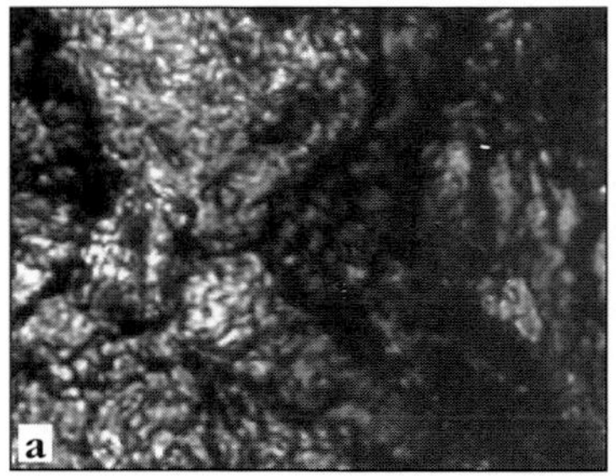

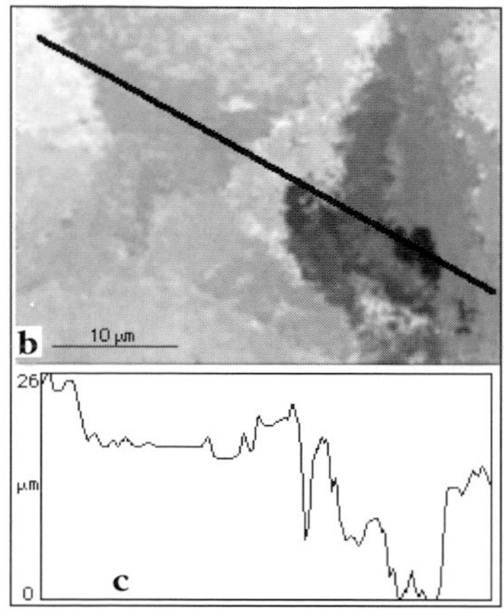

Figure 34. Depth measurement using the confocal scanning light microscope:
a) *extended focus image of an alumina fracture surface obtained by keeping the brightest value from many focal planes at each pixel location;*
b) *range image obtained by assigning a grey scale value to each pixel according to the focal plane image in which the brightest (in focus) reflectance is measured;*
c) *elevation profile along the traverse line shown in figure b.*

One way to generate such a display is to go down columns of the data array (just as in volumetric ray tracing) looking for the maximum voxel value. Keeping only that value produces an image of the entire surface in focus, as was shown in Figures 62, 63, and 64 of Chapter 3. Since the same methods for rotating or shifting the data array to alter the viewing direction can be used, it is also possible to find the maxima along any viewing direction and display the surface as an animation sequence or to construct a stereo pair. **Figure 34** shows the alumina fracture (from Chapter 3, Figures 63 and 64), both as an extended-focus image and as a 2D range image (in which pixel brightness is proportional to elevation). Several presentation modes for range are available images to assist in visualizing the 3D shape of the surface. One, shown in **Figure 34,** is to simply plot the brightness profile along any line across the image. This gives the elevation profile directly.

Figure 35 shows several of the presentation modes for range images. The specimen is a microelectronics chip imaged by reflection CSLM, so both an extended-focus image and a range image can be obtained from the series of focal plane sections. From the range-image data, plotting contour maps, grid or mesh plots, or shaded isometric displays is a straightforward exercise in computer graphics.

One of the classic ways to show surface elevation is a contour map (**Figure 35c**), in which isoelevation lines are drawn, usually at uniform increments of altitude. These lines are of course continuous and closed. This is the way topographic maps are drawn; the same methods are useful at any scale. Since the contour map reduces the pixel data from the original range image to boundary representation, the method for forming the boundaries is the same as discussed in Chapter 5 for segmentation. The lines may be labeled or color-coded to assist in distinguishing elevation.

A shortcut way to draw contour lines on a range image is to present the data as a shaded isometric view, as in **Plate 17**, which

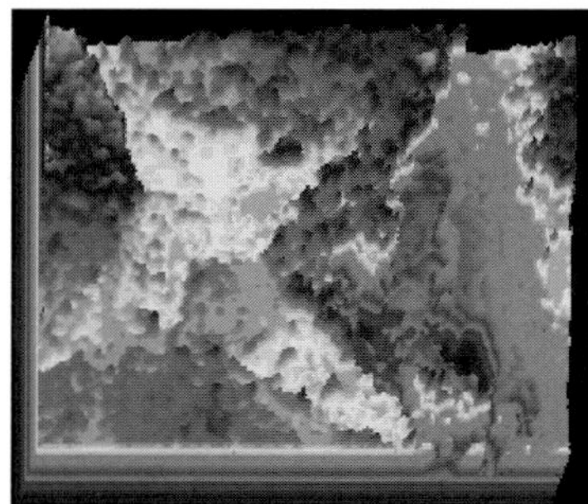

Plate 17. *See color plate, page VIII.*

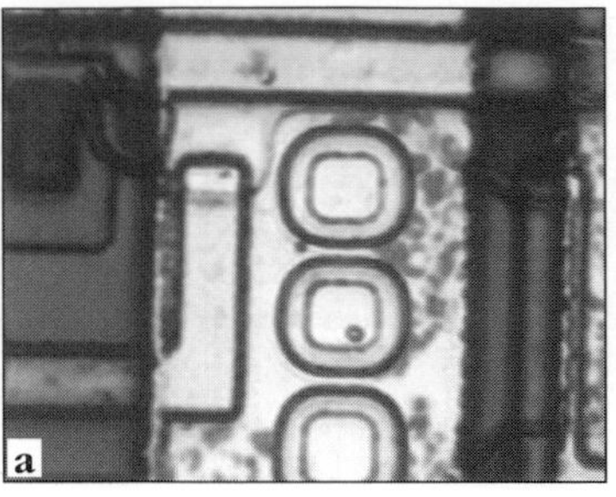

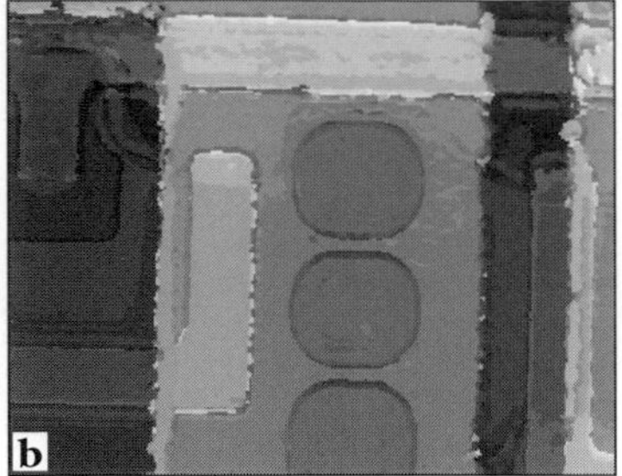

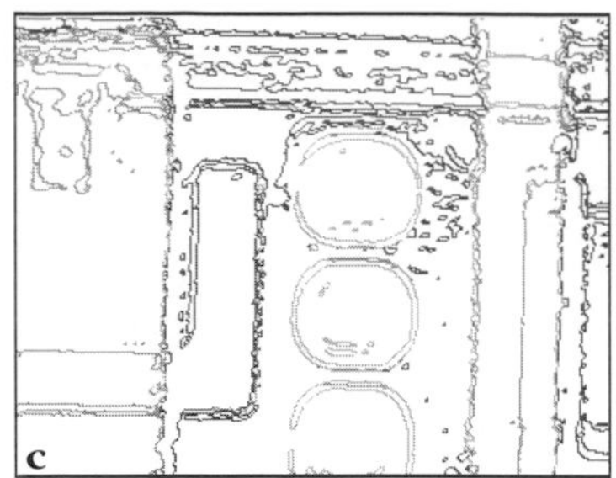

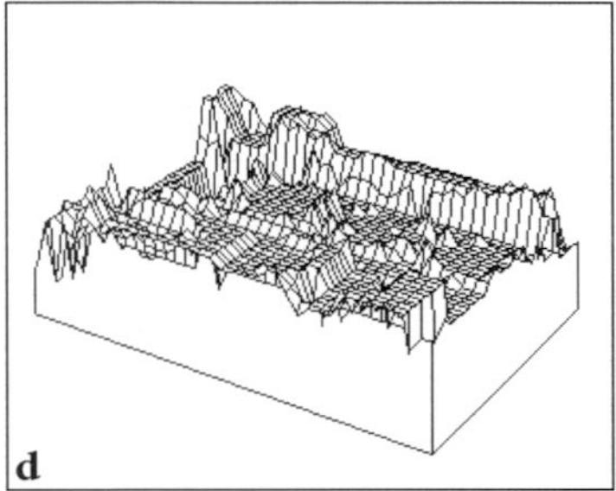

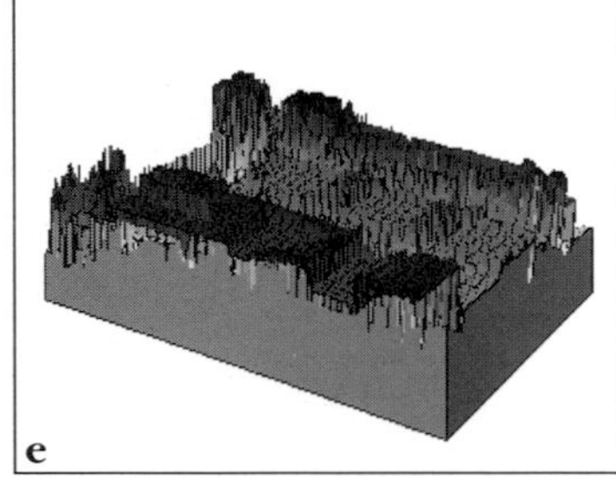

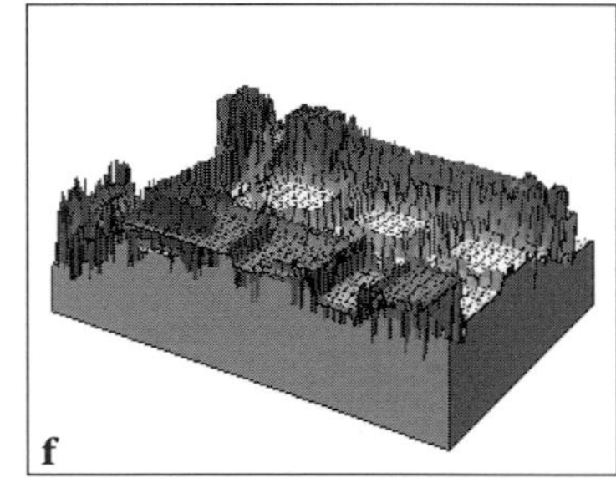

Figure 35. Presentation modes for surface information from the CSLM (specimen is a microelectronics chip):

a) *the in-focus image of the surface reflectance obtained by keeping the brightest value at each pixel address from all of the multiple focal plane images;*

b) *the elevation or range image produced by grey scale encoding the depth at which the brightest pixel was measured for each pixel address;*

c) *contour map of the surface elevation with grey scale coding for the height values;*

d) *isometric grid drawing of the elevation data, with grid spacing equal to 6 pixels;*

e) *the same grid as in figure d with shading to show the elevation values;*

f) *the grid from figure d with the reflectance data from figure a superimposed.*

shows the elevation data for the alumina fracture surface of **Figure 34.** In this image, a 3D representation (without perspective) is used to draw a vertical line for each pixel in the range image to a height proportional to the value. The image is also shaded, so that each point has its grey scale value. Replacing the grey scale values with a pseudo-color table allows the elevations to be communicated in a particularly easy-to-interpret way. Many topographic maps use similar methods to show elevation.

Figure 36 shows an example that looks broadly similar but represents data at a very different scale. It is a 3D view of Ishtar Terra on Venus. The data come from the spacecraft Magellan's side-looking mapping radar. This synthetic-aperture radar bounces 12.5-cm wavelength radar waves off the surface, using the echo time delay for range and the doppler shift to collect signals from points ahead of and behind the direct line of sight. The 2D images obtained by processing the signals are similar in appearance to aerial photographs.

It is also possible to apply brightness values to an isometric display of range data, such as the original reflectivity, texture information, etc., which come from another image of the same area.

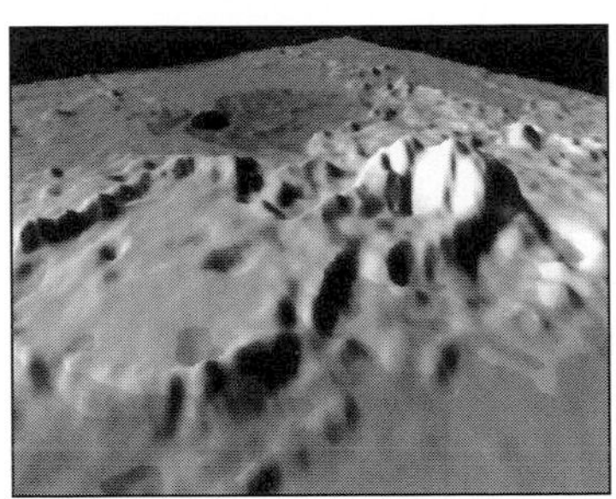

Figure 36. *Reconstructed surface image of Ishtar Terra on Venus, looking northeast across Lakshmi Panum toward Maxwell Montes with an exaggerated vertical scale (Saunders, 1991).*

This is particularly effective when multiband images are recorded. **Figure 35f** shows an example of this display mode.

The surfaces discussed in the preceding section are in fact external physical surfaces of the specimen. Internal surfaces may be defined as boundaries between distinct regions or categorized in more subtle ways. For instance, **Figure 37** shows the data from the SIMS example used above, in which the depth of the voxel having the maximum concentration of silicon at any location is shown. This provides a visualization of the shape of the implanted region. The image is shown as a shaded isometric display, as discussed above.

Surfaces

Surfaces to be examined may be either physical surfaces, revealed directly by reflected light, electrons, or sound waves, or surfaces that are internal to the sample and can be revealed only indirectly after the entire 3D data set has been acquired. The use of computer graphics to display surfaces is closely related to other graphics display modes used in computer-assisted design (CAD), for example. However, the typical CAD object has only a few numbers to describe it, such as the coordinates of borders. Generating the interpolated surfaces and calculating the local orientation and hence the brightness of the image at many points requires a significant amount of computing.

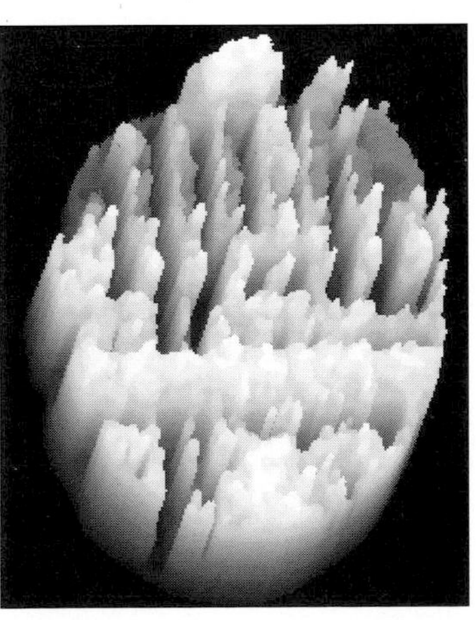

Figure 37. *Isometric display of elevation data within a volume: the height of the maximum concentration on Si in the SIMS voxel array.*

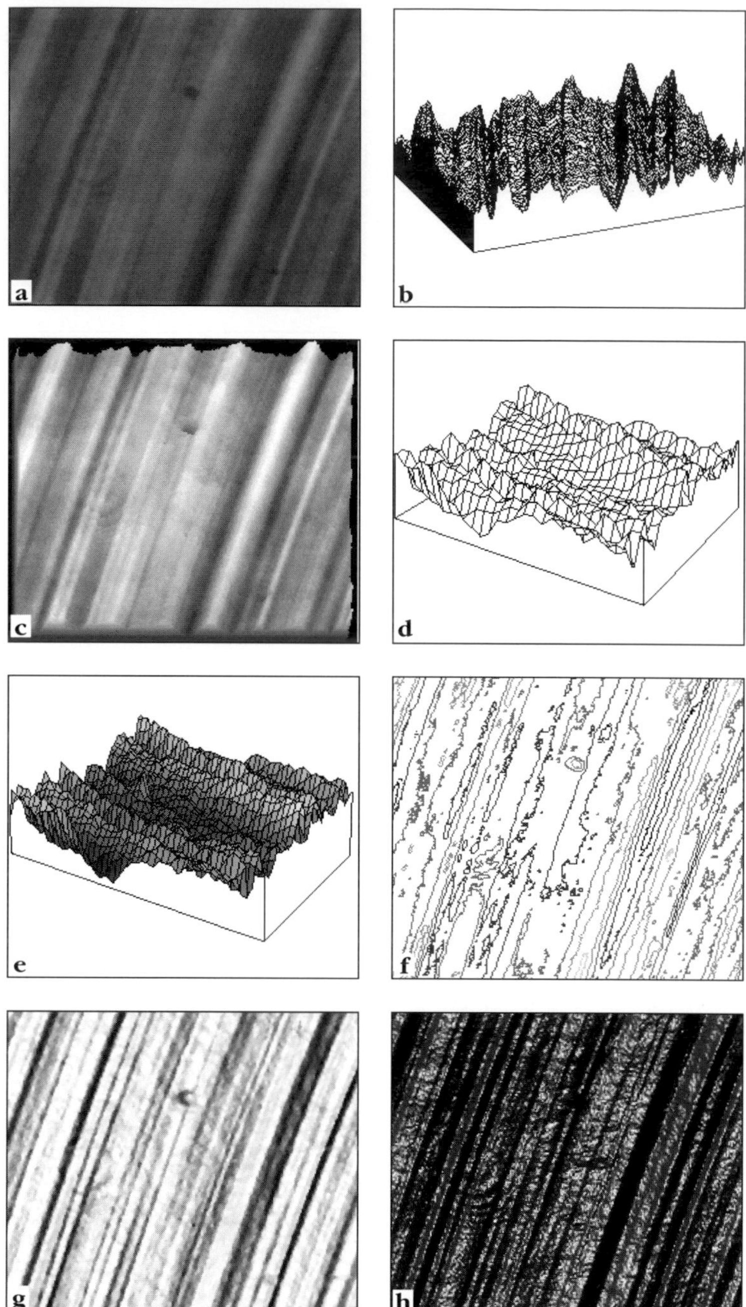

Figure 38. Presentation modes for the surface elevation data from an optical interferometer (specimen is the machined surface of nickel):

a) *original image, in which the grey scale brightness encodes height;*
b) *isometric view produced by drawing multiple line profiles across the surface;*
c) *isometric view with superimposed grey scale values from image a;*
d) *isometric view with a full grid drawn at a spacing of 8 pixels;*
e) *the same grid with shading from figure a;*
f) *a contour map with grey scale shading to indicate the height of lines;*
g) *the surface data rendered as it would appear with a diffuse material;*
h) *the surface data rendered as it would appear with a specular material.*

In contrast, the image data discussed here is typically a complete 3D data set, or at least a complete 2D range image derived from the 3D set. Therefore, there is elevation data at every pixel location in the display image, which allows for extremely rapid image generation. Rendering the surface images shown here took only a few seconds on a desktop computer. Doing the same for a typical CAD object would take many minutes.

Some instruments produce range images directly. Large-scale examples include radar mapping, elevation measurement from stereo pair calculations, and sonar depth ranging. At a finer scale, a standard tool for measuring precision-machined surfaces is interferometry, which produces images as shown in **Figure 38a.** The brightness is a direct measure of elevation and the image can be comprehended more easily in an isometric display, as shown in **Figure 38c.** Notice that the lens artefact (the ring structure at the left side of the image) is not true elevation data and when presented as such looks quite strange.

Displays of surface images (more formally, of range images, since real surfaces may be complex and multivalued, but range images are well-behaved and single-valued) can use any of the techniques described above. These include wire mesh or line profile displays, contour maps, and shaded isometric displays, all compared for the same image data in **Figure 38.** These all involve a certain level of abstraction.

The simple set of line profiles (**Figure 38b**) gives an impression of surface elevation and requires no computation, although the need to space the lines apart results in some loss of detail. Consequently, it is sometimes used as a direct display mode on instruments such as the SEM or STM. Unfortunately, the signal that is displayed in this way may not actually be the elevation, and in this case, the "pseudo-topographic" display can be quite misleading. Adding grid or mesh lines in both directions (**Figure**s **38d** and **38e**) not only requires additional computation, but also increases the effective spacing and decreases the lateral resolution of the display.

Generating an image of a surface that approximates the appearance of a real, physical surface is known generically as rendering and requires more computational effort. Examples are shown in **Figure**s **38g** and **38h.** The physical rules governing the way real surfaces look are simple and are summarized in **Figure 39.** The important variables are the intensity and location of the light source and the location of the viewer. Both are usually given in terms of the angles between the normal vector of the surface and the vectors to the source and the viewer. The absolute reflectivity of the surface (or albedo) must be known; if this varies with wavelength, we say that the surface is colored, because some colors will be reflected more than others.

Finally, the local roughness of the surface controls the degree of variation in the angle of reflection. A very narrow angle for this spread corresponds to a smooth surface, which reflects specularly. A broader angle corresponds to a more diffuse reflection. One of the very common tricks in graphic arts, which you can see any evening in television advertising, is the addition of bright specular reflections to objects, to make them appear metallic and, hopefully, more interesting.

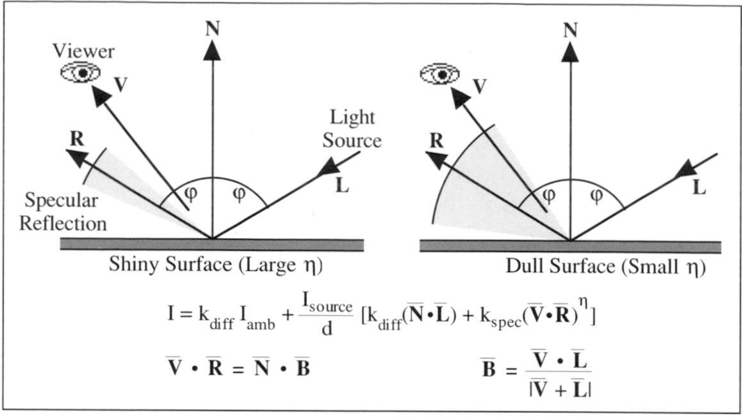

Figure 39. *Lambertian rules for light scattering from surfaces with different specularity. The vectors are N (surface normal), L (light source), R (reflection), and V (viewing direction). The k factors are the diffuse and specular reflection coefficients. The I values are the intensities of the principal and ambient light sources, and h is a constant describing the breadth of the specular reflection, which depends on the fine-scale surface roughness.*

For a typical surface defined by a few points, as in CAD drawings, the surface is broken into facets, often triangular, and the orientation of each facet is calculated with respect to the viewer and light source. The reflected light intensity is then calculated and the result plotted on the display screen or other output device to build the image. This would seem to be a rather fast process with only a small number of facets, but the problem is that such images do not look natural. The large flat facets and the abrupt angles between them do not correspond to the continuous surfaces we encounter in most real objects.

Shading the brightness values between facets (Gouraud shading) can eliminate these abrupt edges and improve the appearance of the image, but it requires considerable interpolation. Better smoothing can be achieved (particularly when there are specular reflections present) by interpolating not the brightness values, but the angles between the centers of the facets. The interpolated angles are then used to generate the brightness values, which vary nonlinearly with angle. This Phong shading is even more computer-intensive.

For continuous pixel images, each set of three pixels can be considered to define a triangular facet, as shown schematically in **Figure 40.** The difference in value (elevation) of the neighboring pixels directly gives the angles of the local surface normal. A precalculated LUT of the image brightness values for a given light source location and surface characteristics completes the solution with minimum calculations. Since this is done at the pixel

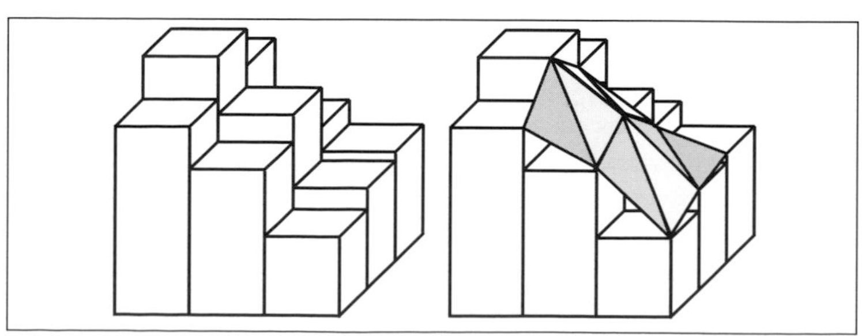

Figure 40. *Diagram showing the construction of a triangular tesselation on a surface formed by discrete height values for an array of pixels.*

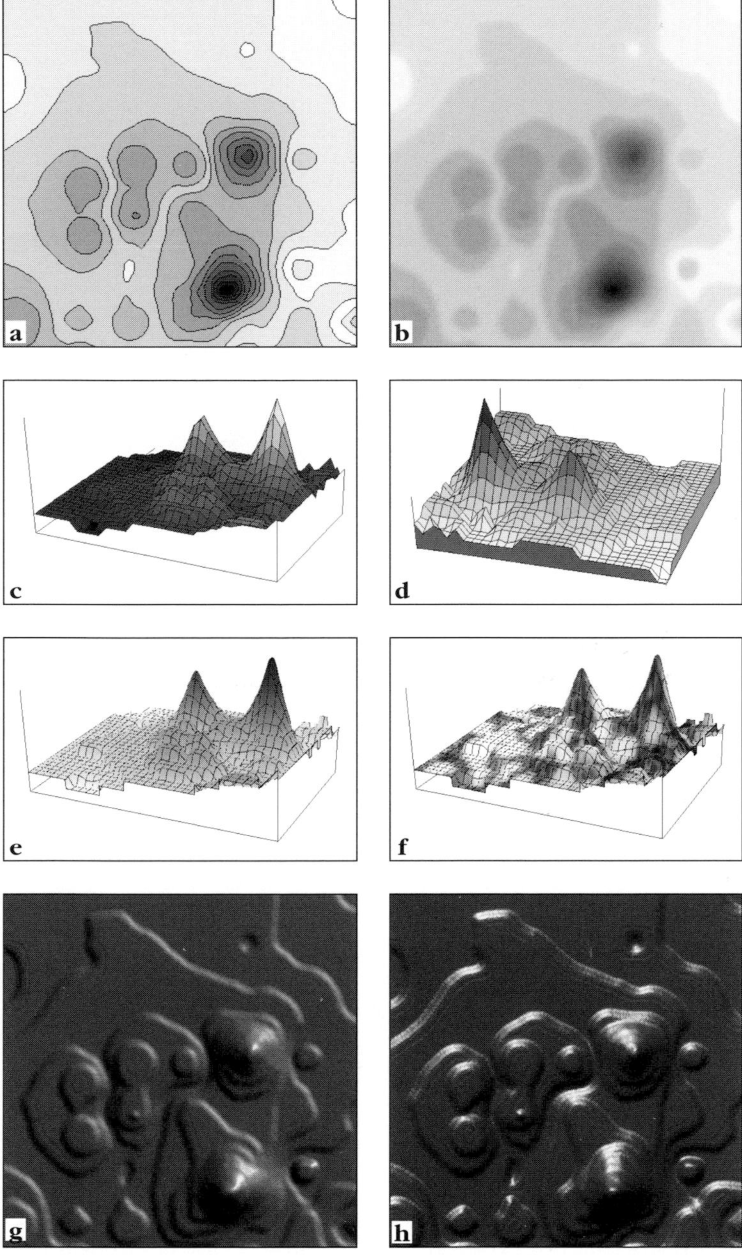

Figure 41. Presentation modes derived from data in an elevation contour map:

a) *the original map, with uniform grey levels shown between the contours to indicate relative height;*

b) *continuous elevation values interpolated between the contour lines by smoothing the grey scale values in figure a;*

c) *perspective view of the surface shown with a shaded grid;*

d) *image c from a different point of view;*

e) *perspective display showing each pixel elevation, shading and a superimposed grid;*

f) *perspective display with a different grey scale image of the same surface superimposed;*

g) *the surface rendered as a diffuse surface;*

h) *the surface rendered as a specular surface with a different location for the light source.*

level in the display, no interpolation of shading is needed. **Figure 41** includes displays of a rendered surface with different light source locations and surface characteristics.

The examples of display modes in **Figure 41** show the reconstruction of a surface from the rather sparse information in a contour map. The map is converted to a range image by applying smoothing, to interpolate values between the contour lines. This can then be shown as an isometric or perspective-corrected grid, with or without superimposed shading. Finally, the facets can be rendered using the relationships of **Figure 39.**

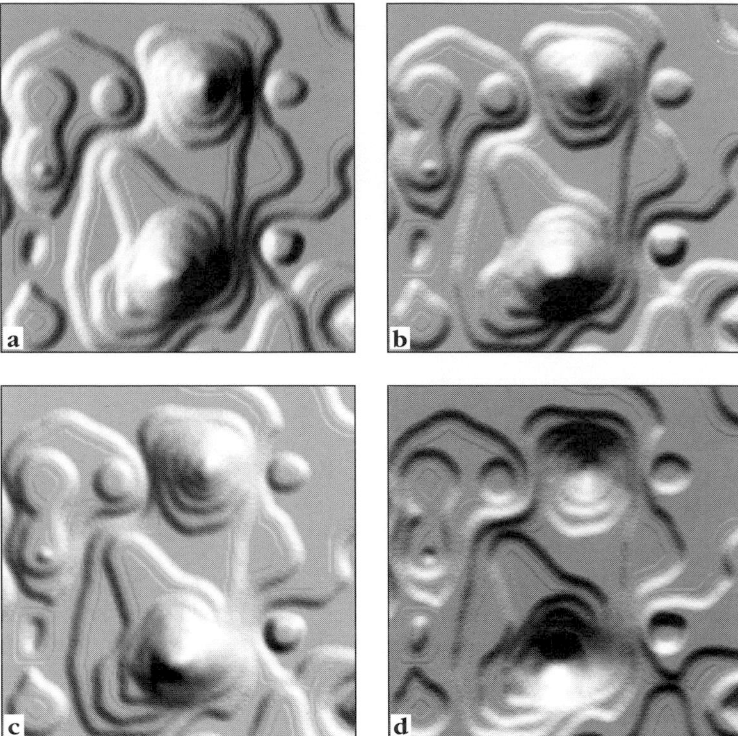

Figure 42. *Rendered surface from Figure 41 with moving light source (four frames from an animation sequence). Notice that when viewed alone, lighting from below (figure d) causes the peaks to appear as valleys.*

Applying image processing operations beforehand to range image data is often used to improve the resulting surface image. Smoothing with kernel operations, which calculate a weighted average, corresponds to Phong shading. Applying a median filter removes noise, which would show up as local spikes or holes in the surface. The names of filters, such as the rolling-ball operator discussed in Chapter 3, come directly from their use on range images. This particular operator tests the difference between the minimum value in two neighborhood regions of different sizes and eliminates points that are too low. The analogy is that the depressions that a ball of defined radius cannot touch as it rolls across the surface are filled in.

Rendering a surface (calculating its brightness according to its orientation with respect to the viewer and light source) using the LUT approach is fast, provided that the appropriate tables for different light source locations and surface characteristics have been calculated beforehand. The tables are not large and can be stored for a reasonable number of cases. This permits a nearly real-time animation of a rendered surface with a moving light source (see **Figure 42**), which is another way to use the dimension of time to reveal 3D spatial information. Changing the surface characteristics, from diffuse to specular or from white reflection to colored, can be used to show multiband data. Obviously, additional surface images are required to specify these characteristics.

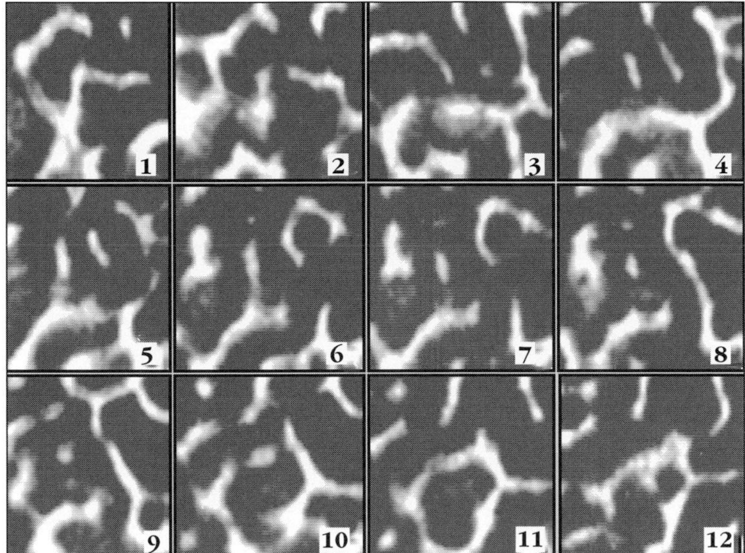

Figure 43. *Sequential images from an ion microscope, showing two-phase structure in an Fe-45% Cr alloy aged 192 hours at 540°C (M. K. Miller, Oak Ridge National Laboratories, Oak Ridge, TN).*

Rendered surfaces from range images have the appearance of real, physical objects, so they communicate easily with the viewer. However, they obscure much of the information present in the original 3D image data set from which they have been extracted. More complex displays, which require real ray tracing, can make surfaces that are partially reflecting and partially transmitting, so that the surface can be combined with volumetric information in the display. This has somewhat the appearance of embedding the solid surface in a partially transparent medium, like fruit in Jello. Such displays can be dramatic in appearance and are useful for communicating complex 3D information, but generating them is too slow to be used to interactively explore complex data sets.

Multiply connected surfaces

Rendering techniques are not restricted, of course, to simple range images. Indeed, 3D image data is most needed for complex, multiply connected surfaces since the topology of such surfaces cannot be studied in 2D images. Rendering more complex surfaces is also possible, but it takes a little longer. **Figure 43** shows a series of 2D planes in a 3D data set from an ion microscope. The sample, a two-phase metal alloy, shows many regions in each image. It is only in the full 3D data set that the connection between all of the regions is evident. In fact, each of the two-phase regions in this specimen is a single, continuous network intimately intertwined with the other. This cannot be seen well even by using resectioning in various directions (**Figure 44**).

Volumetric displays of this data set can show some of the intricacy, especially when the live animation can be viewed as the

__Figure 44.__ ***Section views of the 3D voxel array formed from the images in Figure 43:***

a) *stored brightness values along several arbitrary orthogonal planes;*

b) *stored values on a series of parallel planes with dark voxels made transparent.*

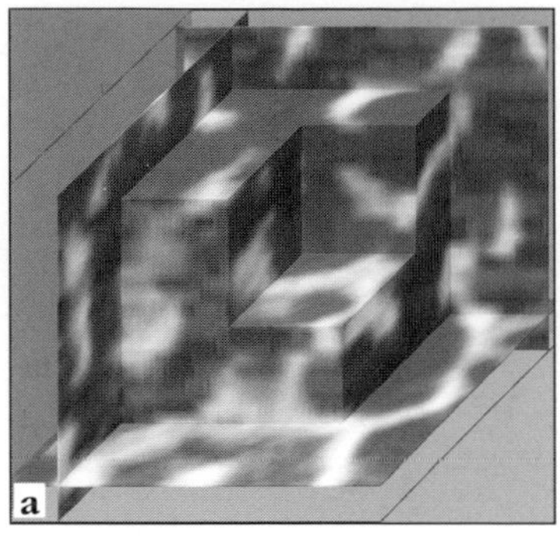

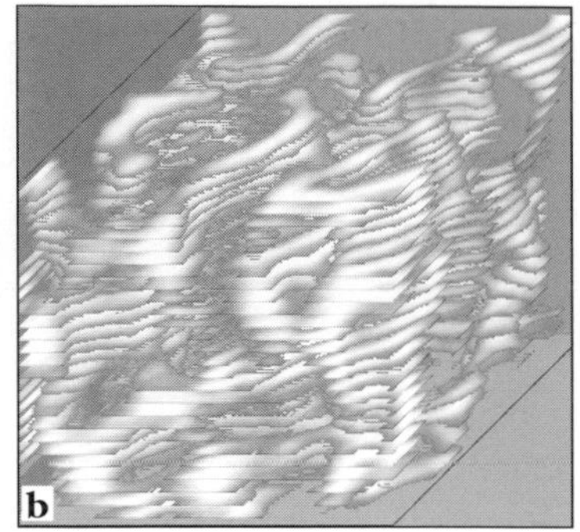

rotation is carried out. **Figure 45** shows a few orientations of the data set using ray tracing to produce a volumetric display; viewed rapidly in sequence, these produce the visual effect of rotation. However, the complexity of this structure and the precedence in which features lie in front and in back of others limits the usefulness of this approach. Isolating the boundary between the two phases allows a rendered surface to be constructed, as shown in **Figure 46.** With the faceting shown, this display can be drawn quickly enough (a few seconds on a desktop computer) to be useful as an analysis tool. A complete smoothed rendering (**Figure 47**) takes much longer (about half an hour on the same computer) or requires access to graphics supercomputers.

Rendering a surface follows the determination of the various surface facets. The simplest kind of facet is a triangle. In the example shown in **Figure 46**, a series of narrow rectangles or trapezoids are used to connect together points along each section outline. For features in which the sections are similar in shape and size, this is fairly straightforward. When the shapes change considerably from section to section, the resulting facets offer a less realistic view of the surface shape.

The greatest difficulty is dealing with splits and merges in the structure. This means that the number of outlines in one section is greater than in the next, so the surface must somehow divide. **Figure 48** shows two ways to address this. In one, the junction actually lies in one of the planes. It may be drawn either by hand or located by various algorithms, such as dividing the feature normal to its moment axis at a point that gives area ratios equal to those of the two features in the next section. The result is fairly easy to draw, since no surface facets intersect.

The second method constructs surface facets from sets of points along the feature boundaries, from the single feature in one section to both of the features in the next section plane. This moves the junction into the space between planes and produces a fairly realistic picture, but it requires more calculation. The intersecting planes must be drawn with a *z*-buffer, a computer graphics technique that records the depth (in the viewing direction) of each

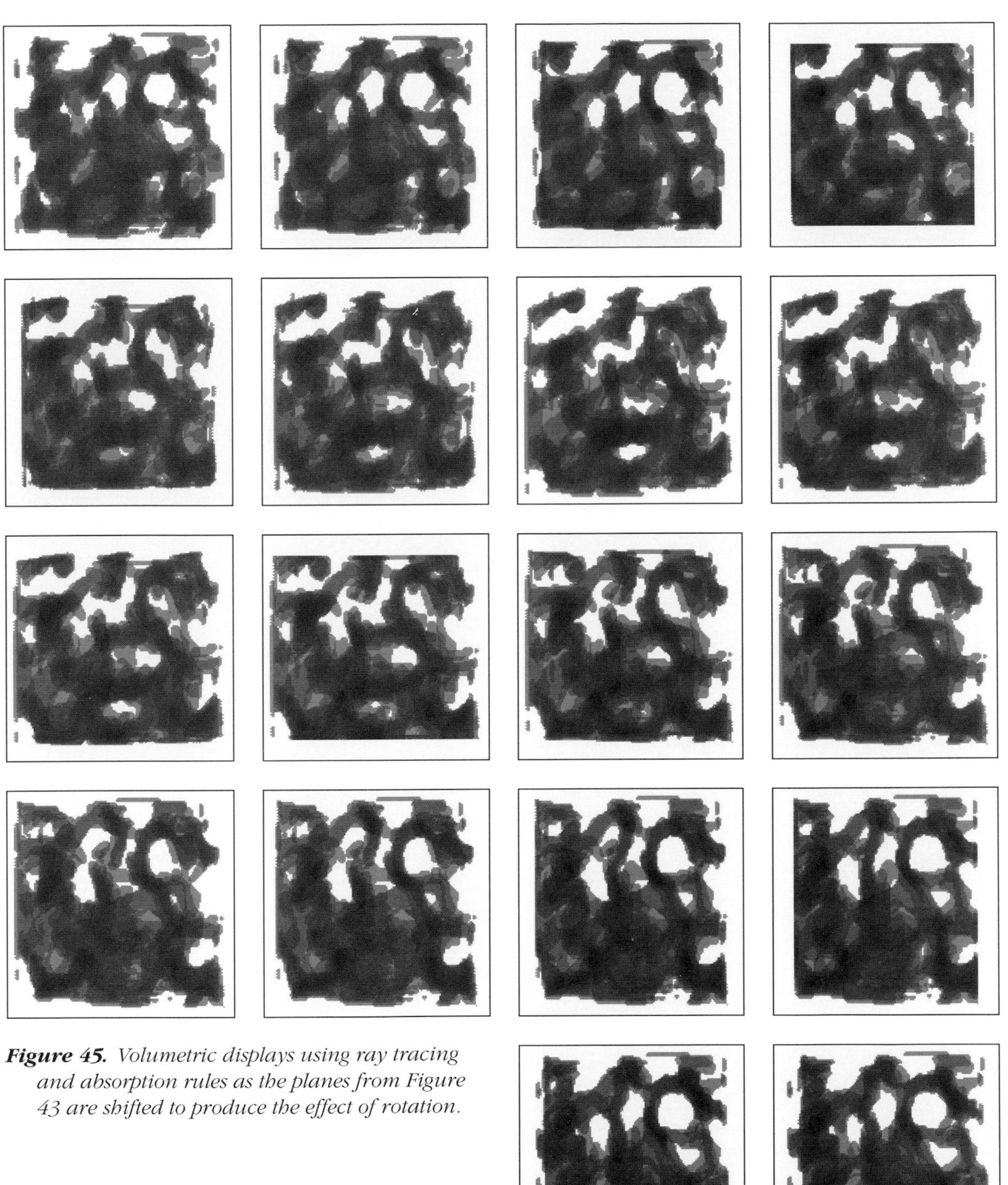

Figure 45. *Volumetric displays using ray tracing and absorption rules as the planes from Figure 43 are shifted to produce the effect of rotation.*

image point and only draws points on one surface where they lie in front of the other.

The major drawback to this kind of surface rendering from serial section outlines is that the surfaces hide what is behind them. Even with rotation, it may not be possible to see all parts of a

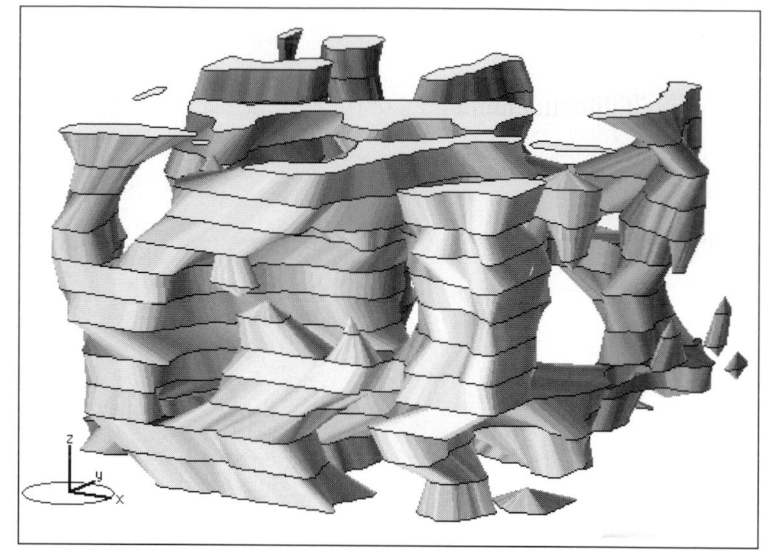

Figure 46. Simple rendering of the boundary surface between the two phases in the specimen from Figure 43, by interpolating planar facets between the planes.

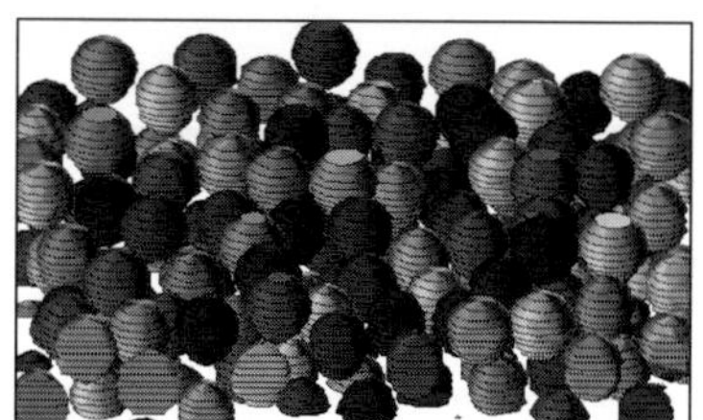

Plate 18. See color plate, page VIII. All color plates appear following page 246.

complex structure. Combining surface rendering with transparency, so that selective features are shown as opaque and others as partially transparent, enabling the hidden structures to become visible, offers a partial solution. **Figure 49** shows an example in which one kind of feature (the spheres) has been given the property to show through any superimposed surface, at a reduced brightness. This allows the spheres to be seen where they lie behind the columns. However, the dimming is not realistic (since the density of the columns is not known) and other structures behind the columns are completely hidden.

In the example shown in **Figure**s **46** and **47,** the boundary was determined by thresholding in each of the 2D image planes, since the plane spacing was not the same as the in-plane resolution. This requires a certain amount of interpolation between the planes, which makes the curvature and roughness of surfaces different in the depth or *z* direction. For data sets with true cubic voxels, for example in the tomographic reconstruction shown in **Figure 15** (and in Chapter 7, Figure 42), the resolution is the same in all directions and greater fidelity can be achieved in the surface rendering. **Plate 18** shows the surface-rendered image from that data set.

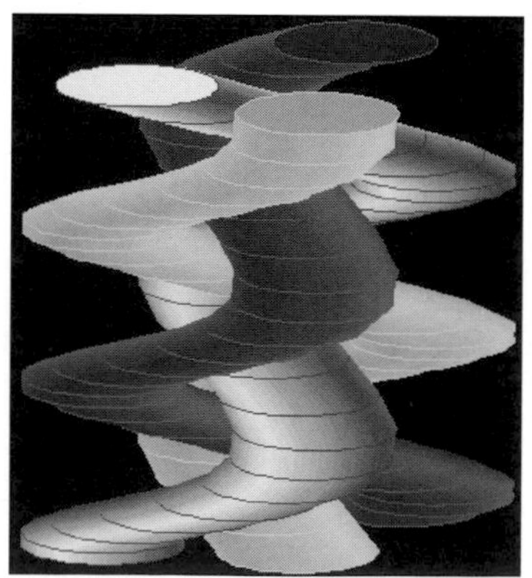

Plate 19. See color plate, page VIII.

Multiple colors are needed to distinguish the many features present (about 200 roughly spherical particles) in this structure. This use of pseudo-color is particularly important to identify the continuity of multiply connected surfaces. **Plate 19** shows another example, in which the structural organization of the braid is much easier to see when each fiber is assigned a unique color palette.

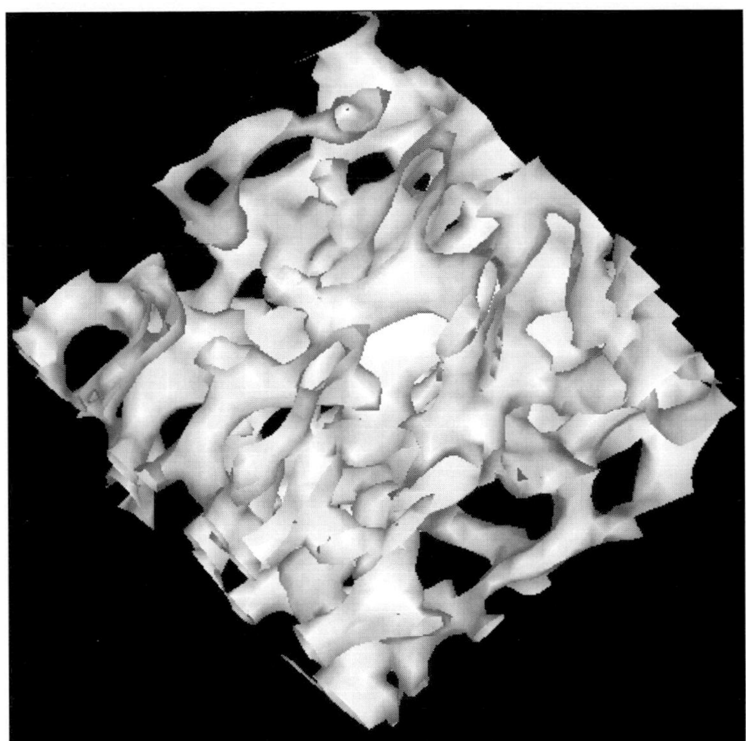

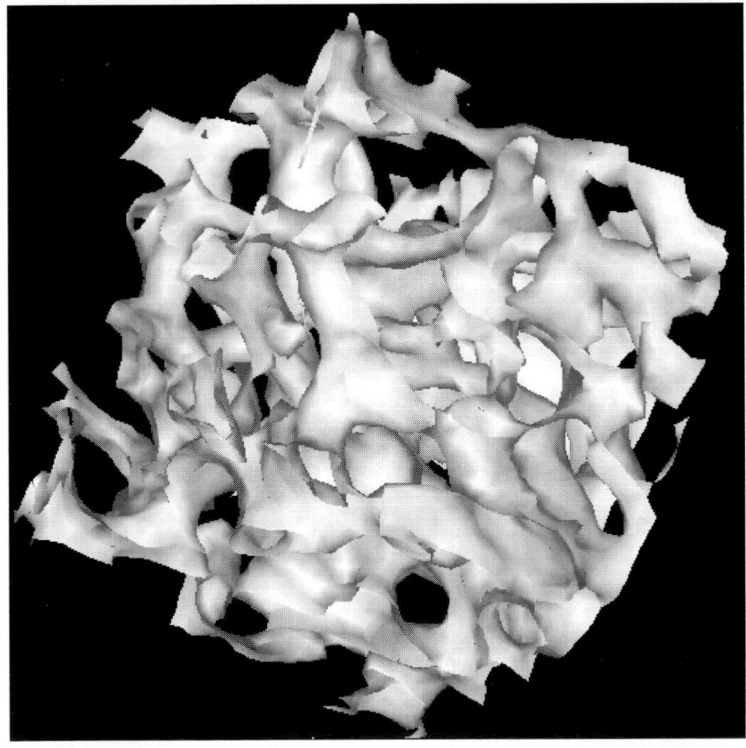

Figure 47. *Two high-resolution rendered views of the boundary surface between the two phases in the specimen from Figures 43 to 46.*

Figure 48. Two ways to render the surface on serial section outlines where splits or merges occur:
a) *dividing one plane into arbitrary regions which correspond to each branch;*
b) *continuous surfaces from each branch to the entire next outline, with intersection between the planes.*

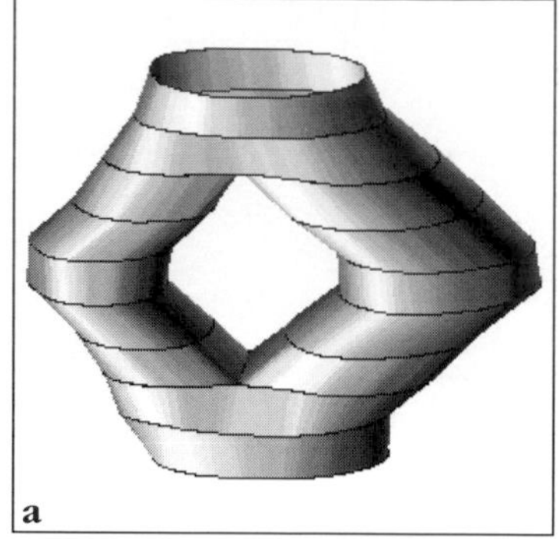

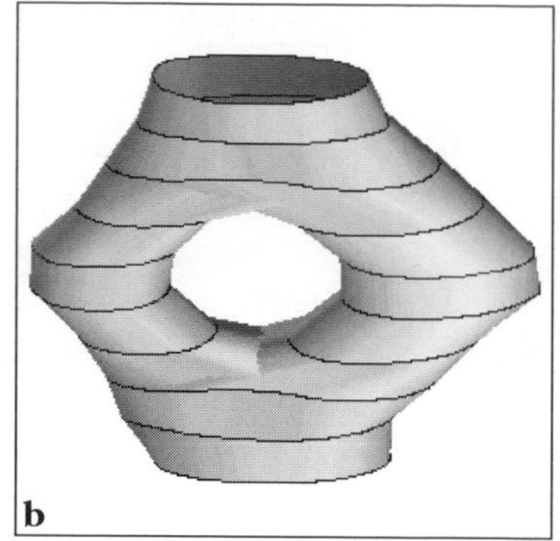

Image processing in 3D

The emphasis so far has been on the display of 3D image data, with little mention of processing. Most of the same processing tools described in the preceding chapters for 2D images can be applied more-or-less directly to 3D images for the same purposes. Arithmetic operations, such as ratios in multiband data, are used in exactly the same way. Each voxel value is divided by the value of the voxel at the same location in the second image. This does not depend on the images having cubic voxels.

However, many processing operations that use neighborhoods, e.g., for kernel multiplication, template matching, rank operations, etc., do require cubic voxel arrays. In a few instances, a kernel may be adapted to non-cubic voxels by adjusting the weight values so that the different distance to the neighbors in the z direction is taken into account. This only works when the difference in z distance as compared to the x, y directions is small (for instance, a factor of 2 or 3 as may be achieved in the CSLM). It will not work well if the image planes are separated by 10 times (or more) the in-plane resolution. Also, any departure

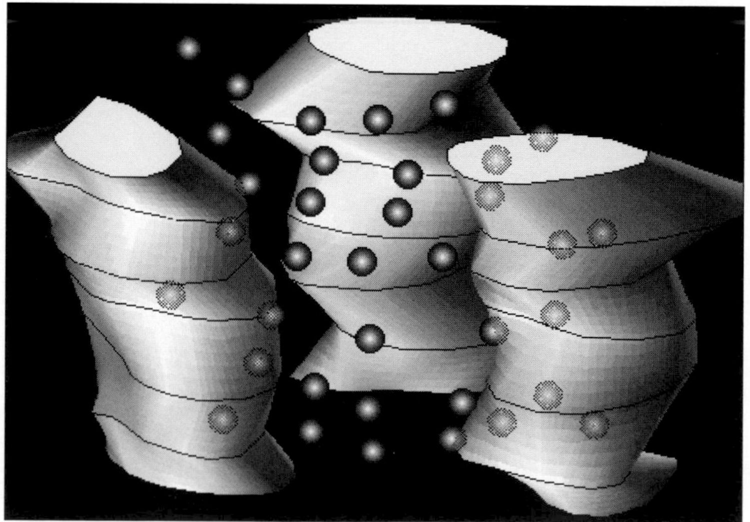

Figure 49. *Combining surface rendering with partial transparency to show structures otherwise hidden by surfaces in front. The spheres which lie behind the frontmost surfaces are dimmed or shown in a different color. Notice that this is only partial transparency in that the front vertical column is completely opaque to the rear one, and the spheres are dimmed uniformly without regard to the actual amount of material in front of them.*

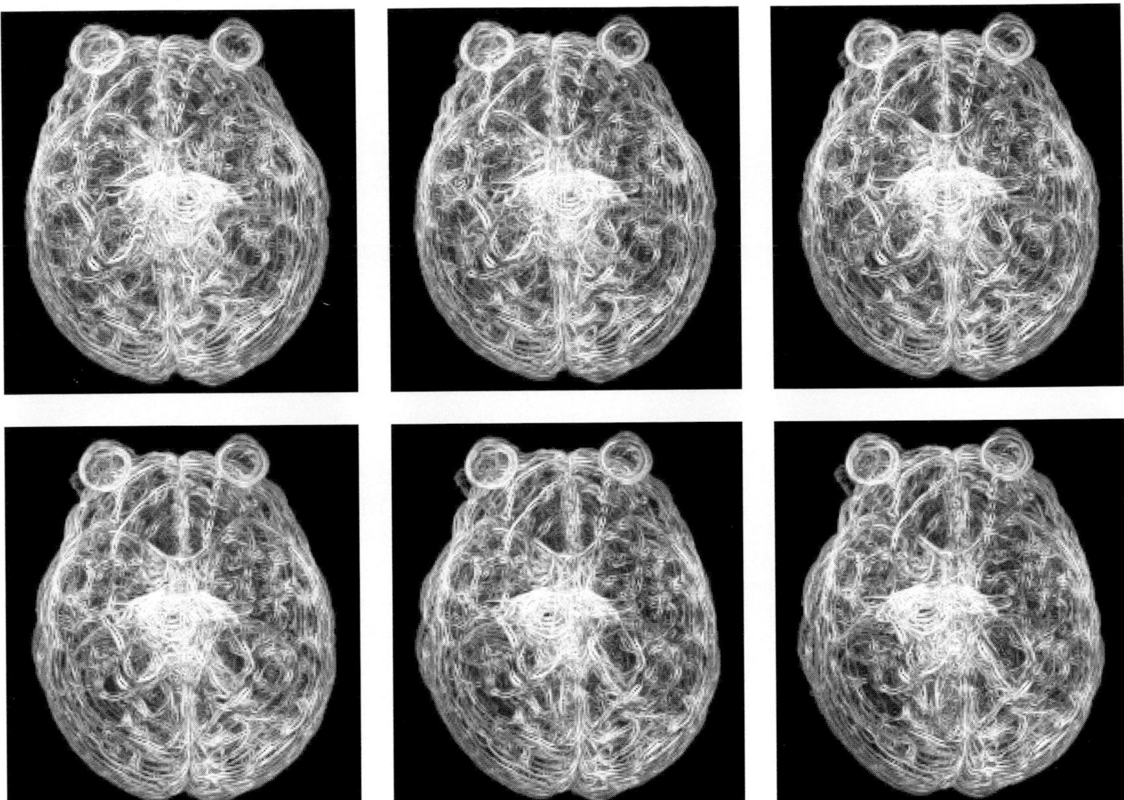

Figure 50. *Several views of the brain from the MRI data set. The skull has been eliminated, individual image planes have been processed with an edge operator, and the resulting values have been used with emission rules to create a volumetric display. Lateral shifting of the planes produces pseudo-rotation. Each pair of images can be viewed in stereo, or the entire sequence used as an animation. Structures are visible from the folds in the top of the brain to the spinal column at the bottom.*

from cubic voxel shape causes serious problems for ranking or template matching operations.

In these cases, it is more common to perform the processing on the individual planes and then form a new 3D image set from the results. **Figure 50** shows a series of pseudo-rotation views of the MRI head images used above. Each slice image has been processed using a Frei and Chen operator to extract edges. This shows the internal structure, as well as the surface wrinkles in the brain. Furthermore, image processing was used to form a mask to delineate the brain (defined as the central bright feature in each slice) and isolate it from other portions of the image. The result is a series of slice images showing only the brain, processed to show the internal edges.

Another display trick has been used here. It is not clear just what volumetric display mode is appropriate for such processed images. Instead of the conventional absorption mode in which transmitted light is passed through the data array, these images use the emission mode, in which each voxel emits light in proportion to its value. Here, that value is the edgeness of the voxel as defined by the Frei and Chen operator. In other words, we see the edges glowing in space. In a live animation, or for those readers who can use image pairs to view the 3D data set stereoscopically, this image creates a fairly strong impression of the 3D structure of the brain. The same type of display of lines in space can be used to display contours within a 3D data set.

This illustration may serve as an indication of the flexibility with which display rules for 3D images can be bent. Non-traditional display modes, particularly for processed images, are often quite effective for showing structural relationships. There are no guidelines here, except the need to simplify the image by eliminating extraneous detail to reveal the structure that is important; an experimental approach is encouraged.

Processing 2D image planes in a 3D data set should be used with some care. It is only justified if the planes have no preferred orientation and are random with respect to the structure or, conversely, if the planes have a very definite but known orientation that matches that of the structure. The latter situation applies to some situations involving coatings. When possible, 3D processing is preferred, even though it imposes a rather significant computing load. The size of neighborhoods increases with the cube of dimension. A kernel of modest size, say 7×7, may be fast enough for practical use in 2D, requiring 49 multiplications and additions for every pixel. In 3D, the same $7 \times 7 \times 7$ kernel requires 343 multiplications and additions per voxel and of course the number of total voxels has also increased dramatically, so processing takes much more time.

For complex neighborhood operations, such as gradient or edge finding in which more than one kernel is used, the problem is further increased because the number of kernels must increase to deal with the higher dimensionality of the data. For instance, the 3D version of the Sobel gradient operator would use the square root of the sum of squares of derivatives in three directions. Since it takes two angles to define a direction in three dimensions, an image of gradient orientation would require two arrays and it is not clear how it would be used.

The Frei and Chen operator (Frei & Chen, 1977), a very useful edge detector in 2D images, can be extended to three dimensions by adding to the size and number of the basis functions. For instance, the first basis function (which measures the gradient in one direction and corresponds to the presence of a boundary) becomes

$$\begin{array}{ccccccccc}
-\sqrt{3}/3 & -\sqrt{2}/2 & -\sqrt{3}/3 & & & & & & \\
-\sqrt{2}/2 & -1 & -\sqrt{2}/2 & 0 & 0 & 0 & & & \\
-\sqrt{3}/3 & -\sqrt{2}/2 & -\sqrt{3}/3 & 0 & 0 & 0 & +\sqrt{3}/3 & +\sqrt{2}/2 & +\sqrt{3}/3 \\
 & & & 0 & 0 & 0 & +\sqrt{2}/2 & +1 & +\sqrt{2}/2 \\
 & & & & & & +\sqrt{3}/3 & +\sqrt{2}/2 & +\sqrt{3}/3
\end{array}$$

It should be noted that in three dimensions, it is possible to construct a set of basis functions to search for lines, as well as surfaces. It remains to find good ways to display the boundaries that these operators find.

3D processing can be used in many ways to enhance the visibility of structures. In **Figure 33,** the boron concentration was shown volumetrically, using emission rules. However, the overlap between front and rear portions of the structure makes it difficult to see all of the details. The surface rendering in **Figure 34** is even worse in this regard. **Figure 51** shows the same structures after 3D processing. Each voxel in the new image has a value proportional to the variance of voxels in a 3×3×3 neighborhood in the original image set. These values are displayed volumetrically as a transmission image. In other words, the absorption of light coming through the 3D array is a measure of the presence of edges; uniform regions appear transparent. The visibility of internal surfaces in this "cellophane" display is much better than in the original and the surfaces do not obscure information behind them, as they would with rendering.

The time requirements for neighborhood operations are even worse for ranking operations. The time required to rank a list of values in order increases not in proportion to the number of entries, as in the kernel multiplication case, but as $N \cdot \log(N)$. This assumes a maximally efficient sorting algorithm and means that ranking operations in very large neighborhoods take quite a long time.

For template-matching operations, such as those used in implementing erosion, dilation, skeletonization, etc., the situation is even worse. The very efficient methods possible in 2D using a LUT or fate table based on the pattern of neighbors will no longer work. In 2D, there are 8 neighbors, so a table with 2^8 or 256 entries can cover all possibilities. In 3D, there are 26 adjacent neighbors and 2^{26} or 67 million entries. Consequently, either fewer neighboring voxels must be considered in determining the result or a different algorithm must be used.

Skeletonization in 3D analogous to that in 2D would remove voxels from a binary image if they touched a background or OFF voxel, unless the touching ON voxels did not all touch each other (Halford & Preston, 1984; Lobregt et al., 1980). If touching is considered to include the corner-to-corner diagonal neighbors as well as edge-to-edge and face-to-face touching, then a minimum skeleton can be constructed. However, if a table for the 26 possible touching neighbors cannot be used, then it is necessary to actually count the touching voxels for each neighbor, which is much slower.

It should be noted that skeletonization in 3D is entirely different than performing a series of skeletonizations in the 2D image planes and combining or connecting them. In 3D, the skeleton

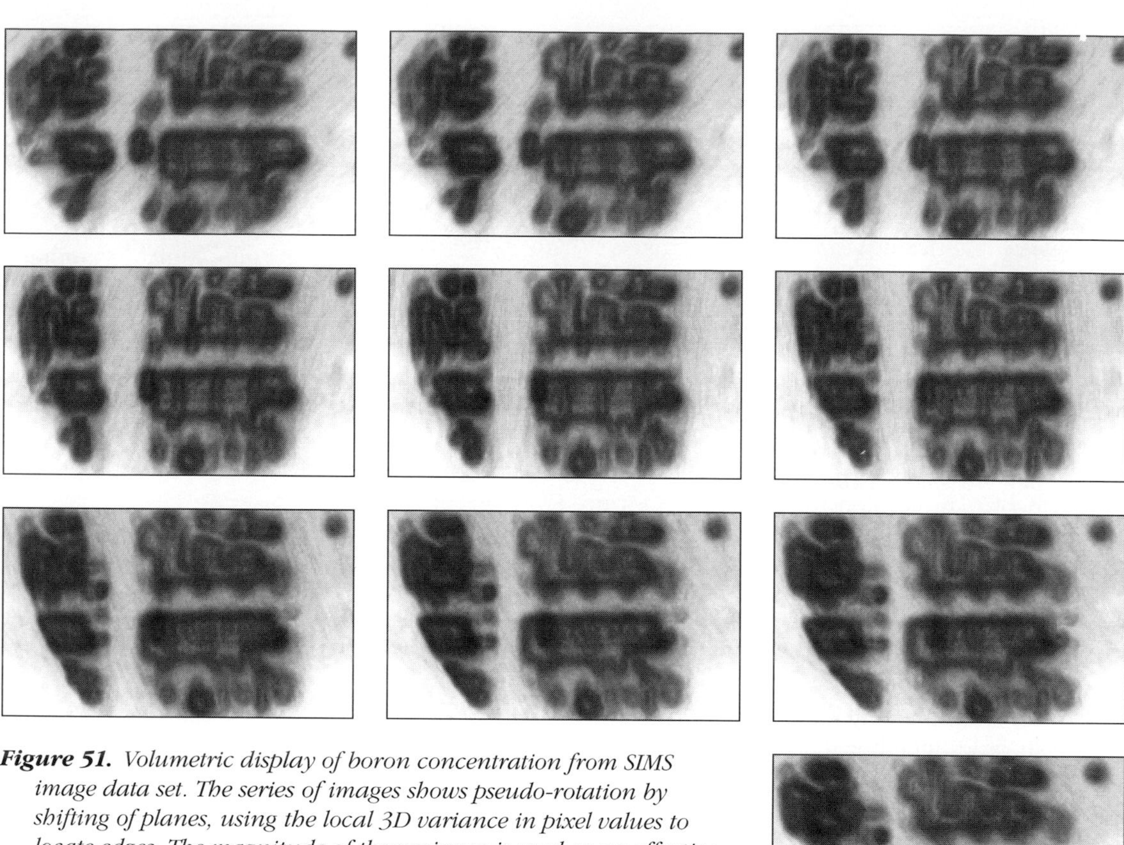

Figure 51. *Volumetric display of boron concentration from SIMS image data set. The series of images shows pseudo-rotation by shifting of planes, using the local 3D variance in pixel values to locate edges. The magnitude of the variance is used as an effective density value to absorb light along rays through the voxel array.*

becomes a series of linear links and branches that correctly depicts the topology of the structure. If the operation is performed in 2D image planes, the skeletons in each plane form a series of sheetlike surfaces that twist through the 3D object and have a different topological relationship to the structure. This is shown schematically in **Figure 52.** The skeleton of linear links and branches in 3D has been formed by connecting the UEPs in each section (see Chapter 6).

Measurements on 3D images

Although the principal thrust of this book is toward image processing rather than measurement, it is clear that one of the reasons for collecting and processing images is to obtain quantitative data from them. This is true for 3D as well as 2D imaging; consequently, some brief comments about the kinds of measurements that can be performed, their practicality, and the accuracy of the results seem appropriate.

Measurements are broadly classified into two categories: feature-specific and global, or scene-based. The best-known global mea-

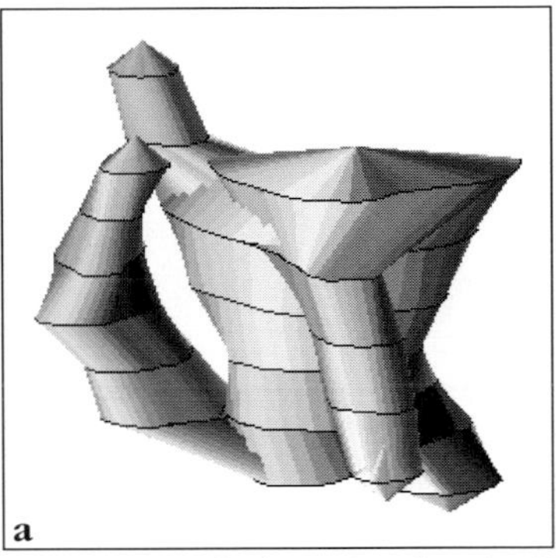

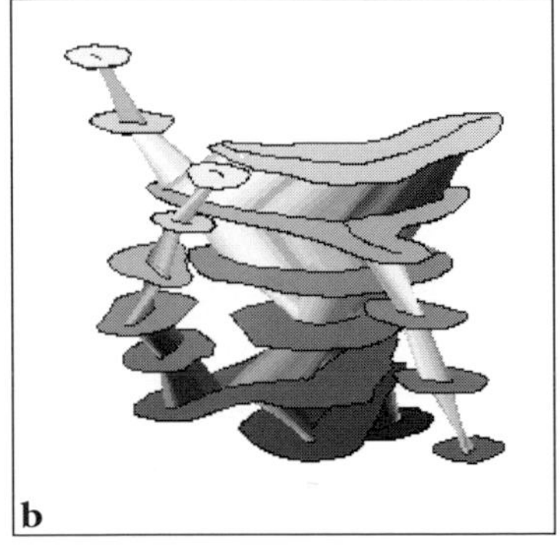

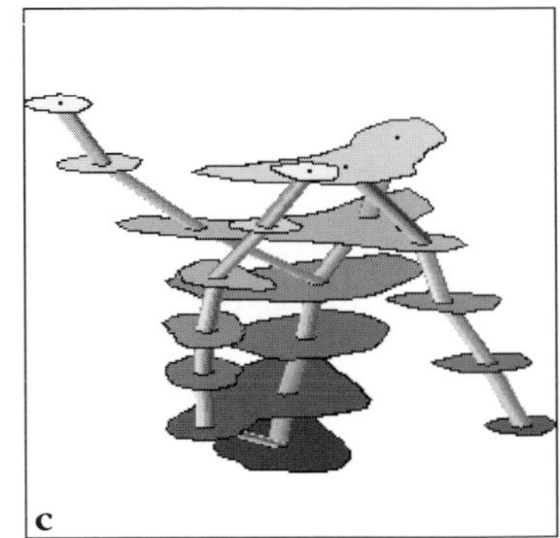

Figure 52. Skeletonization in 3D:
a) *an irregularly shaped solid object represented by planar sections;*
b) *connecting the 2D skeletons of the individual planar intersections;*
c) *3D skeleton formed by connecting the ultimate eroded points of the 2D sections.*

surement is the volume fraction of a selected phase or region. Assuming that the phase can be selected by thresholding, perhaps with processing (as discussed in Chapter 3), then the volume fraction is determined simply by counting the voxels in the phase and dividing by the total number of voxels in the array or in some other separately defined reference volume. The result is independent of whether the voxels are cubic. In fact, the same result can be obtained by counting pixels on image planes and does not depend in any way on the arrangement of the planes into a 3D array.

A second global parameter is the surface area per unit volume of a selected boundary. There are stereological rules for determining this value from measurements on 2D images. One method counts the number of crossings that random lines (for a random structure, the scan lines can be used) make with the boundary. Another method measures the length of the boundary in the 2D image. Each of these values can be used to calculate the 3D surface area.

It might seem that directly measuring the area in the 3D data set would be a superior method without assumptions. In practice, it is not clear whether this is so. First, the resolution of the boundary, particularly if it is irregular and rough, depends critically on the size of pixels or voxels. The practical limitation on the number of voxels that can be dealt with in 3D arrays may force the individual voxels to be larger than desired. It was pointed out before that a 512×512 image in 2D requires 1/4 Meg of storage, while the same storage space can hold only a 64×64×64 3D array.

Using smaller pixels to better define the boundary is not the only advantage of performing measurements in 2D. The summation of boundary area in a 3D array must add up the areas of triangles defined by each set of 3 voxels along the boundary. A table can be constructed giving the area of the triangle in terms of the po-

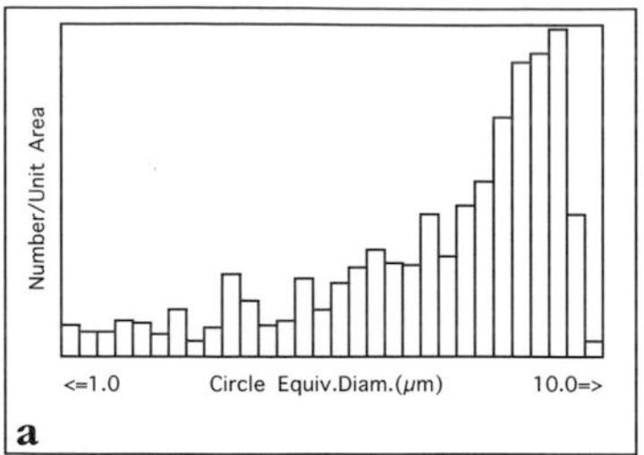

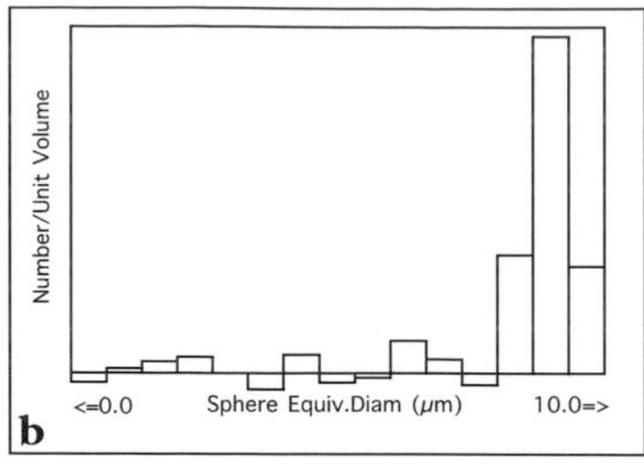

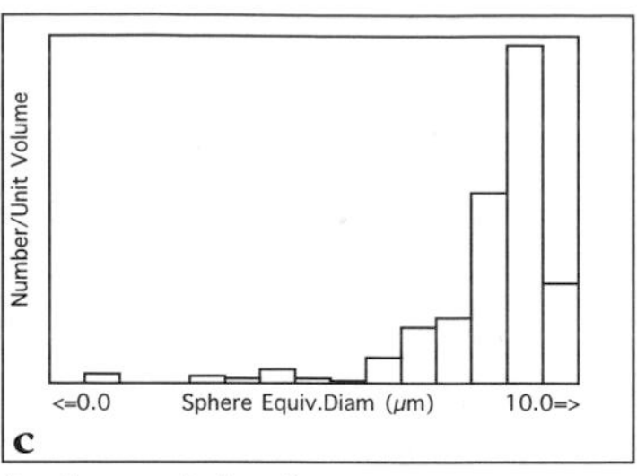

Figure 53. Comparison of 2D and 3D measurement of size of spherical particles in structure shown in Figure 21:

a) *size distribution of circles in 2D plane sections;*

b) *estimated size distribution of spheres by unfolding the circle data in figure a (note negative values);*

c) *directly measured size distribution of spheres from 3D voxel array.*

sition differences of the voxels, but the summation process must be assured of finding all parts of the boundary. There is no unique path that can be followed along a convoluted or multiply connected surface to guarantee finding all of the parts.

For other global properties, such as the length of linear features or the curvature of boundaries, similar considerations apply. The power of unbiased 2D stereological tools for measuring global parameters is such that their efficiency and precision of measurement makes them preferred in most cases.

Feature-specific measurements include measures of size, shape, position, and density. Examples of size measures are volume, surface area, length (maximum dimension), and so forth. In three dimensions, these parameters can be determined by direct counting. The same difficulties for following a boundary in 3D mentioned above still apply. In 2D images, feature measurements must be converted to 3D sizes using relationships from geometric probability. These calculations are based on shape assumptions and are mathematically ill-conditioned. This means that a small error in measurement or assumption is magnified in the calculated size distribution.

Simple shapes, such as spheres, provide good results. **Figure 53** shows the result for the tomographic image of spherical particles shown in **Figure 21.** The measurement on 2D plane slices gives circle areas that must be unfolded to get a distribution of spheres. The result shows some small errors in the distribution, including physically impossible negative counts for some sizes. However, the total number and mean size are in good agreement with the results obtained from direct 3D measurement.

When feature shapes are more complicated or variable, 2D methods simply do not work. If information on the distribution of shapes and sizes is needed, then measurement in 3D, even with the problem of limited resolution, is the only course to follow.

The position of features in 3D is not difficult to determine. Counting pixels and summing moments in three directions provides the location of the centroid and the orientation of the moment axes. Likewise, feature density can be calculated through straightforward summation. These properties can be determined accurately even if the voxels are not square; they are affected only slightly by a reduction in voxel resolution.

Shape is a difficult concept, even in two dimensions. The most common shape parameters are formally dimensionless ratios of size, such as $(\text{volume})^{1/3}/(\text{surface area})^{1/2}$ or length/breadth. Selecting a parameter that has meaning in any particular situation is very ad hoc, based either on the researcher's intuition or on trial and error and regression. In 3D, the values may be less precise because of the poorer voxel resolution, but the accuracy may be better because the size parameters used are less biased. It may be important to the user's intuition to consider 3D shape factors, which are less unfamiliar than 2D ones.

Other approaches to shape in 2D are harmonic analysis, which unrolls feature boundaries and performs a Fourier analysis on the resulting plot, and fractal dimension determination, which was discussed in Chapter 6. Both of these parameters can be determined rather efficiently in two dimensions, but only with great difficulty in three dimensions. Since the 2D results are related stereologically to 3D structure, it is preferable to perform these measurements on the individual 2D image planes.

Closely related to shape is the idea of topology, a non-metric description of the basic geometrical properties of the object or structure. Topological properties include the numbers of loops, nodes, and branches (Aigeltinger et al., 1972). The connectivity per unit volume of a network structure is a topological property directly related to such physical properties as permeability. It is not possible to determine topological properties of 3D structures from 2D images, so these must be measured directly on the 3D data set, perhaps after skeletonization to simplify the structure (Russ & Russ, 1989b).

Conclusion

There is little doubt that 3D imaging will continue to increase in capability and popularity. It offers direct visualization and measurement of complex structures and 3D relationships, which cannot be as satisfactorily studied using 2D imaging. Most of the kinds of imaging modalities that produce 3D images, especially tomographic reconstruction, are well understood, although the hardware will benefit from further development. So will the computers and software. Current display methods are barely adequate for the task of communicating the richness of 3D image data sets to the user. New display algorithms and interface control devices will surely emerge, driven not only by the field of image processing but also by related fields, such as the visualization of super-computer data. The continued increase in computer power and memory is certain. Watching and using these developments offers an exciting prospect for the future.

References

E. H. Aigeltinger, K. R. Craig, R. T. DeHoff (1972) Experimental determination of the topological properties of three dimensional microstructures *J. Microscopy* 95:69-81

N. Baba, M. Naka, Y. Muranaka, S. Nakamura, I. Kino, K. Kanaya (1984) Computer-aided stereographic representation of an object reconstructed from micrographs of serial thin sections *Micron and Microscopica Acta* 15:221-226

N. Baba, M. Baba, M. Imamura, M. Koga, Y. Ohsumi, M. Osumi, K. Kanaya (1989) Serial section reconstruction using a computer graphics system: Application to intracellular structures in yeast cells and to the periodontal structure of dogs' teeth *J. Electron Microscopy Technique* 11:16-26

D. H. Ballard, C. M. Brown (1982) *Computer Vision,* Prentice-Hall, Englewood Cliffs, NJ

F. L. Barnes, S. G. Azavedo, H. E. Martz, G. P. Roberson, D. J. Schneberk, M. F. Skeate (1990) *Geometric Effects in Tomographic Reconstruction* Lawrence Livermore National Laboratory Rep. UCRL-ID-105130

V. Berzins (1984) Accuracy of Laplacian edge detectors *Comput. Vis. Graph. Image Proc.* 27:1955-2010

S. Beucher, C. Lantejoul (1979) *Use of Watersheds in Contour Detection* Proc. Int. Workshop on Image Proc., CCETT, Rennes, France

R. A. S. Blackie, R. Bagby, L. Wright, J. Drinkwater, S. Hart (1987) Reconstruction of three dimensional images of microscopic objects using holography *Proc. Royal Microscopical Society* 22:98

A. Boyde (1973) Quantitative photogrammetric analysis and quantitative stereoscopic analysis of SEM images *J. Microscopy* 98:452

R. N. Bracewell (1984) The fast Hartley transform *Proc. IEEE* 72:8

R. N. Bracewell (1986) *The Hartley Transform* Oxford Univ. Press

R. N. Bracewell (June 1989) The Fourier transform *Scientific American*

L. G. Briarty, P. H. Jenkins (1984) GRIDSS: an integrated suite of microcomputer programs for three-dimensional graphical reconstruction from serial sections *J. Microscopy* 134:121-124

D. S. Bright, E. B. Steel (1986) Bright-field image correction with various image-processing tools, in *Microbeam Analysis 1986* (A.D. Romig, Jr., W.F. Chambers, eds.), San Francisco Press, p. 517-520.

R. K. Bryan, J. Skilling (1980) Deconvolution by maximum entropy, as illustrated by application to the jet of M87 *Mon. Not. R. Ast. Soc.* 191:69-79

I. C. Carlsen (1985) Reconstruction of true surface topographies in scanning electron microscopes using backscattered electrons *Scanning* 7:169-177

K. R. Castleman (1979) *Digital Image Processing* Prentice-Hall, Englewood Cliffs, NJ

R. L. T. Cederberg (1979) Chain-link coding and segmentation for raster scan devices *Comput. Graph. Image Proc.* 10:224-234

Y. Censor (1983) Finite series expansion reconstruction methods *Proc. IEEE* 71:409-419

Y. Censor (1984) Row-action methods for huge and sparse systems and their applications *SIAM Review* 23#4:444-466

J. W. Cooley, J. W. Tukey (1965) An algorithm for the machine calculation of complex Fourier series *Mathematics of Computation*

A. M. Cormack (1963) Representation of a function by its line integrals with some radiological applications *J. Appl. Phys.* 34:2722-2727

A. M. Cormack (1964) Representation of a function by its line integrals with some radiological applications II *J. Appl. Phys.* 35:2908-2913

T. N. Cornsweet (1970) *Visual Perception* Academic Press, New York, NY

M. Coster, J-L. Chermant (1985) *Précis D'Analse D'Images* Éditions du Centre National de la Recherche Scientifique, Paris

P. E. Danielsson (1980) Euclidean distance mapping *Comput. Graph. Image Proc.* 14:227-248

E. R. Davies (1988) On the noise suppression and image enhancement characteristics of the median, truncated median and mode filters *Pattern Recognition Letters* 7:87-97

H. W. Deckman, K. L. D'Amico, J. H. Dunsmuir, B. P. Flannery, S. M. Gruner (1989) *Advances in X-ray Analysis* 32:641

T. R. Edwards (1982) Two-dimensional convolute integers for analytical instrumentation *Anal. Chem.* 54:1519-1524

R. Ehrlich, S. K. Kennedy, S. J. Crabtree, R. L. Cannon (1984) Petrographic image analysis: 1. Analysis of reservoir pore complexes *J. Sed. Petrol.* 54:1365-1378

A. Engel, A. Massalski (1984) 3D reconstruction from electron micrographs: Its potential and practical limitations *Ultramicroscopy* 13:71-84

Y. Fahmy, J. C. Russ, C. Koch (1991) Application of fractal geometry measurements to the evaluation of fracture toughness of brittle intermetallics *J. Mater. Res.* 6:1856-1861

J. Feder (1988) *Fractals* Plenum Press, New York, NY

A. G. Flook (1978) Use of dilation logic on the Quantimet to achieve fractal dimension characterization of texture and structured profiles *Powder Techn.* 21:295-298

J. D. Foley, A. Van Dam (1984) *Fundamentals of Interactive Computer Graphics* Addison Wesley, Reading, MA

H. Freeman (1961) On the encoding of arbitrary geometric configurations *IEEE Trans.* EC-10:260-268

H. Freeman (1974) Computer processing of line-drawing images *Computl. Surveys* 6:57-97

W. Frei, C. C. Chen (1977) Fast boundary detection: A generalization and a new algorithm *IEEE Trans. Comput.* C-26:988-998

B. R. Frieden (1988) A comparison of maximum entropy, maximum *a postiori* and median window restoration algorithms, in *Scanning Microscopy* Suppl. 2 (P. Hawkes, et al., eds.), Scanning Microscopy International, Chicago, p. 107-111

J. P. Frisby (1980) *Vision: Illusion, Brain and Mind* Oxford Univ. Press, Oxford, U.K.

K. S. Fu, J. K. Mui (1981) A survey on image segmentation *Pattern Recognition* 13:3-16

H. Fuchs, S. M. Pizer, L. C. Tsai, S. H. Bloomburg, E. R. Heinz (1982) Adding a true 3-D display to a raster graphics system *IEEE Comput. Graphics Applic.* 2:73-78

K. Fukunaga (1990) *Statistical Pattern Recognition* 2nd Edition, Academic Press, Boston

P. Gaultier, P. Coltelli (1991) A real-time automated system for the analysis of moving images *J. Comput. Assist. Microsc.* 3#1:15-22.

R. C. Gonzalez, P. Wintz (1987) *Digital Image Processing* 2nd Edition, Addison Wesley, Reading, MA

R. Gordon (1974) A tutorial on ART (Algebraic Reconstruction Techniques) *IEEE Trans.* NS-21:78-93

K. J. Halford, K. Preston (1984) 3-D skeletonization of elongated solids *Comput. Vis. Graph. Image Proc.* 27:78-91

R. M. Haralick (1978) *Statistical and structural approaches to texture* Proc. 4th Int. Joint Conf. Patt. Recog., Kyoto, p. 45

R. M. Haralick, I. Dinstein (1975) A spatial clustering procedure for multi-image data *Comput. Graph. Image Proc.* 12:60-73

R. M. Haralick, L. G. Shapiro (1988) Segmentation and its place in machine vision *Scanning Microscopy Supplement* 2:39-54

R. M. Haralick, K. Shanmugam, I. Dinstein (1973) Textural features for image classification *IEEE Trans.* SMC-3:610-621

R. V. L. Hartley (1942) A more symmetrical Fourier analysis applied to transmission problems *Proc. IRE*

D. Hearn, M. P. Baker (1986) *Computer Graphics* Prentice-Hall, Englewood Cliffs, NJ

R. Hegerl (1989) Three-dimensional reconstruction from projections in electron microscopy *European J. Cell Biology* 48 (Supplement 25):135-138

G. T. Herman (1980) *Image Reconstruction from Projections–The Fundamentals of Computerized Tomography* Academic Press, New York

E. C. Hildreth (1983) The detection of intensity changes by computer and biological vision systems *Comput. Vis. Graph. Image Proc.* 22:1-27

B. K. P. Horn (1970) *Shape from shading: A method for obtaining the shape of a smooth opaque object from one view* (AI Tech. Report 79, Project MAC) Mass. Inst. Tech., Cambridge, MA

T. S. Huang (1979) A fast two dimensional median filtering algorithm *IEEE Trans.* ASSP-27:13-18

D. H. Hubel (1988) *Eye, Brain, and Vision* Scientific American Library, W. H. Freeman, New York, NY

H. E. Hurst, R. P. Black, Y. M. Simaika (1965) *Long Term Storage: An Experimental Study* Constable, London

S. Inoue (1986) *Video Microscopy* Plenum Press, New York

A. K. Jain (1989) *Fundamentals of Digital Image Processing* Prentice Hall, London

E. T. Jaynes (1985) Where do we go from here?, in *Maximum Entropy and Bayesian Methods in Inverse Problems* (C. R. Smith, W. T. Grandy, eds.), D. Reidel Publishing Co., Dordrecht, Holland, p. 21-58

J. P. Jernot (1982) Thése de Doctorat és Science, Université de Caen, France

E. M. Johnson, J. J. Capowski (1985) Principles of reconstruction and three-dimensional display of serial sections using a computer, in *The Microcomputer in Cell and Neurobiology Research* (R. R. Mize, ed.), Elsevier, New York, p. 249-263

L. R. Johnson, A. K. Jain (1981) An efficient two-dimensional FFT algorithm *IEEE Trans.* PAMI-3:698-701

Q. C. Johnson, J. H. Kinney, U. Bonse, M. C. Nichols, R. Nusshardt, J. M. Brase (1986) *Micro-Tomography Using Synchrotron Radiation* Lawrence Livermore National Laboratory Preprint UCRL-93538

A. C. Kak, M. Slaney (1988) *Principles of Computerized Tomographic Imaging* IEEE Pub. PC-02071

J. N. Kanpur, P. K. Sahoo, A. K. C. Wong (1985) A new method for grey-level picture thresholding using the entropy of the histogram *Comput. Vis. Graph. Image Proc.* 29:273-285

A. E. Kayaalp, R. C. Jain (1987) Using SEM stereo to extract semiconductor wafer pattern topography *Proc. SPIE* 775:18-26

B. H. Kaye (1986) *Image analysis procedures for characterizing the fractal dimension of fine particles* Proc. Particle Technol. Conf., Nürnberg

J. H. Kinney, Q. C. Johnson, M. C. Nichols, U. Bonse, R. A. Saroyan, R. Nusshardt, R. Pahl (1989) X-ray microtomography on beamline X at SSRL *Rev. Sci. Instrum.* 60(7):2471-4

J. H. Kinney, M. C. Nichols, U. Bonse, S. R. Stock, T. M. Breunig, A. Guvenilir, R. A. Saroyan (1990) *Nondestructive imaging of materials microstructures using X-ray tomographic microscopy* Proc. MRS Symposium on Tomographic Imaging, Boston, MA

R. Kirsch (1971) Computer determination of the constituent structure of biological images *Comput. Biomed. Res.* 4:315-328

C. Lantejoul, S. Beucher (1981) On the use of the geodesic metric in image analysis *J. Microscopy* 121:39

S. Lobregt, P. W. Verbeek, F. C. A. Groen (1980) Three-dimensional skeletonization: principle and algorithm *IEEE Trans.* PAMI-2:75-77

E. Mach (1906) Über den Einfluss räumlich und zeitlich variierender Lichtreize auf die Gesichtswarhrnehmung *S.-B. Akad. Wiss. Wien, Math.-Nat. Kl.* 115:633-648

B. B. Mandelbrot (1982) *The Fractal Geometry of Nature* W. H. Freeman, San Francisco

B. B. Mandelbrot, D. E. Passoja, A. J. Paullay (1984) Fractal character of fracture surfaces of metals *Nature* 308:721

D. Marr (1982) *Vision* W. H. Freeman, San Francisco

D. Marr, E. Hildreth (1980) Theory of edge detection *Proc. R. Soc. Lond.* B207:187-217

D. Marr, T. Poggio (1976) Cooperative computation of stereo disparity *Science* 194:283-287

G. A. Mastin (1985) Adaptive filters for digital image noise smoothing: An evaluation *Comput. Vis. Graph. Image Proc.* 31:102-121

J. J. Mecholsky, D. E. Passoja (1985) Fractals and brittle fracture, in *Fractal Aspects of Materials* Materials Research Society, Pittsburgh, PA

J. J. Mecholsky, T. J. Mackin, D. E. Passoja (1986) Crack propagation in brittle materials as a fractal process, in *Fractal Aspects of Materials II,* Materials Research Society, Pittsburgh, PA

J. J. Mecholsky, D. E. Passoja, K. S. Feinberg-Ringel (1989) Quantitative analysis of brittle fracture surfaces using fractal geometry *J. Am. Ceram. Soc.* 72:60

G. Medioni, R. Nevatia (1985) Segment-based stereo matching *Comput. Vis. Graph. Image Proc.* 31:2-18

D. L. Milgram (1975) Computer methods for creating photomosaics *IEEE Trans.* C-24:1113-1119

D. L. Milgram, M. Herman (1979) Clustering edge values for threshold selection *Comput. Graph. Image Proc.* 10:272-280

M. W. Mitchell, D. A. Bonnell (1990) Quantitative topographic analysis of fractal surfaces by scanning tunneling microscopy *J. Mater. Res.* 5#10:2244-2254

H. P. Moravec (1977) *Towards automatic visual obstacle avoidance* Proc. 5th IJCAI, p. 584

J. C. Mott-Smith (1970) Medial axis transformations, in *Picture Processing and Psychopictorics* (B. S. Lipkin, A. Rosenfeld, eds.), Academic Press, New York

K. S. Nathan, J. C. Curlander (1990) Reducing speckle in one-look SAR images, NASA Tech. Briefs, Feb. 1990, p. 70

A. Nieminen, P. Heinonen, Y. Nuevo (1987) A new class of detail-preserving filters for image processing *IEEE Trans. Patt. Anal. Mach. Intell.* PAMI-9:74-90

J. F. O'Callaghan (1974) Computing the perceptual boundaries of dot patterns *Comput. Graph. Image Proc.* 3(2):141-162

D. P. Panda, A. Rosenfeld (1978) Image segmentation by pixel classification in (gray level, edge value) space *IEEE Trans. Comput.* 27:875-879

T. Pavlidis (1980) A thinning algorithm for discrete binary images *Comput. Graph. Image Proc.* 13:142-157

L. D. Peachey, J. P. Heath (1989) Reconstruction from stereo and multiple electron microscopy images of thick sections of embedded biological specimens using computer graphics methods *J. Microscopy* 153:193-204

S. Peleg, J. Naor, R. Hartley, D. Avnir (1984) Multiple resolution texture analysis and classification *IEEE Trans. Patt. Anal. Mach. Intell.* PAMI-6:518

A. P. Pentland (1983) Fractal-based description of natural scenes *IEEE Trans.* PAMI-6:661

A. P. Pentland, ed. (1986) *From Pixels to Predicates* Ablex, Norwood, NJ

W. K. Pratt (1991) *Digital Image Processing* 2nd Edition, Wiley, New York

T. Prettyman, R. Gardner, J. Russ, K. Verghese (1991) On the performance of a combined transmission and scattering approach to industrial computed tomography, in *Advances in X-ray Analysis* vol 35, Plenum Press, New York, NY

J. M. S. Prewitt, M. L. Mendelsohn (1966) The analysis of cell images *Ann. N.Y. Acad. Sci.* 128:1035-1053

L. Quam, M. J. Hannah (1974) *Stanford automated photogrammetry research* AIM-254, Stanford AI Lab

J. Radon (1917) Über die Bestimmung von Funktionen durch ihre Integralwerte längs gewisser Mannigfaltigkeiten *Berlin Sächsische Akad. Wissen.* 29:262-279

A. A. Reeves *Optimized Fast Hartley Transform with Applications in Image Processing* Thesis, Dartmouth University, March 1990

R. G. Reeves, ed. (1975) *Manual of Remote Sensing* American Society of Photogrammetry, Falls Church, CA

J. P. Rigaut (1988) Automated image segmentation by mathematical morphology and fractal geometry *J. Microscopy* 150:21-30

L. G. Roberts (1965) Machine perception of three-dimensional solids, in *Optical and Electro-Optical Information Processing* (J. T. Tippett, ed.), MIT Press, Cambridge, MA

I. Rock (1984) *Perception* W. H Freeman, New York, NY

A. Rosenfeld, A. C. Kak (1982) *Digital Picture Processing* vol 1 & 2, Academic Press, New York

J. C. Russ (1984) Implementing a new skeletonizing method *J. Microscopy* 136:RP7

J. C. Russ (1986) *Practical Stereology* Plenum Press, New York

J. C. Russ (1988) Differential absorption three-dimensional microtomography *Trans. Amer. Nucl. Soc.* 56(3):14

J. C. Russ (1990a) *Computer Assisted Microscopy* Plenum Press, New York

J. C. Russ (1990b) Surface characterization: Fractal dimensions, Hurst coefficients and frequency transforms *J. Comput. Assist. Microsc.* 2:161-184

J. C. Russ (1990c) Processing images with a local Hurst operator to reveal textural differences *J. Comput. Assist. Microsc.* 2#4:249-257

J. C. Russ, J. C. Russ (1988a) Automatic discrimination of features in grey scale images *J. Microscopy* 148:263-277

J. C. Russ, J. C. Russ (1988b) Improved implementation of a convex segmentation algorithm *Acta Stereologica* 7:33-40

J. C. Russ, J. C. Russ (1989a) Uses of the Euclidean distance map for the measurement of features in images *J. Comput. Assist. Microsc.* 1#4:343

J. C. Russ, J. C. Russ (1989b) Topological measurements on skeletonized three-dimensional networks *J. Comput. Assist. Microsc.* 1:131-150

F. F. Sabins, Jr. (1987) *Remote Sensing: Principles and Interpretation* 2nd Edition, W. H. Freeman, New York

S. Saunders (1991) Magellan: The geologic exploration of Venus *Engineering and Science* Spring:15-27

A. Savitsky, M. J. E. Golay (1964) Smoothing and differentiation of data by simplified least squares procedures *Anal. Chem.* 36:1627-1639

D. J. Schneberk, H. E. Martz, S. G. Azavedo (1991) Multiple energy techniques in industrial computerized tomograhy, in *Review of Progress in Quantitative Nondestructive Evaluation* (D. O. Thompson, D. E. Chimenti, eds.), Plenum Press, New York

H. Schwarz, H. E. Exner (1980) Implementation of the concept of fractal dimensions on a semi-automatic image analyzer *Powder Techn.* 27:107

H. Schwarz, H. E. Exner (1983) The characterization of the arrangement of feature centroids in planes and volumes *J. Microscopy* 129:155

J. Serra (1982) *Image Analysis and Mathematical Morphology* Academic Press, London

L. A. Shepp, B. F. Logan (1974) The Fourier reconstruction of a head section *IEEE Trans.* NS-21:21-43

J. Skilling (1986) Theory of maximum entropy image reconstruction, in *Maximum Entropy and Bayesian Methods in Applied Statistics,* Proc. 4th Max. Entropy Workshop, Univ of Calgary,

1984 (J. H. Justice, ed.), Cambridge Univ. Press, Cambridge, p. 156-178

I. Sobel (1970) Camera models and machine perception AIM-21, Stanford Artificial Intelligence Lab, Palo Alto

S. Srinivasan, J. C. Russ, R. O. Scattergood (1990) Fractal analysis of erosion surfaces *J. Mater. Res.* 5:2616-2619

P. L. Stewart, R. M. Burnett *Seminars in Virology* (in press, 1991), cited in C. J. Mathias Visualization techniques augment lab research into structure of adenovirus *Scientific Computing & Automation* 7#6:51-56

R. G. Summers, C. E. Musial, P-C. Cheng, A. Leith, M. Marko (1991) The use of confocal microscopy and stereoscan reconstructions in the analysis of sea urchin embryonic cell division *J. Electron Microscopy Technique* 18:24-30

M. M. Thompson, ed. (1966) *Manual of Photogrammetry* American Society of Photogrammetry, Falls Church, VA

J. N. Turner, D. H. Szaeowski, K. L. Smith, M. Marko, (1991) Confocal microscopy and three-dimensional reconstruction of electrophysiologically identified neurons in thick brain slices *J. Electron Microscopy Technique* 18:11-23

E. E. Underwood (1970) *Quantitative Stereology* Addison Wesley, Reading, MA

E. E. Underwood, K. Banerji (1986) Fractals in fractography *Materials Science and Engineering* 80:1

R. J. Wall, A. Klinger, K. R. Castleman (1974) *Analysis of Image Histograms* Proc. 2nd Joint Int. Conf. Patt. Recog., IEEE 74CH-0885-4C, p. 341-344

E. R. Weibel (1979) *Stereological Methods* vol I & II, Academic Press, London

J. S. Weszka (1978) A survey of threshold selection techniques *Comput. Graph. Image Proc.* 7:259-265

J. S. Weszka, A. Rosenfeld (1979) Histogram modification for threshold selection *IEEE Trans.* SMC-9:38-52

R. Wilson, M. Spann (1988) *Image Segmentation and Uncertainty* Wiley, New York

G. Wolf (1991) *Usage of global information and a priori knowledge for object isolation* Proc. 8th Int. Congr. for Stereology, Irvine, CA, p. 56

Y. Yakimovsky (1976) Boundary and object detection in real world images *J. Assoc. Comput. Mach.* 23:599-618

G. J. Yang, T. S. Huang (1981) The effect of median filtering on edge location estimation *Comput. Graph. Image Proc.* 15:224-245

S. Zucker (1976) Region growing: Childhood and adolescence *Comput. Graph. Image Proc.* 5:382-399

Index

acoustic microscopy 2, 412
aerial photography 45, 94, 151
algebraic reconstruction 346, 367
alignment..377
animation..396
anti-alias 99, 181
apodization 215
astigmatism..186
astronomy 8, 22, 23, 30
autocorrelation 221
averaging 22, 54, 55, 70, 78
backprojection 343, 366
beam hardening..356
binary images..277
binary mask..284
Boolean 155, 230, 237, 243, 248, 290, 312
boundary representation 251, 268, 392
Butterworth filter 198
charge-coupled device (CCD) 7, 9
classification 274
closing 297
clustering 336
color filtering..37
color images...28, 228
compression...37, 166
confocal scanning light microscope (CSLM) 26, 37, 40, 162, 166, 266, 381, 405, 412
connectedness...270, 286
constraints 349
contour line..265
contour maps 413
contrast expansion...76
convergence 349
convolution 64, 209, 345
correlation 40, 132, 218
custer 314
densitometry 24
derivatives 119
difference of Gaussians (DOG) 131
diffraction 137
dilation 73, 294, 321, 325
distortion 10, 46, 91, 379
edge following 264
edges 119
electron diffraction 3, 182
electronic noise 19
enhancement...101
erosion..72, 294, 325
etching 385
Euclidean distance map (EDM) 322, 337
expansion 102
extended-focus..413
fan-beam 364
fiducial marks..379
fill...288
film 8
filter 202
flat-bed scanners..26
fluorescence................................8, 21, 54, 161, 383
Fourier inversion..366
Fourier transform 166, 342
fractal 147, 190, 302, 332
Frei and Chen 133, 427, 428
frequency transform 63, 82, 166, 245
gamma 9
Gaussian 57
generation 364
grain boundaries 132, 319

halftone 27, 203
Haralick 146
high-pass filter 118, 196
histogram ...14, 24, 78, 106, 151, 226, 249, 252, 260
histogram equalization 105
homomorphic filter 201
hue 34, 37, 231
hue, saturation, and intensity (HSI) 34, 229
human vision 5, 6
Hurst coefficient 148, 191
Hurst texture 243
hybrid median 5, 68, 116, 225
image arithmetic 155
infrared 11, 228
intensity 34, 37, 231
interpolation 97, 395
inverse filter 355
isometric 403
isotropic 299
iteration 305, 323
Joint Photographic Experts Group (JPEG) ...37, 392
kernel 55, 59, 102, 113, 210
Kirsch 126
Laplacian 25, 114, 239, 345
laser printers 27
leveling 45, 80, 156
lookup tables (LUTs) 24, 29, 78, 103, 420, 429
low-pass 196, 239
magnetic resonance imaging (MRI) 42, 291, 339, 394
mask 291, 337
matching 387
maximum entropy 75, 216, 256, 351
medial axis transform 334
median filter 64, 102, 387
morphological 294
mosaic image 96
motion 158, 217
MPEG 392
multiband 233, 401, 411
multiplication 158
noise 254, 294, 354
nonuniform illumination 53
notch filters 204
Olympic filter 70
opening 73, 295, 327
optical sectioning 381
orientation 246
padding 172
parallax 387
periodic noise 194, 209
periodic structure 186, 209
perspective 403
phantom 341, 361
phase 183
pixel-based representation 251, 267
point-spread function 214
polishing 384
polynomial 62, 81, 92, 122
posterization 66, 69
power spectrum 178, 183
preferred orientation 185, 222
profilometers 26
projection 340
pruning 318
pseudo-color 20, 24, 28, 129, 401, 424
Radon transform 341
range images 143, 417
rank filter 205, 212
ranking 64, 84, 135, 303, 429
ray tracing 402, 408
region growing 79, 273
rendering 416
resectioning 398
resolution 17, 23, 55, 353, 377
RGB 33, 35, 229, 277
Roberts' Cross 124
rolling ball filter 140
rotation 91, 96
RS-170 13
run-length encoding 267, 287
satellite images 146, 161, 228, 274
saturation 34, 37, 54, 80, 87, 94, 231, 282
scanning electron microscope (SEM) 20, 25
scanning tunneling microscope (STM) 3, 25, 266
secondary ion mass spectrometer 40
segmentation 35, 225
seismography 368, 412
serial section 40, 95, 377
shading 79
sharpening 115
signal-to-noise 21, 54
SIMS 385
sinogram 341
skeletonization 315, 429
skiz 318, 337
smoothing 57, 113
Sobel 125, 241, 247, 261
split-and-merge 79, 271
statistics 354
stereo 42, 386, 405, 407
stretched 96
subtraction 156
suppression operator 140
TEM 181, 206
template matching 218, 429
texture 143, 239
thickness 380
thresholding 141, 226
time sequence 39
tomography 40, 88, 339, 376
top hat operator 135
topological 315
transfer function 103
translation 91
true color 28, 103
ultimate eroded points 328
unsharp masking 25, 131, 156
variance 132, 144, 240
varifocal mirror 406
video camera 6, 25
videotape 14, 16

vidicon 8, 9
vignetting 10, 80
volumetric display 402
voxels 390
warping 96
watersheds 329
X-ray...............................2, 28, 54, 255, 281, 290, 310
YIQ 31